Hitchhiker's Guide to Internal Medicine

Hitchhiker's Guide to Internal Medicine

ATIF QASIM, MD

Division of Cardiovascular Medicine
University of Pennsylvania School of Medicine
Philadelphia, Pennsylvania

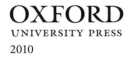

UNIVERSITY PRESS
2010

OXFORD
UNIVERSITY PRESS

Oxford University Press, Inc., publishes works that further
Oxford University's objective of excellence
in research, scholarship, and education.

Oxford   New York
Auckland   Cape Town   Dar es Salaam   Hong Kong   Karachi
Kuala Lumpur   Madrid   Melbourne   Mexico City   Nairobi
New Delhi   Shanghai   Taipei   Toronto

With offices in
Argentina   Austria   Brazil   Chile   Czech Republic   France   Greece
Guatemala   Hungary   Italy   Japan   Poland   Portugal   Singapore
South Korea   Switzerland   Thailand   Turkey   Ukraine   Vietnam

Copyright © 2010 by Oxford University Press, Inc.

Published by Oxford University Press, Inc.
198 Madison Avenue, New York, New York 10016
www.oup.com

Oxford is a registered trademark of Oxford University Press.

Library of Congress Cataloging-in-Publication Data

Qasim, Atif.
Hitchhiker's guide to internal medicine / Atif Qasim.
   p. ; cm.
Includes index.
ISBN 978-0-19-538804-6
1. Internal medicine—Handbooks, manuals, etc. I. Title.
[DNLM: 1. Internal Medicine—Handbooks. WB 39 Q15h 2010]
RC55.Q37 2010
616—dc22   2009045010

9 8 7 6 5 4 3 2 1

Printed in the United States of America
on acid-free paper.

PREFACE

This book represents a major effort over the years as I've gone from a medical student to intern and resident, and then to chief resident and now cardiology fellow. During this time, I've never felt that there was a book specifically directed to medical students or interns to help them put together the information they require to succeed on the wards and also to do well on their shelf exam and USMLE exams. It is my intent, having now worked with many medical students and interns in supervisory and teaching roles, to present a book that will fill that void.

The transition from the classroom learning environment in the first two years of medical school to the inpatient wards is one of the biggest transitions we all make during our medical education. Success in the classroom doesn't necessarily predict success in clinical medicine. This book therefore is intended to help you get the most out of your medicine rotations and to help you prepare the knowledge base needed for the exams you'll have to take.

Each chapter consists of several sections. The first section reviews basic anatomy or physiology. The second section reviews the key features of the physical exam for that area of medicine subspecialty. Thereafter are listed diagnostic tests that are used in the field, followed by a section titled Approach to Common Problems. This latter section covers some of the most common complaints seen in the inpatient setting, such as chest pain, abdominal pain, or change in mental status. So, when you are asked to see and evaluate such a patient, flipping through that particular section in the book may provide guidance concerning what to ask and do until you've seen enough cases to be comfortable in independently evaluating a patient. Finally, the last and largest section of each chapter deals with a systematic approach to medical conditions, in an easy-to-use format that runs through the definition (D), epidemiology (Epi), pathophysiology (P), risk factors (RF), signs and symptoms (SiSx), diagnosis (Dx), and treatment (Tx). While each disease description gives the standard basic information needed at a level appropriate for most medical students and interns, additional reading from the published literature during the work-up of a patients is strongly encouraged—especially given the fast pace of medical advances.

Of course, no book is perfect, so we encourage you to give feedback either on the way the concepts in this book are explained or on new details or facts you feel are invaluable to those in medical school or medicine residency training. This will serve readers of future editions who will also travel along the road of medical education.

Atif Qasim, MD

ACKNOWLEDGMENTS

Writing this book has been a long process. The book was first conceived during my medical school days. Thanks go to many people, first to many of my attending physicians at the Johns Hopkins School of Medicine, particularly Philip Seo, Peter Terry, and H. Franklin Herlong, who looked over initial versions of chapters and provided numerous ideas and input.

In addition, thanks go to many colleagues in medical school and residency, especially Brendan Lucey, David Shook, Nehal Mehta, Raquelle Charles Greer, and Richelle Charles, who provided immensely valuable input for contributions to several sections of the book. At the Hospital of the University of Pennsylvania, I am particularly grateful to Lisa Bellini and Michael Grippe, who helped me fully realize the need to translate my passion for teaching into a publishable book and helped guide me through the process in order to make this a reality.

Finally, special thanks go to my parents and my wife for providing continued support during the long hours that I spent writing the book and who are as happy as I am that it is now finished. Of course, this book would not have been possible without the support of the staff at Oxford University Press, who were very patient and professional in offering advice and help and to whom I'm also forever grateful.

CONTENTS

CONTRIBUTORS

Hugo Aparicio, MD
Department of Neurology
Hospital of the University of Pennsylvania
Philadelphia, PA
Chapter 11: Neurology, Secondary Author

Camille Introcaso, MD
Department of Dermatology
Hospital of the University of Pennsylvania
Philadelphia, PA
Chapter 12: Dermatology, Primary Author

Shin Lin, MD, PhD
Department of Cardiovascular Medicine
Stanford University School of Medicine
Stanford, CA
Chapters 8 and 10: Infectious Diseases and
    Oncology, multiple sections

Caitlin Loomis, MD
Department of Neurology
Hospital of the University of Pennsylvania
Philadelphia, PA
Chapter 11: Neurology, Primary Author

Saeher Muzaffar, MD, MPH
Pulmonary, Allergy, and Critical Care Division
Hospital of the University of Pennsylvania
Philadelphia, PA
Chapter 3: Pulmonology, Pneumoconioses
    section

James Reilly, MD
Renal-Electrolyte and Hypertension Division
Hospital of the University of Pennsylvania
Philadelphia, PA
Chapter 4: Nephrology, section on Renal
    Imaging and Dialysis

REVIEWERS

Valerianna Amorosa, MD
Infectious Diseases Division
Hospital of the University of Pennsylvania
Philadelphia, PA

Serena Cardillo, MD
Division of Endocrinology, Diabetes, and
    Metabolism
Hospital of the University of Pennsylvania
Philadelphia, PA

Jessica Dine, MD
Pulmonary, Allergy, and Critical Care Division
Hospital of the University of Pennsylvania
Philadelphia, PA

Alden Doyle, MD, MPH
Renal-Electrolyte and Hypertension Division
Hospital of the University of Pennsylvania
Philadelphia, PA

Jonathan Dunham, MD
Rheumatology Division
Hospital of the University of Pennsylvania
Philadelphia, PA

Helene Glassberg, MD
Division of Cardiovascular Medicine
Hospital of the University of Pennsylvania
Philadelphia, PA

Jack Goldberg, MD
Department of Hematology-Oncology
Penn Presbyterian Medical Center
Philadelphia, PA

Satish Nagula, MD
Division of Gastroenterology
    and Hepatology
State University of New York at Stony Brook
Stony Brook, NY

Alexander Perl, MD
Department of Hematology-Oncology
Hospital of the University of Pennsylvania
Philadelphia, PA

Raymond Price, MD
Department of Neurology
Hospital of the University of Pennsylvania
Philadelphia, PA

CHAPTER 1

Introduction to Inpatient Medicine Wards

The key to inpatient medicine is the ability to evaluate a patient quickly, but also thoroughly and efficiently. This becomes easier with experience, as residents and attending physicians will focus their clinical questioning on the most pertinent issues necessitating inpatient care, leaving other less urgent issues to be resolved on an outpatient basis. However, when starting out as a medical student, being thorough with respect to all of the patient's medical issues is important both from a learning standpoint and for helping to practice elements of history taking and the physical exam.

TIPS ON WORKING UP AN INPATIENT

Every patient deserves to tell his or her story from the beginning, with several minutes devoted to a generic question such as "What brought you to the emergency room?" or "What brought you to see the doctor today?". Thereafter, more focused questioning should begin on the specific issues at hand. For the medical student, this is the time to obtain a thorough history and perform a complete physical exam. No one else may do such a thorough and detailed job during the admission, although more senior staff may know more about how to elicit certain pertinent points of the history the next day on rounds. There is nothing wrong with going back to ask patients questions you think of later or asking them questions that come up as you find something on the physical exam. For most patients with straightforward problems, a complete history and physical exam should take no more than 1 hour for the trained medical student.

Keeping Track of Patient Information

Everyone has different means of keeping track of patient information: using cards or signouts or copying the histories, physical exam findings, and progress notes into a binder. This may depend on the hospital's charting system and signout system. Find the method that works best for you, depending on your level of comfort with the details, but be sure to pick one method and use it consistently.

Emergency Room (ER) Admissions

If a patient is in the ER, it behooves you to find out all you can about the patient and what has already been done, so spend 5–10 minutes doing a chart biopsy in your computer records and review the laboratory tests. This will help direct your questioning in some cases and help correct information, especially for patients who have a long medical history or who may not be able to recall all of their medical problems. Many patients will be happy to know that you already know a good deal about them before seeing them, especially if they have had most of their care at your hospital. For example, in cases where time is short and you know the patient's complicated past medical history already, it is ok to say during the patient history "Let me tell you what I already know about you based on looking through your prior visits here. Please feel free to correct me if I'm wrong."

Know the shorthand terms for laboratory tests. The most common abbreviations are shown below, though they are being used less and less often with the advent of computerized laboratory reporting systems.

CBC:

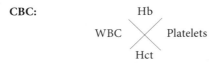

Hb – hemoglobin, Hct – hematocrit

Panel 7:

Na	Cl	BUN	
K	CO_2	Cr	Glucose

Coagulation tests: INR/PT/PTT

Liver function tests are usually not standardized (everyone seems to have a personal method), so these may need to be written out.

PRESENTING ON ROUNDS

Very few people will be following how you work up patients, but everyone will be there to see you present a patient. This is your chance to give all the pertinent details to the covering team and the attending physician for management. It is not necessary to recapitulate every detail stated in your notes. Anyone can read your notes in the chart at any time. Rather, you need to describe the most important features of the presentation and plan and do so in a timely manner.

Without question, the more efficiently you can present the patient, the better your performance will be. Helpful shortcuts include not announcing different parts of the history but just transitioning into them. Most people know the general transition of the history and will understand immediately. So, instead of announcing the family history and social history, you can just state: "Mr. X has no known family history of coronary disease, diabetes, high blood pressure, or cancer. He lives with his wife and three kids and works as a teacher. He has never smoked, drinks on rare occasions, and has never used illicit drugs." You will be better received if your presentations are short and to the point, as this will speed up rounds for the rest of the team.

What are the most common reasons for long presentations, either for a new admission or for a follow-up? One major reason is interruptions by other members, either to ask more questions about the history or to interject a point or two. This can be dealt with in a number of ways. If the question is simple, just answer it and politely ask that other questions be held until the end of your presentation; alternatively, say that you may get to that point in a little while and ask that it be discussed at the time of the assessment and plan.

Another major reason for long presentations is giving information out of order by introducing elements of the assessment and plan upfront as you are reviewing the history of the present illness or the past medical history, interjecting an opinion about what you think is going on. This will invite several questions and lead to a departure from your presentation. Instead, present all of your data objectively and wait until the end to say what you think is going on—inviting discussion with others only at that point.

The last major reason that presentations run too long is that not all of the clinical information is well organized or easily accessible. State just the data that are pertinent, and not all the lab data, unless they are requested (some attending physicians are particular). Make sure to have all relevant data at hand in case you are asked for them, including all past tests and the past history, whether or not it seems pertinent to the presentation at hand.

If you are just starting out, make sure to practice the presentation repeatedly for timing beforehand. A reasonable presentation should take about 10 minutes or less. If your patient has an unusual condition or presentation, it is always helpful to bring some literature for the team, whether you are a medical student or an intern and especially if you are a resident.

Above all, be flexible, and be able to tailor your presentations based on what your attending physician likes or the available time. On any new rotation, it is helpful to find out the preferences of your attending physician on the first day.

WRITING NOTES

Your notes embody much of what you want to communicate to others about your patient and your thought process. They are part of the permanent medical record, unlike what you say on rounds. Admit notes vary slightly in their order but should always contain: History of Present Illness, Review of Systems, Past Medical History, Family History, Social History, Medications, Physical Exam, Data (labs, radiology, and other studies) and Assessment and Plan. Other things that are helpful to have on an admit note include family contact information, code status information, primary care or specialist doctor name and contact information, data from old studies with abnormalities (old CT scans, echocardiograms, and so forth to be complete), and information about the last time patients took their medications.

Follow-up daily progress notes are different. In many places they are called "SOAP" notes since they are written in the following matter:

S: (subjective). State what the patients say about how they are feeling, how their night was; using their own words is preferred.

O: (objective). Here state the vitals and physical exam, list the medications they took, and list any of the lab data that have come back.

A and **P**: (assessment and plan). Here state the patient's problems and for each one give an assessment of their status and then give the plan for what you want to do. This is the most important and mostly widely read section of any note, be it a daily progress note or an admit note. Get into the habit of writing down an assessment and giving a status update of the problem. Do not just state the problem and say you want to change a medication like "Hypertension: increase lisinopril

to 20 mg daily." Instead write "Hypertension: Blood pressure is not well controlled at present at 160/80 mmHg. Patient is currently asymptomatic. Plan to increase the lisinopril from 10 mg to 20 mg daily starting this am." Something as simple as this documents more about your thought process, which is key as a medical student or intern. This of course will be most important with even more complex medical problems.

INTERACTING AS A MEDICINE SERVICE TEAM MEMBER

It is crucial that on a medicine service, team members work well together in evaluating patients and especially in taking care of sick patients. You don't need to know everything or try to appear that you do. It is better to know where or how to get the information. Half of medicine is knowing what to do; the other half is knowing how to find out what to do. More importantly, if you don't know a detail or how to do something, just say so. More often than not, someone will be willing to teach you what you don't know or help you find the necessary information. Just remember that once you are on the wards, the goals have changed. No longer is the focus on the individual, as it may be in the first 2 years of medical school, sitting in lectures or small groups and taking exams. Rather, the focus is on the patient and the well-being of the team. Medical students, interns, and residents who keep this in mind should fare well in all of their rotations.

CHAPTER 2

Cardiology

CARDIAC ANATOMY AND PHYSIOLOGY

Basic Facts

- Under normal resting conditions, a normal cardiac output is 5–8 L/min and can increase to 15–20 L/min during strenuous exercise or other conditions of increased demand.
- The greatest resistance to blood flow and therefore the greatest blood pressure (BP) drop occurs at the level of small arteries and arterioles. This is where regulation of systemic vascular resistance occurs. Most of the blood in the systemic vascular bed is in the venous system at any given time.
- Coronary blood flow is greatest during diastole. Venous blood from the heart drains from cardiac veins into the coronary sinus (posterior structure), which empties into the right atrium.
- Via Frank-Starling mechanisms, increases in preload lead to increases in stroke volume and stroke work because of changes in myocardial fiber length. This leads to increased cardiac output under normal circumstances. Increases in afterload (the pressure against which the heart pumps) causes a decrease in cardiac output under normal circumstances, as the heart has to work harder to eject blood to the rest of the body.
- The major contributors to increased myocardial oxygen demand are increased preload, afterload, increased wall stress (as seen in larger dilated hearts), and increased heart rate.
- Electrical conduction proceeds from the sinoatrial (SA) node in the high right atrium node to the atrioventricular (AV) node through the bundle of His, the right and left

bundles, and then the Purkinje fibers. The vagus nerve carries parasympathetic input to inhibit the SA nodes, AV node, and atrial tissue. The SA and AV node have special types of cells known as pacemaker cells, which have their own automaticity and can generate a rhythm. The SA automaticity is the fastest and is usually what determines the heart rate after being influenced by sympathetic and parasympathetic tone.
- Figure 2-1 shows the heart from an anterior view as it sits in the chest.

Note the different phases of atrial and ventricular contraction, as shown in Figure 2-2.

- Isovolumetric contraction is the period of greatest oxygen consumption. Contraction is starting to occur, but chamber volume is constant. Mitral valve closure and aortic valve opening occur here.
- Valve closure causes normal heart sounds (S_1 and S_2) to occur. Valve opening is usually silent.
- During tachycardia, the time for diastasis shortens.
- Left ventricular end diastolic pressure is defined as the pressure just after atrial contraction when the mitral valve closes.
- There is a slight delay between the recorded electrical and subsequent mechanical activity of the heart. For example, the P wave on the electrocardiogram (ECG), which initiates atrial contraction, occurs just before the mechanical A wave on the jugular venous pressure (JVP) waveform, which represents true atrial contraction. Similarly, the QRS complex occurs just at end diastole, and ventricular contraction follows immediately afterward.

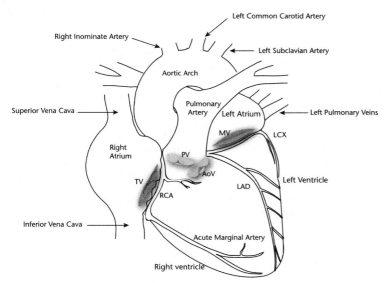

Figure 2-1. Cardiac Anatomy: Anterior View of the Heart. AoV – aortic valve, LAD – left anterior descending artery, LCX – left circumflex artery, MV – mitral valve, TV – tricuspid valve, PV – pulmonic valve, RCA – right coronary artery. Note that the most anterior great vessel of the heart is the pulmonary artery. The right ventricle and right atrium are also anterior structures and are in front of the left atrium and left ventricle. Not easily seen here is the tricuspid valve, a more apical structure than the mitral valve. The tricuspid and mitral valves are not coplanar structures.

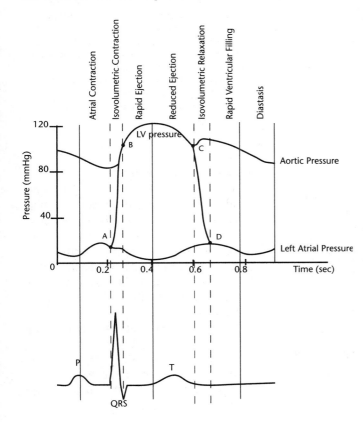

Figure 2-2. Wigger's Diagram. The Wigger's diagram is a simple way to depict several physiologic properties of the heart simultaneously within the context of the timing of the cardiac cycle.
A: mitral valve closes; B: aortic valve opens; C: aortic valve closes; and D: mitral valve opens.

Table 2-1. Blood Supply of the Heart

	Left Coronary Artery (LCA)	Right Coronary Artery (RCA)
Branches	The LCA starts as the left main coronary artery, which divides into the left anterior descending (LAD) and left circumflex (LCX) arteries in most people. Common variants include a third branch, called the ramus intermedius, and separate origins of the LAD and LCX with no left main. The LAD is identified by its downward septal and diagonal branches on the angiogram. It heads toward the apex. The LCX gives off obtuse marginal (OM) branches and lies in the atrioventricular (AV) groove initially. In 10% of patients, it supplies the PDA and thus the posterior wall (termed left dominant circulation).	The RCA courses in the AV groove. Branches include the acute marginal arteries (supply the right ventricle and course along the acute margin of the heart) and the posterior descending artery (PDA). In 85% of patients, the RCA supplies the PDA, which is important for the posterior wall supply (termed right dominant circulation). In 5%, the PDA is supplied by branches of both (termed codominant circulation). Sometimes there are branches after the PDA that supply the posterolateral wall (called posterolateral branches).
Conduction System Supply	Supplies part of the bundle of His, all or most of the left bundle, and part of the right bundle. Hence, in infarction, one may see LBBB. Supplies half of the AV node.	Supplies the sinoatrial (SA) node in most people and usually also half of the AV node, as well as the right bundle and sometimes the right posterior fascicle of the left bundle via the PDA.
Territory Supplied	Supplies 75% of the left ventricle, most of the mitral valve apparatus, and the anterolateral papillary muscle. The LAD supplies the anterior half of the septum and variable amounts of the anterolateral wall. The LCX and its branches supply the lateral wall.	Supplies 25% of the left ventricle, most of the right ventricle, the inferior part of the septum, and the inferior and posterolateral walls. In many people, supplies the posteromedial papillary muscle alone. Possible complications from occlusion include AV heart block, bradycardia, papillary muscle dysfunction (and therefore mitral regurgitation), and right ventricular infarction leading to signs of right-sided heart failure.

Coronary Artery Anatomy

Knowledge of the blood supply to the heart is crucial for understanding acute coronary syndromes. Table 2-1 reviews the major branches of the right and left coronary arteries as well as which structures are supplied. Figure 2-3 shows the basic angiographic views during cardiac catheterization.

THE CARDIOVASCULAR EXAM

Brief Overview of the Cardiovascular Exam

1. Inspection
   - Inspect for cyanosis, pallor, and respiratory distress.

- Assess the JVP (see below).
- Attempt to visualize the point of maximal impulse (PMI) with the patient standing, sitting, or lying supine. Most patients have no visible PMI. A normal PMI is in the midclavicular line near the fourth or fifth intercostal space (ICS). An abnormal PMI is on or below the sixth ICS and lateral to the mid clavicular line.
2. Palpation
   - Feel for the PMI and judge its size. If it is larger than the diameter of a quarter, this is abnormal, signifying hypertrophy. Displacement of the PMI laterally implies dilation. The PMI should be felt during systole. If it is felt during diastole,

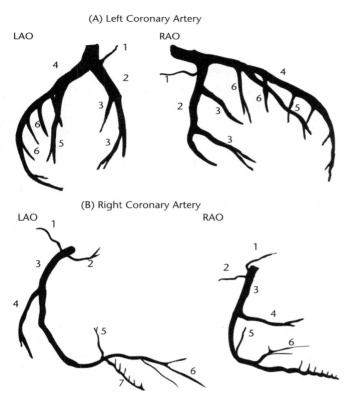

Figure 2-3 (A,B). Left and Right Coronary Anatomy by Common Angiographic Views. These are common angiographic views and refer to the position of the camera in relation to the chest. Additional angulation is provided with caudal or cranial views. LAO - Left Anterior Oblique, RAO - Right Anterior Oblique. (A) 1, atrial branch; 2, left circumflex; 3, obtuse marginals; 4, left anterior descending; 5, diagonal artery; 6, septal perforators. (B) 1, conus artery; 2, SA node artery; 3, right coronary artery; 4, acute marginal artery; 5, AV node artery; 6, posterolateral artery; 7, posterior descending artery.

this suggests left ventricular dysfunction/dyskinesis.

- Experienced observers can feel an S_3 or S_4. Place the end of a tongue depressor on the PMI, leaving the other end in the air to amplify the movement. The vibration from an S_3 or S_4 can then be visualized.
- Feel the left and right parasternal areas for a right ventricle impulse or heave, which implies right ventricular hypertrophy. Place fingers between the third, fourth, and fifth ICS to feel. Lifting the legs may help by increasing right-sided blood return to amplify this finding.

- Feel for thrills over the chest. These are palpable vibrations, usually accompanying grade 4 and higher murmurs.

3. Percussion
   - This is rarely done to determine heart size and in most cases is not necessary, as other means can help judge this property, but it is used to assess for cardiomegaly and pericardial effusions.

4. Auscultation
   - There are five cardinal areas that should be listened to, both with the bell and with the diaphragm. At each station the following should be heard:

□ Right Upper Sternal Border (second ICS)—the aortic area. S_2 is louder here. Aortic stenosis murmurs are heard best here. Listen to the carotid areas for transmission of aortic murmurs if any type of systolic murmur is heard here.

□ Left Upper Sternal Border (second ICS)—the pulmonic area. S_2 is louder here. Compare A_2 and P_2 here and along the entire sternal border if considering increased right-sided pressures.

□ Left Lower Sternal Border (fourth to fifth ICS). S_1 is louder here. This is the best place to listen for an S_3 or S_4 sound with the bell, as these sounds are low-pitched.

□ Right Lower Sternal Border (fourth to fifth ICS)—the tricuspid area. Well-localized tricuspid regurgitation can be heard here. S_1 is louder here. Rubs can also be heard here.

□ Left Lateral Area—the mitral area. Also listen to the axilla or back, if necessary, for radiating murmurs.

5. Other
   • Assess the strength and quality of the peripheral pulses.
   • Listen for carotid and femoral bruits. The carotids are best heard with the bell while the patient is holding his/her breath.
   • Examine the extremities for edema and feel for warmth or coldness. Assess capillary refill time in the nail beds to see if it is sluggish (more than 2 seconds).

More diagnostic hints concerning specific disease entities are discussed later in this chapter.

Pulses and Pressures

Jugular Venous Pressure Assessment

The JVP waveform shown in Figure 2-4 describes the change in right atrial and central venous pressure with time. Estimation of JVP is a surrogate for estimation of right-sided filling pressures, which, in most people, reflects indirectly the left-sided filling pressures and is hence a marker of volume status.

The best way to find the JVP is:

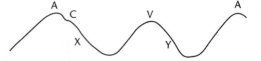

Figure 2-4. Jugular Venous Pressure Waveform.
A wave = atrial contraction.
C wave = isovolumetric ventricular contraction (increased atrial pressure against a closed tricuspid valve).
X descent = atrial relaxation. The right ventricle exerts negative pressure as it contracts, pulling down the bottom of the right atrium as it empties.
V wave = blood entering the atria during atrial diastole and during the rest of active ventricular systole.
Y descent = blood passively fills the ventricle as the tricuspid opens just before atrial contraction.

1. Look for the internal jugular vein at the base of the neck before it rides under the sternocleidomastoid muscle; the external jugular vein is easier to see as it courses through the neck, and while it should not be used for JVP assessment, it can be a helpful adjunct.

2. Place the patient at a 30°–45° angle (or higher in patients with very elevated JVP) and turn the patient's head to either side to view the neck. Alternatively, have the patient look up at the ceiling with the chin up and no neck rotation (this method is more effective in obese patients).

3. Once the internal jugular vein is found, look for the X and Y descents while feeling the pulse. The pulse should occur in between the X and Y descents. Then try to recognize the A wave and V wave in between X and Y, judging their size. Push on the abdomen for 15 to 30 seconds to see if there is any change in the height to help find the JVP as well. (If JVP elevation is sustained after this period of time, as seen in patients with right-sided heart failure, the condition is called *hepatojugular reflux*.) Finally, see which way the neck veins fill by temporarily occluding the external jugular vein and releasing it with pressure. Filling from below indicates high right-sided pressures. Filling from above is normal. Table 2-2 shows examples of abnormal JVP findings.

Table 2-2. Conditions Causing Abnormal Jugular Venous Pressure Findings

Condition	Finding
Tricuspid Regurgitation	Prominent V wave .
Atrial Septal Defects	V wave is much more prominent than A wave.
Atrial Fibrillation	A waves are not visible (concerted atrial contraction is absent).
Constrictive Pericarditis	Steep Y descent, called *Friedreich's sign,* because passive filling is not allowed. There is a marked increase in JVP with inspiration, called *Kussmaul's sign,* where right heart filling is impaired, and JVP increases with inspiration, as opposed to it normally decreasing.
Atrioventricular Dyssynchrony	Large intermittent A waves (Cannon A waves) when the ventricle and atria contract simultaneously (as in atrioventricular nodal reentrant or ventricular tachycardia).

4. Measure the JVP as the vertical distance from the top of the A wave to the sternal angle with the patient lying at any angle; then add 5 cm (the assumed distance from the sternal angle to the chest wall). Alternatively, measure the vertical distance from the sternal angle to the midaxillary line.

Blood Pressure Measurement

- Use a cuff where the bladder portion can circumscribe at least two-thirds of the arm. If the cuff is too large, the BP will be falsely low. If the cuff is too small, it will be falsely high.
- During measurement, the arm should be at the level of the heart (a raised arm will lower the BP) and the patient should be sitting down, without recent strenuous exertion or recent use of coffee/stimulants.
- After feeling the brachial pulse, inflate to well above the expected systolic blood pressure (SBP) and release. Technically, the bell (not the diaphragm) should be over the brachial artery,

as the Korotkoff sounds due to turbulence are low pitched, though this is rarely done in practice. The systolic pressure is the first sound heard during release. The diastolic pressure is heard when the Korotkoff sounds disappear.

The Peripheral Pulse

- This pulse can be used to quickly assess systolic pressure. Rough estimates of the lowest possible BP in normal individuals are: Presence of:

  Carotid pulse—60 mmHg
  Femoral pulse—70–80 mmHg
  Radial pulse—90 mmHg
- Use Doppler ultrasound to assess the peripheral pulse if they are nonpalpable. In patients with suspected peripheral arterial disease, ankle brachial indices (ABIs) can be obtained using the Doppler test to compare the brachial and ankle blood pressure.
- Abnormal findings are shown in Table 2-3.

Table 2-3. Abnormal Peripheral Pulse Findings

Bisferiens Pulse	Two upstrokes are felt. Caused by aortic regurgitation, HOCM, and a patent ductus arteriosus.
Pulsus Alternans	Alternating weak and strong pulses. Associated with severe left ventricular dysfunction and an irregular rhythm.
Waterhammer Pulse	Seen with wide pulse pressure, as in aortic regurgitation or old age.
Parvus et Tardus	A Latin phrase meaning a slow and delayed upstroke, classically seen in aortic stenosis.
Apical Radial Pulse Deficit	Seen in atrial fibrillation. The number of pulses felt at the radial arteries is smaller then the number of S_2 sounds counted by stethoscope since not every pulse is strong enough to generate a palpable radial pulse.

Table 2-4. Abnormalities in the S₁ Heart Sound

Split S₁	Soft S₁ at the Base	Increased S₁ at the Base	Variable S₁ Intensity
1. From delay in tricuspid valve closure as seen in RBBB, tricuspid stenosis, Ebstein's anomaly, left ventricle pacing. 2. Consider if it is an S₄ which will be low pitched. 3. Consider if it is an S₁ plus a systolic ejection click, as in MVP.	1. Mitral regurgitation 2. AV block, since the PR interval is longer when the valve is back in place by the time the ventricle contracts, so the sound isn't as loud. 3. Failing left ventricle with elevated end-diastolic pressure. 4. LBBB.	1. Mitral stenosis. 2. Hyperkinesis. 3. High-output cardiac failure.	1. Mobitz type I but not type II block; there is gradual diminution of the S₁ sound as the PR interval keeps getting longer, as the valves have more time to return to place; then the skip is heard. 2. The only bradycardia with a variable S₁ sound is third-degree AV block. 3. Atrial fibrillation.

Table 2-5. Abnormalities in the S₂ Heart Sound

A. Normal Splitting	B. Single S₂	C. Paradoxical Splitting	D. Wide Fixed Splitting
There is physiologic splitting of S₂ with inspiration as increased preload delays the closure of the pulmonic valve. A₂ and P₂ therefore can be heard as two distinct sounds during inspiration only.	Delayed A₂ such that P₂ movement with inspiration does not allow two distinct sounds to be heard. This is commonly seen in advanced age, causing a delayed A₂, usually from valve abnormalities/calcification.	A₂ comes after P₂ and a split sound is heard even before inspiration. With inspiration, P₂ moves out and only a single sound is heard, the opposite of what is normal. This can be due to a longer left ventricle ejection time (LBBB, ischemic heart disease, aortic stenosis, hypertension). Alternatively, it may be due to premature P₂ closure (patent ductus arteriosus, tricuspid regurgitation, Wolfe-Parkinson-White syndrome).	Here there is a delayed P₂ such that even before inspiration, P₂ follows A₂. Inspiration may only accentuate the difference. Seen in atrial septal defects, RBBB, pulmonic stenosis or atresia, mitral regurgitation, and volume overload of the right heart. Listen closely to make sure that this is not an S₃ or pericardial knock.

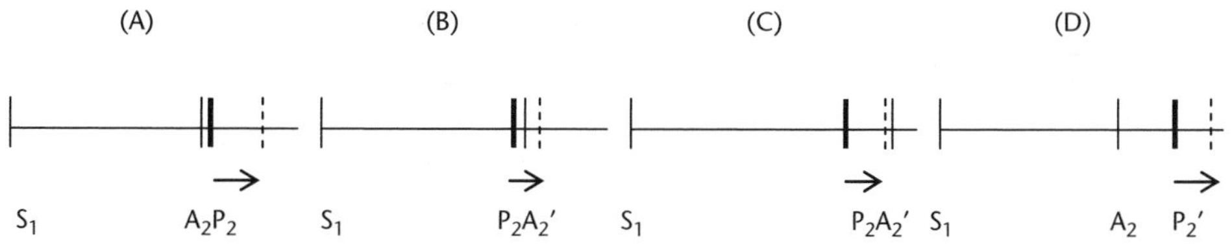

Figure 2-5. Splitting of the Second Heart Sound.

Scenarios A through D correspond to those in Table 2-5. Arrow indicates movement of P₂ with inspiration. Dark vertical lines indicate starting position of P₂, while dashed vertical lines indicate the new position of P₂ during inspiration. Thin vertical lines indicate position of S₁ and A₂ before inspiration. When aortic and pulmonic vertical lines are close together a split in the S₂ sound cannot be heard. Apostrophe indicates abnormality in that component of the second heart sound as the cause.

Heart Sounds

Normal Heart Sounds

Include a crisp S_1 and S_2 with physiological split S_2 during inspiration from increased right-sided pressure. Remember, the valves close in the order of the pneumonic *many things are possible*: *m*itral, *t*ricuspid, *a*ortic, and *p*ulmonary. There are several features of most abnormal heart sounds: abnormal S_1 and S_2, murmurs, gallops, or rubs.

Abnormal S_1 and S_2 Sounds

S_1

Table 2-4 shows several important findings of the S_1 sound that may be heard.

Questions to ask while listening are:

1. Is the S_1 sound single or double?
2. Is the intensity normal (louder at the apex)?
3. Does each beat have the same intensity?

S_2

Table 2-5 and Figure 2-5 also show different important findings for S_2 that may be heard.

Ask:

1. Is it louder at the base?
2. Is it single or double?
3. Is $A_2 < P_2$? Is there inspiratory splitting? (This is best heard in the second or third ICS.)

Murmurs

1. Decide if the murmur is systolic or diastolic by feeling the pulse (systole) when listening for the murmur.
2. Determine in which of the five main listening areas the murmur is loudest and the area to which it radiates.
3. Grade the murmur from 1 to 6 (see Table 2-6).
4. Then note the murmur's shape, radiation, and pitch. Holosystolic murmurs include ventricular septal defects, tricuspid regurgitation, and mitral regurgitation. With crescendo-decrescendo murmurs, decide whether the murmur is late, mid, or early peaking.
5. Assess the response to maneuvers:

Table 2-6. Grading of Systolic Murmurs

Grade	Sound
I	Less than S_1, S_2
II	Equal to S_1, S_2
III	Louder than S_1, S_2
IV	Associated with a palpable thrill
V	Heard with the stethoscope half off the chest
VI	Heard with the stethoscope 1 cm off the chest

- With decreased venous return the sound of most murmurs decreases. Methods to achieve this include (1) the Valsalva maneuver (asking the patient to bear down), which increases intrathoracic pressure, and (2) moving the patient from a supine to a sitting or standing position).
- With increased venous return the sound of most murmurs increases. Methods to achieve this include inspiration, squatting, or the Mueller maneuver, which involves inspiring against a closed glottis.
- Notable exceptions to these rules include hypertrophic obstructive cardiomyopathy (HOCM) and mitral valve prolapse with regurgitation, where murmurs increase with the Valsalva maneuver, since there is less blood flow to the left side, allowing for more relaxation of valvular obstruction and therefore increased blood flow through the valve.

Distinguishing features of different heart murmurs are shown in Table 2-7.

Gallops

Gallops are low-pitched heart sounds best heard with the bell. In tachycardia, they may combine to produce a *summation gallop*—just one sound. Ask the patient to lean on the left side and listen with the bell (used for low-pitched sounds) at the apex and sternum. Causes of gallops are shown in Table 2-8.

Rubs

Generally, a rub is a sign of pericardial irritation. Commonly, it has three phases—atrial

Table 2-7. Differences Among Common Heart Murmurs

Quality	Aortic Stenosis	Aortic Regurgitation	Mitral Stenosis	Mitral Regurgitation
Timing	Systolic	Diastolic	Diastolic	Systolic
Pattern	Crescendo-decrescendo	Decrescendo	Crescendo-decrescendo	Holosystolic usually
Location	Left upper sternal border	Apex	Apex	Apex/back
Radiation	Carotids	Sternal borders	None	Axilla, back
Pitch	Low to high	High to medium	Low to medium	Low to high
Timber	Harsh, coarse	Coarse	Rumbling	Pure

Table 2-8. Gallop Heart Sounds

S_3 (Ventricular Gallop)	S_4 (Atrial Gallop)
Extra sound heard just after S_2. Indicates *subnormal ventricular compliance*. It's diagnostic in older patients until proven otherwise. The blood beats like a mallet against the noncompliant dilated structure.	Due to an atrial kick forcing blood into a stiff poorly compliant ventricle. Seen in LVH with hypertension. Heard just before the S_1.

contraction, ventricular systole, and ventricular filling—but sometimes only two phases are heard. Rubs are best heard with the patient sitting up and listening at the left lower or right lower sternal borders.

Mechanical Valve Sounds

Unlike normal valves, mechanical valves should have *both* an opening *and* a closing sound. Mitral valves open just after S_1 and close at S_2. Aortic valves open just after S_2 and close at S_1. If one cannot hear the opening sound, pathology is present.

When to Get an Echocardiogram for an Abnormal Heart Sound

A benign murmur may be due to physiologic conditions outside the heart (called a *functional murmur*) or to a cardiac condition that is of minimal consequence for the individual involved. The following signs, in combination with other findings, signify that a nonbenign murmur may be present:

- Any and all diastolic murmurs—best heard with the patient sitting forward and on end expiration

- Greater than 3/6 in intensity
- Late-peaking crescendo-decrescendo murmur
- Holosystolic murmurs
- Radiation of the murmur to the axilla/back.
- Unexplained paradoxically split S_2 or a wide fixed split
- Increase in sounds with maneuvers that should decrease preload (consider if there is HOCM or mitral valve prolapse with mitral regurgitation)
- A new murmur in a febrile patient with clinical signs of endocarditis

DIAGNOSTIC AND THERAPEUTIC MODALITIES

Stress Testing

The use of noninvasive stress tests has become common in the evaluation of ischemic heart disease. Table 2-9 shows the reasons for ordering a stress test and the circumstances in which it should be avoided.

- All tests need a *stressor* and a *detector*. These are shown in Tables 2-10 and 2-11, respectively.

Table 2-9.   Indications and Contraindications for Stress Testing

Indications	Relative Contraindications	
1. Confirm a diagnosis of CAD and assess the degree of disease.	1. Acute MI within last 48 hours	5. Recent pulmonary embolism or deep venous thrombosis
2. Give prognostic information in CAD.	2. Severe aortic stenosis	6. Aortic dissection
3. Determine if medical therapy for CAD is working or if the patient is asymptomatic on the current regimen.	3. Decompensated heart failure	7. Uncontrolled severe hypertension
	4. Unstable angina	

Table 2-10.   Stress Testing—Stressors

Stressors	Description	Clinical Use
Exercise Treadmill	Patient walks on treadmill at increased workload (Bruce, Cornell, and Naughton are common protocols). Bruce is the most common protocol, with increases in the speed and grade in stages every 3 minutes. Achieving more than 10 minutes on a Bruce protocol is considered good. Achieving more than 15 minutes is incredible.	Usually the best stressor in a patient who is able to exercise, as it is a good indicator of exercise tolerance/functional capacity and gives useful prognostic information beyond the presence of CAD based on the duration of exercise on or off medications. It has limited use in deconditioned patients and those limited by other factors (peripheral arterial disease, arthritis, lung disease, and so forth). Some labs use hand-powered bicycles when patients cannot walk.
Dipyridamole (Persantine)	Blocks reuptake of adenosine and consequently also acts as a coronary vasodilator. Increases flow only in normal coronary arteries, not in abnormal ones whose arterioles are already quite vasodilated.	Not to be used in patients with active bronchospasm, severe heart block or hypotension, or diffuse multivessel disease (no difference is seen between similarly diseased coronary arteries). Medications such as theophylline, pentoxifylline, and any product with caffeine can interfere with this test and should be held beforehand. In the same way, Persantine can be easily reversed with aminophylline after it has been used in a patient who experiences any side effects.
Adenosine	A direct vasodilator of the small arterioles of the heart, increasing flow only in normal coronary arteries areas more than stenotic areas.	Has a shorter half-life than dipyridamole and its effects are more rapidly reversed after testing, but is much more expensive than dipyridamole. Has the same contraindications as dipyridamole.
Dobutamine	Positive inotrope and chronotrope via β agonist action.	Can cause ischemia by increasing cardiac demand as the heart rate is increased. So, not suitable for someone with a recent acute coronary syndrome, aortic dissection, or tachyarrhythmias. Concomitant β blocker use will make it difficult to reach the target heart rate, and usually should be held prior to testing. Dobutamine can also cause hypotension in some patients (it has some vasodilating activity via β_2 receptors). It is less preferred in patients with LBBB.

Table 2-11. Stress Testing—Detectors

Detectors	Description	Advantages	Disadvantages
ECG	During exercise, continuous 12-lead ECG monitoring is performed, looking for ST segment changes. V_5 has greatest sensitivity. Looks primarily for >1 mm ST segment flattening or 1.5 mm downsloping ST segment changes. Upsloping ST segment changes are nonspecific.	Simple, cheap, and easy to use. Noninvasive. Useful to assess for exercise-induce arrhythmias or symptoms produced with exercise. Commonly used in addition to ECHO or nuclear imaging.	When used alone, sensitivity is lower than that of stress imaging techniques. Any baseline ECG abnormalities (hypertrophy, left bundle branch, ST-T wave abnormalities) make interpretation quite difficult. Does not localize accurately or quantify extent of myocardial damage. Has lower sensitivity in women.
Echocardiography	Performed to look for wall motion abnormalities before and after a stressor is applied.	Same sensitivity/specificity as nuclear imaging studies with experienced readers and technicians. Portable, and results are available immediately. Gives additional parameters such as left ventricular function, size, and thickness, as well as valve function. High sensitivity for LAD and multivessel disease. No radiation used.	Nonstandardized interpretation. Difficult to interpret if wall motion abnormalities already present at rest. Not as useful in patients with poor baseline ECHO images (e.g., those who are extremely obese).
Thallium Nuclear Scintigraphy	Thallium is actively transported into viable cells with active Na-K pumps. The distribution during stressor application is imaged and then again several hours later after redistribution with the patient at rest.	Myocardial uptake is proportional to flow. There is a single injection for both stress and rest images. Considered the gold standard for viability assessment among single-photon agents.	Changes in coronary blood flow can have a large impact on redistribution. Nitrates help facilitate the appearance of thallium redistribution.
Technetium[99] (Tc[99]) Nuclear Scintigraphy Tc[99]: Three Types – Sestamibi, Tetrofosmin, Teboroxime	These are all lipophilic monovalent cations that diffuse passively across the cell membrane and are retained only within viable mitochondria. Initial distribution is proportional to myocardial flow. Redistribution images taken hours later reflect myocardial viability. An initial defect that resolves shows an area that is viable. One that is absent in both cases reflects dead myocardium.	Uptake is not dependent on Na-K pump. Undergoes minimal redistribution over time. Therefore, two injections are done: one at peak stress and one at rest. Can be given to patients with chest pain. Myocardial uptake is proportional to flow. There is minimal redistribution of tracer.	Obesity can interfere with imaging and give false-positive results, especially in women.

(continued)

Table 2-11. Continued

Detectors	Description	Advantages	Disadvantages
Positron-Emission Tomography/ Ultrafast CT	Based on flow and metabolism-dependent uptake of a radioactive tracer (usually Tc^{99}) by living myocardial tissue. Can be used to evaluate perfusion and viability	Can give simultaneous information about perfusion and function; therefore, more useful in patients with known CAD. Allows for evaluation of resting, post-stress, and regional wall motion and thickening Not limited by body habitus	Requires a regular rhythm ECG for gating to be performed Wall motion and thickening can be underestimated in areas where there is previous infarction or ischemia Cannot be performed at peak stress
MRI	New techniques allow for quick imaging with pharmacologic stressors to give high-resolution images showing areas of infarction and ischemia (edema)	High-resolution images also provide structural information regarding the EF, valvular disease, and myocardial disease. Can help classify ischemic versus nonischemic cardiomyopathy	Time required to scan may be long, depending on institution's protocol. Limited use in patients with metal or pacemakers

- A stressor can be functional, such as exercise or dobutamine, which attempts to raise the heart rate to the target level (85% of maximum, or roughly 220 minus the patient's age) for a sustained period of time during which imaging can be performed. Alternatively, a stressor can be an injected agent, such as adenosine or dipyridamole, that vasodilates vessels and increases coronary blood flow. Measures of workload include metabolic equivalents (METS), which are measurements of oxygen consumption (rule of thumb: 4 METS = walking up a flight of stairs; 10 METS = strenuous exercise such as swimming or biking).
- A detector assesses the consequence on the myocardium of either increased workload and oxygen demand or differences in perfusion.
- The specificity and sensitivity of stress testing vary with the experience of the reader and the technical quality of the study, depending on the patient's characteristics.

Cardiac Imaging

Echocardiography (ECHO)

- Echocardiography uses ultrasound to give two- and three-dimensional images of the heart to assess for chamber size, function,

wall motion, ejection fraction (EF), valve structure, congenital abnormalities, intracardiac thrombi, pressure gradients, and the direction of blood flow with Doppler imaging, as well as the presence of effusions.
- A standard ECHO report gives the size of all chambers in addition to the size of the aorta. Valves are reported to have stenosis or regurgitation, quantified as mild, moderate, or severe.
- Pulmonary artery systolic pressure (PASP) can be estimated based on the velocity of tricuspid regurgitation (TR) using the modified Bernoulli equation: PASP = Right Atrial Pressure + 4x (Peak TR Velocity)^2.
- Right atrial pressure is estimated by the degree of inferior vena cava (IVC) collapse upon inspiration; less collapse means higher right atrial pressure.
- Intracardiac shunts can be visualized by a *bubble study* in which contrast material, usually agitated saline bubbles (created by drawing a small amount of air into a saline syringe), is injected into the venous system and then passed from the right heart to the left heart. Early bubbles (within a few heartbeats) suggest intracardiac right-to-left shunts, whereas late bubbles (after more than five beats)

suggest extracardiac shunting from, say, pulmonary arteriovenous malformations.

- M-mode ECHO assesses depth of structures across time along one thin line of ultrasound. It is most accurate for measurements of distances and valve activity.
- Two major basic types of ECHO are commonly used; these are summarized in Table 2-12.

Cardiac Catheterization

This is the gold standard for the identification of obstructive coronary artery disease. Indications are shown in Table 2-13.

- Currently, cardiac catheterization has the highest resolution for coronary artery anatomy as compared to any other imaging modality.
- Cardiac catheterization shows luminal but not extraluminal disease; significant non-obstructive atherosclerosis can still exist, as in positive remodeling, where vessels sometimes expand outward but are highly diseased.

- Patients are lightly sedated, and specially designed catheters are placed via either the femoral or the radial arteries to engage the coronary arteries; contrast dye is injected into the arteries, and cinematographic pictures are taken.
- Common interventions include percutaneous transluminal coronary angioplasty (PTCA), percutaneous coronary intervention (PCI) with either bare metal or drug-eluting stents, valvuloplasty of stenotic valvular lesions, and, more recently, atrial septal defect/patent foramen ovale (ASD/PFO) closure using specially made closure devices.

Cardiac Magnetic Resonance Imaging (C-MRI)

- This method is very precise in discriminating among pericardial diseases, such as in distinguishing constrictive pericarditis from restrictive cardiomyopathy. It can assess for degrees of cardiac fibrosis,

Table 2-12. Features of Transthoracic and Transesophageal Echocardiography

Transthoracic ECHO (TTE)	Transesophageal ECHO (TEE)
Probe across sternum and chest in an awake patient.	Probe inserted through esophagus in anesthetized patient.
Can be used to estimate intracardiac pressures indirectly.	Usually done if TTE is poor or intraoperative assessment is needed. Better used to assess some parts of the aortic arch and valvular vegetations.
Harder to do in postoperative cardiac patients, those with chest tubes, morbidly obese patients, and others who do not have "good windows" for ultrasound.	Carries risk of esophageal injury and sedation.

Table 2-13. Indications and Contraindications for Coronary Angiography

Indications	Relative Contraindications
Stable angina/unstable angina/acute MI (STEMI or high-risk NSTEMI) with a goal to PTCA or pre-CABG	Coagulopathy—needs prior correction
Abnormal stress test in the appropriate clinical setting	Renal failure—limit dye exposure, prevent contrast nephropathy
Ventricular arrhythmia or arrhythmia with no obvious metabolic cause, to assess for CAD	Dye allergy—pretreat with steroids
Left ventricular dysfunction of unclear etiology	Uncontrolled severe hypertension—needs control before arterial puncture
Preoperative assessment in high-risk patients	Decompensated heart failure—treat first, as the patient needs to lie flat for the procedure; intubate the patient in extremis
	Infection—overwhelming sepsis makes catheterization less useful unless a significant cardiogenic component is thought to be present

patterns of which are useful to determine the degree of myocardial viability in specific coronary distributions area as well as helpful in diagnose nonischemic causes of fibrosis, including infiltrative cardiomyopathies such as sarcoidosis.

- C-MRI can also be used to easily assess cardiac chamber volumes and the EF of both ventricles and give cine motion of the heart to assess for wall motion abnormalities.
- C-MRI is useful in identifying ascending aortic dissection in those patients who cannot tolerate contrast computed tomography (CT).
- Disadvantages are that the test can be operator dependent, the patient must be hemodynamically stable and have no relative contraindications (presence of a pacemaker, an implantable cardiac defibrillator [ICD], or other locally embedded metal objects that limit ability to visualize structures), and the patient must be able hold his/her breath.

Coronary CT Angiography

- This is a fast and reliable way to image both heart structure and function.
- Coronary artery imaging is gated to parts of the cardiac cycle, and the best images are acquired at slower heart rates (less motion). Current resolution is still less than that obtained with coronary angiography.
- The amount of intravenous (IV) contrast used is similar to that used in a coronary angiogram and is used to detect putative soft plaques. The CT radiation dosage varies.
- A separate modality without IV contrast performed first provides calcium scores that are useful prognostically. A zero calcium score has a high negative predictive value for coronary artery disease (CAD). A very high calcium score makes it difficult to fully visualize concomitant soft plaques and the CT angiography portion may then be cancelled.
- Coronary CT imaging is commonly used in the ER to identify low- to moderate-risk patients (it has a high negative predictive value).
- It is a good test for patients who cannot undergo preoperative angiography (e.g., someone with

aortic valve endocarditis who will undergo aortic valve surgery and needs a coronary artery assessment beforehand. Cardiac catheterization could disrupt the endocarditic lesion on the aortic valve).

Pacemakers and ICDs

These devices are used to detect abnormal rhythms and pace the heart under a variety of conditions. They are implanted subcutaneously, with electrodes placed within the right atrium and right ventricle via the veins leading into the atria and ventricles, typically the right ventricle (left ventricular leads are placed via the coronary sinus or from a surgically placed epicardial wire).

Pacemakers

Table 2-14 is a reference for basic nomenclature of the pacemaker. Either three or four letters are used to describe a pacemaker device.

Common examples of pacemakers include the following:

VVI—the pacer paces in the ventricle, can sense the native ventricle only, and is inhibited from pacing a ventricular beat when it senses a native ventricular beat.

DDD—atria and ventricles can be paced and are both sensed; the pacer will be inhibited by endogenous beats but will initiate its own beat if it does not sense an endogenous one after a programmed amount of time.

VAT—the pacer paces in the ventricle after it senses the atria, based on the set AV delay.

Common indications for pacemaker insertion include those with symptomatic bradycardia or symptomatic heart block. Complete heart block and Mobitz type II block will need a permanent pacemaker if the cause is not easily reversible, even if the patient is asymptomatic. First-degree AV block and Mobitz type I block do not need a pacemaker in asymptomatic patients. (See the Bradycardias section for the definitions of types of heart block.)

Implantable Cardiac Defibrillators

- The primary function of these devices is to sense for life-threatening fast rhythms and

Table 2-14.   Nomenclature of Pacemaker Modes

First Letter (Chambers That Are *Paced*)	Second Letter (Chambers That Are *Sensed*)	Third Letter (How the Pacemaker *Responds*)	Fourth Letter (Does Pacemaker *Modulate* Heart Rate)
V—ventricles only A—atria only D—both atria and ventricles (dual)	V—ventricles only A—atria only D—both atria and ventricles (dual) O—none	T—triggers pacer to initiate a beat I—inhibits pacer from initiating a beat D—can both trigger and inhibit O—none	R—rate modulated (changes the heart rate based on physical activity levels)

then deliver therapy (either antitachycardia pacing or a shock) to terminate the rhythm if necessary.

- Modern ICDs all have backup pacing in addition to defibrillation in case the heart rate is too slow.
- Two features distinguish ICDs from pacemaker-only devices on a chest X-ray. They are much larger because they need a larger capacitor to provide a shock. They also have a thick shocking coil, which is usually placed in the right ventricle.
- Knowing the brand name is also essential for interrogation; this should be determined before requesting an interrogation.
- Implantation of an ICD for *primary prevention* is for anyone at high risk of sudden cardiac death who has not yet suffered an event. This includes individuals with:
  ◘ Familial syndromes of sudden cardiac death—for example, certain forms of Brugada syndrome.
  ◘ Hypertrophic obstructive cardiomyopathy under certain circumstances (see the HOCM section below).
  ◘ Ischemic and nonischemic cardiomyopathies with an EF < 30%–35% after several months of medical therapy aimed at improving the EF and revascularization as appropriate (these patients are at higher risk of sudden cardiac death).
- Secondary prevention: ICD implantation is for those resuscitated after cardiac arrest from a nonreversible cause (e.g., it is not for acute reversible ischemia or severe electrolyte imbalance).

- After implantation, most devices usually require defibrillator function threshold (DFT) testing to determine how many joules the ICD will need to break ventricular tachycardia (VT) or ventricular fibrillation (VF). This is done by inducing VT/VF by shocking on the T wave and letting the device recover the patient. Many ICDs will also do antitachycardia pacing if the VT is slow enough for the device to pace the heart out of the rhythm.

Criteria for Chronic Resynchronization Therapy (CRT)

- CRT refers to putting in a biventricular pacemaker to allow better synchrony of left and right ventricular contraction. The left ventricular lead is placed down a branch of the coronary sinus and can activate the left ventricle in this fashion.
- Criteria for CRT include: (1) Ejection fraction ≤35%, (2) left ventricular dyssynchrony with QRS >120 msec, (3) moderate to severe congestive heart failure (CHF) symptoms [New York Heart Association (NYHA) class III or IV] despite optimal medial therapy (see Table 2-24).
- Although CRT is not widely recommended for those with class II heart failure, growing evidence suggests it may be useful in select cases with significant evidence of dyssynchrony.
- Whether the patient has a right bundle branch block (RBBB) or a left bundle branch block (LBBB), it is still recommended (most patients in the studies have LBBB).
- This situation is less well studied in patients with atrial fibrillation, though the weight of evidence includes them.

Cardiac Enzymes

- Markers of myocardial cell death specifically used to evaluate for myocardial infarction include troponin, total creatine kinase (CK), and the isoenzyme of creatine kinase with muscle and brain subunits (CK-MB). These are shown in Table 2-15. Older markers used that are much less specific include the aspartate aminotransferase/alanine aminotransferase (AST/ALT) ratio (AST is released from cardiac muscle), the erythrocyte sedimentation rate (ESR), and the white blood cell (WBC) count, which may be elevated in the setting of an acute myocardial infarction (MI).
- Typically, to rule out that an individual has had an actual MI with heart muscle damage, one needs either three sets of negative cardiac enzyme tests (usually both CK and troponin) taken 8 hours apart or two sets of tests taken 12 hours apart in order to assess damage 24 hours after the onset of chest pain. This must be done with serial ECGs as well. Other algorithms may be shorter with newer, more sensitive troponin assays.
- The main difference between these markers of cardiac injury is their sensitivity/specificity for cardiac myocardial injury and half-life. Enzyme tests can be negative initially if they are performed immediately after an event. Figure 2-6 shows the normal time course of each major biomarker.
- Keep in mind that positive cardiac enzyme tests do not always mean MI from an acute coronary syndrome. They can result from cardiac myocyte destruction due to other causes, such as cardiac contusion from trauma, pulmonary embolus

Table 2-15. Use of Cardiac Biomarker in Acute Coronary Syndrome

Enzyme	Timing	Comments
Creatine Kinase (CK)	Rises within 4–8 hours and usually normalizes within 48–72 hours.	Nonspecific because the level may increase after muscle trauma, myocarditis, rhabdomyolysis, polymyositis, and renal injury. Peak level correlates somewhat with infarct size. Usually followed after an MI until the peak value is reached.
CK-MB Fraction	Rises within 4–6 hours of the onset of ACS or MI. Returns to normal within 36 hours, so a better marker for recurrent injury.	Five percent of the total CK is where the upper cutoff limit for possible MI occurs. MB is found in small amounts in healthy adults in skeletal muscle. CK-MB is also increased after cardioversion and cardiac surgery/trauma and from the brain and tongue during seizures.
Troponin I	Rises within 3–6 hours of onset of chest pain and can remain elevated up to 7–10 days afterward.	Cardiac myocyte specific and therefore a very sensitive marker for any cardiac injury. Patients with positive troponins and negative CK or MB may have had an MI several days ago that was not previously diagnosed.
Troponin T	Rises 6 hours after injury and remains elevated for up to 10–14 days.	Similar to troponin I but can be increased falsely in patients with renal failure.
Myoglobin	Earliest positive biomarker.	Positive within 2 hours and quickly returns to normal. Nonspecific because found in skeletal muscle.

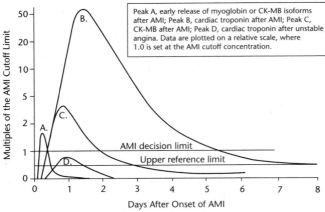

Peak A, early release of myoglobin or CK-MB isoforms after AMI; Peak B, cardiac troponin after AMI; Peak C, CK-MB after AMI; Peak D, cardiac troponin after unstable angina. Data are plotted on a relative scale, where 1.0 is set at the AMI cutoff concentration.

Figure 2-6. Timing of Cardiac Biomarker Release with Acute Myocardial Injury (AMI). Adapted from Wu AHB et al. National Academy of Clinical Biochemistry Standards of Laboratory Practice: Recommendations for the use of cardiac markers in coronary artery diseases. *Clin Chem*. 1999 45:1104–1121.

(PE) with right ventricle strain, demand-related ischemia (a fixed obstructive lesion), or myocarditis, to name a few examples.

APPROACH TO COMMON PROBLEMS

Approach to the Patient with Acute Chest Pain

The approach should always be to rule out the most serious causes first (as shown in Table 2-16) and then focus on other, less serious causes (Table 2-17). In cases where patients are unable to give a history immediately, it is imperative to know how to use your clinical exam to find the cause and your knowledge of known risk factors to risk stratify a patient.

With any critical patient who looks sick and is complaining of chest pain but is unable to give a history, start with the ABCs, do a quick exam, and make sure that an ECG and a set of vital signs is done, using the clues in Table 2-16 to help make a diagnosis.

In stable patients the questions listed in Table 2-18 need to be asked, with a specific focus on symptoms causing serious chest pain.

Approach to the Patient with Acute Coronary Syndrome (ACS)

Acute coronary syndrome includes a spectrum of conditions (unstable angina, non–ST elevation MI, ST elevation MI) that all have the same underlying pathophysiology, namely, *the rupture of a coronary plaque* with ensuing thrombosis and symptomatic partial or complete coronary arterial occlusion. This is in contrast to an atherosclerotic plaque causing luminal occlusion and symptoms on exertion, as seen in stable angina due to supply–demand mismatch. The key to the diagnosis of an acute coronary syndrome is a good history in addition to adjunctive information such as ECG changes and cardiac enzyme tests, each of which alone can give false-positive results in many circumstances. Figure 2-7 provides a practical approach to triage and management.

Approach to the Patient with a Tachyarrhythmia

Basic Advanced Cardiac Life Support (ACLS) guidelines are given elsewhere. The algorithm shown in Figure 2-8 is designed to facilitate the rapid diagnosis of a tachyarrhythmia using a 12-lead ECG with a view to treatment. A more detailed discussion of individual conditions is presented later in this chapter.

Approach to the Patient with Syncope

Syncope is a sudden loss of consciousness (LOC) due to decreased cerebral perfusion pressure followed by spontaneous recovery. Many causes exist, but in up to 30%–50% of cases a cause cannot be identified. Presyncope does not result in LOC but can be due to similar causes as syncope. Questions to ask of anyone with syncope are shown in Table 2-19A, followed by the most common causes, and diagnosis, and treatment in Table 2-19B.

Table 2-16. Causes of Chest Pain Requiring Emergent Intervention

Cause	Signs on Exam/Data to Help Make Immediate Diagnosis
Myocardial Infarction	Inferior MI – Bradycardia, hypotension, nausea, vomiting – Signs of acute right heart failure (elevated JVP, hypotension) Anterior MI – SiSx of left heart failure (pulmonary edema, hypoxia, even cardiogenic shock) – New murmur (mitral regurgitation, aortic insufficiency) Malignant arrhythmia, cardiac arrest
	ECG changes (T wave inversions, ST elevations, a new LBBB), positive cardiac enzymes (later finding) should make the diagnosis.
Massive Pulmonary Embolus	Hypoxic, with minimal improvement in oxygen saturation (implying a large arterial–alveolar gradient) Evidence of deep vein thrombosis (warm, painful calf) Evidence of right heart strain: on ECG (intermittent right bundle), heart sounds: loud P_2 Signs of acute right heart failure Hypotension Patient has multiple risk factors (old age, obesity immobilized, recent trauma)
	PE protocol CT makes the diagnosis. Stat ECHO may show right ventricular strain but is less diagnostic.
Aortic Dissection	Hypotension or hypertension Differential pressures in arms or legs Wide mediastinum may be seen on stat chest X-ray Signs of tamponade and ischemia may be seen from retrograde dissection to coronaries Focal neurologic deficits may be seen from carotid artery dissection or emboli
	Contrast CT, MRA, or transesophageal ECHO of the proximal aorta can make the diagnosis.
Pneumothorax and Tension Pneumothorax	Marked hypoxia Markedly unequal breath sounds; decreased on one side, hypertympanic on the other Tracheal deviation Hypotension
	For tension pneumothorax, needle decompression makes the diagnosis. For pneumothorax, chest X-ray makes the diagnosis.
Cardiac Tamponade	Beck's triad – elevated JVP, distant heart sounds, and hypotension Shock Pulsus paradoxus on exam
	Positive pericardiocentesis makes the diagnosis emergently. ECHO can be used to demonstrate increased pressures if the condition is less emergent.
Esophageal Rupture (rare)	Widened mediastinum on chest X-ray with mediastinal or free peritoneal air Subcutaneous emphysema (crackles heard under the skin)
	Diagnosis is confirmed by a water-soluble contrast study of the esophagus.

Table 2-17. Less Urgent Causes of Chest Pain

Other cardiac causes	Pericarditis; stable angina
Lung	Pleuritis
Musculoskeletal pain	Costochondritis; trauma
Gastrointestinal	Heartburn; esophageal spasm; gastritis; pancreatitis; gallbladder disease; Mallory-Weiss tear
Infectious	Pneumonia; shingles (pain can appear before lesions); abscess
Psychogenic	Anxiety; drug withdrawal

Table 2-18. Questions to Ask the Stable Patient with Chest Pain

	Questions to Ask	Differential Diagnoses
Presentation/ Precipitating Factors	Did the pain come on very suddenly or gradually? Is there anything that brings on the pain (taking a deep breath/walking/ running/lifting/just after a meal/?) Is there anything you do that relieves the pain (changing your position, resting, taking a sublingual nitroglycerin tablet)?	Very sudden onset with associated dyspnea → PE or pneumothorax? Very abrupt onset of excruciating pain through back → aortic dissection? Pain with inspiration → pericardial or pleural inflammation? Pain with exertion and relief with rest → stable angina? Pain after a meal → angina or heartburn? Pain worse lying supine → heartburn or pericarditis. Pericardial pain may be relieved with sitting forward. Pain with pressure on the chest between ribs → costochondritis?
Quality	Is the pain sharp, dull, or burning? Point to the painful area with one finger.	Burning substernal pain may be indicative of heartburn. Cardiac-related chest pain can be dull, aching, or pressure-like but may also be sharp. Pleuritic pain is usually sharp. Focal pinpoint pain is less likely to be cardiac.
Radiation	Does the pain travel anywhere? To your arms/hands? To your neck and jaw? To your back or abdomen?	Radiation to arms, neck, and jaw is indicative of cardiac chest pain. Radiation to back or abdomen should make one consider aortic dissection.
Severity/ Symptoms That Are Associated	How bad is the pain on a scale of 1 to 10? Are there any other things you notice with the pain (problems breathing, nausea, vomiting, sweating, coughing, syncope)?	Intensity of the pain is determined mainly for management and may not help distinguish among many causes. Associated nausea, vomiting, and sweating in addition to shortness of breath are more typical of cardiac chest pain.
Timing	Does the pain come and go? If so, how long does it last? Have you ever had this type of pain before?	Typical acute coronary syndrome cardiac chest pain lasts for 15–30 minutes at a time, not for hours, and is not usually constant but comes and goes unless frank massive infarction has occurred.

Table 2-19A. Important Points to Consider in the History of Syncope

Prodromes	Light-headedness, dizziness, diaphoresis, auras. Was the patient alert enough to break his fall (broken wrist, bruised arm)? Those without a prodrome or with drop attacks are more likely to have a cardiac cause.
Seizure Activity	Bowel, bladder incontinence, tonic-clonic movements, postictal state, duration of LOC? Note that sometimes myoclonus can be seen in syncope, on occasion with prolonged LOC.
Medications	Is the patient taking AV nodal agents, benzodiazepines or other sedating agents, or diuretics?
Activity Just Preceding the Syncope	Extreme exertion inducing syncope may indicate aortic stenosis or ischemia. Vagal-mediated syncope may occur with certain activities.
Comorbidities	Distinguish between young, healthy people (consider situational syncope or congenital structural heart disease, e.g., HOCM) vs. older people with either known structural heart disease or possible neurologic causes.

Table 2-19B. Types of Syncope

Type	Causes	Diagnosis	Treatment
Orthostatic Hypotension	An inappropriate reduction in BP or a heart rate increase in moving from supine to standing condition. May be due to hypovolemia of any cause, autonomic neuropathy, as in patients with severe diabetes, Parkinson's disease, or adrenal insufficiency.	Check orthostatics: Does BP fall >15% in moving from a supine to a standing position, with a rise in heart rate? Patient may be "dry" on exam/laboratory tests (elevated BUN/Cr) or anemic.	Replete fluids in appropriate patients. Treat the underlying condition (e.g., anemia, adrenal insufficiency).
Situational	Increases in vagal tone occur in various physiologic circumstances. Types include those related to • Strained micturition (usually in men). • Prolonged coughing. • Choking or prolonged Valsalva maneuver. • Straining with bowel movements.	The history of what the patient was doing at the time of the event is key to the diagnosis of such types. All of these conditions will require a negative tilt table test on further work-up.	Patient education and prevention of causative situations.
Cardiogenic	• Intrinsic problems of the heart cause hypoperfusion. This type is more serious than other causes in terms of long-term mortality. • *Conduction system disease*—tachyarrhythmias (VT, SVTs, VF, AF), bradyarrhythmias (sinus pause, AV block—called a *Stokes Adams attack* if complete block, sick sinus syndrome). Classically, the LOC is sudden and instantaneous. • *Structural disease*—exertion in patient with HOCM, aortic stenosis, left main coronary disease, severe pulmonary hypertension can cause syncope. Right heart strain from a massive PE can also cause syncope. Rarely, large MIs can cause syncope. • *Carotid sinus disease*—excessive mechanical stimulation by a tight collar or with neck rotation can cause profound bradycardia from pressure leading to reflex arc of increased vasovagal tone.	Conduction system disease is usually seen on ECG or telemetry monitoring or is induced in the EP laboratory. Structural disease and valvular abnormalities are evaluated by ECHO. Carotid sinus hypersensitivity can be assessed with pressure on the carotid bulb. Eliciting a sinus pause of >2 sec is diagnostic. Do not do this in patients with known or suspected carotid stenosis.	Treatment depends on the specific defect found. In general, conduction abnormalities or carotid sinus disease causing syncope may require a pacemaker. Structural and valvular disease may require valve repair and management of the underlying condition.

continued

Table 2-19B. *(continued)*

Type	Causes	Diagnosis	Treatment
Neurologic	Usually due to vertebrobasilar insufficiency, which affects the posterior circulation blood supply to both hemispheres. It is rare for anterior circulation problems to cause LOC, as both hemispheres need to be affected simultaneously for this to occur. Thus, carotid disease is very unlikely to cause syncope but is usually evaluated if the description of syncope or presyncope cannot be distinguished from a transient ischemic attack (TIA).	Evaluation includes an MRI/MRA of the vertebrobasilar system or, at the least, transcranial Doppler scans. Carotid Doppler scans, while useful in working up a cause of TIAs, do not need to be done routinely for syncope unless the patient has risk factors for carotid disease.	Posterior circulation stenting can be done in appropriate patients. Otherwise, keep mean arterial pressure elevated and treat any underlying conditions (e.g., lipid control for atherosclerosis or anticoagulation for hypercoagulable states).
Neurocardiogenic (also called *vasovagal, vasodepressor,* or *neural-mediated syncope*)	1. Increased vagal tone (cardioinhibitory mechanisms) or, less commonly, decreased sympathetic tone (vasodepressor mechanisms) of various causes. 2. Abnormal reflex responses such as those involving the Bezold-Jarisch reflex, where atrial and venous stretch receptors sense volume loading and cause vagal activation. 3. Conditions that cause increased venous pooling and decreased preload with inappropriate compensation can cause the heart to pump faster to increase cardiac output. If the preload is fixed, however, this leads to hypoperfusion. Finally, a problem in central serotonergic pathways has been postulated.	If not clear from the history/exam, consider a tilt table test (the patient is put on a table that is tilted up from horizontal with continuous ECG and BP monitoring). A positive test reproduces syncope or significant changes in BP or heart rate. Provocative testing with isoproterenol or nitroglycerin can be done and the test repeated.	Treatment for those with recurrent symptoms includes β blockers, selective serotonin reuptake inhibitors (SSRIs), and in certain cases fludrocortisone or midodrine, which can decrease venous pooling and increase arterial tone.

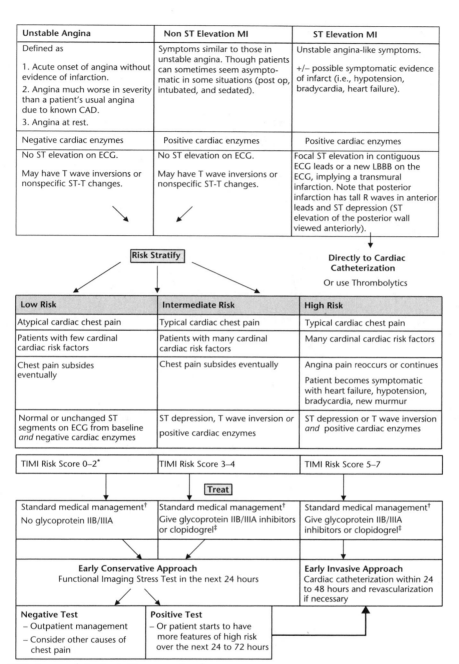

Unstable Angina	Non ST Elevation MI	ST Elevation MI
Defined as 1. Acute onset of angina without evidence of infarction. 2. Angina much worse in severity than a patient's usual angina due to known CAD. 3. Angina at rest.	Symptoms similar to those in unstable angina. Though patients can sometimes seem asymptomatic in some situations (post op, intubated, and sedated).	Unstable angina-like symptoms. +/− possible symptomatic evidence of infarct (i.e., hypotension, bradycardia, heart failure).
Negative cardiac enzymes	Positive cardiac enzymes	Positive cardiac enzymes
No ST elevation on ECG. May have T wave inversions or nonspecific ST-T changes.	No ST elevation on ECG. May have T wave inversions or nonspecific ST-T changes.	Focal ST elevation in contiguous ECG leads or a new LBBB on the ECG, implying a transmural infarction. Note that posterior infarction has tall R waves in anterior leads and ST depression (ST elevation of the posterior wall viewed anteriorly).

Risk Stratify

Directly to Cardiac Catheterization

Or use Thrombolytics

Low Risk	Intermediate Risk	High Risk
Atypical cardiac chest pain	Typical cardiac chest pain	Typical cardiac chest pain
Patients with few cardinal cardiac risk factors	Patients with many cardinal cardiac risk factors	Many cardinal cardiac risk factors
Chest pain subsides eventually	Chest pain subsides eventually	Angina pain reoccurs or continues Patient becomes symptomatic with heart failure, hypotension, bradycardia, new murmur
Normal or unchanged ST segments on ECG from baseline *and* negative cardiac enzymes	ST depression, T wave inversion *or* positive cardiac enzymes	ST depression or T wave inversion *and* positive cardiac enzymes
TIMI Risk Score 0–2*	TIMI Risk Score 3–4	TIMI Risk Score 5–7

Treat

Standard medical management† No glycoprotein IIB/IIIA	Standard medical management† Give glycoprotein IIB/IIIA inhibitors or clopidogrel‡	Standard medical management† Give glycoprotein IIB/IIIA inhibitors or clopidogrel‡

Early Conservative Approach
Functional Imaging Stress Test in the next 24 hours

Early Invasive Approach
Cardiac catheterization within 24 to 48 hours and revascularization if necessary

Negative Test	Positive Test
– Outpatient management – Consider other causes of chest pain	– Or patient starts to have more features of high risk over the next 24 to 72 hours

Figure 2-7. Approach to Acute Coronary Syndrome.
*TIMI Risk Score (one point each)
1. Age> 65; 2. Three or more risk factors for CAD; 3. Prior known stenosis >50%; 4. Two or more anginal events in the past day; 5. Aspirin use in the past 7 days; 6. ST changes on ECG; 7. Positive cardiac markers.

†Standard Medical Management
1. Oxygen; 2. Aspirin; 3. β blocker—avoid in acute heart failure or shock; 4. Heparin or low-molecular-weight heparin; 5. ACE inhibitor; 6. Statin; 7. Nitrates (SLNTG and then nitroglycerin drip); 8. Morphine for continued pain.

‡Clopidogrel is given as a 300-mg or 600-mg loading dose followed by 75 mg daily. It may be held if there is a high likelihood of bleeding or of CABG.

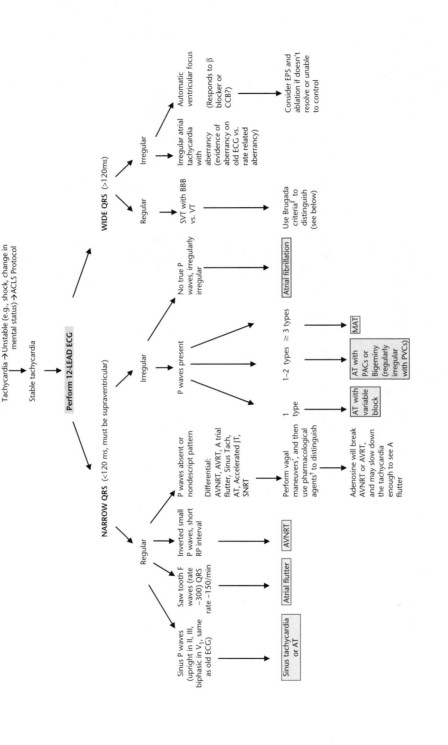

Tachycardia → Unstable (e.g., shock, change in mental status) → ACLS Protocol

Stable tachycardia

Perform 12-LEAD ECG

NARROW QRS (<120 ms, must be supraventricular)

WIDE QRS (>120ms)

Regular

Sinus P waves (upright in II, III, biphasic in V₁, same as old ECG)

Saw tooth F waves (rate ~300) QRS rate ~150/min

Inverted small P waves, short RP interval

P waves absent or nondescript pattern

Differential: AVNRT, AVRT, A trial flutter, Sinus Tach, AT, Accelerated JT, SNRT

Perform vagal maneuvers*, and then use pharmacological agents† to distinguish

Adenosine will break AVNRT or AVRT, and may slow down the tachycardia enough to see A flutter

Sinus tachycardia or AT

Atrial flutter

AVNRT

Irregular

P waves present

1 type

1–2 types

≥ 3 types

AT with variable block

AT with PACs or Bigeminy (regularly irregular with PVCs)

MAT

No true P waves, irregularly irregular

Atrial fibrillation

Regular

SVT with BBB vs. VT

Use Brugada criteria‡ to distinguish (see below)

Irregular

Irregular atrial tachycardia with aberrancy (evidence of aberrancy on old ECG vs. rate related aberrancy)

Automatic ventricular focus

(Responds to β blocker or CCB?)

Consider EPS and ablation if doesn't resolve or unable to control

Figure 2-8. Algorithmic Approach to Patient with a Tachyarrhythmia.

*Vagal maneuvers (carotid sinus massage, Valsalva maneuver)

†Pharmacologic agents:

1. Adenosine 6 mg IV push, then 12 mg IV followed by 12 mg IV while the ECG strip is running. The half-life is short, so it may last only few seconds.

2. Diltiazem, verapamil, or a β blocker can be used for rate control.

‡Brugada algorithm for SVT versus VT

Part One

1. Is there absence of an RS in all precordial leads (assesses for concordance)?

    Yes → VT   No → go to (2)

2. R to S interval >100 msec in one precordial lead?

    Yes → VT   No → go to (3)

3. AV dissociation?

    Yes → VT   No→ go to (4)

4. Morphology criteria for VT present in V_{1-2} and V_6?

    Yes → VT   No→ SVT with aberrant conduction

Note: A new northwest (extreme axis) also strongly suggests VT.

Part Two

Use Morphology criteria for VT
RBBB-like complex (then apply Wellen's criteria):

V_1 monophasic R wave?
        Broad R (>30 msec) with terminal negative forces
        qR pattern?

V_6 rS pattern (r < S), QRS, QR, monophasic R?

LBBB-like complex (apply Kindwell criteria):

V_{1-2} broad R (>30 msec)?
        Notching in downstroke of S wave?
        Interval from onset of R to nadir of S>60 ms?

V_6 QR, QS, QRS, Rr'

AT, atrial tachycardia of any type; AVNRT, atrioventricular nodal reentrant tachycardia; AVRT, atrioventricular reentrant tachycardia; BBB, bundle branch block; CCB, calcium channel blocker; EPS, electrophysiology study; JT, junctional tachycardia; MAT, multifocal atrial tachycardia; PACs, premature atrial contractions; SNRT, sinus nodal reentrant tachycardia; SVT, supraventricular tachycardia.

Approach to the Use and Interpretation of Right Heart (Swan-Ganz) Catheterization

Right heart catheterization can sometimes be an important adjunct to the physical exam in the critically ill patient who has advanced cardiovascular disease. Table 2-20 reviews common indications for its use.

Procedure

The right internal jugular and left subclavian veins are the preferred sites. Femoral vein right heart catheterization is also possible. The catheter is tunneled through the venous system into the right atrium, the right ventricle, and then into the pulmonary artery, where it is placed such that the balloon can be inflated to occlude flow and allow measurement of pressure distally. This pressure is known as the pulmonary capillary wedge pressure (PCWP) and is a surrogate of left atrial pressure, which tells us about the left ventricular end diastolic pressure (LVEDP). Valuable information is obtained during placement as each chamber is traversed, not just after final placement, as shown in Table 2-21.

Table 2-20.   Indications for Right Heart Catheterization

Indications	Contraindications
• To differentiate between different types of shock when this is difficult to do clinically • To assess the hemodynamic response to therapy (e.g., inotropes) • To assess restrictive vs. constrictive vs. tamponade physiology • To assess severity of pulmonary hypertension • To assess for intracardiac shunts	• Profound coagulopathy • Tricuspid or pulmonary valve prosthesis or endocarditis • Right heart or pulmonary artery mass • LBBB (relative), as complete heart block can be caused when RBBB is induced with the catheter in the right ventricle

Note: No study has definitively demonstrated an improved mortality outcome in critically ill patients managed using pulmonary artery catheters.

Table 2-21.   Data Obtained During Right Heart Catheterization

A. Measured Values	Normal Range
Right atrial pressure (RAP) or central venous pressure (CVP)	5 mmHg
Right ventricular systolic/diastolic pressures	25/5 mmHg
Pulmonary artery systolic/diastolic pressures	25/15 mmHg
Pulmonary capillary wedge pressure (PCWP) (assumed equal to left atrial pressure and a surrogate for left ventricular end-diastolic pressure [LVEDP])	6–12 mmHg
Mixed venous oxygen saturation (from the PA)	70%–75%

B. Calculated Values	Calculation	Normal Range
Cardiac output (CO)	By Fick/thermodilution	4–8 L/min
Cardiac index (CI)	CO/body surface area	2.8–4 L/min/m²
Systemic vascular resistance (SVR)	80 x (MAP – RAP)/CO	770–1500 dynes sec/cm²
Pulmonary vascular resistance (PVR)	80 x (mean PAP – PCWP)/CO*	20–120 dynes sec/cm²

MAP, mean arterial pressure; PAP, pulmonary artery pressure.
*Assumes no shunt.

Fick Method for Cardiac Output

$$CO = \frac{VO_2}{(SaO_2 - SvO_2) \times 13.4 \times \text{Hemoglobin}}$$

- VO_2 is the estimated oxygen consumption (assumed from a nomogram or measured).
- SaO_2 is the arterial oxygenation saturation from an arterial blood gas (ABG) determination expressed as a decimal (e.g., 0.98).
- SvO_2 is the mixed venous oxygenation saturation from the Swan-Ganz catheter expressed as a decimal (e.g., 0.75).

Other methods for determining cardiac output, which are based on the use of thermistors and changes in temperature are also available.

Use in Shock

When used to determine the etiology of shock, keep in mind the following:

Septic shock—high cardiac output, low systemic vascular resistance (SVR), low pulmonary capillary wedge pressure (PCWP)
Cardiogenic shock—low cardiac output, low SVR, high PCWP
Hypovolemic shock—low cardiac output, high SVR, low PCWP

DISEASES OF THE CARDIOVASCULAR SYSTEM

Myocardial Diseases

Ischemic Heart Disease (IHD)

D—A condition in which the cardiovascular demand exceeds its oxygen supply, most commonly due to narrowing of coronary arteries from thrombosis or atheromatous plaque accumulation. This encompasses a wide variety of conditions that differ in their pathophysiology, ranging from stable angina to MI.

Epi—Presentations for an MI follows the rule of thirds: one-third of patients present with angina, one-third with evidence of infarction, and one-third with sudden death.

Twenty-five percent of patients with MI do not seek medical attention. Twenty-five percent of MIs are silent and unrecognized and present as new ECG abnormalities or wall motion abnormalities. The so-called *Q-wave infarct* (defined by the presence of Q waves on ECG afterward) has higher in-hospital mortality but the *non-Q-wave infarct* has a higher 12-month reinfarction rate. Mortality due to both types of infarct is equal at 12 months in patients who survive the initial event.

P—The pathophysiology of stable angina is one of a slowly accumulating plaque that causes ischemia with exertion as blood and oxygen flow to the heart, becoming limiting during times of increased myocardial demand. The composition of the plaque varies and can include lipid complexes, calcium, and inflammatory blood components from prior nonocclusive hemorrhage. Conditions in which demand exceeds supply occur during increased wall stress (as seen in heart failure), with an increased heart rate, and under conditions causing increased contractility and stroke work.

Acute coronary syndromes (ACSs), which include unstable angina, non–ST elevation MI (NSTEMI), and ST elevation MI (STEMI), have a different pathophysiology that involves the rupture of a plaque (most often a small, nonocclusive plaque), causing thrombus formation and coronary artery occlusion. There are varying degrees of ischemic damage to the heart, and overt infarction occurs with significant prolonged ischemia. Scar tissue and fibrosis may later form and ultimately may lead to long-term depressed cardiac function and heart failure. Sometimes myocardium can be "stunned" if deprived of its blood supply only briefly after an acute ischemia episode, and can eventually recover full function after reperfusion, which takes hours to days. Hibernating myocardium describes a situation in which there is cardiac muscle dysfunction from a more chronic low blood supply state, which can be reversed with revascularization. There is also a phenomenon called *ischemia at a distance*, in which occlusion of one coronary vessel causes ischemic symptoms in the distribution of another vessel because that vessel already has a high-grade stenosis and collaterals have formed between the two.

RF—The five major risk factors, about which all patients should be questioned, are diabetes, smoking, hypertension, a family history of CAD (first-degree relative affected: male <45 years old, female <55 years old), and hyperlipidemia. Other risk factors include age >55 if male, age >65 if female, obesity, metabolic syndrome, sedentary lifestyle, and glucose intolerance. Other surrogate markers of vascular disease are renal failure, peripheral arterial disease, carotid stenosis, aortic aneurysms, and stroke.

SiSx—Patients may be asymptomatic and found to have ECG changes or positive cardiac enzymes during admission for many other conditions (i.e., heart failure, arrhythmias, sepsis, renal or liver failure). Other patients present with sudden death or cardiac arrest. Classically, symptomatic coronary disease is marked by the presence of angina, of which there are several types (see Table 2-22). The key is to distinguish cardiac symptoms from those due to other causes that can present similarly. Patients who have infarction can present with evidence of left-sided heart failure (pulmonary edema, dyspnea on exertion, S_3 gallop) or right-sided heart failure (increased JVP, lower extremity edema, hepatojugular reflux, bradycardia, and hypotension). In addition, mitral valvular insufficiency can be seen, especially if there is papillary muscle ischemia or infarction.

Dx—The diagnosis of stable IHD can be made simply by the history in the appropriate high-risk patient presenting with symptoms of stable angina. Such patients, however, need to be risk stratified, and after assessing their risk factors for heart disease, stress testing, and/or cardiac catheterization is done to assess the extent of disease and the need for medical or surgical intervention. Patients with sufficiently high risk who have contraindications to stress testing or who present with high-risk ACS may go directly to cardiac catheterization for diagnosis and treatment purposes.

The ECG changes of a developing MI are shown in Figure 2-9.

Tx—Treatment depends on the severity of the disease. Those patients who have subcritical disease (<70% stenosis in a coronary lesion), or who have lesions that are too distal for intervention or who are not suitable for surgery or percutaneous intervention, are managed medically. The normal regimen, in addition to lifestyle changes (diet, exercise, weight loss, smoking cessation), includes aspirin daily, a β blocker, and an angiotensin converting enzyme (ACE) inhibitor or angiotensin receptor blocker (ARB) in all patients with left ventricle dysfunction. In addition, lipid-lowering agents are used with a goal low-density lipoprotein cholesterol (LDL) of <100 mg/dL, and now more commonly <70 mg/dL in those with any additional or uncontrolled risk factor. The high-density lipoprotein cholesterol (HDL) goal is >40 mg/dL. Such medications are titrated to achieve a resting heart rate of 60–70 bpm and a BP of <120/80 mmHg. Short- or long-acting nitrates can be given to patients who continue to experience angina. Occasionally, calcium channel blockers are given for angina or to patients with contraindications to β blockers, but nondihydropyridine calcium channel blockers (diltiazem and verapamil) are discouraged in patients with poor left ventricular function because of data showing an increase in mortality. Patients who also have symptoms of heart failure are managed accordingly with diuretics as well. Those with single or multiple coronary lesions (>70%) generally undergo angioplasty with stent placement if they have symptoms refractory to medications. Stent placement has not been shown to improve mortality in such patients otherwise. Certain patients may be referred for coronary artery bypass grafting (CABG). These typically include patients with left main disease, triple-vessel disease, two-vessel disease with proximal left anterior descending (LAD) stenosis and left ventricular dysfunction, disabling symptoms, and failure on medical therapy. Medical management with percutaneous intervention is now being

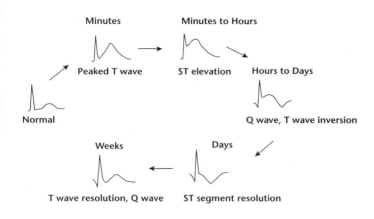

Figure 2-9. ECG Progression of a Q Wave MI.

Table 2-22.   Forms of Angina

Stable Angina	Angina that occurs with exertion and is relieved with rest. Typically, the chest pain is described as a pressure sensation in the chest, lasting 5–20 minutes, worse with exertion, radiating to the arms, neck, jaw or, less commonly, to the back; may be accompanied by shortness of breath, diaphoresis, nausea and vomiting. The response to sublingual nitroglycerin is less specific, but it may relieve pain within 1–2 minutes.
Unstable Angina	Defined as (1) angina chest pain occurring at rest or (2) more frequently or at lower levels of activity than during a previously stable period or (3) of new onset. This is the most alarming type of angina.
Prinzmental's Angina	Chest pain due to coronary spasm. Typically occurs at rest and is one form of unstable angina. ECG changes occur rapidly during an attack but return to baseline rather quickly. The pain lasts for a few seconds to 1 minute.
Angina Decubitus	Chest pain when the patient lies down or is asleep. Usually due to CAD with increased LVEDP such that cardiac perfusion is impaired and subendocardial flow is decreased. Diastolic pressure decreases further when the patient lies down, leading to decreased coronary perfusion and angina.
Anginal Equivalent	Instead of chest pain, the patient presents with other symptoms such as cough, dyspnea, or syncope caused by transient myocardial ischemia and increased oxygen demand. This is more likely to be seen in patients who are older, diabetic, and female.

performed with increasing frequency in these settings as well. Commonly used grafts during bypass surgery are the left internal mammary artery (LIMA) to the LAD (90%–95% patent at 10 years) and saphenous vein grafts (SVGs) to the left circumflex (LCX), obtuse marginal (OM) branches or right coronary artery (RCA) (60% 10-year patency). Graft material from other arteries, such as the radial arteries, can also be used.

Systolic Heart Failure

D—In systolic heart failure, the heart cannot pump sufficiently to meet the metabolic needs of the body while maintaining normal filling pressures. This condition is usually caused by abnormal myocardial contraction and is associated with a reduction in the EF and progressive activation of the neuroendocrine and renin-angiotensin systems. The term *cardiomyopathy*, strictly speaking, applies only to cases not due to ischemia, congenital heart disease, or valvular disease.

Epi—Systolic heart failure affects approximately 4 million people, with 200,000 deaths per year. Of those affected 75% are >65 years of age. It is estimated that 8% of people >75 years of age have heart failure.

P—Systolic heart failure is categorized into (1) right-sided versus left-sided failure,

(2) high-output versus low-output failure, and (3) backward failure (vascular congestion) versus forward failure (inability to perfuse distally). Often there are combinations of elements from these categories. Systolic heart failure is distinguished from diastolic heart failure by a subnormal EF (less than 50%–60%) and is seen in conditions giving rise to a dilated heart (such as chronic volume overload states), structural disease, or decreased myocardial contractility due to other conditions (see Table 2-23). In addition, in cases of chronic heart failure, there is overactivation of the neurohumoral pathways leading to elevation in catecholamines, which causes myocytes to decrease their β receptor density by way of feedback. This decreases intracellular cyclic adenosine monophosphate (cAMP) and reduces contractility over time. Other inflammatory markers, such as tumor necrosis factor alpha (TNF-α), and natriuretic factors, such as atrial natriuretic peptide (ANP) and brain natriuretic peptide (BNP), play an important role as well. Ultimately, because of a reduction in cardiac output, the body attempts to retain sodium and water, resulting in fluid accumulation. Acute heart failure, by contrast, results from an insult to the myocardium that decreases contractility.

SiSx—Systolic heart failure can present differently depending on whether it is acute and uncompensated or chronic and compensated CHF. Patients can have backward failure (pulmonary edema), forward failure (poor perfusion and cold extremities), or a combination of both. Those with compensated chronic heart failure may have no obvious symptoms or complaints but may report fatigue and dyspnea on exertion. Those with acute decompensated heart failure classically have symptoms that can be divided into either right-sided or left-sided heart failure. Symptoms of left-sided heart failure result from pulmonary congestion and include breathlessness, fatigue, orthopnea, paroxysmal nocturnal dyspnea (PND), nocturia, and exertional dyspnea, which are due to pulmonary edema and pulmonic effusions. An S_3 sound may be heard, signifying increased LVEDP. Signs of right-sided heart failure include lower extremity swelling, elevated jugular venous distension (JVD), hepatic congestion and hepatomegaly, and ascites. The degree of symptoms is not always correlated with the EF. The finding of a laterally

Table 2-23.   Cause of Acute Decompensated Heart Failure and Chronic Heart Failure Syndrome

Common Causes of an Acute Heart Failure Exacerbation	Causes of Chronic Systolic Failure
Forgot to take medication/noncompliance (most common in a patient with known heart failure) **A**rrhythmia/anemia **I**schemia/infarct/infection (myocarditis) **L**ifestyle problems (too much salt) **U**pregulation (hyperthyroidism, pregnancy, high-output state) **R**enal failure (causes fluid overload) **E**TOH abuse	Ischemic heart disease Idiopathic Hypertension—long-standing, uncontrolled ("burned-out ventricle") Valvular heart disease (commonly aortic stenosis and mitral regurgitation) Tachycardia mediated (thyroid disease, long-standing AF with rapid rates) Toxin (alcohol, cocaine) or drug related (adriamycin) Inflammatory (viral/bacterial myocarditis/endocarditis/ Lyme disease/HIV) Autoimmune—collagen vascular disease related Infiltrative (sarcoid, amyloid, hemochromatosis) High-output states (peripartum, severe anemia, AVMs, beriberi) Familial Stress myopathies (Takotsubo, sepsis related)—usually reversible with time

displaced PMI suggests dilation and chronic disease. Acute decompensated heart failure can present with dyspnea, hypoxia from vascular congestion, and cardiogenic shock if the insult is large enough. Signs of shock or poor perfusion are hypotension, narrow pulse pressure, cold extremities, and pulsus alternans. Based on the symptoms, one can classify the degree of heart failure by the NYHA classification (Table 2-24). More recently, a heart failure staging system has been used to direct care and treatment (Table 2-25) for chronic heart failure.

Dx—The diagnosis of systolic heart failure is made by history and clinical exam and with demonstration of a depressed EF with an ECHO or other imaging modality. The ECG is variable and may show signs of left ventricular hypertrophy (LVH), or prior infarction with Q waves or poor R wave progression, or

be completely normal. Additional findings include elevated BNP and sometimes elevated transaminases (AST and ALT) due to hepatic congestion from right-sided failure. A chest X-ray may show an enlarged heart, but a normal heart size does not rule out systolic or diastolic dysfunction. In cases of initial presentation, it is important to determine the cause of heart failure by ancillary studies in the appropriate setting. These may include cardiac enzymes, thyroid function tests (TFTs), antinuclear antibody (ANA), complete blood count (CBC), iron studies, the human immunodeficiency virus (HIV) test, and drug level tests. All such patients should either have a stress test or, preferably, left heart catheterization with coronary angiography to rule out or assess the extent of ischemic disease. Right heart catheterization may be warranted at the same time for invasive hemodynamic monitoring in certain patients, to measure intrapulmonary pressures, and to perform endomyocardial biopsy in select cases where the cause of heart failure is unclear or where emergent treatment may be beneficial (as in giant cell myocarditis). Acute decompensated systolic heart failure is diagnosed by the presentation of classic symptoms of left- and/or right-sided heart

Table 2-24.   New York Heart Association (NYHA) Classification of Heart Failure

Class I—structural disease but asymptomatic
Class II—heart failure symptoms with moderate exertion
Class III—heart failure symptoms with minimal exertion
Class IV—heart failure symptoms at rest

Table 2-25.   Classification of Heart Failure by Stage of Disease

Heart Failure Stage	Treatment Goals
Stage A—High risk for developing heart failure, but no symptoms and no structural disease	Treat hypertension, diabetes, hyperlipidemia Smoking cessation
Stage B—Evidence of changes in left ventricle, with evidence of structural disease, no symptoms	ACE inhibitors if there is reduced EF, diabetes, or a history of MI β blockers if there is a history of MI Valvular surgery if needed
Stage C—Decompensated heart failure at least once, with evidence of structural disease	Salt restriction Diuretics ACE inhibitor/angiotensin receptor blockers β blockers +/- Digoxin Spironolactone (class III, IV)
Stage D—Advanced disease refractory to maximum medical treatment; requires transplant.	Inotropic support Intra-aortic balloon pump Ventricular assist devices Heart transplant Hospice care

failure and an abnormal EF. In patients with volume overload, however, it is important to rule out other causes such as primary renal or liver disease.

Tx—Treatment varies for acute decompensations, depending on whether the patient has vascular congestion, poor perfusion, or both. (See Table 2-26.)

Acute Exacerbation

- Use oxygen with a nasal cannula, bi-level positive airway pressure (BiPAP), or mechanical ventilation if necessary.
- Diuresis: place a Foley catheter if needed and keep doubling the IV furosemide every 45 minutes to 1 hour until the patient has good urine output. Start with an IV dose that is double the patient's oral dose at home. In patients taking large doses of furosemide, consider a furosemide drip or give a thiazide diuretic 30 minutes before the loop diuretic dose. Nesiritide (intravenous BNP) can be used in refractory cases if the patient is not hypotensive.
- ACE inhibitors and/or hydralazine can be useful for patients who are vasoconstricted (with a high SVR) to reduce the afterload.
- Nitrates can be used to reduce preload and afterload. They should be used with caution if inferior/right ventricle infarction or right-sided failure is suspected (as the patient will be preload dependent). They are generally used in combination with afterload reduction (ACE inhibitor/hydralazine/intra-aortic balloon pump).
- Consider using inotropes (i.e., dopamine, dobutamine, milrinone) if the patient has evidence of poor peripheral perfusion. These are useful in the short term, but they have been

shown to increase mortality in the long term. They may help increase forward flow enough to facilitate diuresis. Avoid starting new β blockers or calcium channel blockers in a patient with *decompensated* CHF.

- The intra-aortic balloon pump is the ultimate method of afterload reduction when medication fails. The balloon sits in the aorta and inflates during diastole, increasing coronary blood flow. It deflates during systole, reducing aortic pressure and thus afterload.
- When nothing else is effective in treating the patient with shock and volume overload refractory to treatment, consider an emergent ventricular assist device (VAD; a mechanical device that augments cardiac output) or heart transplant in the appropriate patient.

Chronic Heart Failure

General guidelines for patients with systolic heart failure include the following:

- A salt-restricted (<2 g/day) and fluid-restricted (< 2 L/day) diet.
- All patients should also be on loop diuretics, an ACE inhibitor (or, if this cannot be tolerated, an angiotensin receptor blocker), and a β blocker, which is started at a low dose only in someone who has compensated heart failure and then increased as tolerated. These three forms of medication decrease mortality.
- For patients who have significant renal insufficiency or ACE inhibitor or ARB intolerance, hydralazine and nitrates can substitute for the ACE inhibitor or ARB. In cases where there is enough blood pressure room, hydralazine and nitrates can be added to the ACE or ARB. Some data has shown that this combination therapy may be of some benefit in African Americans.

Table 2-26.   Acute Decompensated Heart Failure Exacerbation Treatment Strategy

	Good Perfusion (warm extremities)	Poor Perfusion (cool extremities)
No Vascular Congestion (dry)	This is compensated heart failure. Use standard management for chronic heart failure.	Inotropic support. Management of hypotension.
Vascular Congestion (wet)	Diuresis. Management of hypoxia.	Inotropic support and/or diuresis. Ventricular assist devices. Heart transplant.

- In patients with class III or IV heart failure, addition of spironolactone has been shown to decrease mortality.
- For those with recurrent symptoms or exacerbations, digoxin improves symptoms and exercise tolerance and decreases the risk of hospitalization, but it has no effect on mortality and may even increase mortality in women. It is considered in patients with continued hospital admissions for heart failure.
- Anticoagulation is considered in patients with a low EF (though data for this indication are equivocal) and for the presence of mural thrombi or atrial fibrillation.
- Biventricular pacing may be indicated for those with an EF <35%, NYHA class III or IV heart failure despite optimal medical therapy, and a QRS duration of >120 msec.
- Implantable cardiac defibrillators should be considered for primary prevention of sudden cardiac death in those with an EF <35% after good medical therapy and a life expectancy >1 year.
- Ventricular assist devices can be used for patients with end-stage disease. There are several types, which case be used for the left ventricle or both ventricles. The general principle is that cannulas are inserted in the left ventricle and aorta and then hooked up to an external mechanical pump to generate cardiac output. Heart transplant is the other option in appropriate candidates. Experimental surgical therapies also include the use of constrictive elastic material to cover the heart and prevent further dilatory remodeling, although its benefits are still in question.
- It is important to find the underlying cause and, if possible, treat it to prevent further deterioration. Therefore, patients with CAD should be revascularized when possible. Patients with connective tissue disorders should be treated appropriately to bring their disease under control. Toxic medications and drugs should be discontinued, and hyperthyroidism should be well controlled. Those who have frequent arrhythmias, perhaps leading to tachycardia-mediated myopathy, should be treated as appropriate to suppress the arrhythmias.

Diastolic Heart Failure

D—A condition with signs and symptoms of heart failure due to the inability of the heart to relax properly. Patients may or may not have normal systolic function.

Epi—Anywhere from 40% to 60% of patients have a normal or near-normal EF. Fifty percent of CHF patients >70 years of age have some element of diastolic heart failure.

P—There is impaired relaxation of the ventricle in early diastole due to either decreased compliance of the ventricle or pericardial restraint on the ventricle. Decreased compliance can result from a stiffened ventricle as the result of numerous causes such as long-standing hypertension, infiltrative cardiomyopathies, and so forth. Many patients have a combination of systolic and diastolic heart failure. Because the ventricle cannot relax properly, it is unable to deal well with the changes in preload. Causes of diastolic heart failure are listed in Table 2-27.

RF—Female patients outnumber male ones. Risk factors include increased age, hypertension, obesity, HOCM, African American race, and sleep apnea.

SiSx—Asymptomatic disease is much more common than symptomatic disease. Those with symptoms have dyspnea on exertion and reduced exercise tolerance. With progression, PND, orthopnea, and dyspnea at rest can occur. Patients with severe restrictive or constrictive disease may have symptoms of right-sided heart failure that predominate:

Table 2-27. Causes of Diastolic Failure

Chronic hypertension
Hypertrophic cardiomyopathy
Aortic stenosis
Constrictive pericarditis
Storage diseases (glycogen storage disease, Fabry's disease)
Infiltrative disease (amyloid, sarcoid, hemochromatosis)
Endomyocardial fibrosis
Löffler's cardiomyopathy
Idiopathic restrictive diseases
Post irradiation to the chest
Connective tissue disease associated

lower extremity edema, hepatic congestion, and bloating. Patients are prone to flash pulmonary edema in the setting of very high blood pressure. S_3 and S_4 sounds may be heard on auscultation. Specific conditions such as amyloidosis, sarcoidosis, or hemochromatosis may lead to conduction problems and present with involvement of other organs.

Dx—Diagnosis requires signs of CHF with either normal left ventricular function or evidence of diastolic dysfunction by ECHO, such as E to A reversal (with a greater proportion of left ventricular filling dependent on atrial contraction) or low tissue Doppler velocities (suggesting slow relaxation). Diastolic heart failure should be strongly suspected in a patient with pulmonary congestion, as well as in a patient with signs of heart failure, a normal EF on ECHO, and normal valvular anatomy. Endomyocardial biopsy may be useful if there is strong suspicion of an infiltrative disease that otherwise cannot be identified.

Tx—Treatment goals beyond treating any underlying cause focus on controlling the BP and heart rate, especially in patients with atrial fibrillation (AF). β blockers and calcium channel blockers may be used to help decrease the heart rate and increase the filling time. ACE inhibitors and ARBs may also help reduce the left ventricular mass, although this is not clearly associated with better outcomes. Gentle diuresis in patients with pulmonary congestion and edema is useful; however, as patients are somewhat preload dependent excessive diuresis can decrease preload and cause hypotension. There is thus a narrow therapeutic window. Revascularize and treat appropriately those patients who have ischemia. Poor prognostic signs include severe reduction in exercise tolerance and VT on Holter monitoring. Overall specific treatment for this condition is lacking, and available therapies have not been proven to be as beneficial as those used for systolic heart failure.

Hypertrophic Cardiomyopathy

D—A condition consisting of myocardial hypertrophy without an identifiable cause

that may lead to diastolic dysfunction. When there is significant obstruction of the left ventricular outflow tract (LVOT) the condition is called *hypertrophic obstructive cardiomyopathy* (HOCM) The term *idiopathic hypertrophic subaortic stenosis* (IHSS), a synonym, is now outdated.

P—This is not a single disease but rather a group of diseases, the majority of which are genetic and familial. The most common familial form is autosomal dominant and is due to an amino acid missense mutation in variable parts of sarcomeric genes. A poor prognosis is associated with mutations in β myosin R403Q, R453C, and R719W. Histologic exam shows disarray of cell arrangement and hypertrophy with some fibrosis and disorganized cell architecture. The most common sites of involvement are the septum, followed by the apex and the midventricle. With hypertrophy, some patients will develop LVOT obstruction resulting in LVH and diastolic dysfunction as well as conduction abnormalities. Diastolic dysfunction is caused by impairment of myocardial relaxation such that it takes a long time to transition from systole to diastole. The hypertrophied muscle is also less elastic.

Epi—The prevalence is 1:500 individuals. The condition is most commonly a genetically transmitted cardiovascular disorder. It is the leading cause of sudden death among athletes younger than 35 years.

SiSx—Signs and symptoms depend on the degree of ventricular hypertrophy. Many patients are asymptomatic and are diagnosed on exam. Possible findings include a prominent A wave showing lack of compliance of the right ventricle, as well as a precordial heave. The apical impulse may be diffuse, and an S_4 sound may be palpable and audible. If there is outflow obstruction, a harsh crescendo-decrescendo murmur is heard at the left upper sternal border that does not radiate to the neck or axilla. This *murmur* has different properties than most others with respect to maneuvers; it *increases with lower preload* states (Valsalva maneuver, sitting to standing) because this decreases the size of the left ventricular cavity and causes more obstruction and turbulence to blood flow. Patients who are symptomatic can present with decreased left ventricular compliance leading to pulmonary congestion: dyspnea, dyspnea on exertion, and PND in addition to fatigue. Anything that accelerates the heart rate and decreases the diastolic filling time can make such symptoms worse. Angina from myocardial ischemia can also occur due to a supply–demand mismatch. Decreased cardiac output can lead to syncope and presyncope. Sudden death can also occur from lethal arrhythmias; this is more common among older children and young adults.

Dx—The ECG findings are not pathognomonic, though left axis deviation, biatrial enlargement, and evidence of Q waves in the inferolateral leads from septal hypertrophy can be seen. Echocardiography is the preferred way to make the diagnosis. The diagnosis of a LVOT obstruction in HOCM is based on a resting gradient of >30 mmHg or a provocable gradient of >50 mmHg across the LVOT. Sometimes inappropriate anterior motion of the mitral valve leaflet during systole is also seen, as it is drawn toward the septum by the Venturi effect. Overall, 60% of patients will have structural abnormalities of the mitral valve, usually mitral regurgitation.

Tx—For symptomatic patients, decompensated heart failure should be treated first. Use diuretics with great caution because of dependence on preload for cardiac output. β blockers or calcium channel blockers are first-line therapy even with left ventricular outflow obstruction. Negative inotropic and chronotropic effects allow for diastolic relaxation. Contact sports and continuous heavy physical exertion are to be avoided.

Control of rapid heart rates is important, especially in those who have concomitant AF (seen in up to 10% of patients). Such patients may benefit from AV node ablation and a pacemaker. Pacing causes an effective LBBB, which allows increased filling time. Nonpharmacologic options to reduce outflow obstruction include alcohol septal ablation (selective injection into a septal branch of a coronary artery causes infraction, thinning, and akinesis of part of the hypertrophic segment) and surgical myotomy or myectomy. Finally, transplantation is an option for severely symptomatic patients.

Because of an increased risk of sudden cardiac death in some patients, an ICD is recommended for those with the following risk factors: prior cardiac arrest from VT, a history of sudden cardiac death in an affected family member, nonexertional syncope with no other documented cause, frequent nonsustained ventricular tachycardia (NSVT), a markedly abnormal BP response to exercise, and massive LVH (left ventricle septal wall thickness >3 cm).

Cor Pulmonale

D—Condition consisting of right ventricular dilation, hypertrophy, and failure secondary to pulmonary hypertension that results from pulmonary disease. It can be acute, resulting from extensive PEs, or chronic, which occurs with most other causes.

Epi—It accounts for 5% of adult heart disease in the United States. The 5-year survival is 30% in patients with chronic obstructive pulmonary disease (COPD).

RF—COPD accounts for >50% of cases. Acute massive PE accounts for most cases of acute life-threatening cor pulmonale.

P—Basic mechanisms (1) pulmonary vasoconstriction from chronic or acute alveolar hypoxia, (2) anatomical restriction of lungs, (3) increased blood viscosity, and (4) increased pulmonary blood flow. Causes therefore include anything that causes pulmonary hypertension (except for left-sided heart failure), COPD, chronic restrictive and interstitial lung diseases, idiopathic pulmonary hypertension, chronic PEs, obstructive sleep apnea, and so on. Once there is enough vascular bed destruction, most of the lung space will develop pulmonary hypertension and, over time, cor pulmonale.

SiSx—In chronic cases, signs of right-sided heart failure may be evident: elevated JVP, lower extremity edema, right ventricular heave on exam, right-sided S_4, hepatic congestion, pulsatile liver, and even cirrhosis. Pleural effusions, however, are uncommon. Acute decompensation, as with massive PE, will cause elevated right-sided pressure (usually not a PASP >70 mmHg acutely, as the RV cannot handle such a sudden increase in pressure and this would cause immediate RV failure and death) in addition to hypoxia.

Dx—The ECG may show evidence of right heart strain. Echocardiography will demonstrate a dilated and/or hypertrophied right ventricle and elevated RVSP. A right heart catheter can ultimately demonstrate the degree of pulmonary hypertension. The cause must be lung disease and not left-sided heart failure.

Tx—It is necessary to correct the hypoxia and control hypervolemia. If possible, the underlying disease causing right ventricular dysfunction should be treated. For example, with acute cor pulmonale, as in a massive PE, consider thrombolytic agents or embolectomy surgically. Supplemental oxygen is important, therefore, along with diuresis. Vasodilators may be beneficial in severe pulmonary hypertension. Diuretics may improve the function of both the right and left ventricles; however, diuretics may produce hypotension effects if they are not used cautiously, as these patients are preload dependent and excessive volume depletion can lead to a decline in cardiac output. Phlebotomy is indicated in patients with chronic cor pulmonale and chronic hypoxia causing severe polycythemia, defined as a hematocrit of 65 or more. No surgical treatment exists for most diseases that cause chronic cor pulmonale.

Myocarditis

D—Inflammation of the myocardium.

Epi—The exact incidence is unknown because so many patients are asymptomatic. One percent of all unexplained sudden cardiac death may be due to myocarditis.

P—Most commonly, myocarditis has an infectious cause whether viral (coxsackievirus, echovirus, cytomegalovirus), bacterial, tuberculosis related, or fungal. Noninfectious causes include heavy metals, connective tissue diseases, hypersensitivity reactions to medications, and exposure to toxins. Inflammation can involve all or part of the cardiac chambers. Histologic exam usually shows myocyte necrosis with an interstitial inflammatory cell infiltrate. Giant cell myocarditis is a specific variant that deserves mention since it is potentially treatable. It is rare but is commonly fatal. The cause is unclear but is thought to be autoimmune in part against cardiac skeleton components.

SiSx—Symptoms vary widely and range from excess fatigue, typical cardiac chest pain, sinus tachycardia of unclear origin, acute pericarditis-like symptoms, and conduction problems to florid ventricular failure, cardiogenic shock, and sudden death. Most cases are subclinical, and patients do not seek attention during the acute illness. Fever is seen in 20% of cases. Viral prodromes, if present, occur about 2 weeks earlier.

Dx—There is no gold standard for diagnosis. Endomyocardial biopsy can make the diagnosis in many cases; however, it is rarely performed because management may not be changed. The diagnosis is usually clinical. Cardiac enzyme tests may be positive as a result of myocardial damage. Viral serologic tests can be obtained if a viral cause is suspected; however, their findings will not alter treatment.

Tx—Treatment focuses on the complications (CHF, heart block) and on supportive care. Underlying conditions, if found, should be treated (e.g., remove offending agents, treat tuberculosis and underlying connective tissue disease). Nonsteroidal anti-inflammatory drugs (NSAIDs) are contraindicated, and steroids are of no use for resolution of inflammation in infectious conditions. Giant cell myocarditis should be treated with aggressive immunosuppressive therapy, as this significantly improves survival.

Pericardial Diseases

Acute Pericarditis

D—An inflammation of the pericardial lining due to a variety of causes (infectious, traumatic, and autoimmune). *Dressler's syndrome* is a specific autoimmune pericarditis that develops 2–4 weeks after acute MI or surgery, perhaps due to antigen exposure in which the pericardium was damaged.

Epi—Acute pericarditis is the most common problem involving the pericardium. The diagnosis is usually idiopathic or viral, and a cause is not found.

RF—Risk factors include viral infection, trauma, the post–cardiac surgery state, status post cardiac arrest or MI, and malignancy.

P—The pericardium consists of visceral and parietal layers, between which the potential space of the pericardial cavity normally holds 15 to 30 mL of plasma filtrate. The most common causes of inflammation are idiopathic or viral (echo- and coxsackie-viruses are the most common), bacterial, tuberculosis, uremic, post-MI or postsurgical status, neoplasm related, or a manifestation of a systemic illness like a collagen vascular disease such as lupus.

SiSx—Acute pericarditis usually presents with chest pain that may be pleuritic in nature and exacerbated by inspiration. Pain is classically worse while supine and relieved by sitting up, as there is less friction within the pericardial sac in this position. The pain may radiate to the back, neck, and shoulders. A prodrome of fever, myalgias, or gastrointestinal (GI) distress may precede the symptoms by up to a few weeks. A pericardial friction rub, best heard at the right lower sternal border (RLSB) with the patient leaning forward, may be found and is pathognomonic. Classically, the rub has three components: (1) atrial systole, (2) ventricular systole, and (3) early ventricular diastole. The early ventricular diastole and atrial systole components can combine to produce a diphasic rub. Patients with purulent pericarditis may have acute onset of fever, chills, night sweats, and dyspnea, and chest pain or a rub may not be present. Tuberculous pericarditis can often become constrictive and present similarly to heart failure.

Dx—The diagnosis can be made clinically, based on the history, physical exam, and ECG changes; however, very early in the

Table 2-28. Stages of ECG Changes in Pericarditis

Stage 1—diffuse ST changes across multiple leads and PR depression.
Stage 2—resolution of PR/ST segments to baseline and T wave flattening.
Stage 3—diffuse T wave inversions (TWI).
Stage 4—normalization of the TWIs, which may take days to weeks.

course, there may be neither ECG changes nor a rub on exam. The ECG changes have four stages (see Table 2-28), which are seen in most but not all cases. Diffuse ST elevations and PR depression are classic findings, however. Depending on the cause, troponin leaks may also be seen. An ECHO should be done if tamponade physiology or effusion is suspected, but remember that pericarditis is *not* an ECHO diagnosis. A pericardial tap is used to diagnose purulent or tuberculous pericarditis (which is more likely to be bloody, with positive AFB). Additional tests include the tuberculin purified protein derivative (PPD), antinuclear antibody (ANA), rheumatoid factor, and thyroid function tests (TFTs). A chest X-ray may help determine if there is a large pericardial effusion.

Tx—Viral or idiopathic pericarditis is treated with high-dose NSAIDs. Hospitalization may be warranted to exclude MI if the diagnosis is in doubt or to watch for the development of tamponade, which occurs in up to 15% of patients if there are signs of a significant pericardial effusion. If the patient's symptoms are refractory to NSAIDs, then high-dose steroids are used and tapered over several weeks. Colchicine is another possibility, especially in refractory cases. There is no adverse prognosis associated with Dressler's syndrome. Aspirin or NSAIDs are given first. For uremic pericarditis, dialysis is the treatment of choice, but it is not necessary in patients who are asymptomatic with small effusions.

Pericardial Effusion

D—A condition in which there is a greater than normal amount of fluid in the pericardial space.

P—Any cause of acute or chronic pericarditis can be implicated, including infections (bacterial and viral). The pericardial space normally contains 15–30 mL of fluid; normal pericardial pressure is 0–2 mmHg. An effusion develops from inflammation or injury, and the rise in pericardial pressure depends on the rate of accumulation and the degree of fibrosis of the pericardium. Over time, as much as 2 L of fluid can accumulate without a significant decrease in pressure. Tamponade can occur with rapid accumulation of just 150–200 mL of fluid, however. Hemorrhagic effusions are most commonly caused by local tumor extension.

SiSx—Symptoms are related to the rate of accumulation. Slowly developing effusions are asymptomatic up to a point; then patients may complain of a dull chest pain, dysphagia, dyspnea, hiccups (from phrenic nerve compression), and nausea or abdominal fullness. Large-volume effusions are associated with muffled heart sounds. *Ewart's sign* is dullness to percussion, bronchial breath sounds, and egophony below the angle of the left scapula from a large effusion. Rales can also be heard in the lung field from compression. Additionally, symptoms can occur when there is compression or tamponade physiology (i.e., shock).

Dx—Echocardiography is good way to diagnose and follow pericardial effusions. The ECG may show low voltage and electrical alternans (alternating voltage size in the same lead) if there is a massive effusion. The chest X-ray may show a line exceeding several millimeters from the lower heart border, seen best on the lateral projection. When the cause is unclear or if a purulent pericardial effusion is suspected, diagnostic pericardiocentesis can be done. If a bloody tap is seen, it should be checked for clotting; this would imply a recent bleed, as chronic pericardial fluid has been deprived of clotting factors.

Tx—The underlying condition should be treated. Pericardial drainage may be necessary. If accumulation recurs, a surgical pericardial window, in which an opening in the pericardial sac is made for drainage, may be useful.

This is more commonly used in malignant effusions.

Cardiac Tamponade

D—A fall in cardiac output from compression of the heart by a pericardial effusion where the intrapericardial pressure is elevated.

P—The increase in filling can be due to rapid leakage of blood from the myocardium into the pericardial sac, but it may occur from any type of fluid accumulation (e.g., inflammatory) that eventually is not well compensated for by the heart. There is a reduction in venous return as the pericardial fluid increases, preventing the heart from relaxing properly; cardiac output can fall, and cardiogenic shock can develop. Malignancy is the most common cause, followed by idiopathic pericarditis and bleeding after cardiac surgery or trauma. Acutely, a small amount of fluid can cause tamponade, but if the accumulation occurs over a long period of time, the pericardial sac can accommodate larger amounts of fluid until tamponade-like symptoms are evident.

SiSx—Classically, cardiac tamponade is characterized by *Beck's triad* of hypotension, elevation of JVP, and distant heart sounds. More slowly developing tamponade presents with dyspnea and vague chest discomfort. The JVP in tamponade has a characteristic prominent systolic X descent and a small diastolic Y descent. *Pulsus paradoxus* may also be seen. This is a fall in SBP of >10 mmHg with inspiration. Inspiration normally increases right ventricular filling pressure and causes bulging of the ventricular septum into the left ventricle, causing a small decrease in the left ventricular dimension. Because the pericardium keeps the total heart volume constant, in pathological states such as pericardial tamponade or constrictive pericarditis, the left ventricle will not be able to increase in size and BP falls. Low BP can be a late finding in slowly developing tamponade. A significant pulsus paradoxus can also be seen in restrictive cardiomyopathy, COPD and asthma exacerbation, superior vena cava(SVC) obstruction, and PE, so it is not specific.

Dx—Tamponade is a clinical diagnosis. It is made on the basis of the history and physical exam and is aided by imaging. Echocardiographic findings of increased intrapericardial pressure include an exaggerated respiratory variation of flow across the tricuspid and mitral valves and collapse of the right ventricle and atria in diastole. Right heart catheterization can aid in the diagnosis and may show equalization of diastolic pressures (right atrial pressure, right ventricular diastolic pressure, pulmonary artery diastolic pressure, and pulmonary capillary wedge pressure will be roughly equal). Pericardiocentesis, with measurement of intrapericardial pressure and improvement of hemodynamics after removal of fluid, definitively establishes the diagnosis.

Tx—Urgent pericardiocentesis is required for true tamponade physiology. Volume resuscitation is key in patients with shock. Depending on the underlying cause and location of the fluid surgical decompression may be necessary.

Constrictive Pericarditis

D—A condition in which there is scarring, fibrous thickening, and loss of elasticity of the pericardial sac leading to impairment of ventricular filling.

Epi—The most common causes are idiopathic, radiation therapy related, postsurgical or postmediastinal radiation, postinfectious, and those related to malignancy or post MI. The number of cases from tuberculosis has decreased significantly in the United States but this is still the most common cause worldwide.

P—Constrictive pericarditis can occur after almost any pericardial disease. Both ventricles are affected equally, so the majority of ventricular filling occurs in early diastole. If pericardial inflammation goes on for months, there is resulting fibrosis and fusion of visceral and parietal pericardium, and eventually calcification occurs. Usually the process is symmetric, but it may not be and instead can localize to the right ventricular outflow tract. This can result in a decrease in diastolic filling and an increase in intracardiac pressures. Ultimately, constriction leads to increased venous pressure and progressive right-sided and left-sided heart failure.

SiSx—Early symptoms are malaise, fatigue, and decreased exercise tolerance. With advanced disease there is evidence of left-sided heart failure (pulmonary edema), followed by right-sided heart failure (lower extremity edema, hepatic congestion, elevated JVP). A pericardial knock may be heard. Classically, *Kussmaul's sign* may be seen. There is increased JVP with inspiration. Because of constriction, the right heart cannot accommodate the increased venous preload that normally occurs with inspiration, and therefore, JVP is increased. This sign is not typically seen in tamponade because there is still enough accommodation by the right ventricle in inspiration to allow for an increase in venous return with respiration.

Dx—Echocardiography is not highly sensitive or specific, but it may show pericardial thickening and rapid early diastolic filling that stops abruptly as the heart becomes less compliant (the *square root sign* or dip and plateau sign on hemodynamic tracings). There may also be absence or collapse of the IVC. Sometimes it is difficult to distinguish this condition from restrictive cardiomyopathy, and right and left heart catheterization may be needed. The hemodynamic hallmark is equal diastolic pressures on both sides of the heart and demonstration of inspiratory ventricular interdependence on right heart catheterization (right ventricle and left ventricle pressure tracings vary abnormally with inspiration). Cardiac MRI has been found useful in the appropriate context to look for a thickened pericardium.

Tx—Treat the underlying cause, if possible. Most symptomatic patients, however, will need surgical removal of the pericardium, a procedure called *pericardiectomy*. The procedure has a mortality rate of 5%–10%. Patients who have good initial function can be managed with diuretics, though most will eventually require surgery.

Systemic and Vascular Diseases that Affect the Heart

Infective Endocarditis (IE)

D—An infection of the endocardial surface of the heart. It can involve the heart valves, the valvular apparatus, chordae tendonae, or the site of a septal defect. It is usually classified into acute (days to weeks) and subacute (weeks to months) types and can result in significant valvular disease, embolic phenomena, conduction system disease, and heart failure.

RF—(1) Valvular predisposition: congenital heart disease, prior rheumatic heart disease, mitral valve prolapse (MVP) with regurgitation (a three to eight times increased risk), bicuspid aortic valves, prosthetic valves (greatest risk is in the first 6 weeks), previous endocarditis, surgical shunts, degenerative valvular disease of any other cause; (2) conditions that predispose to bacteremia: intravenous drug use (IVDU; up to a 5% risk per year), immunocompromised states, poor dental hygiene and indwelling catheters or central lines.

Epi—Community-acquired native valve IE has a 5/100,000 incidence. The median age of occurrence is the 40s to 60s. The incidence in the IVDU population, however, is up to 2000/100,000 and even higher in those with already known valvular heart disease. From 25% to 45% of patients have unknown predisposing conditions.

P—With infectious causes, a transient bacteremia or fungemia in the appropriate host allows for the formation of a vegetation—an amorphous mass of platelets and fibrin, microorganisms, and inflammatory cells that the body cannot eradicate. Part of the vegetation can seed other parts of the body, resulting in numerous vascular insults and disease from immune complex deposition. Many simple processes cause transient bacteremia (e.g., brushing teeth, eating); however, it is both the host and the virulence of the organism that determine the formation of vegetation or an abscess. Common types of IE include:

Acute bacterial endocarditis—This is most commonly due to *Staphylococcus aureus* and group B *Streptococcus*. These bacteria are quite aggressive and can infect previously normal valves.

Subacute bacterial endocarditis—This is commonly due to *Streptococcus viridans*, enterococci, and, rarely, the HACEK group of organisms (*Haemophilus* spp., *Actinobacilus, Cardiobacterium, Eikenella, Kingella*), and *Streptococcus bovis* (associated with gastrointestinal malignancy).

Prosthetic valve endocarditis—The organisms causing this disease differ, depending on the amount of time after surgery. Early disease (<60 days) is usually due to *S. aureus*, gram-negative bacteria, and *Candida*. Late disease (>60 days) is usually caused by acquired nosocomial infections with *Staph. epidermidis*, alpha-hemolytic streptococci, or enterococci.

IVDU related—Common organisms include *S. aureus, Strep. pneumoniae*, and then *Pseudomonas, Enterococcus*, and *Candida*. Right-sided lesions valvular lesions (tricuspid and pulmonic valve) are more common because of the method of bacteremia entering the venous system.

Other types of noninfectious endocarditis—These include Libmann Sacks endocarditis (due to systemic lupus erythematosus, autoantibody damage), carcinoid-related disease, and marantic endocarditis (from metastatic disease).

SiSx—There are a variety of presentations:

General—Subacute bacterial endocarditis can present with persistent fevers, chills, sweats, and weight loss. Acute bacterial endocarditis can present with an acutely infectious or septic picture.

Cardiac—A new murmur maybe heard on exam (not seen in all patients). Other presentations include acute heart failure from valvular insufficiency or chordae tendonae rupture, arrhythmias, heart block, and valve ring abscess (one may first see evidence of an increased PR interval, followed by various forms of heart block).

Immunologic—Immune complex deposition can result in glomerulonephritis closely resembling postinfectious glomerulone- phritis and vasculitis. *Osler's nodes* (tender subcutaneous nodules in the pulp of the digits from deposition of immune com- plexes) or Roth spots (oval retinal hemor- rhages) may be seen.

Embolic phenomenon—These include PEs (from right-sided emboli), emboli to extremities, stroke, splenomegaly (emboli to the spleen with immune complex depo- sition), *Janeway lesions* (small, nontender lesion on palms and soles), and *splin- ter hemorrhages* (linear or flame-shaped streaks in the nail beds).

Skin—These consist of petechiae (of the eyes, buccal mucosa, and palatal mucosa).

Dx—Classically, the diagnosis is made by the Duke criteria shown in Table 2-29A and B, which have high sensitivity and specificity.

Tx—Overall mortality is 16%–27% and increases with age, aortic valve involvement, CHF, prosthetic heart valve involvement, and the presence of strokes. Specific organisms also increase mortality: enterobacteriaceae, *Pseudomonas*, and all type of fungi.

Medical Tx

- Prompt antibiotic therapy is critical.
- Drugs that are commonly used empirically until the organism is identified are vancomy- cin (for methicillin-resistant *Staph. aureus*, or *MRSA*) versus oxacillin or nafcillin (for

Table 2-29A.   Duke Criteria for Endocarditis

Major Criteria	Minor Criteria

1. Evidence of organism via one or more of the following:
  a. Positive blood cultures from two separate sets with typical organisms: *Strep. viridans, Staph. aureus, Enterococcus,* HACEK, *Strep. bovis, Strep. pneumoniae*
  b. Persistently positive cultures from cultures drawn more than 12 hours apart, or all of three or a majority of four separate cultures with at least 1 hour between the first and last cultures
  c. Single culture positive for *Coxiella burnetii* (the cause of Q fever) or an antiphase IgG antibody titer >1:800.
2. Evidence of endocardial involvement: positive ECHO for intracardiac mass (TEE recommended for prosthetic valves), abscess, new dehiscence of prosthetic valve, new valvular regurgitation.
	1. Predisposing factors (e.g., IVDU, heart condition)
	2. Fever
	3. Vascular phenomenon (e.g., stroke, emboli, Janeway lesions, conjunctival hemorrhages)
	4. Immunologic phenomenon (e.g., glomerulonephritis, Roth spots, Osler's nodes)
	5. Positive blood cultures not meeting major criteria

Table 2-29B.   Use of the Duke Criteria

Definite Infectious Endocarditis	Probable Infectious Endocarditis	Rejected Infectious Endocarditis
1. Pathologic Criteria: Dx made by culture or by histologic exam of tissue from a vegetation itself, one that has embolized or from an intracardiac abscess. 2. Clinical Criteria (any of the following three combinations): One major and three minor Two major Five minor	Either one major and one minor criterion fulfilled or three minor criteria	Alternative diagnosis is present Resolution of symptoms in 4 days or less No evidence of pathology at surgery or autopsy Clinical criteria not met for above.

Source: Criteria are adapted from *Am J Med.* 1994;96(3):200–209.

methicillin-sensitive *Staph. aureus or MSSA*) plus an aminoglycoside such as gentamicin for synergy. Rifampin is also occasionally added in refractory or high-risk cases. Penicillin with an aminoglycoside can be used for streptococcal and enterococcal endocarditis.

- Ceftriaxone is used for coverage of HACEK organisms.
- Left-sided lesions generally are treated longer (4–6 weeks) than right-sided lesions (2–4 weeks).

Surgical Tx

Indications for surgery include:

- Moderate to severe CHF from valve dysfunction.
- Persistent bacteremia despite antibiotics or inability to treat effectively (fungal disease, *Brucella*, *Pseudomonas* usually).
- Prosthetic valve endocarditis with *S. aureus* or an unstable prosthetic valve.
- Perivalvular extension of infection/abscess formation.
- Recurrent embolic phenomena.

Prophylaxis

For high-risk patients only: those with prosthetic valves, prior IE, congenital heart disease (all cyanotic conditions especially, or any patient with prosthetic material), intracardiac surgery with implantation of a device or a systemic pulmonary shunt of any kind. Previous recommendations for prophylaxis included aortic stenosis, biscuspid aortic valve, MVP with mitral regurgitation, HOCM, and mitral valve repairs; however, these are no longer considered appropriate indications according to the most recently updated guidelines. There are very little data to show by how much antibiotic prophylaxis decreases the incidence of endocarditis in these cases. Prophylaxis is generally provided because of the potentially devastating consequences of IE.

Metabolic Syndrome

D—A condition with a constellation of findings including (1) abdominal obesity, (2) hypertension, (3) diabetes or insulin resistance, (4) low HDL, and (5) hypertriglyceridemia.

Epi—The prevalence is thought to be as high as 22% of the U.S. population and is increasing.

RF—Risk factors include race or ethnic group (more common in African Americans and Mexican Americans), postmenopausal status, elevated body mass index (BMI), physical inactivity, a high-carbohydrate diet, a family history of the disease, and low socioeconomic status.

P—Many factors contribute. The symptoms are interrelated. Abdominal obesity is associated specifically with hypertension and increased TNF-α. Increased insulin resistance can contribute to high BP. Increased androgens may play a role directly related to the amount of abdominal fat. Patients have an increased risk of CAD.

SiSx—Patients are usually asymptomatic but have the previously mentioned constellation of symptoms that often occur together. Some may present with symptoms related to each of the characteristics.

Dx—Specific definitional criteria are needed to satisfy the diagnosis:

1. Abdominal obesity defined as a waist circumference >40 inches in men and >35 inches in women
2. Triglycerides >150 mg/dL
3. HDL <40 mg/dL in men and <50 mg/dL in women
4. Blood pressure >130/>85 mmHg
5. Fasting glucose >100 mg/dL

Tx—The primary goal is usually weight reduction, with a specific focus on abdominal obesity, which should have an impact on the other features of the metabolic syndrome. Treatment of the individual problems is just as important, involving lipid-modifying drugs, ACE inhibitors, oral antihyperglycemics or insulin, with lipid, blood pressure, and hyperglycemia treatment targets similar to those of diabetics.

Essential Hypertension

D—Traditionally defined as elevated BP (>140 mmHg systolic and >90 mmHg diastolic)

Table 2-30.   Joint National Committee-7 Guidelines for Hypertension

	SBP (mmHg)	DBP (mmHg)	Comments
Normal	<120	<80	No treatment needed
Prehypertension	120–139	80–89	No treatment needed unless patient is diabetic or has any form of chronic renal disease; goal is < 130/80 for such patients
Stage I	140–159	90–99	1–2 drug regimen needed for most
Stage II	>160	>100	2+ drug combination needed for most

Source: Adapted from http://www.nhlbi.nih.gov/guidelines/hypertension/.

measured on three separate occasions or elevated BP with evidence of long-standing hypertension as evidenced by end organ damage. Guidelines for definition and treatment are presented in Table 2-30. These will likely be updated in the near future.

Epi—Essential hypertension affects about 60 million people in the United States and 1 billion people worldwide. Normotensive individuals at age 55 have a 90% lifetime risk of developing hypertension. Many are inadequately treated.

P—There are several ways to categorize hypertension:

Essential Hypertension—>90% of all hypertension. There is no identifiable cause, though it is associated with a family history, excess salt intake, inactivity, and obesity.

Secondary Hypertension—There is an identified medical cause. Examples include:

Cardiovascular—coarctation.

Endocardial—Cushing's disease, primary hyperaldosteronism, pheochromocytoma, hyperthyroidism, acromegaly.

Renal—renal artery stenosis, glomerulonephritis, chronic renal disease of almost any cause.

Medications—oral contraceptives, steroids.

Accelerated Hypertension—marked elevation of >130 mmHg diastolic and bilateral retinal hemorrhage and exudates.

Malignant Hypertension—accelerated hypertension with papilledema, in addition to encephalopathy or renal failure.

RF—Risk factors include alcohol use, a family history, obesity, African American race (twofold increased risk), excess salt intake, sleep apnea, advancing age (blood pressure is seen to rise with age in developed countries but not in preindustrial societies with few risk factors).

SiSx—Hypertension is most often asymptomatic and is detected in the medical office. Age-related hypertension causes elevation of systolic BP rather than diastolic BP so there is an increase in pulse pressure (systolic minus diastolic BP). Ultimately, many organ systems can be involved, depending on how long-standing or uncontrolled the condition is. For example:

Central nervous system—predisposes to stroke

Eyes—AV nicking, copper wiring, vision loss

Cardiovascular—hypertrophy, cardiomegaly, diastolic dysfunction, eventually heart failure, predisposes to CAD and arrhythmias

Renal—renal failure, hematuria

Dx—Separate measurements are taken over time as stated in the definition, unless the patient has elevated BP and evidence of end organ damage. Outpatient ambulatory blood pressure monitoring may be needed for those who have "white coat" hypertension and are anxious when they come to the clinic, but it is also useful to see how well treated patients are. The seventh Joint National Committee on Prevention, Detection, Evaluation, and Treatment of High Blood Pressure (JNC-7) classification defines normal blood pressure as shown in Table 2-30. The risk of developing cardiac disease can increase 8- to 10-fold, depending on the person's other risk factors.

Table 2-31. Treatment Options for Hypertension in Specific Cases

Condition	Good Therapy	Questionable Therapy
Prior MI	β blocker and ACE inhibitor or ARB	Calcium channel blockers diltiazem and verapamil when the EF is low.
Stable Angina, Normal EF	β blocker, calcium channel blocker	Vasodilators alone
Systolic Heart Failure	Loop diuretics, ACE inhibitor, β blockers, +/– spironolactone	Calcium channel blockers diltiazem and verapamil
Diabetic	ACE inhibitor or ARB, thiazide diuretics	Some believe that β blockers can mask hypoglycemia, but this is rarely a problem
Peripheral Arterial Disease	ACE inhibitor, β blockers (low dose)	Avoid β blocker if there is severe pain at rest
Gout	β blocker and ACE inhibitor or ARB	Thiazide diuretics
Osteoporosis	Thiazide diuretics	Loop diuretics (promote loss of Ca^{2+})
Pregnancy	Methyldopa, hydralazine, β blockers, calcium channel blockers	ACE inhibitors/ARBs are teratogenic
Pheochromocytoma	Phenoxybenzamine (α blocker) before β blockers	B blockers alone
Migraines	β blockers, calcium channel blockers	–
Hyperthyroid States	β blockers	–

Each 20 mmHg pressure increase doubles the risk of cardiac disease.

Tx—Treatment depends on the severity of hypertension, the stage, and the comorbidities. For essential hypertension, weight loss is perhaps the most important nonpharmacologic intervention in obese patients, in addition to salt restriction and smoking cessation. First-line drug therapy depends on the associated conditions but usually includes ethiazide diuretics, ACE inhibitors, or calcium channel blockers. β blockers and clonidine are usually adjunctive therapies in most patients. Those with newly diagnosed stage II hypertension should start therapy with two agents initially, one of which should be a diuretic such as hydrochlorothiazide (HCTZ) if appropriate. See Table 2-31 for some basic guidelines.

Hypertensive Crisis

D—A condition in which there is a severe elevation of BP that has the potential to become life-threatening. It is called a hypertensive emergency if there is a sign of end organ damage requiring immediate BP control. It is called hypertensive urgency if there is no sign of new end organ damage, but the patient's BP is markedly elevated and has the potential to lead to end organ damage. Distinguishing characteristics are shown in Table 2-32.

Epi—A total of 500,000 people are affected each year. Hypertensive crisis occurs in 1% of all hypertensive adults, and 50% of such patients have uncontrolled primary hypertension. The peak period of incidence is 40 to 50 years.

P—The distinction between urgency and emergency is not absolute. Depending on the underlying reason for the patient's hypertension, there can be many causes. Most often, it is a result of noncompliance with the BP medication regimen. In other cases, it is due to prolonged elevated BP that can lead to an acute event (i.e., aortic dissection, MI, stroke), onset of a catecholamine surge that leads to symptoms (i.e., pheochromocytoma, thyrotoxicosis), or secondary to the use of drugs (i.e., monoamine oxidase inhibitors, tricyclic antidepressants, cocaine, amphetamines). In patients with chronic hypertension there is autoregulation by the kidneys, which adapt over time to keep vital organs well perfused

Table 2-32. Hypertensive Urgency versus Emergency

Condition	Hypertensive Urgency	Hypertensive Emergency
Example	Elevated BP and either asymptomatic or moderate symptoms (headache, chest pain, syncope)	Elevated BP and evidence of end-organ damage: • Renal: acute renal failure, hematuria • Neurologic: hypertensive encephalopathy (headache, change in mental status), stroke, subarachnoid hemorrhage, hypertension s/p head trauma • Cardiovascular: MI, acute left ventricular failure, pulmonary edema, aortic dissection • Other: eclampsia, malignant hypertension
Treatment Time Course	BP should be reduced over 1 to 3 hours with oral agents. IV agents in refractory cases and therefore admission to ICU.	Treat in ICU with IV agents *Decrease the MAP by 25% in 1 hour* Then to normal in 24 hours Exceptions include acute MI or aortic dissection, in which case one should reduce BP as close as possible to normal with the patient still mentating
Agents of Choice	Captopril Clonidine Labetalol Nifedipine Change to IV agents if patient is nonresponsive.	Labetalol (for most patients except those with left ventricular failure) Nitroglycerin (myocardial ischemia, left ventricular failure; not for right ventricular infarction) Nitroprusside (for most emergencies except left ventricular failure) Enalapril (for left ventricle failure) Captopril (scleroderma crisis) Phentolamine (for pheochromocytoma) Hydralazine (for eclampsia)

at the higher BP. This is the reason for not correcting the BP too rapidly, especially in the setting of stroke. In hypertensive emergency, it is the degree of end organ damage that determines the severity of disease, not the absolute BP.

RF—Risk factors include male sex, African American race, tobacco use, cocaine use, low socioeconomic status, and medical noncompliance.

SiSx—The presentation varies. Patients with hypertensive urgency can be asymptomatic. Patients with hypertensive emergency may complain of cardiac-like chest pain, have hypertension encephalopathy (a combination of headache and change in mental status from a sudden increase in BP due to cerebral edema), and show signs of new heart failure, stroke, malignant hypertension, or renal failure.

Dx—All patients should have BP checked in all extremities. Diagnosis is made by evidence of end organ damage (see below). All patients should have complete and focused neurologic and cardiac exams, including an ECG, blood urea nitrogen (BUN), creatinine, and urinalysis (U/A) sent. Other tests are ordered thereafter based on the setting: cardiac enzymes if there is concern for ischemia, a head CT scan if there is concern about subarachnoid hemorrhage or stroke, electrolytes if there is a change in mental status, a chest X-ray to look for additional signs of heart failure and assess the mediastinum, and a chest CT scan with contrast or magnetic resonance angiography (MRA) to assess for aortic dissection. A work-up for secondary causes of hypertension is appropriate in most patients, looking for such conditions as hyperaldosteronism, hyperthyroidism, pheochromocytoma, renal artery stenosis, or other renal disease.

Tx—Admission to an intensive care unit is required for all cases of hypertensive emergency. Admission to the hospital may be required for some but not all cases of hypertensive urgency if the BP cannot be brought down with oral medication in the clinic.

Aortic Dissection

D—A condition in which a tear occurs between the intima and media of the aorta, where blood accumulates.

P—An aortic intimal tear is the inciting event, whether caused by trauma or by a predisposed and weakened aortic wall. Blood enters the tear and separates the intima from the media and adventitia, creating a so-called false lumen (not lined by endothelium). Progression can occur, and multiple communications between the true and false lumen can be found. This tear can increase along the plane of the aorta and progress in either direction, causing vascular compromise of distal branches and cardiac and neurologic sequelae. Dissection is exacerbated by increased pulse pressure. It is also possible to have a reentry tear somewhere distal, so that the false lumen is decompressed back into the true lumen. The most common location for dissection is several centimeters above the aortic root and just distal to the left subclavian artery.

Epi—Mortality is classically 25% in 24 hours, 50% in 48 hours, and 80% in the first week.

RF—Hypertension but not atherosclerosis is an independent risk factor. It generally occurs in 50- to 70-year-old males, but if it occurs in younger people, consider Marfan's or Ehlers-Danlos syndrome, bicuspid aortic valve, coarctation of the aorta with or without Turner's syndrome, pregnancy, and trauma. One should also consider cystic medial degeneration from infectious causes (e.g., syphilis).

SiSx—Classically, aortic dissection is described as an intense ripping, tearing, or stabbing chest pain that is likely to radiate to the back. Pain begins suddenly and reaches its greatest peak in minutes; it may resolve but usually does not. Complications include tamponade and MI from retrograde dissection, occlusion of the brachiocephalic artery, and stroke.

Dx—Diagnosis is made by CT with IV contrast or, alternatively, by MRA, angiography, or even ECHO (if dissection at the root or arch is suspected). On the physical exam, one may find, elevated JVP, an aortic insufficiency murmur, and differential BPs between the arms or the arms and legs (a classic finding, though it is not common). The ECG may rule out other causes, but it is not diagnostic unless the dissection involves the coronary arteries. Classically, the chest X-ray shows a widened mediastinum, although this sign is not very specific.

Tx—Treatment depends on where the dissection has occurred (see Figure 2-10). For dissection involving the ascending aorta (Stanford A type) immediate surgical treatment is needed, usually involving replacement of the aorta with long-lasting graft material (Dacron or Gortex) and possible valve replacement, if needed. For a dissection involving the descending aorta only (Stanford B type) medical management is used initially, including BP control with IV β blockers to decrease pulse pressure. Vasodilators such as nitroprusside prevent reflex tachycardia.

Aortic Aneurysm

D—An abnormal dilation of the aorta that can occur along any part of its course.

Epi—It occurs in 1%–5% of the population; 75% of aortic aneurysms are confined to the abdomen. They are most commonly infrarenal.

P—The normal aorta is about 3 cm wide in the ascending area and 2 cm near the kidneys. True aneurysms involve all three layers of the artery wall, whereas pseudoaneurysms, which have only a thick fibrous capsule, involve only parts of the wall. Aneurysms can be fusiform (circumferential dilatation) or saccular (as a bud off one side) in shape. As wall stress is equal to pressure times radius divided by tension (law of Laplace), a larger radius increases wall stress. Causes of dilatation include atherosclerosis (not necessarily hypertension), cystic medial degeneration, Marfan's syndrome, Ehlers-Danlos syndrome, infection (syphilis, for example), and trauma. It is not uncommon

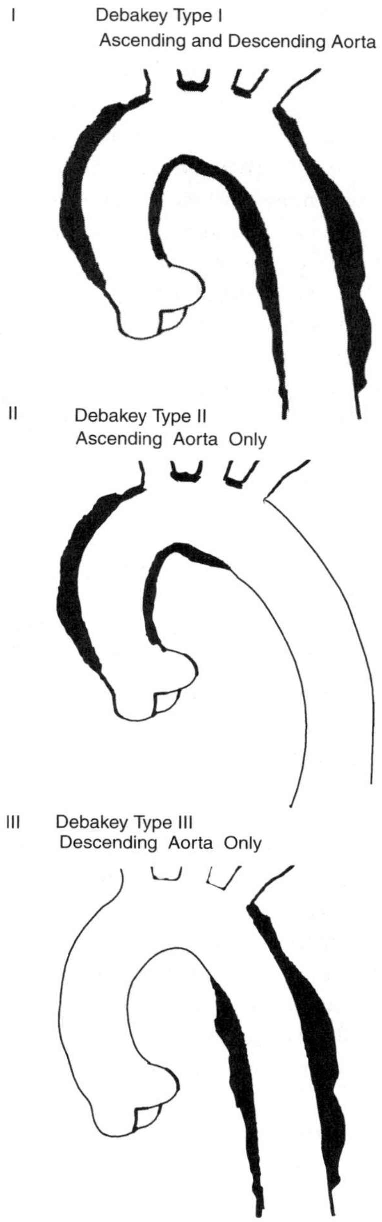

I   Debakey Type I
     Ascending and Descending Aorta

II   Debakey Type II
     Ascending Aorta Only

III Debakey Type III
     Descending Aorta Only

Figure 2-10. Classification of Aortic Dissection.

Debakey Type I	Debakey Type II	Debakey Type III
Ascending and descending aorta	Ascending aorta only	Descending aorta only
Stanford A—Any proximal		Stanford B—Distal only

for the patient to have additional aneurysms, such as iliac or popliteal aneurysms.

RF—Risk factors include older age, CAD, Marfan's or Ehlers-Danlos syndrome, or other related large-vessel genetic conditions.

SiSx—Most aneurysms are asymptomatic and are picked up on exam or on screening for another cause. Twenty percent of patients may have symptoms of pain or tenderness. Patients with a ruptured abdominal aortic aneurysm (AAA) may have the classic triad of abdominal/back pain, hypotension, and a pulsating mass. Popliteal and femoral aneurysms rarely rupture, but at a size of greater than 2 cm present a risk for thrombus formation.

Dx—Most aneurysms, as noted above, are found incidentally as part of the work-up of another complaint. Diagnosis is made first by ultrasound and then by contrast CT, if necessary, to delineate the extent of disease and the presence of additional aneurysms.

Tx—Treatment consists of watchful waiting versus surgery, depending on the aneurysm's size and rate of growth. The average growth rate is about 0.3–0.4 cm/yr. A 4 cm aneurysm has a 5%/yr risk of rupture, and a 6 cm aneurysm has a 15%/yr risk. Therefore, the approximate average cutoff for surgical intervention is roughly 5 cm, depending on how rapidly the aneurysm has been increasing, its location, and the underlying condition. Patients with Marfan's syndrome have stricter criteria overall for surgical repair, and surgery is generally performed even earlier. Surgical repair involves the use of a large amount of graft material to replace the aorta, with anastomosis of all the appropriate branches. If there is involvement of the aortic root, a composite graft with the aortic valve as well can be placed. Isolated abdominal AAAs are approached through retroperitoneal incisions, with proximal and distal clamps, and by covering the graft with the original sack. Perioperative and postoperative complications include postoperative MI, neurological damage (from failure to get a good blood supply to the spinal cord), renal failure, embolization to distal arteries, and colonic ischemia.

For patients with infrarenal disease alone, an endoluminal stent can be placed without surgical repair, which fits inside the aneurysm and closes it off. Thoracic aortic aneurysms, depending on their location, can also be treated with stent grafts on occasion.

Peripheral Artery Occlusive Disease

D—A condition of chronic atherosclerotic disease in the peripheral arteries similar to that found elsewhere in the body, such as the coronary arteries.

P—Most common locations for disease are (1) the superficial femoral artery, (2) the aortoiliac area, mostly seen in 40- to 60-year-olds, and (3) the anterior tibial artery and the area distal to it especially in people with diabetes and advanced renal disease. The change in resistance to flow is proportional to $1/radius^4$, so when the radius of the artery is decreased 50%, the resistance is increased significantly. A vessel can adapt initially, but it soon reaches the point of no return. People who exercise may build collateral flow. The affected muscle groups are always distal to the level of pain, so calf pain implies popliteal involvement and buttock pain implies aortoiliac artery involvement. *Leriche's syndrome* is a triad of impotence, lack of femoral pulses, and gluteal muscle wasting in addition to claudication due to proximal arterial occlusive disease.

RF—The risk factors are the same as those for cardinal cardiac risk factors (diabetes, hypertension, a family history, tobacco use, hyperlipidemia) and other, less common cardiac risk factors. Other factors include (1) Buerger's disease or thromboangiitis obliterans (see Chapter 6), (2) cystic adventitial disease, and (3) popliteal entrapment syndrome (from muscle compression)

SiSx—Symptoms usually progress through several stages:

1. Claudication—increased pain in areas of arterial insufficiency that occurs with exercise and is relieved with rest. It is similar to the pain of stable angina from heart disease. It is seen in about 10% of patients over 70 years old.

2. Rest pain—most commonly seen in the metatarsal area and commonly occurs at night. Classically, patients report that the pain is relieved with the limb hanging over the end of the bed. This is similar to the unstable angina of heart disease and signifies more advanced disease because gravitational pressure is necessary to allow for adequate perfusion.

3. Skin ulcer—indicating arterial insufficiency with trauma. It is usually painful except in diabetics.

4. Gangrene—If it is *wet gangrene*, the ulcer has become infected with gas-forming bacteria. This is deadly in diabetics and is a definite indication for amputation. If it is *dry gangrene* (in which case there is no infection), mummification of the digit occurs and it falls off by itself.

Dx—The history and physical exam can usually make the diagnosis. A more quantitative measure is the ankle-brachial index (ABI), where the BP is measured in the upper extremity and then in the lower extremity with Doppler. A ratio of lower extremity to upper extremity SBP of 0.7–0.9 indicates mild disease, 0.4–0.7 is moderate disease, and <0.4 is severe disease. False results are seen in older individuals with stiff, calcified vessels.

Tx—For those with claudication only, medical treatment is typically considered:

1. Risk factor modifications are similar to those of patients with CAD (stop smoking, limit alcohol use, and control of hypertension, hyperlipidemia, and diabetes).

2. Exercise rehabilitation is instituted to form collaterals.

3. Antiplatelet agents (aspirin, dipyridamole) and rheologic modifiers such as pentoxifylline are used. This increases red blood cell (RBC) deformity and decreases the fibrinogen concentration, platelet adhesiveness, and blood viscosity (however, data for their use are limited).

For those with rest pain, revascularization via surgery may be an option, depending on the flow rate. A preoperative angiogram is necessary to qualify the extent of disease. Surgical

Table 2-33. Mechanisms of Tachyarrhythmias

Type	Description	Example(s)
Reentry	Cardiac impulses reexcite an area through which it has already passed. This is the *most common type*.	AF, atrial flutter, AVNRT, AVRT, SNRT
Enhanced Automaticity	SA or AV node changes with sympathetic tone or ectopic activity in atrial or ventricular tissues.	Sinus tachycardia
Triggered Activity	An afterpotential triggers another action potential. Associated with increases in Ca^{2+} flux and long QT.	MAT

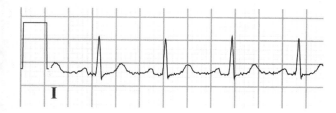

Figure 2-11. Sinus Tachycardia. Courtesy of Ralph Verdino, M.D., Hospital of the University of Pennsylvania.

options include a synthetic or venous graft. If blood flow is poor and gangrene is present, amputation may be necessary. Overall, of those patients presenting initially with claudication alone, the amputation rate at 5 years is only 5%; the mainstay of treatment is exercise to build up collaterals. Fifty percent of patients with rest pain may ultimately need amputation.

Tachyarrhythmias

These are conditions in which the heart rate is persistently >100 bpm. There are three known mechanisms for all tachycardias, as shown in Table 2-33.

Sinus Tachycardia

D—Increased heart rate with normal sinus rhythm. See Figure 2-11.

Epi—This is the most common tachycardia.

P—The cause is increased levels of catecholamines. If it persists for weeks, it can produce damage by causing a tachycardia-induced cardiomyopathy. The differential diagnosis is quite varied (see Table 2-34).

SiSx—Symptoms depend on the underlying etiology. Many patients are asymptomatic.

Assess the BP if it is low; then consider volume loss and shock.

Dx—The ECG shows a regular tachycardia with p waves preceding every QRS. The key point is that P waves are upright in ECG leads I and II and are biphasic (part above and part below the baseline) in V1. The maximum rate is about 220 bpm—the patient's age. A rate higher than this should lead to consideration of an alternative diagnosis, especially if the patient has no obvious reason to be in sinus tachycardia. Work up the underlying cause if it is not obvious.

Table 2-34. Causes of Sinus Tachycardia

Stress
Exercise
Hypovolemia
Fever
Chronic infection
Anemia
Hyperthyroidism
Hypoxia
Pulmonary embolus
Medications (e.g., β agonists)
High-output states (pregnancy, arteriovenous malformations)

Tx—Treat the underlying cause (replace volume if the patient is hypovolemic or blood if the patient is anemic, treat fevers, etc.).

Multifocal Atrial Tachycardia (MAT)

D—Condition in which multiple atrial foci are independently triggering ventricular beats through the AV node. At least three P wave morphologies are needed for the condition to be called MAT (see Figure 2-12).

RF—This is usually seen in severe pulmonary disease such as COPD or with illness causing hypoxemia. Advanced age is another risk factor.

SiSx—Patients may be asymptomatic or may experience palpitations. Typically, the heart rate is not very fast.

Dx—Diagnosis is made by an ECG showing an irregular rhythm with p waves of at least three different morphologies, each followed by a QRS complex. When the heart rate is <100 bpm, the condition is called *wandering atrial pacemaker*. The heart rate is commonly 100–130 bpm, with R-R intervals that are variable.

Tx—Treat the underlying illness. There is little role for antiarrhythmics; however, if necessary, calcium channel blockers and/or amiodarone are used.

Sinus Node Reentrant Tachycardia

D—Condition in which a reentrant circuit forms in the AV node, resulting in tachycardia.

Epi—It accounts for <5% of all SVTs.

RF—Risk factors include structural heart disease and CAD status/post inferior MI.

P—Reentry occurs within the sinus node, and impulses go down the normal conduction pathway. The p waves are identical to the sinus rhythm. Wenckebach block often occurs with this rhythm.

SiSx—The heart rate varies from 80 to 200 bpm; patients are asymptomatic or have palpitations. Patients with structural heart disease may decompensate at high heart rates.

Dx—The ECG will show what looks like sinus tachycardia, except perhaps that the rate is much faster and the patient has no obvious reason to be in sinus tachycardia. The diagnosis may be made post facto after breaking the rhythm with adenosine.

Tx—Vagal maneuvers or adenosine can terminate this rhythm. Atrioventricular blocking agents such as β blockers, calcium channel blockers, and digoxin can prevent its recurrence.

Atrial Fibrillation (AF)

D—Disorganized atrial activity resulting in a very high rate (>400 bpm) of irregular, poorly coordinated atrial contractions. Different types are recognized and are shown in Table 2-35.

Table 2-35. Types of Atrial Fibrillation

Type	Definition
Paroxysmal AF (PAF)	Terminates on its own in <7 days. Most cases usually last <24 hours.
Persistent AF	Lasts >7 days. May eventually terminate spontaneously or with cardioversion. Thereafter, the patient can have episodes of PAF or more episodes of persistent AF.
Permanent	Lasts >1 year. Cardioversion either failed or was never tried.
Lone AF	Any of the above types of AF without any evidence of structural heart disease in young patients <60 years; considered to be at low risk for stroke.

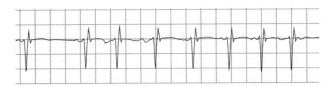

Figure 2-12. Multifocal Atrial Tachycardia.
Courtesy of Ralph Verdino, M.D., Hospital of the University of Pennsylvania.

P—This condition usually involves four or more reentrants circuits. Ultimately, either from structural heart disease or systemic disease, the atria develop multiple foci of waves of depolarization in several different directions at a high rate. Recently, it has been found that many of these waves originate in the pulmonary veins. Fortunately, the AV node is not able to conduct all of these impulses, resulting in an irregularly irregular conduction pattern and heart rate.

RF—Hypertension and advanced age are the most common risk factors for AF. Others risk factors include structural heart disease, rheumatic heart disease, hyperthyroidism, valvular disease (especially mitral regurgitation and mitral stenosis), CAD, pericardial disease, postcardiac surgery states (especially after valve repairs), an acute alcohol "holiday heart" following binge drinking, pulmonary disease, and systemic illness. Atrial fibrillation may be seen in ACS, but this is not a common cause. Common causes of AF are shown in Table 2-36.

Table 2-36. Causes of Atrial Fibrillation

Pulmonary disease/Pulmonary embolus/
  pericarditis
Infection, ischemia
Rheumatic heart disease
Age related
Thyroid disease
Etoh intoxication/withdrawal
Sick sinus syndrome/sleep apnea

Epi—It is seen in 10% of patients >80 years of age. The median age of onset is 75 years.

SiSx—Most patients are asymptomatic and are diagnosed on a routine exam or an abnormal ECG. Some may present with palpitations, light-headedness, chest pain, syncope, or confusion. The most common finding is an irregularly irregular pulse. An apical pulse deficit may be present (the differential in heart rate is counted via the radial pulse and with the stethoscope over the heart, as not every auscultated ventricular beat is forceful enough to reach the extremities). Jugular venous waveform shows loss of A waves.

Dx—An ECG should be enough to make the diagnosis unless the heart rate is too fast to allow it to be distinguished from other SVTs, though the fact that it is irregular should narrow the diagnosis considerably. There are no visible organized P waves; instead, there is either a flat baseline (fine AF) or many fibrillatory waves causing a wavy baseline (coarse AF), as shown in Figure 2-13. Holter monitoring can be helpful to determine the frequency and duration if the condition is paroxysmal atrial fibrillation (PAF). The most basic work-up beyond the history and exam should include thyroid stimulating hormone (TSH), a chest X-ray, and ECHO to look for structural heart disease and to assess the size of the atria.

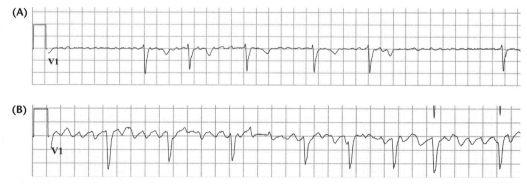

Figure 2-13. Atrial Fibrillation (A) Fine atrial fibrillation; (B) Coarse atrial fibrillation.
Courtesy of Ralph Verdino, M.D., Hospital of the University of Pennsylvania.

Tx—Treatment depends on the patient's age, comorbidities, the cause of AF, and how symptomatic the patient is. If the condition is acute and the patient is unstable (hypotension, change in mental status, heart failure, MI), immediate cardioversion is necessary. Underlying conditions that are reversible (e.g., thyroid disease, infection leading to AF) need to be treated concomitantly. Otherwise, the principles of therapy are rate control, anticoagulation, and rhythm control (medical or surgical) if appropriate.

- *Rate control*—Agents used are β blockers, AV nodal calcium channel blockers, and digoxin. Patients who remain tachycardic for a long period of time are subject to the development of tachycardia-mediated cardiomyopathy. In extreme cases, those refractory to rate control may require AV node ablation and placement of a pacemaker if they have chronic AF.

- *Anticoagulation*—This is considered for any AF lasting for >24 hours as well as for PAF. Paroxysmal atrial fibrillation and persistent AF carry a similar risk of stroke. Assess the risk of stroke (see Table 2-37 for a common scoring system used) compared to the risk of bleeding (which is increased in those with prior intracerebral hemorrhage, active GI bleeds, increased fall risk, and poor medical compliance or follow-up). In general, for nonrheumatic heart disease–related AF, anticoagulate with heparin initially and then with warfarin to an international normalized ratio (INR) of 2.0–3.0 if the CHADS$_2$ score >1. Weigh the risks and benefits if the CHADS$_2$ score ≤1. Patients <65 years of age without any risk factors may be managed with a full dose of aspirin. (See Table 2-37.)

- *Rhythm control*—Consider this strongly in patient with AF who are symptomatic (i.e., decompensated CHF, those who need AV synchrony). In asymptomatic patients with compensated heart failure, data suggest that rate control may be just as good as rhythm control. However, some argue

Table 2-37. The CHADS$_2$ Score for Paroxysmal Atrial Fibrillation

Feature	Points
CHF (any history)	1
Hypertension History	1
Age >75	1
Diabetes	1
Stroke/TIA (prior)	2

Points	Stroke Risk/yr (%)
0	0.5
1	1.5
2	2.5
3	5.3
4	6.0
5 or 6	6.9

Source: JAMA 2001;285(22):2864–2870.

that everyone should have a chance at rhythm control at some point in their course.

To this end, guidelines suggest that for new-onset AF of <48 hours' duration, perform medical or electrical cardioversion and continue anticoagulation for 4–6 weeks afterward (the atria still have a high risk of clot formation in this period) if there are no contraindications.

For new-onset AF of >48 hours' duration or of unknown duration, one can perform TEE to rule out an intracardiac thrombus (the most common location is the left atrial appendage) and then, if the TEE is unremarkable, perform cardioversion with continued anticoagulation. Alternatively, one can use rate-controlling agents and anticoagulate for 4–6 weeks, then perform cardioversion without a TEE.

Agents used for chemical cardioversion with varying success are Vaughan-Williams antiarrhythmic classification III agents (see Table 2-38 for this classification scheme): amiodarone (avoid this in young patients and in those with liver disease

Table 2-38. Vaughan-Williams Classification of Antiarrhythmic Drugs

Class	Basic Function	Examples	Uses
Ia	Sodium channel blocker—moderate	Quinidine Procainamide Disopyramide	Ventricular arrhythmias, PAF with Wolfe-Parkinson-White syndrome
Ib	Sodium channel blocker—weak	Lidocaine Mexiletine Phenytoin	Ventricular tachycardia, AF
Ic	Sodium channel blocker—strong	Flecanide Propafenone Moricizine	Paroxysmal AF, in those without ischemic heart disease.
II	β blocker	Metoprolol Atenolol Esmolol Bisoprolol	After myocardial infarction, Rate control in AF, Useful in most types of tachyarrhythmias
III	Potassium channel blocker	Amiodarone Sotalol Dofetilide Dronedarone	Ventricular tachycardia, AF, Supraventricular tachycardias (but not as a first choice)
IV	Calcium channel blocker	Verapamil Diltiazem	Rate control in AF, Supraventricular tachycardias
V	Direct nodal inhibition	Digoxin Adenosine	Supraventricular tachycardias

AF, atrial fibrillation.

or thyroid disease), sotalol (avoid this in patients with renal failure), and dofetilide. (Class Ic) agents include flecanide and propafenone (avoid these agents in patients with structural heart disease or CAD, as they increases mortality), which are used in otherwise healthy patients who are symptomatic with AF.

Patients with significant structural heart disease as a contributing factor (e.g., left atrial size over 5 cm) may be difficult to cardiovert and maintain in sinus rhythm. Nonpharmacologic options include ablation of the pulmonary vein foci (success rates of 60%–80%) in the electrophysiology (EP) laboratory or a surgical technique called the *MAZE procedure*, in which multiple surgical incisions block multidirectional depolarization.

Atrial Flutter

D—Condition in which there is one large macro-reentrant circuit in the atria, usually at a rate near 300 bpm.

RF—Risk factors are very similar to those of AF. They include underlying structural heart disease (especially left atrial enlargement or biventricular failure), congenital heart disease, rheumatic heart disease, COPD, the presence of AF, thyrotoxicosis, pericarditis, pulmonary embolism, and cardiac surgery.

Epi—There are 200,000 new cases per year. The condition is 2.5-fold more common in men than in women.

P—This is a macro-reentrant arrhythmia, typically in the right atrium, circulating at about 300 bpm (atrial rate) to reach the AV node. There is more organized contraction of the atria compared to AF; however, it occurs at such a fast rate that appropriate atrial filling does not occur.

SiSx—Symptoms include palpitations, fatigue, light-headedness, and dyspnea. As in AF, many patients are asymptomatic.

Dx—The ECG makes the diagnosis. One sees the appearance of classic sawtooth waves called *flutter waves* (*f waves*) most clearly in

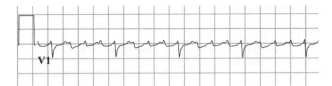

Figure 2-14. Atrial Flutter. Courtesy of Ralph Verdino, M.D., Hospital of the University of Pennsylvania.

the inferior leads (see Figure 2-14). The ventricular response rate is classically one half or one third of the atrial rate (150 or 100 bpm), though this can vary if the patient is taking antiarrhythmic drugs or has large atria. There are two types of flutter waves:

Type I (typical, common)—f waves (240–340 bpm). These waves have a larger circuit than type II waves. They are more negative than positive in inferior leads.

Type II (atypical, quite uncommon)—faster f waves (340–440 bpm). They have a smaller circuit than type I waves. They are more positive than negative in inferior leads.

Tx—Treat any underlying condition or precipitant if found. The treatment course is very similar to that of AF (see above), except that the rhythm and rate control are much more difficult and there is much more success with ablation of the circuit in the EP lab compared to AF. Typical principles include the following: cardiovert if the patient is unstable, as in AF, and treat any underlying exacerbating condition. Control the ventricular rate with β blockers, calcium channel blockers, or digoxin in patients with a rapid heart rate, using first IV and then oral medications. Patients with high-degree AV block and a normal ventricular rate do not need rate control. Anticoagulate patients at high risk for stroke (less well studied, but these patients have a stroke risk similar to that of patients in AF). Most clinicians will try cardioversion at least once if it is the first episode, using a TEE to assess for atrial clot with guidelines similar to those of AF (see above). Antiarrhythmic drugs such as Ia, Ic, and class III agents can be tried (see Table 2-38), but in general they are not very successful. Many patients are offered ablation of the flutter in the EP lab if rate control is difficult to achieve with medication. The success rate is >90% for ablation.

Atrioventricular Nodal Reentrant Tachycardia (AVNRT)

D—Condition in which a reentrant circuit is set up within the AV node itself, leading to tachycardia.

RF—This is generally seen in people without structural heart disease.

Epi—It accounts for 70% of the rarer types of tachycardia.

P—There are several conditions that must be met for AVNRT to develop. (1) Two functional conduction pathways have to exist in the AV node: one is faster in conduction, the other slower (this can occur congenitally or after ischemic disease or other injuries to the AV node). An intrinsic property of these pathways is that those faster in conduction have long refractory periods and those slower in conduction have short refractory periods. (2) Initiation of the typical reentrant circuit must occur, usually with an extra beat, either a premature atrial contraction (PAC) or premature ventricular contraction (PVC). (See Figure 2-15.)

SiSx—Symptoms include palpitations, angina, CHF, and rarely even shock if the patient has underlying structural heart disease that depends on an increased filling time and a slower heart rate. The patient may note multiple episodes of palpitations that resolved with coughing or vagal maneuvers. Syncope is seen from rapid rates or from the aftereffect of bradycardia/asystole when it terminates. Cannon A waves (very large A waves) may be seen from atria and ventricles contracting simultaneously.

Dx—The ECG shows tachycardia. The rate of AVNRT is usually 150–250 bpm and is quite regular, with little variance. Classically there are inverted and narrow P waves occurring

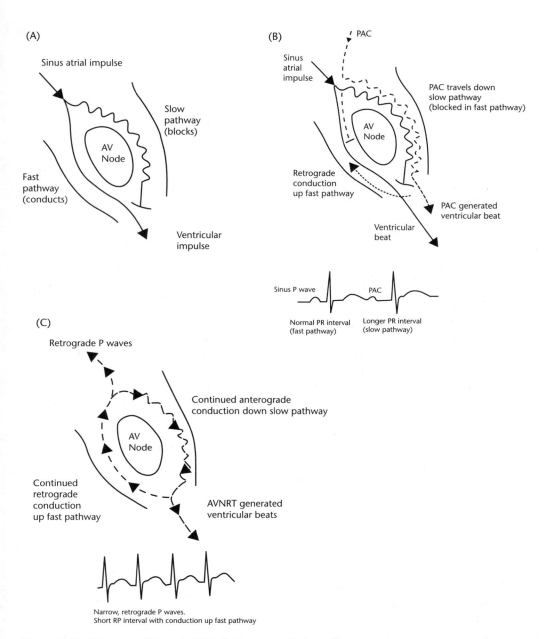

Figure 2-15. Diagram of Typical AV Node Reentrant Tachycardia.

(A) With normal conduction, an atrial pulse travels down the fast and slow pathways, but only the fast pathway conducts a ventricular beat, as the slow pathway arrives later and sees refractory tissue. Therefore, the slow pathway is normally clinically silent.

(B) An abnormal rhythm is initiated when an early atrial beat or PAC (dashed lines) occurs. It is blocked at the fast pathway, which is still refractory, and instead goes down the slow pathway, which has quickly recovered (has a shorter refractory period). This time the slow pathway impulse not only can activate the ventricles but also can now travel back up the AV node retrograde through the fast pathway, which by this time has recovered.

(C) The impulse continues in a loop back down the slow pathway, activating the ventricles again and traveling up the fast pathway in a cycle. Retrograde P waves are generated as the atria are now activated from the AV node (these may be seen before or after the QRS or may be obscured in the QRS complex), always in a 1:1 ratio with ventricular activation.

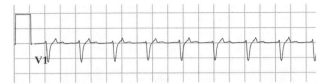

just before or just after the QRS, as shown in Figure 2-16. The P waves are inverted because of activation from the AV node upward. They are narrow because the right and left atria are activated simultaneously from the AV node as opposed to sinus rhythm where the right atrium is activated first (the sinus node lives there) and then the left atrium afterwards. The initiating PAC will have a longer PR because it uses the slow pathway. Many times P waves are not seen because they are buried within the QRS, making diagnose difficult without use of vagal maneuvers/pharmacologic agents to slow down the heart rate or brake the rhythm. When the P wave is seen, the RP interval (distance from the R wave to the next visible P wave following it) is short because the AV node activates the atria and ventricles almost simultaneously. In rare cases, one can have atypical AVNRT in which a PVC generates the rhythm which goes up going up to the atria via the slow pathway and down via the fast pathway, causing a longer delay between ventricular activation and atrial activation and a long RP interval.

Tx—Vagal maneuvers, carotid sinus massage, and IV adenosine can both increase acetylcholine and make the fast pathway more refractory so that the slow pulse goes down the ventricle only once. This can stop the rhythm. Calcium channel blockers and β blockers can also be used chronically for management. For patients who are refractory or unwilling to take medications over the long term, there has been good success with ablation of the circuit in the EP lab (>95%).

Atrioventricular Reciprocating Tachycardia (AVRT)

D—*Atrioventricular reciprocating tachycardia* is a generalized term for tachycardia involving an accessory pathway. Subsets include conditions involving preexcitation of the ventricles, the most famous of which is the Wolfe-Parkinson-White (WPW) syndrome in which there is pre-excitation via an accessory pathway, as well as an associated supraventricular tachycardia.

Epi—It is one-third as common as AVNRT.

P—A large reentrant circuit occurs in this rhythm that uses an accessory conduction pathway called a *bypass tract*. This is a passageway for impulse conduction from atria to ventricles that is independent of the AV node and the His-Purkinje system. If the impulse travels down the AV node/His-Purkinje system and then back up the accessory pathway to the atria, it is called an *orthodromic reciprocating tachycardia* (ORT, See Figure 2-17), which is most common. If the impulse first

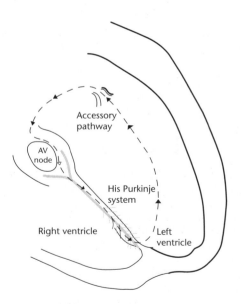

Figure 2-17. Diagram of Atrioventricular Reciprocating Tachycardia.

travels down the accessory pathway and then up the AV node to the atria, it is called an *antidromic reciprocating tachycardia* (ART). In ART, preexcitation of the ventricle occurs though the accessory pathway first, as conduction down to the ventricles via the accessory pathway is faster than through the AV node. This causes a delta wave on the ECG as part of the ventricle is depolarized right before the His-Purkinje activation. Orthodromic reciprocating tachycardia is initiated when a PVC occurs after a sinus beat and conducts upward toward the atria through the accessory pathway (because the AV node is refractory) and then down the AV node to the ventricles and back again in a cycle. P waves may be seen buried in the T waves and are best seen in lead AVL. Antidromic reciprocating tachycardia is initiated by a PAC occurring after a sinus beat that goes through the accessory pathway (because the AV node is refractory) and uses the His-Purkinje system on the way back up to the atria. There is a wide complex QRS and or delta wave from preexcitation. Some accessory pathways can function only in one direction. If they function only in the retrograde (ventricle-to-atria) direction, this is a called a *concealed bypass tract* since there will be no evidence of preexcitation on the ECG.

SiSx—Patients may be asymptomatic or have palpitations, chest pain, angina, or syncope.

Dx—The ORT type of AVRT is hard to distinguish from AVNRT in many cases, as both may break with adenosine. In general, ORT behaves as a longer RP tachycardia, as the P wave/atrial activity will occur later than the ventricular activity, since the atria have to be activated in retrograde fashion via a bypass tract. Definitive diagnosis is made in the EP lab, assessing for the presence of a bypass tract. For ART, the ECG may show evidence of preexcitation and a widened QRS complex. Provocative testing can be done with adenosine infusions (decreases conduction through the AV node and favors the bypass tract) and procainamide (decreases conduction through the bypass tract and favors the AV node) as

well as a treadmill exercise (increases conduction through the AV node, causing less preexcitation in some individuals). In other patients, use of IV isoproterenol can unmask catecholamine-facilitated bypass tracts. In a patient with a known bypass tract and SVT, procainamide (rather than adenosine) is usually the drug of choice initially.

Tx—Acute treatment can involve vagal maneuvers and adenosine (interrupts the circuit in the AV node) or preferably procainamide (decreases conduction in the bypass tract). If a patient goes into AF with an accessory pathway, this can cause VT or VF, necessitating electrical cardioversion. Therefore, ablating the bridge is necessary. In WPW, treatment (i.e., ablation) is required if the patient is ever symptomatic.

Ventricular Tachycardia (VT)

D—Defined as three or more consecutive PVCs at a rate >100 bpm. It can be sustained (>30 seconds or associated with hemodynamic collapse) or nonsustained VT (NSVT) (<30 seconds, no associated hemodynamic effects).

P—May types and varieties exist, most commonly due to reentry and less commonly to triggered activity. It commonly occurs post-MI and is polymorphic (Figure 2-18), with active ischemia or, more commonly, is monomorphic if it is scar-based VT (Figure 2-19). It can be a sequela of a long QT and is exacerbated in the setting of low magnesium and potassium. Ventricular tachycardia can originate in one of the fascicles of the left bundle (fascicular VT) or along the outflow tracts (left ventricular outflow tract VT or right ventricular outflow tract VT); all of these conditions are more amenable to ablation. Less commonly, VT it can be catecholamine induced.

RF—Risk factors include CAD, MI, structural heart disease, myocarditis, and disease of conduction system. Nonsustained VT can be caused by electrolyte abnormalities, by systemic infections, by hypovolemia with or without structural heart disease, and finally, by anything that causes a long QT (drugs most commonly or congenital conditions).

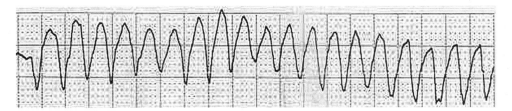

Figure 2-18. Polymorphic VT. Courtesy of Joshua Cooper, M.D., Hospital of the University of Pennsylvania.

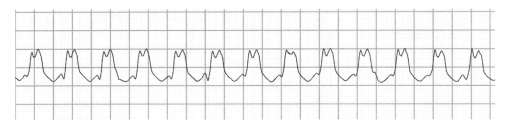

Figure 2-19. Monomorphic VT. Courtesy of Ralph Verdino, M.D., Hospital of the University of Pennsylvania.

SiSx—The presentation varies from asymptomatic tachycardia to syncope and sudden death. Heart rates <150 bpm are well tolerated by most patients in the short term. Virtually all patients with heart rates >200 bpm have symptoms.

Dx—The ECG or the telemetry monitor will show a wide-complex tachycardia. It must be distinguished from SVT with aberrant conduction causing a wide QRS. This is done using the Brugada criteria (see the Approach to the Patient with a Tachyarrhythmia section). Simple indications that are highly suggestive of VT on a 12-lead ECG include:

1. A *northwest axis*, meaning extreme axis deviation;
2. The presence of capture or fusion beats where occasionally the sinus beat captures or partially captures the ventricle;
3. Atrioventricular dissociation in which the P waves are slower and have nothing to do with the QRS complexes;
4. Concordance, meaning that the QRS complexes are all positive or all negative (absence of an RS complex); and finally,

5. Whether or not the QRS complex looks like a normal RBBB or LBBB.

The bottom line, however, is that if a patient has known CAD and a wide-complex tachycardia, the condition is VT until proven otherwise. Try also to distinguish between polymorphic VT (most commonly from ischemic and/or a long QT) and monomorphic VT (typically scar-based post-MI or in an area of fibrosis in a dilated cardiomyopathy).

Tx—If the patient is unstable, one follows the ACLS protocol with prompt defibrillation. Patients with stable, sustained VT can be rate controlled with β blockers, calcium channel blockers, or amiodarone if they are asymptomatic until the underlying cause is discovered, or they can be cardioverted. Other antiarrhythmics can be used as well such as mexiletine or procainamide. Ventricular tachycardia refractory to medication may require ablation in the EP laboratory. This can be done using either an endocardial or epicardial approach, depending on the origin of the arrhythmia. Patients with no easily reversible cause should have an ICD placed for prevention of sudden cardiac death.

Ventricular Fibrillation (VF)

D—A chaotic and rapidly fatal ventricular rhythm with no organized electrical activity that results in little to no cardiac output. In many cases, this rhythm is preceded by VT.

Epi—Seventy-five percent of patients with cardiac arrest have VF as their initial rhythm. Those who survive have an increased risk of sudden death. Predictors of an increased risk of sudden cardiac death include evidence of ischemia, a decreased EF, many PVCs on telemetry >10/hr, inducible VT, advanced age, and traditional risk factors for CAD.

RF—All the risk factors for VT apply to VF.

SiSx—Patients are nonresponsive and have no palpable pulse or blood pressure.

Dx—Diagnosis is performed by telemetry monitoring leads showing unorganized fibrillatory waves (Figure 2-20).

Tx—Ventricular fibrillation is fatal within 5 to 10 minutes without resuscitation. It virtually never terminates spontaneously. Initiate the ACLS protocol, which includes primarily cardiopulmonary resuscitation (CPR) and electrical defibrillation. If the patient recovers, work on reversing the underlying cause (treatment for a long QT, derangement of electrolytes, active ischemia, and so forth).

Accelerated Idioventricular Rhythm (AIVR)

D—A type of VT seen almost exclusively in ischemic heart disease during an MI, usually after reperfusion of the occluded vessel. The patient may or may not have a heart rate >100 bpm.

P—An ectopic ventricular focus competes with the sinus node and takes over the ventricular rate when any type of AV block occurs or the sinus rate slows for any reason. This rhythm is also seen with digitalis toxicity in addition to reperfusion from ischemia.

SiSx—The patient is usually asymptomatic but has a wide, complex rhythm on the telemetry monitor.

Dx—Diagnosis is made by ECG or telemetry (which shows a wide, complex ventricular rhythm that is faster than the typical ventricular escape beat of 20 to 40 bpm with AV dissociation; see Figure 2-21); however, there are more QRS complexes than p waves (which distinguishes AIVR from complete heart block). Typically, AIVR is not very tachycardic.

Tx—Treatment is rarely necessary. Atropine can accelerate the sinus rhythm to suppress

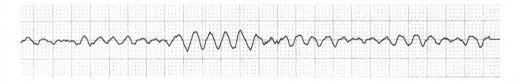

Figure 2-20. Ventricular Fibrillation.
Courtesy of Joshua Cooper, M.D., Hospital of the University of Pennsylvania.

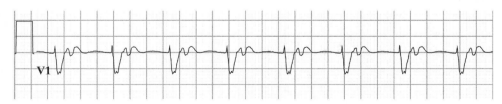

Figure 2-21. Accelerated Idioventricular Rhythm.
Courtesy of Ralph Verdino, M.D., Hospital of the University of Pennsylvania.

AIVR. There can be loss of AV synchrony, and the condition can progress to VT or VF in rare cases. Usually AIVR resolves on its own.

Torsade de Pointes (TdP)

D—A polymorphic VT associated with delayed myocardial depolarization and a long QT interval.

P—QT prolongation strongly predisposes to this condition and can be congenital or acquired. Patients who are bradycardic with this predisposition may be at higher risk of developing TdP.

RF—Acquired forms are drug induced. Other risk factors are electrolyte abnormalities (most commonly hypokalemia and hypomagnesemia), hypothyroidism, stroke, MI, organophosphate poisoning, myocarditis, severe CHF, and mitral valve prolapse. Class Ia drugs and, less commonly, class III agents are associated with TdP.

SiSx—Episodes are usually brief (<20 seconds) but can be sustained and degenerate into VF. Some patients lose consciousness; others are quite symptomatic and feel palpitations before the rhythm breaks.

Dx—Telemetry monitoring shows a fast polymorphic wide complex tachycardia with a heart rate usually >200 bpm. The QRS axis twists around the electrical axis (see Figure 2-22).

Tx—If TdP is sustained, defibrillate the patient. Correct hypokalemia, giving Mg^{2+} and CA^{2+} empirically. Bradycardia, if present, can be corrected with isoproterenol or temporary transvenous pacing. This is important, as bradycardia can prolong the QT and cause these episodes to be more frequent. Keeping the heart rate high can shorten the QT temporarily until the underlying cause is treated or corrected.

Bradycardias

These are defined as a heart rate <60 bpm. Mechanisms include:

- Abnormal impulse formation
  - Sinus node pacemaker malfunction (e.g., sick sinus syndrome)
- Abnormal conduction
  - Fibrosis (seen in inflammatory conditions, cardiomyopathies)
  - Ischemia
  - Infiltration (amyloidosis, sarcoidosis, hemochromatosis)
  - Medication related (β blocker, calcium channel blockers)
  - Infection (endocarditis with abscess, erosion of the conducting tissue)
- Normal conditions
  - High vagal tone (e.g., in athletes)

Atrioventricular Conduction Block

D—A condition in which not all impulses generated in the atria travel down via the AV node to the His-Purkinje system to cause ventricular activation.

RF—Risk factors include ischemia, drugs (especially AV nodal blockers such as digoxin, calcium channel blockers, amiodarone, and β blockers), increased vagal tone, post– cardiac surgery status, CAD, familial heart block, HOCM, infiltrative disease, neuromuscular disease, and cardiac tumors.

P—There are three main types. The AV node in general is the slowest part of conduction because of the inherent properties of its cells. The escape rhythm of its pacemaker cells, in

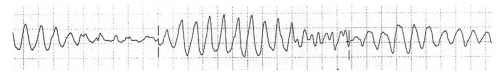

Figure 2-22. Torsade de Pointes. Courtesy of Joshua Cooper, M.D., Hospital of the University of Pennsylvania.

the absence of a sinus beat, is about 40 to 60 bpm. In patients with very fast atrial rates (>200 bpm), the AV node's slow conduction and refractoriness are protective and AV block is therefore physiologic. In diseases states, however, AV block occurs, causing a ventricular rate <60 bpm, and it can be symptomatic. Classically, there are three types of AV block: first degree, second degree, and third degree, as shown in Table 2-39 and Figure 2-23.

Table 2-39. Types of Atrioventricular Block (AVB)

Type of Block	ECG Features	Comments
First-Degree AVB	Long PR interval (>200 msec). Always 1:1 ratio of P to QRS, no dropped beats.	Usually from high vagal tone or AV nodal blocking drugs.
Second-Degree AVB	Always a dropped beat such that the P: QRS ratio is not 1:1. Type I (Wenkebach)—PR intervals are nonuniform. They keep prolonging until a dropped beat occurs. This appears as "grouped beating" on the ECG (implies *disease in the AV node*). Type II (Mobitz)—P intervals are regularly spaced (implies *disease below the AV node*).	Seen in patients with structurally abnormal hearts, in those with RBBB or LBBB, and in those on AV nodal blocking agents (calcium channel blockers, β blockers, or digoxin). Nomenclature is 2:1, 3:1, 4:1 (the number of P:QRSs) in high-grade block or 4:3, 5:4 (the number of P:QRSs before each dropped beat). *With a 2:1 block, it is hard to tell types I and II apart.*
Third-Degree AVB	Complete AV dissociation. The P waves march out on their own, as do the QRSs. There must be more P waves than QRS complexes (otherwise, one can argue that there is just a faster ventricular escape).	Consider this when the QRS rate is very slow (40 bpm) Also, realize that the escape rhythm can be narrow (escape in the junction) or wide (an escape in the ventricle), depending on where the escape pacemaker is located.

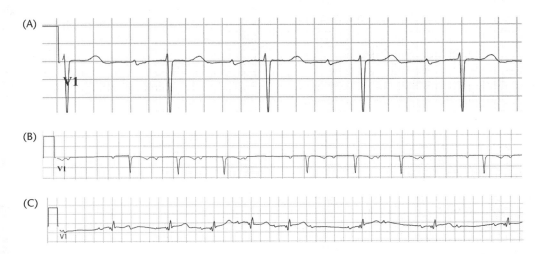

Figure 2-23 (A–C). Rhythm Strips of Different Forms of Heart Block.
(A) First-degree AV block. Courtesy of Ralph Verdino, M.D., Hospital of the University of Pennsylvania.
(B) Second-degree type I AV block. Courtesy of Ralph Verdino, M.D., Hospital of the University of Pennsylvania.
(C) Second-degree type II AV block. Courtesy of Joshua Cooper, M.D., Hospital of the University of Pennsylvania.

SiSx—Patients may be asymptomatic, depending on the degree of AV block, or have syncope, dyspnea, or chest pain. They may also have symptoms on exertion due to the inability to raise their heart rate as needed.

Dx—Diagnosis is made by telemetry and the ECG, showing the classic characteristics outlined above.

Tx—First-degree and type I second-degree AV block usually need no treatment except for removal of offending agents if the patient is symptomatic. Type II and third-degree heart block require either permanent pacemaker or temporary pacing wire if the condition is temporary (e.g., post inferior MI heart block) as they suggest infranodal disease.

Sick Sinus Syndrome (Tachy-Brady Syndrome)

D—A condition of abnormal sinus function characterized by:

1. Chronic inappropriate bradycardia
2. Sinus pauses, arrest, and no appropriate escape rhythm
3. Atrioventricular conduction disturbances
4. Carotid sinus hypersensitivity
5. Occasional SVTs (see in over 50% of patients), atrial fibrillation being the most common

Epi—The median age of incidence is the mid-70s. There is 80% survival at 3 years.

P—Any disease that affects the SA node can be a precipitant. Most commonly, the SA node is replaced with fibrous tissue and there is fibrosis of the rest of the conduction system. Disease of the SA nodal artery (CAD, inflammation, emboli) can lead to sick sinus syndrome. Infiltrative disorders and drugs (antiarrhythmics), in addition to trauma or surgery, are other exacerbating factors.

Dx—Diagnosis is made by the ECG and the history, showing the characteristics in the definition.

Tx—In general, most patients need a pacemaker. This condition accounts for half of the pacemakers placed for symptomatic bradycardia. The tachyarrhythmias can be controlled with AV nodal agents, and backup pacing can then be used to prevent bradycardia. If AF is also present, then anticoagulation should be done in appropriate patients.

Carotid Sinus Hypersensitivity

D—Sinus pauses of >3 sec with a drop in BP of 50 mmHg or more after carotid sinus massage. This condition is called *carotid sinus syndrome* when accompanied by syncope or near syncope.

Epi—It affects up to one-third of elderly men with CAD. It may explain up to 40% of syncope in elderly patients.

P—Two types exist: cardioinhibitory and vasodepressive responses. In most cases, the function of the baroreceptor apparatus is intact.

Dx—Carotid sinus massage should be performed in a controlled environment in the supine and erect positions to elicit the findings mentioned in the definition. One should look for either a fall in BP (classified as a vasodepressor response) and a pause or asystole (classified as a cardioinhibitory response). This procedure is not typically done, however, if the patient has a carotid bruit or stent or a prior stroke/transient ischemic attack (TIA).

Tx—No therapy is needed unless this condition is thought to be the cause of syncope or near syncope. For cardioinhibitory types, the treatment of choice is a pacemaker. For vasodepressive types, the treatment is unclear. Selective serotonin reuptake inhibitors (SSRIs) have been used with limited success.

Valvular Heart Disease

Aortic Stenosis (AS)

D—A condition in which there is progressive stenosis of the aortic valve with narrowing of the valve orifice.

Epi—It is the most common cause of valvular left ventricular outflow obstruction. Patients who present with angina have a 50% survival rate at 5 years; those who present with syncope have a 50% survival rate at 3 years; and those who present with heart failure have a 50% survival rate at 1 year.

P—Common causes are (1) congenital (e.g., sequelae of a bicuspid valve; 10% of such patients will also have a coarctation), (2) acquired rheumatic valve disease, or (3) the most common in the United States: degenerative calcific AS from abnormal calcification, which is usually seen in patients in their 70s and 80s. Whatever the cause, there is a progressive narrowing of the valve orifice. The left ventricle faces an increased afterload as the valve area decreases and develops higher systolic pressures as a consequence, causing LVH, a less compliant ventricle and increased importance of atrial contraction in filling. The greater left ventricular muscle mass also increases the myocardial oxygen demand. Once symptoms develop, the survival rate decreases dramatically unless patients are surgically treated.

SiSx—Classically, a RUSB crescendo-decrescendo murmur that radiates to the carotids is heard. Many patients may have no symptoms at presentation. Symptoms are classically found in three forms—angina, syncope, or heart failure—and indicate the AS is severe, needing treatment. Angina usually results from the increased myocardial demand. There is a strong association with CAD in this population. Syncope can occur from the fixed outflow obstruction during an episode of increased demand, causing hypoperfusion to the brain in addition to hypotension. Heart failure from both diastolic and systolic dysfunction can be seen. The classic findings on the exam include a pulsus *parvus et tardus* (a weak, slow carotid pulse from the delayed upstroke). A systolic thrill over the carotid arteries may be palpable in severe AS. The apical impulse on exam is nondisplaced but diffuse and sustained. A double impulse implies a palpable A wave. The intensity of the murmur does not relate to the severity of the stenosis. The later the murmur starts in systole, however, the greater the degree of stenosis, as it takes longer to open the valve. S_2 also becomes softer, and an absent A_2 (single, non split S_2) is a sign of severe or critical AS. Aortic stenosis is often accompanied by aortic regurgitation with calcific immobile valve leaflets, which neither open nor close properly. The *Gallavardin phenomenon* occurs in severe calcific AS; in this condition, high-frequency parts of the murmur radiate to the apex. Aortic sclerosis is a mild form of this condition in which the valves move well but are calcified and there is no large reduction in valve area.

Dx—Diagnosis is made by the physical exam initially, and is quantified by ECHO and then by left and right heart catheterization (the gold standard). Important parameters are the degree of left ventricular hypertrophy, the aortic valve area (a normal valve is 2–3 cm², moderate stenosis is <1.5 cm², severe stenosis is <1.0 cm², and critical AS is <0.7 cm²), and the mean pressure gradient between the aorta and the left ventricle. Mean gradients of 40–50 mmHg across the valve suggest severe stenosis. Echocardiography uses the continuity equation, measuring the area and velocity of blood going into the valve and the velocity of blood across the valve to determine the area of the valve. Left heart catheterization uses a special catheter to measure pressures simultaneously in the left ventricle and aorta and, using the cardiac output from the right heart catheterization, calculates the valve area. In patients with a low EF and low cardiac output, both methods can underestimate the degree of AS. In such cases, challenge with dobutamine can be done, and valve gradients are remeasured.

Tx—Medical management is used for patients who are completely asymptomatic and without signs of left ventricular dysfunction or elevated left-sided pressures. The goals are CAD prevention and BP and heart rate control. Nitrates are avoided because of the risk of cerebral hypoperfusion, and vasodilators are avoided because they can cause hypotension (the heart cannot increase cardiac output after vasodilation to maintain blood pressure because of the aortic valve obstruction). For any patient who has symptoms from AS or has left ventricular dysfunction as a result of AS, surgical treatment with a prosthetic or metallic valve is needed. In non surgical patients percutaneous aortic balloon valvuloplasty can be performed palliatively.

More recently, percutaneously placed aortic valves have been used and may be more readily available in the future. These valves are inflated inside and over the original calcified valve. Surgical options in younger patients may include the Ross procedure (in which the pulmonary valve is placed in the aortic position and a prosthetic pulmonic valve is used) for calcific AS. Replacement of the valve is often preferred over repair, as removal of calcific areas results in leaflet fibrosis and retraction with time. For noncalcific AS, repair may be possible. In patients without CAD and a normal EF, the mortality due to repair is 2%–3% and 10-year survival is 85%.

Aortic Regurgitation (AR)

D—Condition in which aortic valve incompetence allows blood to flow back into the ventricle. This is also called aortic insufficiency.

P—Common causes include (1) the presence of a bicuspid valve, (2) myxomatous valves, (3) endocarditis, (4) rheumatic heart disease, and (5) Marfan's or Ehlers-Danlos syndrome with aortic root dilation. Acute AR is usually caused by infection, dissection, and trauma and may be a surgical emergency. Chronic AR is due to diseased valve cusps or dilation of the aortic root. Conditions of chronic volume overload lead to left ventricular dilation and eccentric hypertrophy, causing AR.

SiSx—Acute AR can present as cardiogenic shock. Patients with chronic AR may be asymptomatic for a long time. Symptoms can reflect right heart failure or left heart failure. Angina can develop from decreased diastolic pressure and filling of the coronaries. The exam may reveal a diastolic soft, rumbling murmur. There may also be a systolic murmur from the increased flow across the aortic valve due to the increased left ventricular diastolic volume. A second diastolic murmur called the *Austin Flint murmur* can also be heard, in which the mitral valve closes prematurely because of a rise in diastolic pressure. When the AR is severe and wide open, a murmur may not be heard; one may hear just an S_3. Other clues in the exam are a large

pulse pressure producing a so-called water hammer pulse. Classic signs, none of which are specific, include *Duroziez's sign*, where compression at the femoral artery causes a systolic murmur but increased compression causes a very early diastolic decrescendo murmur too; *Hill's sign*, where leg pressures are lower than arm pressures; *De Musset's sign*, which is head bobbing with each aortic pulsation; *Rosenbach's sign* of hepatic pulsation; *Becker's sign* of retinal arteriole pulsation; *Mueller's sign* of uvular pulsation; and *Quincke's sign* of capillary pulses visible in the nail beds. Maneuvers such as standing from a squatting position will decrease the murmur as preload is decreased. Once symptoms develop, there is usually a rapid decline in functional status.

Dx—Most cases are discovered on exam and then confirmed with ECHO showing aortic insufficiency.

Tx—Severe acute AR is a surgical emergency. An intra-aortic balloon pump will not help in this case and will increase the degree of AR (it inflates in diastole). Surgical treatment is the definitive therapy in chronic AR in patients who are good candidates. Surgery should be considered in those who have severe symptomatic AR, and for those who have started to develop ventricular dilation or reduced EF because of the AR. Medical therapy for chronic AR consists of management of the changes in the left ventricle (dilation) and complications of elevated left-sided pressures. Angiotensin converting enzyme inhibitors and/or hydralazine also slow the progression of left ventricular dysfunction; nifedipine has been shown to slow the progression of left ventricular dysfunction and delays the time to surgical treatment. β blockers should be given if AR is from aortic dissection acutely and the patient is hemodynamically stable.

Mitral Stenosis (MS)

D—Condition in which there is outflow obstruction through the mitral valve orifice due to valvular disease.

P—Rheumatic heart disease is by far the most common cause worldwide, though many patients are not aware of having had rheumatic fever. Acute rheumatic fever can cause mitral regurgitation, but stenosis develops decades later. Characteristic thickening of leaflets occurs with fibrous obliteration. There is also commissural fusion, chordal fusion and shortening, and calcium deposition on the leaflets, chordae, and annulus. Other causes of MS include congenital mitral stenosis, myxomatous disease, thrombus accumulation, valvulitis from systemic lupus erythematosus, amyloid, or carcinoid, infiltration from mucopolysaccharidosis, and infection of mitral annular calcification with encroachment on leaflets. Increased left atrial pressure occurs and is transmitted to the pulmonary vasculature and then to the right heart structures.

SiSx—A long asymptomatic course at first is common. When symptoms start, they usually reflect increased pulmonary venous congestion (dyspnea, fatigue, orthopnea) or structural atrial disease from enlargement such as atrial fibrillation. Hemoptysis can occur, with rupture of small bronchial veins due to high left-sided pressure. Hoarseness occurs when the dilated left atrium impinges on the recurrent laryngeal nerve (Ortner's syndrome). Embolization is also a possibility, as is endocarditis. Right ventricular failure eventually occurs from high pulmonary pressure. The exam may show a diastolic rumble murmur, which increases with exercise and is heard best in the left lateral decubitus position. One may hear an opening snap; the closer to A_2 it is, the tighter the valve.

Dx—Echocardiography makes the diagnosis. One may also see left atrial dilation, high pulmonary artery pressure, and a pressure gradient between the left atrium and left ventricle during systole. A normal mitral valve area is 4 to 6 cm². When the area is less than 2 cm², a pressure gradient can develop. Disease is considered to be severe when the area is <1.0 cm², moderate when it is 1.0 to 1.4 cm² and mild when it is <2.0 cm². Right and left heart catheterization can also be used to estimate the valve area using the cardiac output and pressure gradient from the left atrium (measured by the PCWP) and the left ventricle.

Tx—Medical treatment includes salt restriction, diuretics, and other drugs as appropriate for structural heart disease and concomitant arrhythmias. Anticoagulation is recommended in any patient who has had a prior stroke or TIA or who has atrial fibrillation. It should probably also be used for those with a high risk of stroke (when an enlarged left atrium or spontaneous ECHO smoke is seen), although the data are less well established. Surgical options include valve commissurotomy, which has a 10% rate of restenosis, percutaneous balloon valvuloplasty/valvotomy, and mitral valve repair or replacement, depending on the etiology. Heavily calcified valves are less ideal candidates for percutaneous valvuloplasty because the valve can be torn. Mitral surgery has an 80% survival at 10 years in appropriate candidates. Mitral valve surgery or valvuloplasty should be considered in asymptomatic patients who have moderate to severe MS with pulmonary hypertension (PASP >50 mmHg at rest or 60 mmHg with exercise).

Mitral Regurgitation (MR)

D—Condition in which there is retrograde flow through the mitral valve as a result of dysfunction of the valve leaflets, chordae tendonae, papillary muscles, left ventricle, and/or mitral annulus.

P—Myxomatous change is more common than rheumatic causes in the United States. Acute MR can be caused by ischemic damage to the papillary muscles or endocarditis. Chronic causes include any cause of left ventricular dilation over time leading to widening of the valve leaflets.

SiSx—Symptoms depend on whether the condition is acute or chronic. Acute MR presents with pulmonary congestion, PND, dyspnea on exertion, and cardiogenic shock in some cases. Chronic MR can be asymptomatic for years; the first symptoms usually are decreased exercise tolerance and exertional dyspnea. Long-standing MR can cause pulmonary hypertension. The exam may show a holosystolic murmur that classically radiates to the axilla or back (if the anterior leaflet is disrupted).

Dx—The diagnosis is made by ECHO to assess the severity of MR, the mechanism, and associated cardiac abnormalities. Transesophageal echocardiography may be necessary to further define disease severity and pathologic valve abnormalities and to determine if valve repair is possible or replacement is needed.

Tx—Treat chronic MR with salt restriction, diuretics, endocarditis prophylaxis, and afterload-reducing agents. Surgery is done when medical treatment fails, though it is difficult in patients with a severely dilated left ventricle and pulmonary hypertension. Criteria for surgical correction in chronic MR include those with severe symptomatic MR, and those who have a low EF, left ventricular dilation, or significant pulmonary hypertension as a result of the MR.

Treat acute MR with the intra-aortic balloon pump and consider using IV nitrates. Surgery should be performed to correct the regurgitation with repair or mitral valve replacement (MVR).

Mitral Valve Prolapse (MVP)

D—Condition in which the mitral leaflets bow back into the atrium past the annulus during ventricular systole.

Epi—It is the most common form of valvular disease in the United States Despite prior reports suggesting a higher prevalence in women, MVP actually appears to have equal prevalence in men and women of 2.5%.

P—The condition can be primary or secondary. There can be normal valvular structures but disproportion between the leaflet size and the left ventricular cavity. The primary form is due to myxomatous proliferation of the leaflets, usually with a prominent middle layer of the leaflet. Mitral valve prolapse can be hereditary or associated with connective tissue diseases, Marfan's syndrome, Ehlers-Danlos syndrome, or myotonic dystrophy.

SiSx—Most patients have no symptoms, and the diagnosis is made on routine exam or ECHO for another reason. Associated symptoms, however described, include palpitations, easy fatigability, and postural light-headedness. On exam, one may hear a mid to late systolic ejection click. Maneuvers that shrink the left ventricular cavity (i.e., decreased preload or afterload such as caused by sitting or standing up) cause the click to occur earlier. Raising the legs and increasing the preload causes it to occur later. This is in fact sufficient for the diagnosis of MVP. Many types of SVTs, VT, and even bradyarrhythmias have been reported to be associated with MVP. There is also an increased incidence of bypass tracts. Transient ischemic attacks have also been reported.

Dx—The diagnosis can be reasonably made by exam and maneuvers. Echocardiography can confirm the diagnosis by showing prolapse of one or both mitral valve leaflets.

Tx—For patients with a history of TIAs, aspirin therapy is indicated. Palpitations can be treated with β blockers, and EP testing can be done for more serious arrhythmias. Antibiotic prophylaxis for endocarditis is no longer recommended for these patients, although it was used in the past.

Adult Congenital Heart Diseases

Adult congenital heart disease is a complex topic and includes a number of conditions. Treatment has advanced such that many patients are surviving to adulthood. Table 2-40 briefly summarizes some of the most common entities that may be seen in adult patients.

Table 2-40. Common Congenital Heart Conditions

Common Condition	Definition	Signs/Symptoms	Diagnosis	Treatment
Atrial Septal Defect (ASD)	Communication between the two atria: can be of three types: secundum defect (80%), primum defect (10%), or sinus venosus defect (10%).	Depends on the size of the shunt. If it is large, the patient may have pulmonary hypertension, dyspnea, right heart failure, dyspnea on exertion, and eventually Eisenmenger's syndrome with cyanosis and right-to-left shunting. Atrial arrhythmias and stroke from paradoxical embolism can occur.	Exam may show fixed split S_2 in large left-to-right shunts. Pulmonic valve systolic murmur from increased flow and right ventricular lift. ECHO with a bubble study or TEE showing communication between the atria makes the diagnosis.	Small shunts—watch and wait if patient is asymptomatic. Usually for large shunt fractions (pulmonary to systemic blood flow ratio of >1.5:1) or if symptoms such as stroke merit closure. Primum defect—surgical closure. Secundum—surgical or percutaneous closure. Sinus venosus—surgical closure.
Ventricular Septal Defects (VSDs)	A communication between the ventricles. Can be either membranous VSD (in the upper membranous part of the interventricular septum) or muscular VSD.	Most adults are asymptomatic. Can cause dyspnea on exertion with larger shunts, pulmonary hypertension, and cyanosis. Endocarditis can occur with smaller shunts.	Exam: holosystolic murmur at the left sternal border that radiates rightward. ECHO makes the diagnosis.	Many close early in childhood; large VSDs can cause heart failure in childhood and are surgically closed. In most adults, the diagnosis has already been made. Muscular VSDs may be closed percutaneously. Surgery is contraindicated in Eisenmenger's syndrome.
Coarctation of the Aorta	Narrowing of the thoracic descending aorta, most commonly below the ductus arteriosis (95%) and left subclavian artery, usually with collateral development elsewhere. Association with bicuspid aortic valve.	May be asymptomatic or present with hypertension or murmur. Headache, leg cramps, muscle weakness may be present.	Systolic BP may be >10 mmHg higher in the arms than in the legs. An ejection murmur may be heard over the chest and upper back along the spine. Chest X-ray may show rib notching (from dilated collateral vessels). ECHO, catheterization, or MRA can make the diagnosis and estimate the gradient across the coarctation.	Surgical correction usually for gradients >20 mmHg or with CHF symptoms. Surgical repair may include end-to-end anastomosis, bypass graft, or prosthetic patch. Balloon angioplasty and stent placement can also be done in select patients.

continued

Table 2-40. (continued)

Common Condition	Definition	Signs/Symptoms	Diagnosis	Treatment
Ebstein's Anomaly	Deformity of the tricuspid valve with apical displacement of the septal and posterior leaflets and adhesion to the right ventricular free wall. A significant portion of the right ventricle can be atrialized and thin.	Atypical chest pain, dyspnea on exertion, arrhythmias. Concomitant ASD is common. Cyanosis is seen early if there is a comcomitant ASD or PFO and significant tricuspid regurgitation is present.	Right parasternal left, split S_1 wide, tricuspid regurgitation murmur without an increase during inspiration (noncompliant right ventricle). ECHO can make the diagnosis.	Fifty percent of patients survive to age 50. Management of arrhythmias, tricuspid valve replacement, or annuloplasty may be required. A palliative Fontan procedure may be needed in other patients. ASD closure may be needed in some patients.
Tetrology of Fallot	One abnormality causing four conditions: 1. VSD. 2. Right ventricular outflow (infundibular) and obstruction. Pulmonary stenosis may occur. 3. Right ventricular hypertrophy. 4. Overriding aorta that is dilated; 25% have a right-sided aortic arch.	Arrhythmias (atrial flutter and ventricular tachycardia) are common. This is the most common form of cyanotic congenital heart disease and is usually seen at birth.	ECHO shows RVH, a gradient across the right ventricular outflow tract, and a VSD. Pulmonary stenosis usually protects against the development of pulmonary hypertension.	Most patients die in childhood without surgical correction. They can have a right ventricular outflow patch and VSD closure. Often severe pulmonary regurgitation is left as a result.
Transposition of the Great Arteries	Condition in which the great arteries are discordant with the aorta arising from the right ventricle and the pulmonary artery arising from the left ventricle.	Usually cyanosis occurs at birth. A shunt (PDA, ASD) is necessary for survival.	Diagnosed at birth, usually with cyanosis. ECHO makes the diagnosis, showing discordant great vessels.	Requires corrective surgery with the atrial switch or arterial switch procedure.

| Patent Ductus Arteriosus (PDA) | Failure of the embryonic ductus arteriosus to close, causing a shunt from the aorta to the pulmonary artery. Usually the origin is at the left PA. | Small or moderate- sized PDAs are usually asymptomatic up to middle age. Large PDAs cause pulmonary hypertension and eventually Eisenmenger's physiology. | Symptoms of pulmonary hypertension or right-sided failure. Hyperdynamic apical impulse. Wide pulse pressures. Continuous, rough machinery murmur is heard with a thrill in the upper chest. Cyanosis is seen in advanced disease. ECHO is useful, but MRI or CT or angiography makes the diagnosis. | Small shunts are compatible with better survival until patients develop CHF. Large shunts should be corrected early if caught. Surgical ligation or transcatheter closure with coils or occluder devices can be done. Closure is usually contraindicated in Eisenmenger's physiology. |

CHAPTER 3

Pulmonology

PULMONARY ANATOMY AND PHYSIOLOGY

- Note in Figure 3-1 that the right lung has three lobes and the left lung two lobes. On the lateral view, note that the left upper lobe is mostly an anterior structure and the right middle lobe is completely anterior. This is important to note while reading chest X-rays for infiltrates or pneumothoraces.
- The main function of the lungs is to facilitate gas exchange of oxygen and carbon dioxide (CO_2). They also metabolize and filter compounds in the blood and, at times, act as a blood reservoir.
- Each lung has over 300 million alveoli, the smallest unit of gas exchange. After the trachea, the airways branch considerably. At a certain point in this branching, gas exchange begins to occur. The conducting airways (from the trachea all the way to the *terminal bronchioles*) are not involved in gas change. Gas exchange starts with the *respiratory bronchioles*, which have alveolar buds.
- Type I pneumocytes occupy most of the alveolar surface epithelial layer and are joined by tight junctions. Their main function is to form specialized thin layers with capillaries to facilitate gas transfusion.
- Type II pneumocytes are fewer in number and line part of the alveoli. They secrete surfactant, which lowers the surface tension, allowing the alveoli to stay open. They can also differentiate into Type I cells after lung injury.
- Mucus is secreted by goblet cells and mucous glands to help remove small particles. The mixture is then propelled upward by cilia (mucociliary clearance).
- The blood supply of the lungs is via the pulmonary arteries, in addition to the bronchial arteries that come off the descending aorta. Venous drainage is via the pulmonary veins.

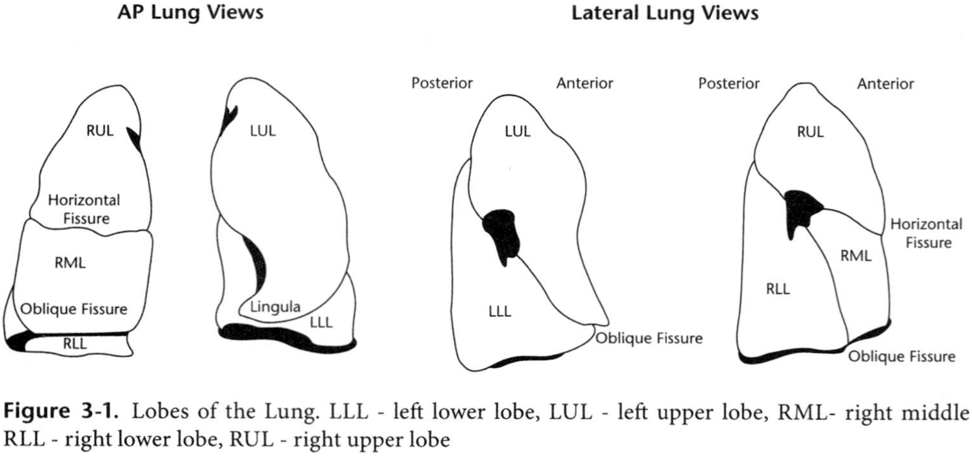

Figure 3-1. Lobes of the Lung. LLL - left lower lobe, LUL - left upper lobe, RML- right middle lobe, RLL - right lower lobe, RUL - right upper lobe

THE PULMONARY PHYSICAL EXAM

1. Look for clubbing, respiratory distress, accessory muscle use, cyanosis, and cough and listen for hoarseness.
2. Visualize the position of the trachea. One will see displacement away from the side with a pneumothorax or large pleural effusion, but shifted toward the side of atelectasis.
3. Assess for symmetrical inspiratory expansion by looking at the back or feeling the flanks during a full inspiration and expiration.
4. Percuss posteriorly to determine the position of the diaphragms. There should be dullness below the diaphragms.
5. Listen to breath sounds posteriorly and anteriorly. Most commonly missed findings are in the right middle lobe, heard best laterally and anteriorly. Apices can be listened to above the clavicles.
6. Specific physical findings and techniques are listed in Tables 3-1 and 3-2.

Table 3-1. Pulmonary Physical Exam Findings

Findings	Description	Examples
Bronchial Breath Sounds	As opposed to normal or *vesicular breath* sounds, in this condition expiratory sounds are as loud and long as inspiratory sounds (similar to sounds over the trachea). Caused by turbulent flow in central airways through consolidated, stiff, or dense lungs.	Heard in patients predominantly with pneumonia, but also in atelectasis with an open airway and advanced pulmonary fibrosis.
Dullness to Percussion	Instead of resonant sounds during percussion, dullness is heard. Due to lack of normal air-filled lung.	Consider consolidation or atelectatic lung, fluid-filled lung, large mass, elevated diaphragm, or chest wall abnormality that prevents sustained vibration after chest is struck.
Hyperresonant Percussion	Percussion sound is more resonant than expected compared to other parts of the lung fields. Due to loss of the dampening effect by the normal lung.	Pneumothorax, severe emphysema, and hyperinflation, as in severe asthma.
Decreased Intensity of Breath Sounds	Inspiratory or expiratory sounds are muffled.	From decreased production of respiratory motions or decreased transmission from large airways because of an obstruction. Seen in emphysema. There may also be an interruption between the airway and chest wall allowing another means for air outlet.
Broncophony	Voice sounds (but not actual words) are transmitted clearly through the lung fields. Normally, one does not hear words exactly as they are spoken; they should be somewhat muffled.	Occurs over a lung area where the alveoli are filled with fluid or replaced by solid tissue. It may be heard in pneumonia, in atelectasis, or with lung masses.
Pectoriloquy	Literally, "chest speaking." Like bronchophony, but one *can hear identifiable words* a patient speaks or whispers while listening to peripheral lung zones.	Second most sensitive finding of consolidation after egophony.
Egophony	Asking the person to say *eeeee*, which sounds like *aaaa* over part of a lung field.	In areas of compressed lung from consolidation, from atelectasis, or in the area of lung compression from a large pleural effusion. This muffles the transmission of sound.
Wheezes	Discrete high-pitched musical sounds usually heard in expiration, secondary to vibration of airway walls with flow limitation.	Think primarily of asthma and bronchitis.

continued

Table 3.1 *(continued)*

Findings	Description	Examples
Ronchi	Low-pitched vibratory sounds heard in inspiration and expiration.	Usually secondary to mucus, which can be abolished with a cough.
Squeak	A very brief, high-pitched musical sound in mid/late inspiration.	Often transient; may be heard in bronchiolitis obliterans organizing pneumonia (BOOP).
Fine Crackles	Momentary clicking from opening and closing of small airways. Usually end-inspiratory or pan-inspiratory.	Common in patients with an early pneumonia or, more commonly, in interstitial lung disease of any kind.
Coarse Crackles	More muffled; individual clicking sounds are louder and fewer in number.	More early inspiratory crackles are common in COPD, whereas more pan-inspiratory crackles occur in congestive heart failure (CHF).
Abnormal Fremitus	With the palms of the hands placed flat on the back, ask the person to say *toy* while feeling for vibrations with vocalization (*99* does not emulate the original German *neun und neunzig* used when this finding was first described. It sounds more like the word *toy*).	Increased fremitus can be seen in the presence of significant fluid, a solid lung mass, or consolidation. Decreased fremitus may be seen in emphysema, effusions, or massive pulmonary edema.
Clubbing	A blunting of the Lovibond angle between the nailbed and the nailfold. Putting the fingernails of the opposite hands together normally makes a diamond shape. This is not present here.	Seen in advanced lung disease, bronchiectasis, CF, and nonpulmonary conditions such as cyanotic congenital heart disease or inflammatory bowel disease. May also be familial. Usually associated with a shunt.

Table 3-2. Distinguishing Characteristics of Common Pulmonary Conditions

	Pneumothorax	Consolidation	Effusion
Decreased Breath Sounds	+++	+	++
Dullness to Percussion	Hyperresonant	+	+
Egophony	−	++	−

DIAGNOSTIC AND THERAPEUTIC MODALITIES

Numerous diagnostic techniques exist for invasive and noninvasive evaluation of the lungs. These are shown in Table 3-3.

Pulmonary Function Tests (PFTs)

Pulmonary function tests are a quantitative way to assess both static and dynamic lung volumes as well as mechanical gas exchange properties of the lung. They include the following types of studies: spirometry, flow volume loops, lung volume measurements, and measurement of the diffusion capacity of carbon monoxide.

The three major categories of abnormalities are (1) obstructive defects, (2) restrictive defects, and (3) gas exchange defects. It is useful to know the volumes and capacities for interpreting these tests as shown in Figure 3-2.

The mostly commonly used PFTs are:

1. *Spirometry*: This is ordered with all PFTs to assess the basic degree of obstruction or restriction or to follow the progression of a disease. The patient inhales completely and then exhales as forcefully and rapidly as possible while lung volume versus time is graphed (see Figure 3-2). Forced expiratory volume at 1 second (FEV_1), forced vital capacity (FVC), the FEV_1/FVC ratio, and vital capacity (VC) are obtained, along with percentages

Table 3-3. Invasive and Noninvasive Studies of the Lung

Chest X-Ray	The most important initial imaging tool. From 10% to 15% of symptomatic patients with infiltrative lung disease will have no findings. Routine films include PA and lateral films, although an AP film may be done in patients who cannot stand for the former. Decubitus films may be done to assess for pleural effusion. See Appendix B for more detail on interpretation.
Standard Chest CT	The most helpful supplement to chest X-ray, which effectively separates the lung, mediastinum, pleura, and chest wall. It is useful in distinguishing interstitial and alveolar diseases, staging lung cancer, assessing mediastinal and hilar lesions, and distinguishing diffuse lung disease and pleural disease. It is also useful to evaluate solitary pulmonary nodules. Normal cuts are 2- to 5-mm slices. IV contrast is useful when attempting to distinguish adenopathy from other tissue, specifically vessels.
High-Resolution CT (HRCT)	Best used to evaluate parenchymal diseases causing pulmonary fibrosis, with representative samples cut at high resolution up to 0.15 mm in different parts of the lung. Good for examining diseases such as IPF or pulmonary bronchiectasis. Not ideal for evaluating for the presence of a solitary pulmonary nodule or masses since only sampled cuts are done at varied levels, and not fine imaging cuts along the entire lung.
PE Protocol CT	Most CT scans today are spiral. There is a special protocol for PE with timed IV dye injection. It is generally good at detecting pulmonary artery clots that are larger and more proximal. Also used to assess lower extremity vasculature for clot.
MRI	Good for lesions at the lung apices when coronal sections are needed. It may also show vascular malformations and lymphatic structures, and is useful for evaluation of the pericardium, superior sulcus tumors, and neurogenic tumors. It is superior to CT in evaluation of chest wall masses and small, occult mediastinal neoplasms and also when patients are allergic to CT contrast.
Ventilation/ Perfusion (V/Q) Scan	This test is used to detect pulmonary emboli by looking for mismatch between areas of the lung that are ventilated and perfused. Results are given as high probability (90% chance of PE), intermediate probability (20–60%), and low probability (<5% chance of PE). It is also used in patients getting pulmonary resection who have poor functional reserve to see which good areas of the lung to leave intact. Finally, it can assess for the presence of macrovascular shunting.
Pulmonary Angiography	Contrast dye is infused into the pulmonary artery tree and a picture of the branching pattern is obtained to look for abnormalities. It is the gold standard for detecting PE and is also useful to diagnose pulmonary arteriovenous malformations. This procedure is necessary if embolectomy is planned.
Bronchial Angiography	Similar to pulmonary angiography, but the bronchial arteries are visualized as they come off the aorta. This is commonly done while looking for sources of pulmonary hemorrhage in a patient with hemoptysis. It is necessary before embolotherapy is done to stop bleeding.
Bronchoscopy	A scope is put down the trachea after sedation and allows visualization of the bronchial tree up to the level of subsegemental bronchi. Bronchoalveolar lavage can be done, in which 100–150 mL of saline is instilled and aspirated to be analyzed. Biopsies of mediastinal lymph nodes can also be obtained, as well as samples of lung parenchyma and pleura.
VATS (Video-Assisted Thorascopic Surgery)	Small holes are made in the chest usually in order to biopsy a larger piece of lung tissue or pleura under direct camera visualization. Can also be used for resection of peripheral pulmonary nodules and bullous lung disease.
Endobronchial Ultrasound (EBUS)	Minimally invasive procedure that uses ultrasound on the bronchoscope that can show real-time imaging of airways, vessels, lungs, and lymph nodes. It can be used to help view hard-to-reach areas and gain access to lymph nodes for biopsy or aspiration.

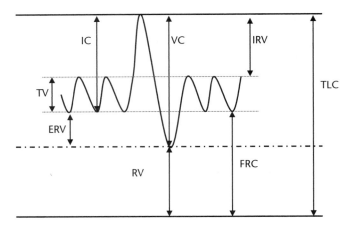

Figure 3-2. Lung Volumes and Capacities in Normal Ventilation.
Notes: Volumes are the smallest units of measurement, and capacities are made by summating volumes.
Special values that may be seen in PFTs are FVC—same as VC but done as forcefully and rapidly as possible,
causing the airways to narrow and slowing the rate of expiration; FEV_1—volume forcefully expired in the first
second after a maximal breath. It reflects the status of large airways.
ERV, expiratory reserve volume; FRC, functional residual capacity; IC, inspiratory capacity; IRV, inspiratory
reserve volume; RV, residual volume (volume of air left that cannot be expired); TLC, total lung capacity; TV,
tidal volume (at rest); VC, vital capacity (maximal air expelled from lungs after a maximal inspiration).

compared to normal population standards.
The test is very reproducible if done correctly
and can be repeated after the use of a bronchodilator or a bronchoconstrictor such as
methacholine to test for airway hyperreactivity. The quality of the study is defined as good
(rapid volume upstroke with little hesitation
and breathing proceeds until there is a long
plateau in the air velocity), fair, or poor.

2. *Flow volume loops*: These tests are usually
ordered when a fixed obstructive defect is
suspected. Cases A–D shown in Figure 3-3
highlight different possible findings.

3. *Lung volumes*: These tests are used to obtain
data on additional volumes and capacities
that simple spirometry cannot give, such as
the residual volume. There are two methods:

a. *Helium dilution method*: The patient is given
a known concentration of helium to breathe
in, and all the expired gas is collected using
a unidirectional breathing mask with a
bag. This is done until an equilibrium concentration of helium is reached that is the
same within the collecting bag and lungs.
This expired gas now has a different helium

concentration from the starting amount
after gas exchange in the lung, and by the
gas law equation, the lung volumes involved
in gas exchange can be calculated. Note that
this technique *only measures those areas
involved in gas exchange*.

b. *Body plethysmography*: The patient is
placed in an airtight chamber, through a
tube connected to the outside, and then
exhales to the functional residual capacity (FRC). After equilibration measurements are made, the patient inhales deeply
causing chest volume expansion. Because
it is a closed system, as the patient's chest
expands, there is a subsequent decrease
in the volume of air inside the chamber
and an increase in chamber air pressure,
which can be measured. Using Boyle's
law ($Pressure_1 \times Volume_1 = Pressure_2
\times Volume_2$), the total lung volume with
inspiration can be calculated. This method
therefore also *measures areas in the lung
not involved with gas exchange* since it
takes into account pressure differences.
It is most appropriate for patients with air

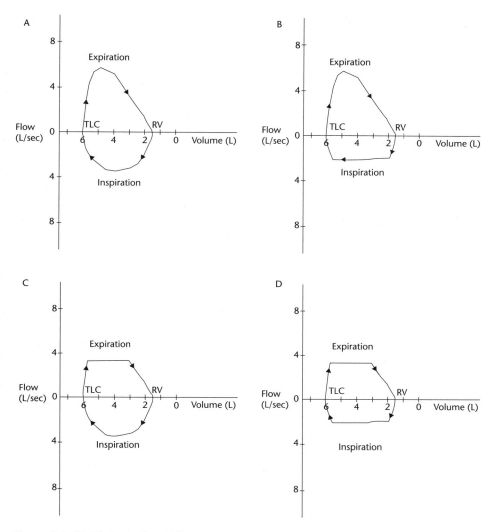

Figure 3-3 (A–D). Basic Flow Volume Loops.
In each figure, the Y axis is flow (negative is flow inward and positive is flow outward) and the X axis is volume, with the rightward end being zero. In normal people, the inspiratory amplitude should be *less* than the expiratory amplitude (A). If the inspiratory amplitude is blunted, consider an extrathoracic obstruction (B), which would mean that something is prohibiting the patient from taking a deep inspiratory breath. If the expiratory amplitude is blunted (C), consider an intrathoracic obstruction prohibiting full exhalation. If both the inspiratory and expiratory amplitudes are blunted, think of an upper airways obstruction preventing both (D). RV, residual volume; TLC, total lung capacity.

spaces that do not communicate with the bronchial tree such as bullae or blebs. It is more commonly used than the helium dilution method, as it is more reliable, although it is limited by marked obesity.

4. *Diffusion capacity of carbon monoxide* (D_LCO): This is a test of the integrity of gas exchange at the alveolar/capillary membrane. It may be ordered to help distinguish between asthma, bronchitis, and emphysema, to determine the severity of emphysema, or to monitor the progression of an interstitial lung disease. Abnormalities in gas exchange should be suspected when the

patient has a history of becoming hypoxic with exercise. The patient inhales a known small amount of carbon monoxide (considered an analogue of oxygen, which has a similar molecular weight but 200 times the affinity to hemoglobin), and it is measured in the blood. The diffusion capacity is proportional to the surface area of gas exchange and the difference in partial pressures of gas across the diffusion barrier. It is inversely proportional to the thickness of the barrier (lung parenchyma). Patients with values less than 40% have a high 3-year mortality. At 40% and below, most, if not all, patients will need home oxygen. Causes of increased and decreased $D_L CO$ are shown in Table 3-4.

A simple algorithm for interpretation of PFTs is as follows:

1. Look at the patient's height and weight to help guide the interpretation. The FRC will be lower in obese patients, and obesity may produce a more restrictive pattern.
2. Look at the VC first to see if it is within normal limits. Then look at the FEV_1. If both of these parameters are within normal limits, there is no obstructive or restrictive defect. If either or both are reduced, then look at the FEV_1/VC ratio.
3. First, look for obstruction: Is the FEV_1/VC ratio lower than the normal limit? If it is, then the severity of the obstructive defect is roughly determined by the absolute value of the FEV_1. An $FEV_1 > 2.0$ L is a mild defect; 1–2 L is a moderate defect; and <1 L is a severe obstructive defect.

4. Second, look for the presence of restriction by using the total lung capacity (TLC) test. If the TLC is decreased, restrictive lung disease is present. Assess the severity of restriction by determining how much the TLC is reduced (80%–90% of the predicted value is borderline restriction, 65–80% is a mild restriction, 50–65% is a moderate restriction, and <50% is a severe restrictive defect). In pure restrictive lung disease the FEV_1/VC ratio should be normal as both FEV_1 and VC are reduced by a similar amount. With a mixed obstructive and restrictive picture, both FEV_1/VC ratio and TLC are reduced. Increased TLC and RV, on the other hand, suggest hyperinflation (as seen in COPD or asthma when other evidence points to an obstructive picture).
5. Look at the RV, which is indicative of air trapping. If it is >120% of the predicted value, then the condition is more consistent with an obstructive picture.
6. Finally, look at the $D_L CO$. If it is <80%, then it is considered abnormal and a gas transfer defect exists; 65–80% is considered a mild defect; 50–65% is a moderate defect; and <50% is a severe diffusion defect. Values greater than 100% will be seen in the cases outlined in Table 3-4.

Common PFT abnormalities are summarized in Table 3-5.

Table 3-4.   Causes of Abnormal Diffusion Capacity of Carbon Monoxide ($D_L CO$)

Decreased $D_L CO$	Increased $D_L CO$
Emphysema, interstitial fibrosis, multiple pulmonary emboli, pulmonary edema, sarcoidosis, pulmonary alveolar proteinosis, anemia, pulmonary hypertension	Pulmonary hemorrhage, left-to-right intracardiac shunts, vascular congestion, polycythemia vera, diffuse lung disease when lung volume is normal

Table 3-5.   Review of Common Pulmonary Function Test Abnormalities

Obstructive Defect	Restrictive Defect	Gas Transfer Defect
Decreased FEV_1/VC ratio. TLC is normal or increased.	Decreased TLC. FEV_1/VC ratio usually normal or increased.	Decreased $D_L CO$.
Severity judged by decrease in absolute FEV_1.	Severity judged by amount of decrease in TLC.	Severity judged by percent decrease in diffusing capacity.

APPROACH TO COMMON PROBLEMS

Approach to Acute Dyspnea

Dyspnea is defined as shortness of breath or as an uncomfortable awareness of breathing. It is important to consider the differential diagnosis in categories of pulmonary disease, heart disease, or central nervous system (CNS) disease, the first two being the most common. First, one must distinguish between acute (minutes to hours) and chronic dyspnea (days to weeks or months).

Acute Dyspnea

Table 3-6 lists the differential diagnoses, clues that may be found in the history or on physical exam, and treatment to help stabilize the patient. More specific information about individual disease processes is found in other sections of this chapter.

Approach to Chronic Cough

This is defined as a cough that persists for more than 6–8 weeks. It is the fifth most common complaint at outpatient centers in the United States. The cough reflex is initiated by stimulation of receptors in the airway or lung interstitium, which then travel through cranial nerves IX and X to the cough center in the medulla. Efferent signals travel to the diaphragm and other respiratory muscles.

All patients should be questioned for the following:

- Duration of the cough.
- Productive sputum and its color.
- Associated fever, chills, weight loss, or other symptoms.
- Recent upper respiratory infection.
- Symptoms of gastroesophageal reflux disease (GERD), postnasal drip, or aspiration.
- Medications (specifically, ACE inhibitors) and drugs of abuse.
- History of asthma or allergies and triggers for these conditions.
- Tobacco use, past or present.
- Other chronic illnesses (heart or lung disease such as congestive heart failure [CHF], COPD).
- Tuberculosis exposure.

Table 3-6. Common Causes of Acute Dyspnea

Condition		Classical Findings in History or Exam	General Treatment
Respiratory	Bronchospasm	Wheezing, history of smoking. Personal or family history of asthma, eczema. Environmental triggers to dyspnea such as an inhalant, pollen, exercise, or pets. Accompanying cough.	Trial of albuterol, atrovent, and/or inhaled or parenteral steroids.
	Pulmonary Embolus	Very acute onset of SOB, possibly with fever, tachycardia, and risk factors for clot formation. An A-a gradient may be present.	Start anticoagulation. Confirm with V/Q scan, chest CT.
	Pneumothorax	Sudden onset of SOB, hyperresonant to percussion and decreased breath sounds on one part of chest. Tension pneumothorax may have tracheal deviation.	Chest tube. Immediate needle decompression if tension pneumothorax is suspected. Give 100% oxygen.
	Acute Respiratory Infection	Fever, productive cough with purulent sputum, malaise, focal crackles, and signs of consolidation on exam and infiltrate on chest X-ray.	Antibiotics if bacterial origin suspected.
	Aspiration	History of being found down at the scene; history of alcoholism; inability to protect airway for any reason. Usually lower lobe infiltrates on chest X-ray, right > left side. Aspiration may be silent in some cases.	Antibiotics as needed. Prevention of recurrence.

continued

Table 3-6.   *(continued)*

Condition		Classical Findings in History or Exam	General Treatment
	Anaphylactic Response	Allergic reaction following administration of drug, IV contrast, or bee/wasp sting. Look for wheezing and rash or swelling as well.	Give subcutaneous epinephrine if serious; otherwise, give antihistamine and steroids.
Cardiovascular	MI	Chest pain lasting 15 to 30 minutes with nausea, vomiting, diaphoresis, and radiation to arm or jaw, as well as ECG changes.	Assess severity. Give aspirin, β blocker, heparin, and consider emergent catheterization.
	CHF	History of cardiomyopathy, crackles in lung fields. SOB is worse when supine. Lower extremity edema, hepatomegaly. Dyspnea mainly with exertion.	Aggressive diuresis.
	Tamponade	Elevated JVP, distant heart sounds, hypotension. History of trauma or chest pain. Echocardiography will confirm the diagnosis.	Emergent pericardiocentesis
CNS Related	Drug Overdose	History of drug abuse; pinpoint pupils may suggest opiate overdose.	Trial of nalaxone (Narcan). Serum or urine toxin screen. Salicylate level for aspirin toxicity.
	Panic Attack	History of anxiety or psychiatric disorder. Absence of other pathology. Sense of impending doom, tachycardia, shaking, choking, trembling, and dizziness.	Usually resolves on its own. Long-term treatment includes behavioral therapy and/or SSRIs.

Table 3-7.   Common Causes of Chronic Cough

Condition	Diagnostic Hints	Treatment
Postnasal Drip	Can be allergic, nonallergic, vasomotor rhinitis, or sinusitis related. Environmental trigger may be present.	Use an antihistamine/decongestant and inhaled nasal steroids. A change should be seen in 1 week. Order a sinus CT scan to demonstrate chronic sinusitis if suspected, which may be treated with an antibiotic and a nasal decongestant.
Asthma	In cough variant asthma this can be the presenting sign. It may occur more often at night or in the early morning. Patient may have a history of atopy (atopic dermatitis or allergies). Diagnose with PFTs the methacholine challenge test or empiric therapy.	Inhaled bronchodilators and possibly inhaled steroids, depending on severity.
GERD	Cough occurs while lying supine or after eating certain foods. May be associated with a sour taste in the mouth or abdominal/chest pain. Can have no associated symptoms except for a cough.	Avoid causative foods. Stop smoking. Elevate the head of the bed. Use and H_2 receptor blocker or a protein pump inhibitor (PPI). Avoid meals 3 hours before sleeping. Avoid late night snacks.
Post URI	Recent viral illness. History of asthma or allergy.	If there is evidence of bronchospasm, an inhaled β agonist may be of use. Nonspecific therapy for chronic nonproductive cough includes antitussives such as dextromethorphan.

Evaluation may include chest X-ray, purified protein derivative (PPD), and sputum culture with Gram stain, depending on the patient.

For all patients, the most common causes of chronic cough are postnasal drip, asthma, GERD, and postviral bronchospasm. One or more of these conditions is most likely to be the cause in nonsmoking patients who are otherwise healthy and not on ACE inhibitors. The presenting features and treatment of chronic cough are described in Table 3-7.

Approach to Acute Respiratory Failure

This is defined as the inability to maintain normal arterial gas tensions. There are two types that have to be distinguished:

1. *Hypoxemic respiratory failure*—hypoxia without CO_2 retention, meaning a PaO_2 <50 mmHg.
2. *Hypercarbic respiratory failure or ventilatory failure*—hypoxia with CO_2 retention, meaning a partial pressure of oxygen in arterial blood (PaO_2) <50 mmHg *and* a partial pressure of CO_2 in arterial blood ($PaCO_2$) >45 mmHg.

Each type is treated separately.

Hypoxemic Respiratory Failure

Alveolar ventilation is maintained but in most cases there is marked ventilation-perfusion (V/Q) mismatch, with altered amounts of perfusion and ventilation in different parts of the lung. Common diseases involved include acute pulmonary edema from heart disease, acute respiratory distress syndrome (ARDS), diffuse viral or bacterial pneumonia, aspiration pneumonitis, and, very rarely, fat embolism after fractures.

Hypercapnic Respiratory Failure

There is both V/Q mismatch *and* inadequate alveolar ventilation.

The main causes of inadequate ventilation are grouped as follows:

1. Intrinsic lung disease (e.g., COPD, cystic fibrosis, asthma).
2. Neuromuscular disorders (polymyositis, myasthenia gravis, Guillain-Barré syndrome).

3. Central nervous system disorders that affect respiratory control (e.g., drug overdose, stroke), leading to hypoventilation.
4. Chest wall disorders or trauma.

Treatment is based on the underlying cause. In all patients with hypoxemia there are generally five causes, as shown in Table 3-8.

DISEASES OF THE PULMONARY SYSTEM

Diseases of Obstruction

Chronic Obstructive Pulmonary Disease (COPD)

D—A progressive condition in which there is irreversible airflow obstruction on forced expiration. It primarily includes two disease entities: (1) emphysema and (2) chronic bronchitis. Many patients have both coexisting conditions. Asthma generally is excluded, as by definition it is mostly a reversible airflow obstruction; however, COPD patients also may have some reversibility or airway hyperreactivity, as seen in asthma.

1. *Emphysema* is a condition defined histologically by enlarged, dilated air spaces because alveolar septa are destroyed. Mild types have only microscopic changes, but advanced disease has larger air spaces known as blebs and bullae.
2. *Chronic bronchitis* is defined clinically by a chronic productive cough occurring for 3 months of the year for at least 2 years without any other defined cause. In most *but not all* cases, it leads to chronic airflow obstruction. Thus, not all cases of chronic bronchitis may be considered COPD. If a component of reversibility is present, the condition is called *asthmatic bronchitis*.

Epi—Chronic obstructive pulmonary disease is the fourth leading cause of death in the United States. Fifty percent of patients die within 10 years after diagnosis. Ninety percent of all COPD is attributed to smoking; however, only one-seventh of smokers develop COPD. The mortality rate has doubled every 5 years

Table 3-8. Features of Different Causes of Hypoxemia

Causes of Hypoxemia	Description	Treatment	Example
V/Q Mismatch	There is variation throughout the lung, so some areas are better ventilated than perfused, and vice versa. On a global scale this results in hypoxemia.	Treat the underlying cause and give supplementary oxygen.	Acute exacerbation of chronic bronchitis.
Shunt	Blood that enters the pulmonary arterial system is not ventilated. This does not increase PCO_2; it just decreases PaO_2.	Supplementary oxygen is most necessary in this case, but improvement in oxygenation is less than expected or not complete. Find and correct the underlying condition.	Intracardiac shunts—defect the presence of an atrial septal defect with right-to-left shunting. Intrapulmonary shunts— pulmonary embolus, ar*teriovenous malformation.*
Hypoventilation	Patient is not taking enough breaths or is breathing at low tidal volume such that minute ventilation is low. By definition, this causes hypercapnia as well as hypoxemia.	Depending on the cause, get the patient to breathe faster by reversal of respiratory depression or through mechanical ventilation. Supplemental oxygen rapidly increases oxygenation in these patients.	Sleep apnea with hypoventilation. Oversedation
Diffusion Impairment	Conditions that decrease D_LCO cause diffusion impairment, which typically causes hypoxemia with exertion.	Supplemental oxygen; transfusion in an anemic patient and diuresis in a patient with heart failure. Treatment of the underlying condition if the patient has restrictive lung disease.	Exacerbation of a restrictive lung disease. Acute pulmonary edema.
Low Inspired PO_2	At high altitude, PaO_2 is lower.	Body naturally will compensate with secondary polycythemia by increasing 2,3 bisphosphoglycerate (BPG). Alternatively, supplemental oxygen can be used.	Travel to high altitude quickly without supplemental oxygen.

for the past two decades, and there has been a 70% increase in incidence over the last 20 years. Most patients are over age 50 and have smoked for decades.

RF—Risk factors include cigarette smoking, male gender, a history of multiple childhood upper respiratory illnesses, low socioeconomic status, a family history of the disease, and α1-antitrypsin deficiency (there should be a high degree of suspicion in examining younger individuals).

P—Disease generally begins in the small airways and progresses. Tobacco and other environmental pollutants cause inflammation in the peripheral airways; cells infiltrate and release cytokines and proteolytic enzymes. In bronchitis there is mucous plugging with impacted secretions, peribronchiolar fibrosis, and narrowing with obliteration of airways. In emphysema, lung elastin is destroyed by proteolytic forces, as cigarette smoke also inactivates antiprotease enzymes. Garden-variety emphysema produces destruction in a centrolobular pattern since it follows the path of ventilation, and destruction occurs in upper lung zones first and lower lung zones later. In α1-antitrypsin deficiency, destruction occurs in a panacinar pattern because it follows the distribution of blood flow and therefore involves the lower lung zones more than the apex. In either case, alveolar destruction leads to V/Q mismatch, inflammation, fibrosis, and hyperinflation of the lung. With prolonged hypoxemia, pulmonary hypertension develops, which can ultimately lead to right heart failure, a condition called *cor pulmonale*. Patients with COPD also have an accelerated decline in pulmonary function. The normal decline in FEV_1 is 30 mL/yr, but smokers have accelerated decline of 80 mL/yr, which can be slowed with smoking cessation.

SiSx—Symptoms vary widely, depending on when patients come to medical attention. Bronchitic patients may present with only a chronic smoker's cough. Others patients may present with acute respiratory failure requiring intubation and ventilator support during a severe exacerbation.

There are two extreme presentations, which are shown in Table 3-9. Most patients fall somewhere in between these categories.

Dx—The diagnosis is made by the exam, the history, and a few diagnostic tests. On exam one may find decreased breath sounds, prolonged expiration to more than three times the duration of inspiration in severe cases, an increased anteroposterior (AP) diameter with elevation of clavicles, and increased resonance on percussion. Patients should not have clubbing unless there is some other pathology (i.e., shunt or malignancy).

Chest X-ray has poor sensitivity/specificity for screening. It may show hyperinflation with flat diaphragms, enlarged anterior and retrocardiac spaces, a paucity of vessels, a long, narrow cardiac silhouette, and perhaps markings only in the lower lung zones.

Pulmonary function tests are diagnostic, showing a decreased FEV_1/FVC ratio, with the stage or severity of functional impairment determined from the FEV_1 (the most important mortality predictor). When FEV_1 falls to 50% of the predicted value,

Table 3-9. Differences in the Two Major Forms of COPD

Emphysematous COPD (called *pink puffers*)	Bronchitic COPD (called *blue bloaters*)
Presents at older ages.	Presents at younger ages.
Progressive dyspnea, weight loss, and little or no cough.	Weight gain, prominent cough, wheezing, and ronchi.
Asthenic person with well-developed neck and abdominal muscles. Dyspneic, with pursed lip breathing or grunting expressions. Speech punctuated by frequent inspirations, called *telegraphic speech*. May lean forward to breathe in the "tripod position" on elbows to stabilize the shoulder girdle and allow the accessory muscles to help maximally.	Obese individual with less dyspnea. May seem sluggish or drowsy and complain of headaches in the morning because of hypercapnia.
1. Mild hypoxemia because V/Q mismatch is proportional and patient breathes faster to compensate as well.	1. More marked hypoxia because of severe V/Q mismatch.
2. *Hypocapnic* because of tachypnea (hypercarbia is more common in later stages and is a poor prognostic sign).	2. *Hypercarbia* causing reduced central respiratory drive and further arterial desaturation. Peripheral cyanosis and polycythemia can result. Patient is more likely to have chronic respiratory failure. Edema can be present if right heart failure occurs.
3. Decreased D_LCO.	3. Usually normal or increased D_LCO.
Little/no improvement with bronchodilators.	Some improvement with bronchodilators.

the patient may have exertional breathlessness, and chest infection and acute bronchitis are more common. When FEV_1 is 30% of the predicted value, SOB may start to interfere with normal activities of daily living (ADLs). The absolute value of FVC is reduced because of the increased air trapped in the lung and the increased RV. In addition, D_LCO, is decreased in emphysema but not in chronic bronchitis/asthma, and when D_LCO is less than 50%, many patients will desaturate with exercise.

Tx—It is necessary to assess the severity of disease and exclude other causes of breathlessness. Treatment should include smoking cessation (perhaps the most important treatment and prevention), regular exercise, and prophylactic influenza and pneumococcus vaccines. Bronchodilators, specifically anticholinergics like ipratropium are useful in stable COPD along with β agonists. This combination is synergistic. Systemic steroids are used in acute exacerbations along with more frequent use of bronchodilators. Inhaled steroids can improve symptoms and decrease clinic visits. Acute chest infections during exacerbations must be treated aggressively. Antibiotics can be given when there is increased sputum or a change in the quality of sputum. In general, mucolytics and chest physical therapy have no role in COPD. Continuous low-flow oxygen is the treatment of choice in hypoxemic patients and has been shown to decreased mortality. Ultimately, those refractory to therapy and in acute respiratory failure may need to be intubated. Lung transplantation should be considered in suitable candidates with severe disease, as should lung volume reduction surgery (especially in those with hyperexpanded lungs that have large areas that are not effective in gas exchange).

Asthma

D—A chronic obstructive disease of the small and medium-sized airways characterized by:

1. Obstruction to airflow from *reversible* narrowing of airways, either from smooth muscle contraction, hypersecretion of mucus, or airway edema.

2. Bronchial hyperactivity and constriction from a variety of stimuli, including allergens, chemicals, exercise, cold air, and cigarette smoke that otherwise would not cause the same response in normal individuals.

3. Inflammation of small and medium-sized airways.

Several variants exist with different sets of triggers. Patients can have more than one distinct type:

Allergic asthma: This is an immune-mediated response via type I hypersensitivity, which is precipitated by exposure to allergens such as seasonal pollens, ragweed, or pets. It accounts for 10% of all asthma and usually begins during childhood. Allergic asthma is associated with rhinitis, eczema, urticaria, and a positive family history.

Intrinsic nonallergic asthma: This is the most common type of asthma. It occurs in reaction to specific stimuli but is non-immune-mediated and not due to an allergic cause. The cause is not entirely clear; theories include a combination of nonspecific bronchial muscle hyperreactivity from abnormalities such as an overactive parasympathetic or deficient sympathetic nervous system allowing overreaction to inhalation of irritants. There is persistent airway hyperreactivity, and symptoms begin usually in adulthood. It is commonly seen after a viral respiratory infection.

Occupational asthma: This occurs in occupational settings without an immunologic basis. Bronchospasm occurs in reaction to metal fumes, smoke, wood, grain, dusts, or industrial chemicals.

Exercise-induced asthma: Asthma is precipitated with exercise. It usually resolves within 30 minutes after stopping the activity and is thought to be related to heat and water loss from the airway, changes in the osmolarity of secretions, and induction of release of inflammatory mediators. Running in cold weather is even more likely to cause this condition. Usually the asthma is worse right after exercise and then improves.

Aspirin sensitivity asthma: Nonsteroidal anti-inflammatory drugs can precipitate asthma in 5% of asthmatics. This form is associated with nasal polyps (Samter's triad of aspirin sensitivity, asthma, and nasal polyps). It is more common in women than in men. It is thought to be due to excessive production of leukotrienes from inhibition of the COX enzyme pathway. Asthma begins 2 hours after aspirin ingestion and may result in respiratory failure. It usually improves after desensitization.

Epi—Asthma affects 5% of the population. Its incidence has been increasing since the 1980s. There are 4000 deaths per year despite advances in treatment options.

SiSx—Symptoms can change during the course of an attack, depending on how long it lasts. Between attacks, the person can have completely normal pulmonary function and be asymptomatic; therefore, it is a good idea to ask about the variance of breathing patterns. Classically, one sees episodic bouts of coughing with dyspnea, expiratory wheezing and chest tightness, and breathing with a prolonged expiratory phase. Tachypneic patients with prolonged expiratory phases are unable to exhale all the air before the next breath and breath stacking can occur, impairing ventilation.

Severe attacks are accompanied by tachypnea, extensive accessory muscle use, and inability to talk in full sentences.

Later, cyanosis, hypotension, and bradycardia, along with a marked pulsus paradoxus, occurs in addition to mental status changes. The severity of the attack can also be judged by the patient's ability to use the peak flow meter (<150 L/min generally indicates a severe attack). During a prolonged attack, if muscle fatigue occurs with tachypnea, respiratory failure is possible.

Dx—The clinical history and family history are important in making the diagnosis. A response to empiric treatment with bronchodilators and anti-inflammatories suggests reversible airway obstruction. However, to make the diagnosis, spirometry is the gold standard. It shows an obstructive ventilatory defect when the patient is symptomatic that corrects with bronchodilator use.

Asymptomatic patients may undergo provocation tests with bronchoconstrictors, such as in the methacholine challenge test. A decrease in FEV_1 of >25% is indicative of the condition. This test, however, is better used to rule out asthma (sensitivity) than to rule it in (specificity) since people without asthma can have a positive test. In the asthmatic patient's sputum, classic findings are active inflammatory cells, Creola bodies (desquamated aggregates of epithelial cells), Curschmann's spirals (mucous casts of the small airways), and Charcot Leyden crystals (lysophospholipase from the eosinophil granules).

Tx—For the acute asthma attack:

1. First, give oxygen and bronchodilators (β agonists such as albuterol and anticholinergics such as ipratropium). In those who do not show an immediate response or whose symptoms are not well controlled after 48 hours, systemic steroids are indicated. They have a peak effect after 6 hours. They decrease inflammation and the chance of an acute exacerbation. Patients should continue to receive these drugs for at least the next several days, although the exact dosage and time of use or taper are controversial. Inhaled steroids have no role in acute exacerbations. They take 3–5 days to start working, so they are started before discharge and overlapped with oral steroids. They help prevent further attacks. Second-line agents for acute attacks include magnesium sulfate and theophylline; the latter drug is usually discouraged in this circumstance for lack of good data. Subcutaneous terbutaline or epinephrine is most useful in children with status asthmaticus from allergic asthma that is refractory to other treatment. It is less commonly used in adults.

2. The decision for changes in treatment depends on how stable the patient is. Arterial blood gases (ABGs) should be obtained in all but the mildest attacks. In mild asthma, one sees a respiratory alkalosis with decreased partial pressure of oxygen (PO_2) (hypoxemia is due to V/Q mismatch and responds readily to oxygen). A normal ABG with a normal pH and PCO_2

in someone who is having an attack and is clearly tachypneic is a poor sign, as the patient should be hypocapnic if he or she is breathing heavily. As the PCO_2 increases above normal and the pH falls because respiratory acidosis occurs, this suggests that the patient is tiring and it is time to consider intubation.

3. For outpatient management, commonly used agents include:
   a. Short-acting β agonists and longer-acting agents such as salmeterol.
   b. Inhaled steroids to prevent inflammation and fibrosis.
   c. Mast cell inhibitors (cromolyn), which are only preventive.
   d. Antileukotriene drugs such as monteleukast and zafirlukast (leukotriene receptor inhibitors), and zileuton (a 5-lipoxygenase inhibitor that produces leukotrienes). They also are only preventive for bronchospasm and work in up to 70% of patients.
   e. Anti-IgE therapy such as subcutaneuous omalizumab (Xolair) can be used in select patients with moderate to severe allergic asthma with elevated IgE levels and a positive allergen skin test. Response rates are 30%–50%.

The decision about how to treat depends on the severity of the asthma. Table 3-10 shows some different treatment options based on the severity of the condition.

Bronchiectasis

D—An irreversible and abnormal dilation of the bronchi, either focal or diffuse, with thickening of the bronchial walls.

P—Infectious and noninfectious conditions destroy the bronchial walls, and normal elements are replaced by fibrous tissue. This occurs at the level of medium-sized airways (segmental and subsegmental bronchi). Dilated airways tend to accrue material that cannot be cleared well, and the walls become thickened with peribronchial inflammation. Causative agents are mostly infectious, such as repeated bacterial pneumonias or viral infections, TB, and *Mycobacterium avium-intracellulare* (MAI) or allergic bronchopulmonary aspergillosis (ABPA). Noninfectious causes include cystic fibrosis, collagen-vascular diseases, toxic inhalant exposure, chronic aspiration, and, rarely, inflammatory conditions [e.g., ulcerative colitis (UC) or rheumatoid arthritis (RA)]. Three different types of bronchiectasis can occur—cylindrical, varicose, and cystic—which describe the appearance of dilated bronchi.

Epi—The most common cause is recurrent bacterial pneumonias.

RF—Risk factors include immunodeficiency, cystic fibrosis (CF), congenital cysts, bronchial stenosis, α1-antitrypsin deficiency, disorders of mucociliary clearance such as Kartagener's syndrome, yellow nail syndrome (hypoplasia

Table 3-10. Treatment of Asthma Based on Severity

Asthma Severity	Symptoms	Medications
Mild Intermittent	Less than 2x/week Brief flares (rare) Activity not limited	None or prn β agonist
Mild Persistent	More than 2x/week Flares on a weekly basis Mildly limited activity	1. β agonist prn *and* scheduled low-dose inhaled steroid *or* 2. Mast cell inhibitor or 3. Leukotriene modifier
Moderate Persistent	Daily symptoms Flares more than 2x/week Moderately limited activity	1. Intermediate-dose scheduled inhaled steroid 2. Long-acting inhaled β2 agonist *or* other controller
Severe Persistent	Symptoms constant Flares frequent, prolonged Activity severely limited Frequent symptoms at night	High-dose inhaled steroids and long-acting inhaled β2 agonist and other controllers

of lymphatics), or frequent pulmonary infections for any reason.

SiSx—Symptoms include persistent chronic cough of purulent sputum, recurrent chest colds, and hemoptysis in as many as 50%–70% of patients, as the airway erodes into a blood vessel. This is usually manifested as blood-tinged sputum, not frank large-volume hemoptysis. If, however, a bronchial artery is eroded into, there can be significant bleeding. Pleuritic pain also may be described. In more advanced cases, hypoxic patients exhibit cyanosis, clubbing, and cor pulmonale. The exam can show any combination of rhonchi, rales and wheezing.

Dx—Pulmonary function tests are normal in mild cases, but usually obstruction is present in many severe cases. The chest X-ray may show evidence of peribronchial fibrosis and possible segmental lung collapse, while patients with cystic bronchiectasis have large air spaces indistinguishable from bullae. The chest X-ray shows ring shadows, which are the dilated, thick-walled airways, next to vessels. Longitudinally on a CT scan, they appear as "train tracks" and dilated airways will extend to the periphery of the lung fields, where they normally are not seen. High-resolution CT can suggest a cause: proximal bronchiectasis is more common in ABPA, and multiple nodules suggest MAI.

Tx—Treatment includes antibiotics, especially inhaled tobramycin if there is increased sputum production on a regular basis, as patients are colonized with *Pseudomonas* and other organisms. Surgical resection is generally not helpful but is a last resort. Bronchodilation and oxygen therapy can be helpful, especially if the patient is hypoxic. Chest physical therapy is helpful to clear secretions, as are flutter valves. Mucolytic agents like deoxyribonucleases (DNAses) have not been proven to have significant benefit in non-CF patients; however, they are still commonly used. For large-volume hemoptysis, bronchial artery embolization may be necessary. Bronchial arteries can become tortuous and hypertrophied, form collaterals in patients with long-standing bronchiectasis, and may appear in unexpected locations. Hence, initial bronchography is important for treatment.

Cystic Fibrosis (CF)

D—An autosomal recessive disorder due to a mutation in the CFTR gene characterized by widespread exocrine gland dysfunction involving mainly the lungs, GI tract, and pancreas.

Epi—It is one of the most common severe genetic diseases in the United States. Five percent of Caucasians are carriers. The disease affects males and females equally. Approximately 30,000 individuals with CF are living in the United States. Ninety-nine percent of deaths are from respiratory failure, with the rest from portal hypertension secondary to biliary cirrhosis. This is the most common cause of obstructive airway disease among people under age 30. Ten percent of patients are actually diagnosed in adolescence. Nearly 50% of patients survive to age 25. Of note, these patients are less likely to get certain GI infections such as *Clostridium difficile*.

P—Multiple mutations exist in CFTR on chromosome 7 (Δ508 is the most common), but most lead to chloride impermeability and increased resorption of Na^+, causing viscous mucus that leads to obstruction of organs served by exocrine glands.

SiSx—Pulmonary symptoms begin with plugged bronchi, causing airway obstruction and recurrent pulmonary infections, most commonly with *Pseudomonas, Staphylococcus aureus, and Haemophilus influenzae*. Proressive parenchymal destruction ensues, affecting primarily the upper lobes first. Bronchiectasis results, with hemoptysis from a bronchial artery after erosion into an airway. Over the longer term, one sees cyanosis and cor pulmonale. Digital clubbing and nasal polyps are also prominent. As for GI-related symptoms, 15% of infants present with meconium ileus. Patients can have greasy stools and flatulence, malabsorption from pancreatic exocrine insufficiency along with fat-soluble vitamin (A, D, E, and K) deficiencies, fatty infiltration of the liver, and focal biliary cirrhosis. Many have abnormal glucose tolerance. Fifty percent of infant patients present with failure to thrive. Ninety-five percent of affected males are infertile, but affected females generally are not.

Dx—The sweat chloride test is abnormal in almost all cases of CF. Pilocarpine is applied to the arm, and the amount of sweat produced is measured. Na^+ and Cl^- are elevated drastically in the sweat of CF patients. A test is considered abnormal if >60 mEq/L is seen in a patient under 20 years old and >80 mEq/L in an adult. Genetic testing can also be done and can be used to help screen future pregnancies or other family members. Ultimately, the diagnosis of CF can be made with a positive sweat test and either a positive family history, and the presence of obstructive pulmonary disease, or pancreatic insufficiency. Pulmonary function tests may show an obstructive pattern, with D_LCO usually within normal limits. The chest X-ray shows hyperinflation, bronchiectasis, and reticulonodular fibrosis, depending on the time course.

Tx—Complete eradication of colonizing organisms is impossible. Deoxyribonuclease (pulmozyme), which hydrolyzes intracellular DNA and makes sputum less viscous, has been shown to decrease the chance of infection and improve respiratory function. Chest physical therapy, bronchodilators, and anti-inflammatory agents are also helpful. Antipseudomonal antibiotics such as β-lactams and aminoglycosides should be used for acute infections and inhaled antibiotics for chronic maintenance if patients are still culture positive and have productive sputum. Replacement of pancreatic enzymes can be done with oral pills, and supplement fat-soluble vitamins. It is virtually impossible to prevent disease progression in most patients, however, and lung transplant will eventually be necessary. Survival after transplantation is similar to survival for those receiving lungs for other indications (80% survival at 1 year). Hemoptysis from bronchial artery communication with airways must be treated with embolization if it fails to stop on its own. Note that there are numerous collaterals from other vessels besides the bronchial arteries that can cause bleeding.

α1-Antitrypsin Deficiency

D—An autosomal recessive disease affecting mainly the lung, the liver, and sometimes the skin through a deficiency in a secretory glycoprotein made by hepatocytes whose normal function is to inhibit proteolytic autodestruction.

P—The AAT protein is an inhibitor of the proteolytic enzyme elastase. The most common family of alleles for the corresponding gene is as follows: normals are MM, heterozygotes are MZ, and homozygotes are ZZ; then there is a mutation in which there is no detectable protein (null mutation). Emphysema in the lungs is thought to be due to excess neutrophil elastase, which destroys elastin the lung. In the liver, disease occurs through a different mechanism. Here there is polymerization of the variant AAT protein that accumulates in hepatocytes, causing damage and loss of normal function. Biopsy therefore shows strongly periodic acid–Schiff (PAS)–positive staining of material resistant to digestion by enzymes. Liver disease therefore is *not* observed in null mutation patients. For the lung, there is a minimum plasma threshold below which there is insufficient AAT for protection (approximately 80 mg/dL); this usually occurs in the ZZ phenotype.

Epi—The disorder affects is 1/3000 people with a prevalence in the United States of 80,000–100,000. Up to 10% of homozygotes do not develop the lung disease. The disease is thought to be commonly underrecognized.

RF—The family history is important. Men are at greater risk for lung disease. Smoking causes emphysema to develop earlier.

SiSx

Lung—similar to emphysematous COPD but earlier onset (<50 years of age) presenting with dyspnea, cough, phlegm, and wheezing. Breath sounds may be decreased markedly in the lower lung fields, as opposed to the upper lung fields, as in garden-variety emphysema. Many patients have chronic upper respiratory infections.

In nonsmokers, lung function decreases on average after age 50. Severe deficiency is associated with bronchiectasis.

Liver—evidence of cirrhosis may be seen, as well as liver synthetic dysfunction (see Chapter 5) in certain patients. Progression to hepatocellular carcinoma can also occur.

Skin—panniculitis may be seen where there are inflammatory lesions. This is very rare.

Dx—The association of lung and liver pathology in a young patient should suggest this disease. On a chest X-ray or CT scan, the difference from classical emphysema may be seen in that bullous changes appear at the bases first rather than at the apices. Pulmonary function tests may show evidence of obstruction and liver biopsy findings in certain patients are consistent with the description above. Ultimately, the genetic test for the allele can be done for diagnosis in suspected patients.

Tx—In the first two decades of life, liver disease, not lung disease, is the most common cause of morbidity. The goal of treatment is to raise AAT levels above the protective threshold in those patients who are not completely deficient. Intravenous infusion of pooled human AAT can augment levels and is safe and well tolerated, though randomized controlled trials (RCTs) have not been done. Aerosolized forms have also been administered, but there are no current clinical studies favoring their use. To increase endogenous amounts of AAT in those who do not have null mutations, danazol, tamoxifen, and estrogen/progesterone combinations have been used. The success of gene therapy is at present unclear. Symptomatic treatment, as in emphysema, is otherwise useful, with supplemental oxygen if necessary. Treatment of hepatic complications such as ascites and encephalopathy is the same as that from other causes (see Chapter 5). Ultimately, lung and liver transplantation can be attempted. It is not yet clear whether lung transplant patients need AAT augmentation therapy thereafter since recurrent emphysema would take a while to occur, longer than expected after transplant survival in most cases. Therefore, it should be done only if radiographic changes develop in the new lung.

Bronchiolitis Obliterans (BO)

D—Considered to be an obstructive disease and most commonly seen as a manifestation of posttransplant chronic rejection. It can also present after a poorly resolving pneumonitis.

RF—It is seen in collagen vascular disease (especially RA) and after bone marrow transplantation. If it is seen following lung transplantation, it is considered to be part of chronic rejection.

P—The pathophysiology is unclear; viral infection may be implicated.

SiSx—Patients may present with subacute exertional dyspnea; an obstructive pattern is seen in PFTs. The exam is usually normal.

Dx—In early stages, BO is hard to distinguish from other diseases. A chest X-ray and exam are used to rule out other causes. Sputum cultures are sterile. More advanced disease features abnormal chest expansion with end inspiratory squeaks, and the chest X-ray or CT scan will show bronchiectasis and hyperinflation or air trapping. Persistent patchy bilateral ground glass opacities in the lower lung fields with hyperinflation are typically also seen.

Tx—The disease is generally progressive and steroid nonresponsive. There is no good treatment per se. In cases of rejection, retransplant may be necessary. Macrolides such as azithromycin may decrease inflammation.

Allergic Bronchopulmonary Aspergillosis

D—A hypersensitivity reaction in which asthmatic symptoms occur after bronchi are colonized by *Aspergillus* or a similar fungus.

Epi—More than 95% of patients have extrinsic asthma. The disease occurs in 2%–10% of patients with CF.

RF—Atopic individuals with asthma are at risk. The disease is more common in adults than in children.

P—*Aspergillus* colonization of susceptible individuals occurs through inhalation exposure and leads to a strong IgE and IgG immune-mediated response. Other fungi have also been reported, but this is the most common. Despite this, the fungus continues to colonize the airway and leads to recurrent symptoms. Further damage to the airways from proteolytic fungal enzymes can result in bronchiectasis. There are two main features: marked eosinophilic infiltration of the lungs in patients with features of eosinophilic pneumonia and mucous plugging of the airway with heavy infiltration by hyphae.

SiSx—The disease usually presents as asthma exacerbation that is refractory to treatment in a patient who was previously under good control. Classically, brownish mucous plugs are expectorated. Peripheral blood eosinophilia, fever, and malaise may also be seen. Only about 10% of patients have systemic symptoms such as fever, malaise, and night sweats.

Dx—Diagnosis requires a high degree of clinical suspicion. The chest X-ray can show either infiltrates or bronchiectasis, usually in the proximal upper lobes, atelectasis, or classical signs such as "train lines" (shadows from thick but nondilated bronchi). High-resolution CT may show diffuse cylindrical bronchiectasis. Pulmonary function tests will show obstruction with air trapping, but only one-half of patients may have a positive response to bronchodilatory therapy. The minimum diagnostic criteria are (1) a history of asthma, (2) elevated total serum IgE, (3) central bronchiectasis, and (4) immediate skin-type sensitive to *Aspergillus fumigatus*. Other noteworthy laboratory test findings are elevated specific serum IgE and IgG against *A. fumigatus* and a positive sputum culture. A negative skin prick and negative intradermal reactivity to *Aspergillus* antigen virtually exclude the diagnosis.

Tx—Steroids that are tapered over 3 to 6 months are usually effective in controlling symptoms and limiting progressive injury. Inhaled steroids do not appear to have benefit in acute episodes. Serial measurements of IgE can be done, which correlate with disease activity. Antifungal agents generally are not recommended. The prognosis depends on the stage of lung disease.

Sleep Apnea

D—Intermittent cessation of breathing during sleep. It can be central or obstructive. Central apnea is complete cessation of airflow and respiratory effort for at least 10 seconds ("won't breathe"). Obstructive apnea is cessation of airflow despite continued respiratory effort by the CNS ("can't breathe"). In mixed apnea, there is a combination of the two.

P—During sleep, normal cortical activity is removed and the brain stem assumes a greater role in breathing. The two main abnormal breathing patterns that can be seen during sleep are (1) apnea and hypopneas—lack of breathing—and (2) Cheyne-Stokes respirations—alternating hyperventilation and hypoventilation, which is seen mostly in cases of central apnea. The periodicity of the apneas is proportional to the severity of the underlying disease.

RF—Risk factors include obesity, postmenopausal status, and increased age.

SiSx—Patients complain of daytime sleepiness caused by the recurrent nighttime arousals. They can have loud snoring with punctuated apneas, which may awaken them for 5–10 seconds, or feel a choking or gasping sensation at this time. They may complain of waking up on the floor or the spouse will complain of flailing movements of his or her partner. Patients may also complain of lower extremity edema upon waking or of nocturia unrelated to right heart failure. When apnea is infrequent, sleepiness occurs only during sedentary activities. When it is more severe, patients can fall asleep even while talking or driving. Patients can also present with arrhythmias during periods of desaturation such as bradycardias or atrial fibrillation. These conditions imply chronic sleep apnea. Pulmonary hypertension may be seen in patients with or without daytime hypoxemia (usually milder when it occurs without hypoxemia). The exam is generally normal.

Dx—If the history is suspicious, one makes the diagnosis by a sleep study in which polygraphic recordings are made. The study measures the electroencephalogram (EEG) to stage sleep, an ECG, oximetry, and respiratory effort. A positive test demonstrates multiple apneic episodes

Tx—The goals is to reverse the airway obstruction in patients without CNS dysfunction.

Many patients need to lose weight and avoid sedatives, although these two things alone are not always helpful. More severe apnea may require continuous positive airway pressure (CPAP) at night applied to the upper airway to prevent collapse and eliminate apneas. If this is unsuccessful, surgical reconstruction of the upper airway may be necessary and the patient may need a tracheostomy. In Cheyne-Stokes-type breathing from CNS-related conditions or heart failure, supplemental oxygen can be helpful, but treatment of the underlying chronic condition is required.

Diseases of Restriction

Interstitial Lung Diseases

These conditions are characterized by disease of the lung interstitium, as opposed to alveolar diseases, which involve the air spaces. Characteristically, they share features of a restrictive pattern on spirometry and a gas transfer defect may be present, depending on the severity of disease. Because of the overwhelming number of interstitial lung diseases, there is sometimes confusion in classification, especially among the idiopathic causes. Table 3-11 outlines broad categories to help organize them. The idiopathic interstitial pneumonias are by far the most common; of the diseases in this category, idiopathic pulmonary fibrosis (IPF) occurs most often.

Idiopathic Interstitial Pneumonia

D—Condition of diffuse infiltration of the lung parenchyma, alveolar walls, and air spaces of unknown causes. There are four types, which are classified based on histologic and clinical findings, of which usual interstitial pneumonia (UIP) is by far the most common. Table 3-12 shows how to distinguish the different types.

Environmental Lung Diseases (Pneumoconioses)

These are a group of interstitial lung conditions related to inhalation of environmental agents and result from the body's response over time. Patients are often asymptomatic for many years before developing clinical disease. Several well-described conditions are compared in Table 3-13.

Hypersensitivity Pneumonitis (Extrinsic Allergic Alveolitis)

D—A condition in which repeated inhalation of various organic agents leads to an immune-mediated inflammation of the terminal airways, alveoli, and lung parenchyma. Different names are given based on the inhalant. Examples include:

Farmer's lung—mold hay's thermophilic *Actinomyces*, *Micropolyspora*, or *Aspergillus* species.

Bird breeder's disease—protein in avian droppings.

Chemical worker's lung—simple chemicals such as isocyanates.

Plastic worker's lung—paint-hardened plastic curing agents.

RF—Employment in a field such as those above is a risk factor.

Epi—Farmer's lung is the most common of these conditions in the United States.

P—Lymphocytes and monocytes react to inhaled chemicals or organic dusts. There is also an immune complex reaction leading to parenchymal and airways disease.

SiSx—All symptoms present similarly to those of interstitial pneumonitis but vary with the intensity of the exposure and therefore can be acute or chronic in nature. The acute form of this disease is characterized by cough, fever, chills, and malaise soon after exposure and should resolve as long as no further exposure is present. The subacute form appears over weeks, includes cough and dyspnea, and can progress. It may also persist with continued antigen exposure and can be transformed into the chronic type, which can be hard to distinguish from IPF. Exam may show fine crackles and exertional dyspnea necessitating oxygen. Clubbing and pulmonary hypertension, and even respiratory failure, can also be seen.

Dx—A high degree of clinical suspicion is needed. Examining for serum precipitants against suspected antigens should be done as

Table 3-11. Categorization of Interstitial Lung Disease

Collagen Vascular Disease-Related Causes	Drug-Related Causes	Idiopathic Interstitial Pneumonias	Environmental or Occupational Related Causes	Rare Known Causes
Rheumatoid Arthritis SLE Sjögren's Scleroderma Polymyositis Dermatomyositis MCTD Churg-Strauss syndrome Goodpasture's syndrome Wegener's granulomatosis	Amiodarone Methotrexate Bleomycin Phenytoin Heroin Nitrofurantoin Radiation	Idiopathic pulmonary fibrosis (IPF) UIP is seen on histology Non-IPF interstitial pneumonias Classified by histology into several types • DIP • AIP • NSIP • RBILD • COP	Asbestosis Silicosis Coal workers' pneumonitis Hypersensitivity pneumonitis Beryliosis	Lymphangioleiomyomatosis (LAM) Pulmonary Langerhans' cell histiocytosis Eosinophilic pneumonia Bronchiolitis obliterans organizing pneumonia (BOOP) Amyloidosis Pulmonary alveolar proteinosis

SLE, systemic lupus erythematosus; MCTD, mixed connective tissue disease; DIP, desquamative interstitial pneumonia; AIP, acute interstitial pneumonia; NSIP, nonspecific interstitial pneumonia; RBILD, respiratory bronchiolitis-associated interstitial lung disease; COP, cryptogenic organizing pneumonia.

Table 3-12. Distinguishing Characteristics of the Major Forms of Idiopathic Interstitial Pneumonia

Condition	Idiopathic Pulmonary Fibrosis (IPF)	Other Idiopathic Interstitial Pneumonias (Categorized by Histologic Class)				
		Desquamative Interstitial Pneumonia (DIP)	Acute Interstitial Pneumonia (AIP)	Nonspecific Interstitial Pneumonia (NSIP)	Respiratory Bronchiolitis-Associated Interstitial Lung Disease (RBILD)	Cryptogenic Organizing Pneumonia (COP)
Histologic Classification	Usual Interstitial Pneumonia (UIP) Usually required for a diagnosis of IPF.	A misnomer for what were earlier thought to be desquamated pneumocytes.	Also called Hamman-Rich syndrome	A catchall term for all other mixed categories.	Considered to be a smoker's bronchiolitis.	The idiopathic form of bronchiolitis obliterans organizing pneumonia.
Epi	Male > female by 2:1. More common in middle aged patients 50 to 60 years old.	Male > female by 2:1. Mean age is 10 years less than UIP (40s to 50s).	Male = female. Mean age of onset is about 50 years.	Female > male slightly. Mean age of onset is about 50 years.	Female > male slightly. Mean age of onset is 30–40s.	Male = female. Mean age of onset is 50–60s.

	The most common interstitial lung disease.	Found almost exclusively in smokers.	85% are smokers.	Associated with occult collagen vascular disease in 10%–20% of cases, most commonly dermatomyositis and polymyositis.	Almost all patients are current or prior heavy smokers.	No association with tobacco use.
SiSx	Subacute progressive exertional dyspnea, nonproductive cough. Exam may show fine basilar crackles. Onset is generally insidious.	Similar to IPF.	Explosive onset of symptoms and more rapid progression to respiratory failure, almost mimicking ARDS in time course.	Similar to IPF, though associated symptoms of collagen vascular disease may be seen. Associated fever may be seen in up to one-third of patients.	Subacute cough, dyspnea. Acute respiratory failure is rare. Coarse rales found on exam.	Most are symptomatic for <2 months prior to diagnosis. Very similar to community-acquired pneumonia with flu-like illness, but also with persistent nonproductive cough, dyspnea, and weight loss.
Dx	HRCT may show the classic pattern of peripheral (subpleural) and bibasilar reticulonodular opacities and honeycomb change, which can sometimes make the diagnosis with clinical information.	CT will show a so-called geographic distribution of ground glass infiltrates. There are no reticulonodular opacities, as in IPF. All lesions look the same temporally.	Chest X-rays are normal in as many as one-fifth of patients but otherwise may show bilateral infiltrates, as in ARDS. The acute nature of this idiopathic entity helps distinguish it from the other conditions.	CT shows no honeycombing; ground glass infiltrates are more common.	Chest X-ray shows diffuse reticulonodular interstitial infiltrates. Lung volumes are normal. CT may show fine nodules and air trapping as well as ground glass infiltrates.	CT shows peripheral patchy distribution of opacities in the lower lung zones and disease is usually bilateral. Fifty percent have recurrent or migratory opacities. Honeycombing is rare at initial presentation. Effusions, pleural thickening, and cavitation can be seen.
	Lung biopsy classically shows patchy, nonuniform, alternating zones of fibroblast proliferation, with a leading edge of collagen deposition, and honeycomb cysts with mucoid material.	Lung biopsy shows an increased number of macrophages. There are no honeycomb lesions, but there are thickened alveolar septa lined by cuboidal pneumocytes. Most characteristic is	Lung biopsy shows distinct very thick alveolar wall from significant fibroblast proliferation and hyperplastic type II pneumocytes. It resembles the diffuse alveolar damage seen in ARDS. There are few inflammatory cells.	Lung biopsy shows only foci of isolated disease that have mixed characteristics and may resemble UIP or DIP.	Laboratory tests are not helpful. Pulmonary function tests (PFTs) may show mixed obstruction-restriction.	Biopsy shows proliferation of granulations tissue within small airways and chronic inflammatory changes surrounding the alveoli.

continued

Table 3-12. (continued)

Condition	Idiopathic Pulmonary Fibrosis (IPF)	Other Idiopathic Interstitial Pneumonias (Categorized by Histologic Class)				
	The key is that there is great *temporal variance* in the lesions seen: some are new, and others are old and fibrotic. This is thought to be due to gradual multiple microscopic insults over time.	the presence of numerous pigmented macrophages in the distal air spaces, which are not desquamated pneumocytes, as originally thought. All lesions are uniform in time and are about the same age.	Changes are temporarily uniform.	Positive ANA and other serologic titers may be found if there is an associated CTD.	Biopsy shows mononuclear infiltrate in the respiratory bronchioles with fibrous scarring. There are many tan-brown-pigmented macrophages as well.	There is no severe derangement of the lung architecture. ESR is typically quite elevated >100. Autoantibodies are usually negative.
Tx	Poor response to steroid and cytoxic therapies, which are the mainstays before lung transplant Mean survival is 3 to 5 years, with death from respiratory failure.	Steroids are useful in the majority of patients. Overall survival is about 70% after 10 years and 27% survival at 12 years.	Prognosis is just as poor as that of ARDS. Few patients respond to therapy. Most die of respiratory failure within a few months.	Good response to steroid and cytotoxic therapy.	No specific therapy. Smoking cessation, steroid therapy, and immunosuppressive therapy have not proven to be of benefit. Long-term survival is common.	Steroids are the mainstay usually up to 100 mg/day. Two-thirds of patients usually recover. Recurrence is common, and one-third have persistent disease. Cyclophosphamide can also be used as a steroid-sparing agent. Overall prognosis is good.

Table 3-13. Comparison of Commonly Described Pneumoconioses

Condition	Asbestosis	Silicosis	Coal Worker's Pneumoconiosis (CWP)	Berylliosis
D	Interstitial pulmonary fibrosis resulting from inhalation of asbestos fibers. Other nonmalignant and malignant asbestos-related lung diseases may also be present.	A nodular fibrotic disease of the lungs caused by chronic exposure to silica dust.	A condition caused by long-term exposure to and inhalation of coal dust.	A disease due to exposure to beryllium dust used in high-tech metallurgy. It has both acute and chronic forms. The chronic form arises after sensitization to beryllium and causes a systemic granulomatous disease similar to sarcoidosis. The acute form, a pneumonitis, results after intense exposures, which are now rare.
Epi	About 1.3 milllion workers in United States exposed; now more common in newly industrializing countries. Associated with bronchogenic cancer, particularly in smokers. Mesotheliomas are also associated with long-term asbestos exposure.	About 1 million people in the United States are exposed. Those with silicosis have about a 30 times higher risk of developing TB infection.	Over 10,000 coal miners have died in the last decade from this condition. The incidence has increased recently. Most patients are >50 years old.	Relatively uncommon disease in the United States.
RF	Seen in mining and milling, and commonly used in old buildings because of its insulation properties; therefore, more common in people involved in such work. Use is still common for pipe and boiler insulation and friction surfaces (brake pads).	More commonly seen in people doing sandblasting, mining, glassworking, and pottery. Pulmonary fibrosis occurs in a dose–response fashion to the exposure.	Working in coal mines. Generally requires at least 20 years of heavy dust exposure.	Occurs as a result of work with old fluorescent lights, beryllium metal products (alloys, ceramics, and radiographic and vacuum tubes), aerospace components, electronics, ceramics, scrap metal, and nuclear reactors.

continued

Table 3-13. (*continued*)

Condition	Asbestosis	Silicosis	Coal Worker's Pneumoconiosis (CWP)	Berylliosis
SiSx	Symptoms are directly related to the duration of exposure, usually 20 years before disease is manifest. Restrictive lung disease with pulmonary fibrosis eventually is seen after heavy exposure and presents with dyspnea and dry cough.	There are three clinical forms: acute, accelerated, and chronic silicosis. Acute silicosis presents like a pneumonia within weeks to 5 years in people with intense exposures. Accelerated and chronic silicosis require 5–10 years of exposure. Symptoms include dyspnea, dry cough, or respiratory failure in advanced disease; otherwise, patients may remain asymptomatic.	Many patients are asymptomatic initially. Dyspnea develops eventually. Like silicosis, progressive massive fibrosis occurs in a minority, with resulting deterioration in lung function and development of pulmonary hypertension and cor pulmonale.	Acute disease symptoms include cough, chest pain, bloody sputum, and crackles along with patchy air space on the chest X-ray, which usually resolve within 1 year. The chronic form is similar to sarcoidosis with dyspnea, cough, chest pain, arthralgias, weight loss and fatigue, and with a latency of months to many years after exposure. Extrapulmonary symptoms are less common than in sarcoidosis. Chronic disease may progress to pulmonary fibrosis if left untreated.
Dx	Asbestosis strictly refers to interstitial lung disease appearing on the chest X-ray as linear opacities mostly at the *lung bases*, the diaphragm, and the cardiac border. Early CT changes show ground glass infiltrates and later fibrosis. Imaging commonly reveals other asbestos-related disease such as calcified pleural plaques or effusions. Less often, mesothelioma may be present and is often heralded by chest wall pain. Spirometry shows a restrictive or mixed restrictive/obstructive pattern. Without symptoms, these lesions only imply exposure, not disease, and may be incidental findings.	Acute silicosis results in consolidation or ground glass opacities bilaterally. Classically, small, rounded nodular opacities are seen in *upper lobes* with hilar adenopathy, usually in chronic silicosis. Calcification of hilar nodes may be seen and described as "egg shell" calcification. Rarely, progressive massive fibrosis occurs when silicotic nodules form conglomerates with a diameter >1 cm.	Characteristics spots are seen on the chest X-ray or CT scan in a patient with the appropriate history. First seen are usually small, rounded opacities mostly in the *upper lobes*. Larger nodules suggest more complex disease, as does significant fibrosis. Calcified hilar nodes are not seen unless silica is present. Caplan's syndrome may arise in miners with rheumatoid arthritis and is manifest by rounded, rapidly progressing, and often cavitary densities on chest X-ray.	Chronic disease manifests with nodular or irregular opacities usually in upper lobes and hilar adenopathy. Lung biopsy will show noncaseating granulomas that are indistinguishable from those of sarcoidosis. Exposure is established on the basis of the history or environmental sampling. Diagnosis requires a history of exposure; biopsy as above; and positive blood or bronchoalveolar lavage LPT (lymphocyte proliferation test), which exposes the patient's lymphocytes to beryllium in vitro. It may also be possible to show the presence of beryllium in the lung, lymph nodes, or urine.

Tx			
Symptomatic treatment for dyspnea unless condition continues. Removal of further exposure to asbestos is key. Treatment for mesothelioma entails surgery and chemotherapy; outcomes are poor.	Treatment involves removing the offending agent. There is no specific treatment for silicosis otherwise, except symptomatic treatment with cough suppression, bronchodilators, and oxygen if needed. Patients are at increased risk of developing TB infection, so perform annual TB test. Progressive massive fibrosis most often culminates in respiratory failure and death.	No specific treatment aside from avoidance of continued exposure and symptomatic care. Follow-up for progression of disease is important.	The most important step in management is complete cessation of further exposure to beryllium. Steroid therapy has been recommended in chronic beryllium disease, and long-term steroid therapy is believed to alter the course of the disease favorably, although there are no reports of permanent cure.

part of the work-up in any patient with ILD with a suggestive history. There is no specific chest X-ray or CT pattern, and findings range from diffuse reticulonodular infiltrates to honeycombing and effusions. Pulmonary function tests will show a restrictive pattern and abnormal D_LCO in chronic cases. Bronchoalveolar lavage can show a marked lymphocytic infiltrate, and lung biopsy may be diagnostic. Finally, an inhalation challenge test can be done at a specialized center.

Tx—Identification of the antigen and removal of the cause is most important to prevent progression of disease. The chronic form may be irreversible. In acute patients or subacute patients with physical impairment, steroids are given. There is no need for long-term therapy if there is no further exposure to the antigen.

Bronchiolitis Obliterans Organizing Pneumonia (BOOP)

D—A syndrome defined by the presence of granulation tissue in small bronchiolar airways and alveolar ducts. Granulation tissue fills the lumens of terminal and respiratory bronchioles in addition to alveoli, unlike the pattern seen in BO. Idiopathic cases are sometimes confused with cryptogenic organizing pneumonia, a similar condition that rapidly resolves with steroid administration.

Epi—It is thought to represent 25% of all cases of chronic infiltrative lung disease.

RF—Half of the cases are idiopathic, but associated causes are infectious (viral, mycoplasma, atypical bacterial most commonly), drug reactions (minocycline, gold, sulfasalazine, among many others), rheumatologic (RA, IBD, SLE), and postradiation therapy of the lung.

SiSx—The disease usually presents as a subacute flu-like illness with low-grade fever over several months, including a mild nonproductive cough, dyspnea, malaise, and weight loss. Rarely, one may see pleuritic chest pain and hemoptysis. Crackles may be heard in up to two-thirds of patients. Clubbing is unusual.

Dx—The chest X-ray shows bilateral diffuse alveolar opacities. Small nodules are seen in one-half of patients. The CT scan shows patchy ground glass infiltrates in a subpleural or peribronchovascular distribution. There may also be bilateral airspace consolidation and mediastinal lymphadenopathy. Pulmonary function tests will show a *restrictive* defect. Lung biopsy via video-assisted thorascopic surgery (VATS) or open surgery is the only way to make a definitive diagnosis. Computed tomography classically shows sparing of the most peripheral lung fields with ground glass infiltrates. It is rare to see effusions or cavitations. Linear opacities at the bases are associated with a poor prognosis. The D_LCO is mildly to moderately decreased in almost all patients; the ESR is invariably increased.

Tx—Overall mortality is 10%, and two-thirds of patients given steroids will have a complete recovery. Prednisone for several months or up to a year is necessary; otherwise, there can be recurrence, in which case retreatment with steroids is necessary.

Idiopathic Diseases of the Lung

Sarcoidosis

D—A multiorgan disease of unknown cause characterized by noncaseating granulomas that can affect any organ but primarily the lungs, lymph nodes, eyes, and skin.

Epi—The prevalence is 10/100,000 to 20/100,000. It is more common in African Americans, who have a lifetime risk of 2.4%. Most cases present between 10 and 40 years of age. Half of the patients have disease detected by chest X-ray before the onset of symptoms.

RF—There is an increased incidence in young adults and African American women. African Americans are affected more acutely than other racial groups and have more severe disease. Spontaneous remissions are common in mild disease. Activated macrophages and CD4 cells accumulate in discrete granulomas.

SiSx

Pulmonary: Presenting symptoms vary and can range from asymptomatic to SOB, cough, and chest discomfort, to chronic infections from bronchiectasis, as seen in fibrocystic sarcoid, in which hemoptysis can also occur. Rarely, one sees pleural effusions or hears crackles, and the chest X-ray generally "looks much worse than symptoms." See below for classification.

Dermatologic: There are protean manifestations that can imitate almost anything; those most commonly seen are maculopapular eruption of the nares, lips, eyelids, forehead, and neck, as well as at previous trauma sites (surgical scars). Pink waxy nodular lesions (erythema nodosum) can be seen on the arms and legs. A violaceous discoloration of the nose, cheeks, chin, and ears is termed *lupus pernio*.

Ophthalmologic: Symptoms are seen in up to 20% of patients and are the presenting symptoms in 5%. Iridocyclitis, chorioretinitis, and keratoconjunctivitis are usually seen.

Cardiovascular: Ventricular arrhythmias causing sudden death are the classic electrical abnormality and may be seen with a restrictive cardiomyopathy in long-standing disease. Conduction abnormalities, however, may be the earliest presenting manifestation of cardiac sarcoid, including varying forms of heart block.

Reticuloendothelial system: There is hepatomegaly in 20% of patients with abnormal LFTs, peripheral lymphadenopathy, and splenomegaly with resulting anemia. Leukopenia and thrombocytopenia can also be seen.

Musculoskeletal: Muscle aches are common. Acute polyarthritis usually occurs in the ankles; chronic arthritis may also develop.

Renal: Calcium metabolism is affected due to extrarenal production of calcitriol by activated sarcoid macrophages leading to hypercalcemia.

Neurologic: Protean manifestations include cranial nerve palsies (facial nerve usually) and central diabetes insipidus and are seen in about 5% of patients.

Other symptoms: Painless swelling of the salivary and lacrimal glands may be seen.

Dx—Diagnosis generally is made by the demonstration of noncaseating granulomas from the involved organ that is easiest to biopsy—usually the skin, but the conjunctivae, transbronchial lymph nodes, the lungs, and cutaneous lymph nodes may also be biopsied.

There are several identified classes of lung disease based on the chest X-ray findings that have prognostic significance. These are shown in Table 3-14.

Tx—Ninety percent of patients respond to steroids acutely and are controlled on 10–15 mg of prednisone on average. Steroids are generally not given initially for Class I or Class II lung disease. However, they are used for CNS, cardiac, or severe eye disease and if PFTs show decreased lung function. If no symptoms exist, one can observe rather than start steroid therapy immediately. Alternatives to steroids include numerous cytotoxic agents, such as methotrexate and azathioprine. Chloroquine/hydroxychloroquine may also be helpful in mucocutaneous sarcoidosis.

Table 3-14.   Classes of Sarcoidosis Based on Chest X-Ray

Class	Description	Rate of Spontaneous Regression
Class I	Bilateral hilar lymphadenopathy with normal lung parenchyma	80%
Class II	Bilateral hilar lymphadenopathy and parenchymal infiltrates mainly in upper lung zones	60%
Class III	Interstitial fibrosis and infiltrates, more in upper lung zones with shrinking nodes	30%
Class IV	Cystic nodular lesions and/or advanced fibrosis	0%

Pulmonary Langerhans' Cell Histiocytosis

D—A groups of disorders with fibrosis and non-malignant infiltration of the lung by histiocytes (macrophages) and eosinophils. There are several variants, depending on whether the disease is localized (eosinophilic granuloma—usually in the bone or lung) or diffuse (as in Letterer-Siwe disease or Hand-Schueller-Christian syndrome). This condition was also formerly known as histiocytosis X.

Epi—The disease is rare, occurring almost exclusively in whites who are 20–40 years old.

RF—Smoking is the most important risk factor in adults.

P—It is caused by proliferation of Langerhans cells (cells from bone marrow, capable of migrating from skin to lymph nodes) into lung interstitium and airspaces.

SiSx—Symptoms include cough, chest pain, fever, and spontaneous pneumothorax. The triad of lytic bone lesions, exophthalmos, and diabetes insipidus is sometimes seen.

Dx—The chest X-ray or CT scan shows that pulmonary histiocytosis produces bilateral reticulonodular infiltrates, most commonly in the upper lobes, with a tendency to form cysts and progress to fibrosis and honeycombing. A definitive diagnosis requires biopsy of the lesion and exam of bronchoalveolar lavage fluid. Histologic exam of the organ in question reveals proliferating histiocytes with cytoplasmic inclusions known as *X bodies*. Pulmonary function tests will show restriction and impaired gas exchange.

Tx—Steroids are given for pulmonary manifestations, but their efficacy is not clear. Surgery or radiotherapy can be used for localized bone disease. In some patients, the disease remits.

Pulmonary Alveolar Proteinosis

D—A rare condition in which alveoli accumulate phospholipids and protein-rich fluid without any known underlying disease or other organ involvement.

Epi—More males than females are affected. The condition appears in all age groups.

P—A phospholipid- and protein-rich substance very much like surfactant accumulates in alveoli, perhaps as a result of impaired clearance. The interstitium is spared. There are few inflammatory cells. Secondary causes of impaired clearance have been linked to HIV, lymphoproliferative disorders, and TB.

SiSx—Symptoms include dyspnea, nonproductive cough, and possibly cyanosis. Rales are found on exam. Patients are predisposed to unusual forms of infection, especially *Nocardia* and fungal infections. Pulmonary fibrosis may be a late manifestation.

Dx—There is a characteristic bilateral alveolar infiltrative pattern in a perihilar distribution on the chest X-ray. Bronchoalveolar lavage returns proteinaceous material, and lung biopsy shows PAS-positive material in the alveoli.

Tx—Observation is needed in patients with minimal symptoms. Otherwise, bronchoalveolar lavage with whole lung lavage can be used to help reverse the abnormality. Steroids can increase the risk of infection. The prognosis depends on the cause, whether primary or secondary. Overall, one-third of patients have spontaneous remission not requiring therapy, one-third need whole lung lavage, and one-third have progressive disease despite treatment.

Lymphangioleiomyomatosis (LAM)

D—Uncommon lung condition of pulmonary smooth muscle and cyst formation causing small airway obstruction, effusion, and pneumothoraces.

Epi—The sporadic form mostly affects women of childbearing age. The disease is seen mostly in Caucasians. There is some association with the tuberous sclerosis complex.

P—The primary pathologic abnormality is proliferation of smooth muscle cells around bronchovascular structures and cystic dilatation of terminal airspaces. Eventually, many cysts up to several centimeters in diameter can be seen. The etiology is unclear; however, estrogen appears to play an important role, as this condition does not present prior to menarche and only rarely after menopause, usually in those taking estrogen.

SiSx—It may present as small airway disease with dyspnea, cough, wheezing, and mild to moderate hemoptysis. Spontaneous pneumothorax is the presenting sign in many patients, occurring in up to 50%. Chylothorax is seen but overall is rare. Lymphangioleiomyomas may be seen elsewhere, such as the abdomen, causing bloating and abdominal pain. Meningiomas are seen more frequently in these patients, as are renal angiomyolipomas, which can grow quite large.

Dx—The disease is usually misdiagnosed as asthma. This diagnosis should be suspected in young women with early-onset emphysema, recurrent pneumothoraces, or a chylous pleural effusion. High-resolution CT can help make the diagnosis and can show the numerous cysts. Ultimately, lung biopsy is done for confirmation. It shows the characteristic findings of smooth muscle proliferation and cystic dilation of air spaces.

Tx—There is no proven therapy. Progestins and gonadotropin releasing hormone agonists are sometimes partially successful. Lung transplant can be considered; posttransplant survival is similar to that in patients with pulmonary fibrosis and emphysema.

Vascular and Structural Diseases of the Lung

Pulmonary Embolism (PE)

D—A condition in which a venous blood clot forms elsewhere in the body and travels into the pulmonary arterial vasculature, causing obstruction of blood flow. The great majority of clots are derived from deep venous thromboses.

Epi—Five million people have venous thrombosis each year, 10% of these have a PE, and 10% of those patients die. The diagnosis is missed in many, and mortality is as high as 30%.

P—Formation and dissolution of venous clots is common in many people. However, under normal circumstances, it is unusual for these clots to cause disease. Most clots form in the venous networks of the pelvis and legs (90% of the time) and are called deep venous thromboses (DVTs). Those from the upper venous systems occur in the setting of central lines or IVDU. Commonly, they originate as a platelet nidus on the undersurface of valves. Turbulence under the valves can damage endothelium, and venous hypertension can stretch the walls. When part of the clot dislodges, it travels through the IVC to the heart and into the pulmonary arterial system, becoming trapped in various locations. Large clots can cause a saddle embolus that straddles the bifurcation of the right and left pulmonary arteries. When 50%–60% of the pulmonary perfusion is obstructed, RV strain and cardiac failure can ensue. Hypoxic vasoconstriction can also occur throughout the rest of the lung. Infarction can occur, but this is rare since there are two other sources of oxygen (airways and bronchial circulation). The primary physiologic consequence is V/Q mismatch from ventilated but underperfused areas (dead space).

RF—Risk factors, classically described by Virchow's triad, include (1) venous stasis (due to immobilization, hospitalization, or varicosities), (2) injury to veins (from trauma, peripheral venous disease such as thrombophlebitis, chronic cardiopulmonary disease, or recent surgery—especially orthopedic surgery), and (3) a hypercoagulable state caused by any of a number of factors such as oral contraceptive pill (OCP) use, malignancy, and inherited hypercoagulable disorders. Other, less specific risk factors include age (exponential increase after age 50), obesity, tobacco use, and major trauma.

SiSx—Most classical PE symptoms are sudden onset of SOB, pleuritic pain, with tachypnea, tachycardia and dyspnea, cough, and chest pain. Low-grade fever may be present. The exam may be normal unless the patient is quite sick. Hypotension, shock, and syncope are ominous signs. Patients with a DVT may complain of an aching, painful leg with muscle tenderness. Swelling, and pitting edema may be present. Low-yield but classical signs for a DVT are:

Homan's sign: sensation of tightening and pain during foot dorsiflexion.

Moses' *sign*: tenderness on anteroposterior and not lateral calf compression.

Lowenberg's sign: calf tenderness on 180 degree circumferential compression of calf.

Peabody's sign: spasm of the calf muscle with leg elevation and extension of the foot.

Pratt's sign: distension of pretibial veins when the patient is supine.

Dx—Diagnosis requires a high degree of clinical suspicion. The chest X-ray is usually normal or shows some plate-like atelectasis or a small pleural effusion. Though rare, classical chest X-ray signs are *Hampton's hump* (a wedge-shaped peripheral infarct) and *Westermark's sign* (decreased vascular markings of the pulmonary arteries centrally). The ECG may show sinus tachycardia or signs of right heart strain (a new right bundle branch) or the less commonly seen $S_I Q_{III} T_{III}$ *pattern* of right heart strain (an S wave in lead I, a Q wave and an inverted T in lead III). The most common finding is nonspecific ST and T wave changes. An ABG test may show some hypoxia and respiratory alkalosis because of tachypnea, and the alveolar-arterial or A-a oxygen gradient may be enlarged. Remember, however, that a normal A-a gradient does not rule out the diagnosis but merely makes it less likely.

The main tests currently used to diagnose a PE are a V/Q scan or a PE protocol CT (see Figure 3-4). The latter test can be performed with venous "runoff" to look for DVTs in the

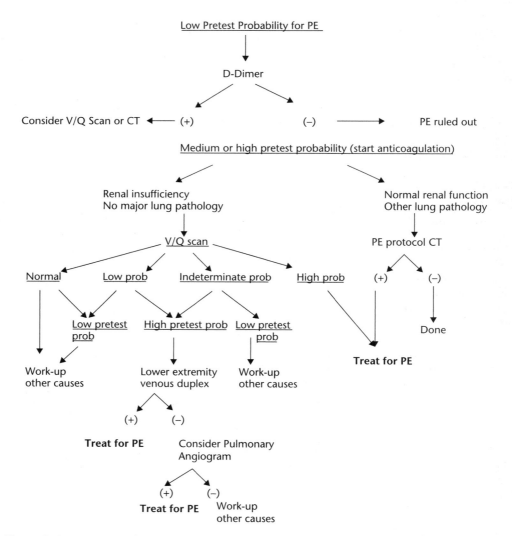

Figure 3-4. Diagnostic Algorithm for Pulmonary Embolism Based on Pretest Probability.

lower extremities at the same time. The gold standard, pulmonary angiography, is rarely used today. Its use depends on the pretest probability of PE. In general, CT is best for large-vessel PEs; it may miss smaller peripheral PEs. The V/Q scan is more useful in showing areas of segmental mismatch.

If the V/Q scan is completely normal, it generally rules out a PE; more commonly, however, the probability of PE is given based on the findings. A high-probability scan indicates a 90% chance of PE. A low-probability scan doesn't rule out PE if there is high clinical suspicion. A positive D dimer is sensitive but not specific and is therefore when negative it can be used to rule out a PE or DVT only when the pretest probability is low. For DVTs, venography is the gold standard, but it is no longer performed. Bilateral B-mode compression ultrasound is used instead, and is 97% sensitive and specific when the patient has symptoms; it is only 50% sensitive and 98% specific in asymptomatic patients. These studies demonstrate if the vein is compressible or a clot is visible. All other added modalities do not provide much additional sensitivity or specificity.

Tx—Anticoagulation is used to prevent further clots as the body resorbs or recannulates the ones that are already present. It can take up to weeks or months for clots to resolve. Current recommendations are to anticoagulate with IV heparin to an activated partial thromboplastin time (aPTT) of 60–80 seconds for the first 5 days and use warfarin with a goal international normalized ratio (INR) of 2–3 for at least 6 months after the reversal of the predisposing event that caused the PE, though a longer duration of anticoagulation may be recommended after considering the supposed etiology and/or severity of the insult. For example, some argue that life threatening, massive PEs of unclear etiology after extensive work-up may require lifelong anticoagulation because of a presumed hypercoagulable state. Tissue plasminogen activator (TPA) with or without surgery may be used for a large embolus that is causing hemodynamic compromise. In patients with recurrent disease despite anticoagulation, with a contraindication to anticoagulation (GI bleed or hemorrhagic stone), or with a large PE such that additional PEs would be nearly fatal, placement of an inferior vena cava (IVC) filter may be recommended.

Pulmonary Hypertension

D—Elevated mean pulmonary artery pressure (PAP) that can be primary, as in idiopathic pulmonary arterial hypertension (IPAH), or secondary to multiple causes. In general, the PAP exceeds 25 mmHg at rest or 30 mmHg during exercise, though these are only rough values, as PAP increases with age. Concomitantly, many patients who have a primary lung etiology may also have increased pulmonary vascular resistance.

P—Several general mechanisms are associated with increased pulmonary pressure and are not necessarily mutually exclusive. As pressure = flow x resistance, increased PAP can result from increased pulmonary blood flow (e.g., systemic to pulmonary shunts) or increased pulmonary vascular resistance— either from intrinsic lung conditions, such as chronic hypoxic vasoconstriction or pulmonary vascular bed destruction, or extrinsic conditions that increase pulmonary venous pressure, such as left ventricular failure. Pulmonary hypertension is categorized by the World Health Organization (WHO) scheme shown in Table 3-15.

RF—Pulmonary hypertension is associated with anorectogenic agents, specifically fenfluriamine appetite suppressant use, cocaine, amphetamine use, portal hypertension, and HIV infection. Many of these factors are associated in general with pulmonary hypertension. In certain cases, the family history is important.

Epi—By far the most common cause is related to COPD.

SiSx—Symptoms can be relatively nonspecific, but patients may present with exertional dyspnea or fatigue since they cannot increase their cardiac output during exertion. Small-volume hemoptysis or a cough may also be

Table 3-15. Classification of Pulmonary Hypertension

Group 1	Group 2	Group 3	Group 4	Group 5
Directly increased pulmonary arterial pressures	Secondary to increased pulmonary venous pressure	Secondary to hypoxemia or parenchymal lung diseases	From thrombotic or embolic disease	Inflammatory, mechanical and extrinsic compression or idiopathic
Idiopathic pulmonary arterial hypertension (IPAH)	Left-sided heart failure	COPD	Chronic thromboem-bolic disease	Histiocytosis X
Collagen vascular disease related	Valvular disease	Any ILD		Sarcoidosis
Portopulmonary hypertension (with cirrhosis)	Pulmonary veno-occlusive disease	Sleep-disordered breathing		Fibrosing mediastinitis
Anorectogens	Compression of the central pulmonary veins as by tumor, lymphadenopathy, or mediastinitis			
HIV related				
Congenital systemic-to-pulmonary shunts				

seen. When significant right ventricular failure develops, patients may feel chest pain (usually from right ventricular strain) or have exertional syncope in addition to lower extremity edema and abdominal bloating. A very dilated artery can cause hoarseness from recurrent laryngeal nerve compression or chest pain from dynamic compression of the left main coronary artery, though these conditions are rare. Exam may reveal a louder P_2 component of the second heart sound or a split second heart sound, a palpable right ventricular heave, right-sided S_3, elevated neck veins, and lower extremity edema.

Dx—Echocardiography, the least invasive method, can estimate the pulmonary artery systolic pressure (PASP) only if a tricuspid regurgitation jet is visible. It uses the Bernoulli equation and several assumptions (PASP = four times the square of tricuspid regurgitation jet velocity added to the estimated right atrial pressure). Right atrial pressure is estimated based on the amount of inferior vena cava collapse. If the images or measurements are not adequate, then the estimate can be significantly off. The gold standard for measurement of PASP is right heart catheterization (see Chapter 2), in which a catheter is inserted via the superior vena cava or inferior vena cava into the pulmonary artery to make precise measurements. Once the diagnosis is made, one should search for the underlying cause(s). A comprehensive evaluation in an individual with significant pulmonary hypertension without an obvious cause (such as left heart disease) may include:

1. Right heart catheterization to document the degree of pulmonary hypertension and assess for any component of left-sided heart failure.
2. V/Q scan to assess for thromboembolic disease.
3. Sleep study to assess for sleep apnea.
4. Laboratory tests for certain connective tissue diseases [antinuclear antibody (ANA), rheumatoid factor, antineutrophil cytoplasmic antibody (ANCA)], liver function tests, and the HIV test.
5. High-resolution CT scan to assess for interstitial lung disease.
6. Pulmonary function tests may also be useful to document the degree of any obstructive or restrictive lung disease.

It is important to know that acutely the right ventricle can only generate peak systolic pressures of

45–50 mmHg; higher values suggest a chronic or acute-on-chronic process. Patients who complain of exercise-induced symptoms and have normal or high normal PA pressures at rest can have an ECHO during exercise to see if PA pressures increase (PA pressures normally increases with exercise, but this response will be exaggerated in patients with early pulmonary hypertension).

Tx—Most important is to find or rule out the causes of reversible pulmonary hypertension in order to treat them. Otherwise, the use of pulmonary vasodilators may be indicated in the appropriate situation (see the following section on idiopathic pulmonary arterial hypertension).

Idiopathic Pulmonary Arterial Hypertension (IPAH)

D—An idiopathic condition characterized by elevated PA pressure due to precapillary pulmonary hypertension or pulmonary arterial hypertension (PAH) for which no other cause has been found.

Epi—This rare condition has an incidence of 2/1,000,000 worldwide. Female patients outnumber male patients by as much as 9:1. Most patients present in their 30s to 40s, but they can present at any age.

P—A familial form of IPAH accounts for 10% of cases and is due to an autosomal dominant mutation in the BMP2 receptor. Generally, however, the cause is not known and the condition is thought to be due to inappropriate vasoconstriction of pulmonary artery smooth muscle, either via potassium channel abnormalities or by an imbalance between vasoconstrictive and vasodilatory mediators. The final common pathway leads to increased resistance to blood flow and elevation of PAP. Over time, this can lead to failure of the right ventricle and ultimately decreased cardiac output. The pulmonary capillary wedge pressure (PCWP) remains normal until the late stages, when impaired left ventricular diastolic filling occurs with an intruding interventricular septum from right ventricular hypertrophy (RVH). The right ventricle eventually fails, and right atrial and right ventricular end-diastolic pressures rise to compensate.

As the PAP increases, thrombotic pulmonary arteriopathy occurs, involving thrombosis of small muscular pulmonary arteries. Eventually this can lead to so-called *plexogenic pulmonary arteriopathy*, in which there is remodeling and intimal fibrosis of the vasculature.

SiSx—Classically, the presentation is one of gradual onset of dyspnea that progresses to marked dyspnea with minimal activity over a period of about 2 to 3 years. Fatigue, angina from right ventricular ischemia, and syncope or presyncope may be signs of right ventricular failure, as are elevated JVP, reduced carotid pulse, tricuspid regurgitation murmur, and a palpable right ventricular lift. Additionally, one may hear an increased P_2. Clubbing is unusual.

Dx—The diagnostic criteria for IPAH include demonstration of a resting mean PAP >25 mmHg and the absence of significant parenchymal lung disease, chronic thromboembolic disease, left-sided valvular or myocardial disease, congenital heart disease, or systemic connective tissue disease. At a minimum, after documentation of high PA pressures is made by ECHO, the work-up involves an ANA, thyroid function tests (TFTs), LFTs, an HIV test, sleep study, V/Q scan, and a right heart catheterization. The right heart catheterization is needed to document the degree of pulmonary hypertension and to rule out underlying cardiac disease such as a shunt or left heart failure. Right heart catheterization is also useful to test the response to pulmonary vasodilators.

Non specific findings of pulmonary hypertension on the chest X-ray are enlarged pulmonary arteries with clear lung fields. The ECG may show right axis deviation and RVH. In addition to high PA pressures, the ECHO may show an enlarged right ventricle, perhaps compressing the left ventricular and an abnormal, flattened septum because of the RVH. Pulmonary function tests may show a mild restrictive pattern. Hypoxemia is seen due to V/Q mismatch and decreased cardiac output. The D_LCO is also decreased. A high resolution chest CT may be needed to assess for interstitial lung disease in some cases.

Tx—Anticoagulation is important with advances disease because of a predisposition to clot with pulmonary disease and in situ thrombosis. Diuretics for control of edema should be given with caution, as too much fluid removal will reduce the preload, which is dangerous in right heart failure.

All patients in whom IPAH is confirmed should be tested to see if they respond to short-acting pulmonary vasodilators such as adenosine, nitric oxide, or prostacyclin, and to see if they have additional pulmonary reserve [defined as a decrease in PAP by >10% or a decreased in pulmonary vascular resistance (PVR) by >25%]. Responders may be candidates for vasodilatory therapy, which includes oral calcium channel blockers, epoprostenol (a prostacyclin analogue approved for functional New York Heart Association [NYHA] class III and IV failure), and other vasodilators such as bosentan (an endothelin receptor antagonist). Additional therapies include phosphodiesterase inhibitors such as sildenafil as an orally administered agent. The routine use of digoxin for heart failure in IPAH is controversial. Sometimes a right-to-left shunt can be created by balloon atrial septostomy to increase systemic blood flow in patients with syncope or severe right heart failure. Patients who fall into NYHA classes III and IV and who do not respond to pulmonary vasodilator testing, and patients who deteriorate while taking chronic oral vasodilators, should also be considered for transplantation. Otherwise, supportive care, including supplemental oxygen, should be used if necessary. The mean survival is about 3 years from the time of diagnosis, and most patients ultimately need heart and lung transplants (because of severe irreversible right sided heart failure) if they are healthy enough for this procedure to be performed.

Acute Respiratory Distress Syndrome (ARDS)

D—A condition of acute hypoxic hypocapnic respiratory failure with loss of lung compliance and pulmonary edema.

Epi—Seventy-five percent of cases of ARDS are due to sepsis, trauma, and aspiration. Forty percent of patients with sepsis develop ARDS. Ninety percent require mechanical ventilation within 3 days.

RF—Risk factors include overwhelming infection, sepsis, disseminated intravascular coagulation (DIC), burns, trauma, pancreatitis, heroin overdose, blood transfusion, aspiration, and liver disease.

P—For unclear reasons, endothelial permeability is increased and protein-rich fluid enters the interstitium at an increased rate, beyond the clearance rate by lymphatics, causing capillary edema. Hypoxemia results from severe V/Q mismatch rather than from diffusion impairment. The increased work of breathing eventually leads to respiratory fatigue and failure.

SiSx—Early on, there may be a latency period without signs or symptoms. These can develop within 24 to 48 hours of the insult. Tachypnea develops, with resulting hypocapnea and mild hypoxemia at first. As ARDS progresses, the patient may develop frothy pink or red sputum, diffuse rales, and widespread infiltrates. Many become cyanotic as respiratory failure ensues.

Dx—Classical criteria are for ARDS are (1) acute onset of severe dyspnea, (2) diffuse bilateral alveolar infiltrations seen on chest X-ray, (3) a PaO_2 (in mmHg) $/F_IO_2$ (in decimal form) ratio <200, and (4) a PCWP <18 mmHg (meaning that this occurs in the absence of heart failure). Sometimes it is difficult to distinguish ARDS from left heart failure, though ARDS usually occurs in the absence of cardiomegaly, perihilar alveolar infiltrates, and pleural effusions, as may be seen in left heart failure. Infiltrates are also more peripheral and have more air bronchograms.

Tx—The key to treatment is intubation followed by low tidal volume mechanical ventilation (6–8 mL/kg vs. the normal 10–15 mL/kg) with permissive hypercapnia. This involves ventilating the patient at a lower than normal tidal volume, allowing some degree of hypercapnia to occur. The idea is that in ARDS, alveolar flooding is nonuniform and one does not want to overdistend the normally functioning alveoli that are still working to promote recovery. During this time the underlying cause, if found, is treated. Nonetheless, most patients do not recover. Mortality is 60%–70%, with one-third of patients dying within the first 3 days.

Pneumothorax

D—Accumulation of air in the pleural space, which can cause compression of the underlying lung parenchyma. There are several types.

Primary pneumothorax: arises from rupture of small subpleural apical blebs and is more common in tall, thin, young males.

Secondary pneumothorax: occurs in condition such as COPD (where blebs may be present), trauma, or TB pleural disease, or may be iatrogenic from placement of central lines or thoracentesis.

Tension pneumothorax: occurs when the chest wall defect acts as a one-way valve drawing air into the chest cavity with each inspiration but not letting it out. This is a medical emergency and requires immediate decompression.

SiSx—In unilateral pneumothorax, patients may complain of sudden onset of pleuritic chest pain and dyspnea. The exam will show diminished/absent breath sounds and hyperresonance to percussion with decreased tactile fremitus.

Dx—The chest X-ray is used primarily to make the diagnosis. Ideally, the diagnosis of tension pneumothorax should be made clinically.

Tx—Small pneumothoraces will resolve on their own; larger ones need chest tubes with the tips positioned toward the apices where air will go. Pleurodesis (injecting an irritant to scar the pleura and lung together) can be done in patients with recurrent pneumothoraces due to anatomic conditions. Tension pneumothorax requires immediate needle decompression and then chest tube placement.

Bullous Lung Disease

D—The presence of small apical blebs or bullae in otherwise healthy individuals. It can be congenital or acquired.

Epi—Patients have an increased incidence of lung cancer.

SiSx—Patients can be asymptomatic. Complications can include pneumothorax, infection and formation of a lung abscess, bleeding into bullae and lung compression, and COPD-like symptoms.

Dx—A chest X-ray showing the findings and an otherwise unremarkable history can make the diagnosis.

Tx—Surgical treatment may improve lung function; in most cases, no treatment is needed.

Bronchopulmonary Sequestration

D—A developmental disorder of the lung in which there is a region of lung parenchyma that has an incomplete or no connection with the airways and is supplied by aberrant arteries arising off the aorta. The sequestration can be intralobar (has the same visceral pleura as adjacent lung tissue) or extralobar (has its own pleural lining to separate it from other lung tissue).

Epi—Extralobar sequestration is less common (25% of cases) than the intralobar form but is more common in men. Many patients have other congenital abnormalities such as diaphragmatic hernia.

P—Extralobar sequestrations may communicate with the stomach. They are located in the lower chest and occur twice as often on the left as on the right. Sequestrations rarely contain air because they do not have communication with the airways. Venous return is usually through the azygous system rather through the pulmonary veins. Intralobar sequestrations have pulmonary venous drainage.

SiSx—Most sequestrations are asymptomatic and are discovered incidentally by chest X-ray. Large ones can cause respiratory distress in the neonate.

Dx—The diagnosis of bronchopulmonary sequestration is made from a chest X-ray showing a basilar density that does not fill during bronchography (contrast opacification of the airways seen on X-ray) and cannot be visualized by bronchoscopy. The CT scan delineates the anatomy, and the diagnosis is confirmed by angiography showing the aberrant artery.

Tx—Preoperative localization of the abnormal blood supply is key to avoid bleeding during resection. Extralobar sequestrations are usually removed without damage to surrounding normal lung tissue; lobectomy is needed for intralobar sequestrations, and those patients who undergo resection have a good prognosis if there are no surgical complications.

Diseases of the Pleura

Pleural Effusion

D—Fluid collection in the pleural space between the parietal and visceral pleura. It is not a disease but a sign of an underlying disease that must be determined.

P—Pleural effusion may accompany any process that causes inflammation of the parietal pleura or compression of the lung. The pleural space normally contains a small amount of transudative fluid from the parietal pleural surface that is removed through lymphatics. The visceral pleural surface is supplied by the bronchial circulation with drainage into the pulmonary veins. Therefore, there can be either obstruction of lymph flow away from the pleura, via increased systemic venous pressure or pulmonary hypertension, or increased plasma oncotic pressure causing an effusion. Much of the lymph drainage of the abdomen passes via the diaphragm, so ascites commonly creates a right-sided pleural effusion. The causes of pleural effusion are listed in Table 3-16.

SiSx—Pleurisy is often present with a small inflammatory effusion, and sometime a friction rub can be heard. Large bilateral pleural effusions can cause dyspnea, but orthopnea is uncommon. Dyspnea may seem disproportionate in patients who have heart disease or COPD, but removing even small amounts of fluid can improve the symptoms considerably. Accumulation starts at the bases of the lungs. A dull to flat percussion note is found over the area and accompanies absent/decreased breath sounds. There is decreased fremitus. If there is a compressed lung, one may hear bronchial breath sounds. Once the effusion becomes very large, there can be decreased chest expansion. The mediastinum is usually shifted away from the side of effusion in this case.

Dx—When there are no adhesions between pleura, the earliest sign is blunting of the costophrenic angle on the lateral view of the chest X-ray, since fluid will accumulate posteriorly in a standing patient. When costophrenic angle blunting is seen on the PA chest X-ray, more than 300 mL of fluid is present in an average-sized person. With larger amounts of fluid, there is opacification of the lower lung base on the chest X-ray. Lateral decubitus films can be very helpful, since they can recognize up to 15 mL of fluid along the chest wall. A CT scan is also a good way to diagnose free pleural fluid because it can separate pleural and parenchymal densities. The effusion may lie within a fissure (interlobular effusion), most commonly the right major fissure. A loculated effusion may also produce a shadow that lies flat against the lateral surfaces and bulges into the lung field in one or more locations.

Unless a cause has been established, the effusion should be drained by thoracentesis to establish a diagnosis. Therapeutic thoracentesis (removing large amounts of fluid) is helpful in large effusions to improve symptoms, but no more than 1–2 L should be removed at a time to prevent excessive fluid shifts.

At a minimum, one should determine the total protein, lactic dehydrogenase (LDH), differential cell count, culture, pH, glucose, and perhaps amylase. When an inflammatory effusion is suspected, a needle biopsy of the pleura may be done.

Tx—This varies based on the underlying disease. Infectious causes are treated with antibiotics and a chest tube. Malignant effusions generally have a poor prognosis, as they are indicative of late-stage disease. Congestive heart failure is treated with diuresis. See Table 3-16.

Table 3-16. Distinguishing Characteristics of Pleural Effusions

Type of Effusion	Transudative Effusion	Exudative Effusion
Fluid characteristics (Ratios are for pleural fluid divided by serum values)	Protein concentration < 3 g/dL Lactic dehydrogenase (LDH) ratio <0.6 Protein ratio <0.5	Protein >3 g/dL LDH ratio >0.6 Protein ratio >0.5 Pleural fluid LDH > two-thirds normal upper limit for serum Pleural fluid cholesterol >45 mg/dL (need any one of the above to call it exudative)
Diagnostic hints	History of heart disease, abnormal LFTs, hepatomegaly, renal dysfunction, anasarca, pedal edema, bilateral crackles.	If gross blood is seen, consider a traumatic tap, PE, tumor or hemothorax. A low glucose level implies empyema, RA (if very low), or TB. If pH <7.3, consider infection. A high protein content implies TB (almost always >4.0 mg/dL), multiple myeloma, or Waldenström's macroglobulinemia (both usually >7.0 mg/dL). Elevated amylase can be due to acute or chronic pancreatitis, esophageal rupture, or malignancy. The presence of both air and fluid in the pleural cavity indicates a possible bronchopleural fistula. A WBC count >2500 per microliter implies an inflammatory lesion.
Causes	CHF, cirrhosis, nephrotic syndrome, superior vena cava obstruction, hypoalbuminemia, protein-losing enteropathy, constrictive pericarditis.	Parapneumonic, TB, lung cancer, PE, hypothyroidism, viral infection, pancreatitis, splenic infarction (left-sided), collagen vascular disease, traumatic tap, hemothorax, asbestosis, and many other causes.
Treatment	Treat the underlying condition (e.g., diuresis, protein replacement), consider therapeutic thoracentesis.	If the condition is malignant, consider pleurodesis (injection of irritant material to make the pleural layers scar together) if chemotherapy or radiation therapy does not work. Place a chest tube for drainage in infections along with antibiotics for empyema.

CHAPTER 4

Nephrology

RENAL ANATOMY AND PHYSIOLOGY

- The normal adult kidney is 11.0 to 12.0 cm in length, 5.0 to 7.5 cm in width, and 2.5 to 3.0 cm in thickness. The right kidney lies lower than the left and under the liver. The two kidneys filter approximately 180 L of fluid and excrete ~1 to 1.5 L each day. Normal urine output is >30 mL/hr. Figure 4-1 shows the gross anatomy of the kidney.
- The functional unit is the nephron (500,000 to 1 million per kidney), as shown in Figure 4-2.
- The blood supply for each kidney is provided by a single renal artery off of the aorta, though additional accessory renal arteries are common.
- Both renal veins drain into the inferior vena cava (IVC), but only the left one meets the left testicular or the ovarian vein beforehand. This is clinically important, as sometimes a left varicocele can signify renal cancer.
- Each component of the nephron has a specific function, as shown in Table 4-1.

DIAGNOSTIC AND THERAPEUTIC MODALITIES

Urinalysis

Simple and cost effective, urinalysis is perhaps the most effective test to assess renal disease. The major findings of a basic dipstick analysis are shown in Table 4-2.

Urine Microscopy

Take 10 mL of fresh collected urine (e.g., not collecting in a Foley catheter for a while), centrifuge for 5 minutes, and remove 9 mL of supernatant, leaving 1 mL. Use this amount to resuspend the pellet. Put a drop on a slide with a coverslip and view it. Urine casts conform to the shape of the renal tubule in which they formed and are therefore cylindrical, with regular margins. All casts have a matrix composed of the Tamm-Horsfall mucoprotein. Urine crystals are varied and in certain cases point to specific diseases or conditions (see Table 4-3 and Figure 4-3).

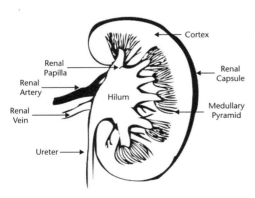

Figure 4-1. Gross Anatomic Structures of the Kidney.

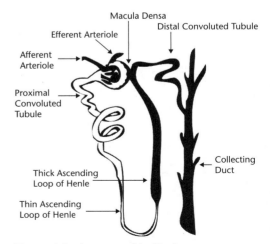

Figure 4-2. Anatomy of the Nephron.

Table 4-1. Components of the Nephron

Location	Function	Site of Action of Medication/ Endogenous Molecules
Glomerulus (Bowman's capsule and capillary tufts)	Filtration and GFR regulation via juxtaglomerular apparatus and renin–angiotensin system. When flow is low, as in hypotension, renin is released, causing angiotensin II–mediated efferent arteriole constriction.	*Afferent Arteriole:* Epinephrine constricts via α_1 receptors and decreases urine output. NSAIDs prevent dilation via prostaglandins. *Efferent Arteriole:* ACE inhibitors and angiotensin receptor blockers prevent constriction and lower blood pressure.
Proximal Convoluted Tubule (PCT)	From 50% to 65% of total solutes and water are reabsorbed (NaCl, glucose, amino acids, organic acids, phosphate, etc). Organic solutes are secreted.	Carbonic anhydrase inhibitors such as acetazolamide act as diuretics. Dopamine inhibits reabsorption here. Renal-mediated drug secretion occurs here.
Thin Ascending Loop of Henle (tALH)	Water is reabsorbed.	None.
Thick Ascending Loop of Henle (TALH)	25% of Na^+ is reabsorbed via the Na^+-K^+-$2Cl^-$ channel.	Loop diuretics such as furosemide and bumetanide block the Na^+-K^+-$2Cl^-$ channel.
Distal Collecting Tubule (DCT)	~5% more Na^+ and Cl^- are also resorbed via Na^+ and Cl transporters.	Thiazide diuretics such as hydrochlorothiazide block the Na^+-Cl^- cotransporter.
Collecting Tubule	~5% more Na^+ is reabsorbed; K^+ and H^+ are excreted.	Potassium-sparing diuretics such as spironolactone, amiloride, and triamterene block aldosterone-sensitive sodium channels. Aldosterone acts physiologically to cause Na^+ reabsorption and K^+ and H^+ excretion.
Collecting Duct	Antidiuretic hormone (ADH) acts to reabsorb water by facilitating aquaporin water channel function. Atrial natriuretic peptide (ANP) works to halt Na^+ reabsorption.	Exogenous ADH is given in central diabetes insipidus. Exogenous BNP.

Table 4-2. Dipstick Analysis

Specific Gravity Normal: 1.005–1.030 g/mL	A reading of 1.010 g/mL indicates isosthenuria, which is the specific gravity of normal plasma. The inability to raise (concentrate) or lower (dilute) urine suggests tubular dysfunction. A reading greater than 1.020 g/mL is consistent with prerenal physiology.
pH: Normal 4.5 and 7	Persistently alkaline urine is unusual but is seen in UTIs with urease-producing organisms such as *Klebsiella* and *Proteus*.
Leukocyte Esterase	Usually positive in the setting of pyuria and suggests activated leukocytes; specific but not sensitive.
Nitrite	Positive in the presence of urease-producing organisms such as *Klebsiella* and *Proteus*.
Protein	Measures only albumin. Adding sulfosalicylic acid (SSA) to a urine specimen will precipitate all proteins. A positive SSA test in the setting of a negative dipstick strongly suggests a urinary paraprotein.
Blood	Measures the presence of heme; is positive in hematuria but also in myoglobinuria from rhabdomyolysis or free heme liberated by RBC lysis in the blood.

Table 4-3. Findings on Urine Microscopy

Finding	Conditions
Hyaline Casts	Not specific for renal disease. Seen in dehydration, prerenal states, and concentrated urine.
Red Cell Casts	Highly indicative of some form of glomerulonephritis.
White Cell Casts	Usually indicative of infection or inflammation such as pyelonephritis or interstitial nephritis.
Epithelial Cell Casts	Seen in acute tubular necrosis and interstitial nephritis.
Fatty Casts	Seen in patients with significant proteinuria with breakdown of lipid-rich epithelial cells. Droplets have cholesterol esters and cholesterol. Polarized light reveals the classical "Maltese cross" shape, a property of esterified cholesterol in a liquid crystal state.
Coarse Granular Casts	Nonspecific but may represent acute tubular necrosis.
Broad Waxy Casts	Seen in chronic renal failure. They indicate stasis in poorly functioning and enlarged collecting tubules.
Calcium Oxalate Crystals	Mostly without clinical meaning as seen in acidic or neutral urine but can indicate calcium oxalate stones in the appropriate clinical setting. However, can be seen in excess in ethylene glycol ingestion if the clinical picture is consistent (acute renal failure, acidosis). The crystals appear in two shapes. Classically, they are octahedral, or envelope-shaped (dihydrate), but they can also be needle-shaped (monohydrate). Seen in acidic or neutral urine.
Struvite Crystals (also called triple phosphate crystals)	Struvite stone formation occurs only if excess ammonia is made and pH increases, which makes phosphate less soluble. Seen in UTIs such as with urease-producing organisms (*Proteus* or *Klebsiella*).
Uric Acid	Found in acidic urine. Has many shapes and sizes. May be seen in excess in acute renal failure and ongoing tumor lysis syndrome.
Cysteine Crystals	Characteristic hexagonal shape. Seen in cystinuria, an inherited autosomal recessive disorder.

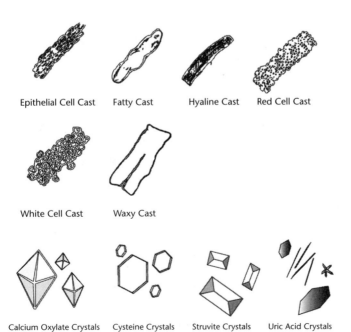

Epithelial Cell Cast   Fatty Cast   Hyaline Cast   Red Cell Cast

White Cell Cast   Waxy Cast

Calcium Oxalate Crystals   Cysteine Crystals   Struvite Crystals   Uric Acid Crystals

Figure 4-3. Findings on Urine Microscopy.

Renal Imaging

There are numerous modalities for renal imaging, each of which is most useful in specific circumstances. Table 4-4 discusses the use of each modality.

Dialysis

This is the most common mechanical intervention in nephrology and is a renal replacement therapy. It is used to remove toxic waste materials, regulate electrolytes, and optimize the intravascular volume status. It is used both acutely and chronically and can be a temporary or permanent treatment, depending on the nature of the renal failure and the likelihood of renal recovery. The different forms of dialysis are compared in Table 4-5.

Indications for Acute Hemodialysis

A—Severe acidosis that is refractory to medical therapy and hyperventilation, especially if complications such as arrhythmias or hypotension develop.

E—Electrolyte abnormalities, particularly hyperkalemia.

I—Intoxication (small molecules such as lithium, aspirin, methanol, and ethylene glycol can be removed); remember that digoxin and phenytoin cannot be removed by dialysis.

O—Overload of volume (if the patient cannot tolerate diuretics).

U—Uremia (most emergent if encephalopathy causing seizures or pericarditis with effusion occurs).

Renal Biopsy

- Routine evaluation of specimens includes light microscopy, immunofluorescence, and electron microscopy, each providing some important information.

Indications for biopsy vary but may include the following:

- Acute nephritic syndrome, when due to a suspected systemic disease in which renal biopsy can make the diagnosis and guide treatment. However, many conditions, such as microscopic polyangiitis, Wegener's granulomatosis, and anti-glomerular basement membrane (GBM) disease, need urgent treatment before a biopsy diagnosis is made. Hence, treatment may be started on the basis of additional clinical or laboratory evidence of disease.

- Suspected lupus nephritis, with acute renal insufficiency and active sediment to help determine the prognosis and guide therapy. Repeat biopsy may be needed after treatment or during a flare to distinguish active lupus from other causes.

- Biopsies of transplanted kidneys are performed for changes in renal function to look for rejection, infection, recurrent disease, and the degree of scarring in the appropriate clinical scenario.

- In general, there is no important reason to do renal biopsies for isolated asymptomatic glomerular hematuria and isolated nonnephritic proteinuria.

Relative contraindications that may increase the patient's risk/benefit ratio include:

- Small, hyperechoic kidneys suggestive of chronic irreversible disease.

- A solitary native kidney (complications of biopsy can cause loss of all remaining renal function).

- Multiple renal cysts.

- Uncontrollable bleeding diathesis.

- Uncontrollable hypertension.

- Hydronephrosis.

- Active renal infection.

Complications can include:

- Bleeding is the main complication and can occur (1) under the renal capsule, leading to painful tamponade, (2) in the collecting system, leading to hematuria, and (3) into the perinephric space, leading to hematoma. Most bleeding occurs within 24 hours after the procedure.
  - Microscopic bleeding is seen in almost all patients.
  - Macroscopic bleeding is seen in roughly 10% of patients.
  - Intrarenal arteriovenous fistula formation is seen in up to 15%.

- A decrease in hemoglobin level of 1 g/dL postprocedure is not unexpected.

- A transjugular renal biopsy can be done to reduce the risk of perinephric bleeding in select patients.

Table 4-4. Commonly Used Renal Imaging Modalities

Modality	Common Uses

Renal Ultrasound	• Most commonly used radiographic screening tool for kidneys and the rest of the genitourinary (GU) system
	• No exposure to radiation or contrast
	• Detects size and location of kidney
	  • Most kidneys measure 9–12 cm
	    • Large kidneys may indicate acute inflammation
	    • Small kidneys imply a chronic, fibrotic process
	      • Echogenecity implies chronicity and irreversibility
	    • Asymmetric kidney size (>1.5-cm difference) implies a local lesion, perhaps unilateral renal artery stenosis; evaluate further
	      • Doppler evaluation of arteries can show increased resistive index
	• Sensitive for obstruction (hydronephrosis) and can often localize the lesion
	  • Bilateral vs. unilateral; evaluates for urinary bladder distension
	• Useful to detect and characterize lesions 1 cm or greater
	  • Able to distinguish between simple cysts and complex lesions requiring further investigation
	  • Can detect ureteral or perinephric fluid collections (such as abscesses)
	• Can detect nephrolithiasis, but CT is more sensitive
	• Useful to localize the kidney in real time for increased safety in biopsy

Plain Film of the Abdomen (KUB)	• Limited role in evaluation of kidney disease • May detect calcium-containing stones; sometimes can visualize struvite or cysteine stones • Uric acid stones are radiolucent and require CT for evaluation • Lucency or lack thereof may give clues to the composition of the stone

CT Scanning	• *Noncontrast* helical scanning ("stone protocol") is the gold standard to detect renal and ureteral stones
	• Contrast studies are the next step in evaluation of complex lesions found on screening ultrasound
	  • Sensitive in the detection of renal cell carcinoma
	• CT angiography may detect renal artery stenosis and/or renal vein thrombosis
	• Able to detect hydronephrosis but less informative regarding chronicity compared to ultrasound
	  • Can detect level of ureteronephrosis more precisely than ultrasound

MRI	• Magnetic resonance angiography (MRA) increasing in favor as first-line evaluation for renovascular disease • More useful for atherosclerotic disease; less useful for fibromuscular disease • Useful adjunct in radiographic evaluation of renal cell carcinoma • Controversy remains regarding use of gadolinium contrast in patients with reduced GFR and risks of nephrogenic systemic fibrosis; practice at present is to avoid gadolinium exposure except under guidance of nephrologists
Intravenous Pyelogram (IVP)	• Able to detect gross abnormalities in renal, ureteral, and bladder anatomy • Relatively contraindicated in patients with reduced GFR because of increased risk of contrast nephropathy and relatively poor image quality (contrast uptake is GFR-dependent) • Intravenous pyelography (IVP) less commonly used now but can be the imaging modality of choice for acute stones, as it is often both diagnostic and therapeutic

Radionuclide Scanning	• Used primarily to assess renal function instead of anatomy
	• Injection of radionuclide with gamma scanning over both kidneys:
	  • Technetium-based agents most often used for GFR evaluation
	    • Filtered, not reabsorbed
	  • Hippuran scan evaluates renal blood flow
	    • Secreted into the tubules
	• Delay in elimination can be caused by parenchymal disease or obstruction, evaluated by furosemide administration
	  • Furosemide does not augment elimination in cases of obstruction
	• Captopril can be used to assess for dynamic renal artery stenosis
	  • Much less sensitive than newer CT and MRA exams
	• Useful in differentiation of function between kidneys
	  • Predicts the effects of unilateral nephrectomy on overall GFR
	• Can be used to differentiate perfusion defects, tubular dysfunction, and obstruction in kidney transplants with postoperative delayed graft function

Table 4-5. Differentiation Between Forms of Renal Dialysis

	Peritoneal Dialysis (PD)	Intermittent Hemodialysis (HD)	Continuous HD
Description	Dialysate fluid (usually a concentrated glucose solution) is instilled into the patient's peritoneum and removed after an equilibration period. Waste and excess fluid are removed, mainly by an osmotic and oncotic gradient across the peritoneal membrane between splanchnic circulation and the peritoneum.	The patient's blood is run through an artificial membrane that filters waste and regulates electrolytes before returning it to the patient. Transmembrane pressures can be altered independently of dialysis to remove excess plasma volume (called *ultrafiltration*).	Similar to HD except done continuously at a slower blood flow to reduce significant fluid shifts. This is particularly useful in patients who are already hemodynamically unstable and unlikely to tolerate intermittent HD. As in intermittent HD, waste removal and volume removal can be independently adjusted.
Common Regimens	• *Continuous/Ambulatory (CAPD):* Regularly scheduled exchanges at prescribed times. • *Automated (APD):* Exchanges performed with a "cycler" machine. • *Nocturnal/Intermittent (NIPD):* Machine exchanges occur only at night, with patient "dry" during waking hours. *Note:* Most outpatient regimens are hybrids of these models, tailored to the patient.	*Inpatient:* Sessions are 2–4 hours, three to seven times weekly at the nephrologist's discretion. *Outpatient:* At HD centers, usually three times weekly for 3–4 hours per session. Some patients perform daily dialysis at home.	Continuous dialysis for patients in a hospital setting, almost always in an ICU.
Access	Surgically placed, tunneled peritoneal catheter. Can be used immediately, but ideally one should wait 2 weeks for the catheter to stabilize in the skin tunnel.	• AV shunt, usually in an upper extremity. Either surgically created fistula or a plastic implant (graft). These take several weeks to mature. OR • Large-bore double-lumen central venous catheter (preferably jugular or femoral). Catheters can be made permanent by creating a tunnel through the skin.	Catheters are preferred even in patients who already have arteriovenous shunts, to avoid patient and health care worker safety issues that are associated with long-term cannulation (e.g. decannulation, needle injuries, and vascular damage).
Advantages	• Gentler form of dialysis for chronically hypotensive patients (e.g., those with CHF). • Patient-centered therapy that allows patient to maintain a normal lifestyle and dialyze at home. • Avoids indwelling vascular access.	• Most efficient form of dialysis; considered the gold standard. • Able to titrate solute clearance and volume removal independently.	• Best option for hemodynamically unstable patients. • Continuous nature allows greater ultrafiltration on a daily basis (such as in decompensated cirrhosis or CHF).

continued

Table 4-5. *(continued)*

	Peritoneal Dialysis (PD)	Intermittent Hemodialysis (HD)	Continuous HD
Disadvantages	• Volume removal and solute clearance cannot be titrated independently. • Less efficient than HD; requires some residual function. Many patients eventually convert to HD as residual function fades. • Requires patient or caretaker to take on significant responsibility. • Previous abdominal surgery is a relative contraindication.	• Requires indwelling vascular access; catheter-related bacteremia has significant morbidity and mortality. • AV shunts require 2–4 weeks or longer to mature after placement. • In-center HD requires a large time commitment.	• Costly; requires intensive nursing care and laboratory monitoring. • Continuous nature limits patient mobility.
Complications	• Peritonitis (rarely life-threatening). • Hyperglycemia. • Hypoalbuminemia. • Pleural effusions related to ascites.	• Access infections (catheter-related bacteremia can be fatal). • Hypotension. • Access-related bleeding or clot. • Hemolysis (rare). • Allergic reactions to membrane (rare).	• Similar to HD.

APPROACH TO COMMON PROBLEMS

Approach to the Hypovolemic Patient

Hypovolemia is defined by a decrease in total body water, but patients are generally symptomatic only when this results in a low circulating plasma volume. In dealing with a patient with a disorder of body volume, it is important to keep in mind the following proportions:

• Total body water (TBW) is considered to be approximately 60% of weight in men and 50% of weight in women (see Figure 4-4).

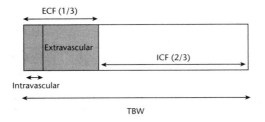

Figure 4-4. Distribution of Total Body Water. ECF, extracellular fluid; TBW, total body water.

• Two-thirds of TBW is in the intracellular fluid (ICF) compartment and one-third is extracellular fluid (ECF).
• Of the ECF, three-quarters of water is extravascular (interstitial) and one-quarter is intravascular (in plasma).
• Therefore, 1/12th of TBW is intravascular.

In the hypovolemic patient, the history, exam, and laboratory tests may show the following classic signs:

• Thirst.
• Dry mucous membranes.
• Flat neck veins.
• Tachycardia.
• Poor skin turgor (takes longer than usual for pinched skin on the dorsum of the hand to resume its flattened shape).
• Decreased urine output as the kidneys try to conserve water.
• Rapid weight loss in a patient over a few days is typical of water loss, as it is hard to lose weight rapidly in any other fashion.
• Orthostatic hypotension (measure blood pressure and pulse with the patient supine

and then after 2 minutes with the patient standing; in general, blood pressure will drop >20 mmHg or the pulse will increase >20 bpm).

- High BUN/Cr ratio and increased hematocrit due to hemoconcentration.

In approaching the possible causes, consider the broad categories of the differential diagnosis in the work-up:

- Renal causes—diuretics, diabetes mellitus or diabetes insipidus (both with polyuria), adrenal insufficiency.
- Extracellular fluid sequestration—burns, pancreatitis, peritonitis, conditions causing extravasation of fluid out of the vasculature and into the interstitium (third spacing) and a lower circulating plasma volume.
- Gastrointestinal losses—vomiting, diarrhea.
- Vascular—hemorrhage.
- Other insensible losses—sweating, fever, intense exercise, increased breathing. These are typically more subacute than acute.

Treatment depends on the acuity and severity of the condition. For instance, unstable patients who are hemorrhaging need immediate fluid resuscitation. Those who are stable need only replacement and maintenance fluids. Generally, one would correct the underlying cause and provide fluid replacement with approximation of the water deficit, which is equal to $0.6 \times \text{Weight} \times [([\text{Na}^+] / 140) - 1]$. Pressors are used in severe cases. Table 4-6 describes common resuscitation and maintenance fluids.

Note the following:

- Common maintenance fluids are D_5NS or D_5 ½NS since glucose should be given to prevent muscle breakdown in patients who are NPO; 20 to 40 mEq K^+ is also added in most cases. However, boluses of fluid should never have K^+ because of the potential for hyperkalemia.
- The rate of infusion for maintenance in someone who is NPO is calculated using the 4 2 1 rule: Give 4 mL/kg for the first 10 kg, 2 mL/kg for the next 10 kg, and 1 mL/kg for every kilogram thereafter. Thus, a 70-kg man would require 110 mL/hr for maintenance: (40 + 20 + 50) mL/hr.

Approach to the Hypervolemic Patient

Hypervolemia is defined as an increase in total body water that is generally driven by abnormal salt balance rather than problems with water homeostasis. In some patients, TBW can be increased and, at the same time, intravascular volume can be decreased because of excess fluid loss from the vasculature into the interstitium, known as *third spacing*. This perpetuates ongoing mechanisms to retain more sodium and

Table 4-6. Fluid Resuscitation and Maintenance

Common IV Solutions	Components	Common Uses
Lactated Ringer's (LR)	130 mEq Na^+ 110 mEq Cl 28 mEq lactate 4 mEq K^+ 3 mEq Ca^{2+}	Fluid resuscitation in trauma. Cannot be used as a maintenance fluid because lactate is converted to HCO_3^- and the patient would become alkalotic. Helps buffer blood if acidosis is present.
Normal Saline (NS)	154 mEq Na^+, 154 mEq Cl	Isotonic to body fluids. Can also be used as acute rehydration solution.
½ NS	77 mEq Na^+, 77 mEq Cl	More commonly used for acute rehydration in patients with hyperchloremic metabolic acidosis and as IV fluid in children.
¼ NS	39 mEq Na^+, 39 mEq Cl	D5 ¼ NS is a common pediatric maintenance fluid.
D_5W	5 g dextrose (50 g) in 1 L of water	Isotonic. Sugar helps prevent muscle breakdown. Also commonly used to replace free water deficits.

water, increasing the circulating intravascular volume.

Clues to hypervolemia on exam are better viewed as a constellation since each individual symptom is not by itself definitive. In fact, sometimes one cannot easily determine the patient's volume status. Therefore, for the purpose of careful monitoring, a right heart catheter can be used to measure central venous pressure and pulmonary capillary wedge pressure (see Chapter 2):

Pulmonary: shortness of breath, dyspnea on exertion (DOE), orthopnea, bilateral inspiratory crackles, evidence of pulmonary edema or pleural effusions on chest X-ray.

Cardiovascular: elevated JVP, S_3, lower extremity pitting edema, elevated blood pressure.

Gastrointestinal: enlarged liver (from congestion), ascites, sacral edema.

Extremities: pitting edema, anasarca.

Other: marked weight gain over a short period of time.

The main mechanisms to think of in the differential diagnosis in such patients should include:

- Excessive intravenous (IV) fluid (in hospitalized patients).
- Heart failure.
- Nephrotic syndrome.
- Cirrhosis with portal hypertension.
- Renal failure—acute or chronic.
- Hypoproteinemia.

Treatment depends on the underlying causes. Diuresis with medication is usually the first line of treatment for most causes, though it is harder to perform in patients with elevated creatinine (Cr) or low albumin; in these cases, dialysis can be used acutely if the condition is severe. It also must be used with caution, as it can cause hypotension in patients with significantly low intravascular volume.

Therapeutic paracentesis may be helpful in certain causes of ascites (see Chapter 5), and therapeutic thoracentesis may be necessary in patients with large pleural effusions.

The method of diuresis varies, but for an acute presentation of hypervolemia in a patient with CHF, for example, with preserved renal function, keep doubling the IV furosemide dose every hour until adequate urine output occurs. For patients refractory to diuresis, a thiazide such as metolazone can be added one-half hour before the next furosemide dose. It blocks distal sodium resorption and allows for more diuresis even though normally thiazides work poorly at a high glomerular filtration rate (GFR). For patients with ascites from cirrhosis, spironolactone is the diuretic of choice. The uses of different diuretics are described in Table 4-7.

Approach to Acid-Base Disorders

These are conditions in which the body's normal acid-base balance is disrupted. They may be acute or chronic and with or without appropriate compensation. Multiple acid-base disorders can also occur together.

By definition, serum pH <7.4 constitutes *acidemia*; the term *acidosis* refers to processes that decrease pH. Similarly, serum pH >7.4 constitutes *alkalemia*, and *alkalosis* refers to processes that increase pH.

There are four major categories with the following characteristics, as shown in Table 4-8.

Combinations of disorders are common. The following five-step algorithm can be used to determine all the acid-base disorders that are present in a clinical scenario.

Step 1: Is the patient alkalemic (pH >7.45) or acidemic (pH <7.35)? A normal blood pH is between 7.35 and 7.45.

Step 2: What is at least one primary disorder? (See the chart in Figure 4-5.) Check the bicarbonate level first to determine if there is a metabolic process. Then look at the CO_2 level to see if there is a respiratory process. You may find two processes here if there is a mixed condition [for instance, with a low pH, a low bicarbonate level (metabolic acidosis) and a low CO_2 level (respiratory alkalosis) would be a mixed condition].

Table 4-7.   Characteristics and Uses of Common Diuretics

Agent	Mechanism	Uses
Carbonic Anhydrase Inhibitors Acetazolamide	Inhibits the activity of carbonic anhydrase, which causes both NaCl and $NaHCO_3$ loss. A net diuresis does not occur, as excess fluid and ions are reabsorbed in more distal segments.	Not used for diuresis in general, but can be used to alkalinize the urine and counter contraction alkalosis.
Loop Diuretics Furosemide Bumetanide Toresemide Ethacrynic acid	Competes for the chloride site on the Na-K-2Cl carrier in the TALH and decreases net Na^+ reabsorption. This also leads to decrease in paracellular Ca^{2+} absorption that depends on this gradient, causing increased calciuria. At the maximum dose, can lead to excretion of 20–25% of filtered sodium at the peak response.	Useful for almost all edematous states where fluid removal is the primary concern.
Thiazide Diuretics Chlorothiazide Hydrochlorothiazide Chlorthalidone Indapamide Metolazone	Inhibits the Na-Cl cotransporter in the distal tubule and at maximum dosage inhibits reabsorption of 3–5% of filtered Na^+. By an independent mechanism, these diuretics are able to increase the reabsorption of calcium as well.	Less useful in edematous states; better used for hypertension where marked fluid loss is not necessary. Useful in the treatment of kidney stones.
Potassium-Sparing Diuretics Amiloride Spironolactone Triamterene Eplerenone	Amiloride and triamterene act directly to inhibit the aldosterone-sensitive Na^+ channels in the collecting tubule. Potassium which normally leaves cells to balance the lumen's negative charge created by reabsorbed Na^+, is not excreted when these drugs are used. Spironolactone competitively inhibits aldosterone. Eplerenone is a newer agent that does not have the estrogen-like side effects of spironolactone.	Leads to maximal excretion of 1 to 2% of the filtered Na^+. Used with a loop or thiazide diuretic commonly in refractory edema. Spironolactone is especially useful for ascites in cirrhosis, in part because, unlike most diuretics, it does not require renal delivery to the sites of action (which are impaired in many edema-associated diseases).
Osmotic Diuretic Mannitol	A nonabsorbable polysaccharide that inhibits salt and water.	Produces a relative free water diuresis. Used in postischemic acute renal failure to prevent progression to ATN.

Table 4-8.   Types of Primary Acid-Base Disorders

Condition	pH (7.40)	$PaCO_2$ (40 mmHg)	HCO_3^- (24 mEq/L)
Metabolic Acidosis	Low	Normal to low	Low
Respiratory Acidosis	Low	High	Normal to high
Respiratory Alkalosis	High	Low	Normal to low
Metabolic Alkalosis	High	Normal to low	High

Note: Normal reference values are in parentheses.

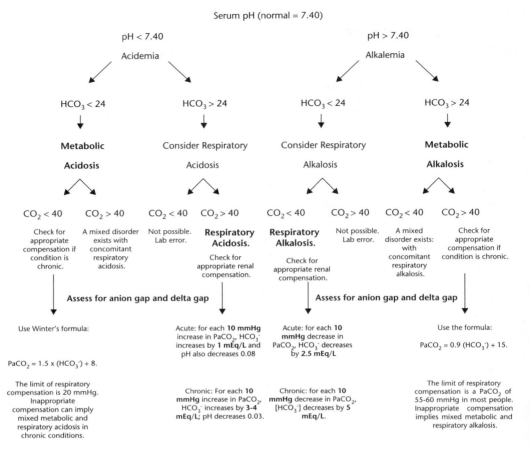

Figure 4-5. Process for Determining Primary and Secondary Acid Base Disorders.

Step 3: Calculate the anion gap [(Sodium) – (Bicarbonate + Chloride)]. This is always useful even if the pH is elevated; if there is a gap, you have found an underlying metabolic acidosis that is being masked. Stop here if you have already found three acid-base disturbances.

Step 4: Calculate the Δ-gap to see if another nongap acidosis or metabolic alkalosis is present (see the section on Metabolic Acidosis). The Δ-gap = Anion Gap – 12 + HCO_3. (It is 24 if all of the acidosis is from a decrease in the body's HCO_3^-.) If the Δ-gap is >31, a metabolic alkalosis also present. If it is <21, a nonanion gap acidosis is also present.

Step 5: If necessary, look for appropriate compensation using the formulas shown in Figure 4-5.

The work-up and treatment of various disorders are described elsewhere in this chapter.

Be sure to keep in mind the following rules while going through the steps:

Rule 1: A gap metabolic acidosis is always considered a primary process.

Rule 2: You cannot overcompensate for a primary process with a secondary process and overcorrect the pH.

Rule 3: You cannot have more than three acid-base disorders at the same time; so, if you find three, then you can stop looking for more.

Rule 4: Occasionally, two primary processes can occur simultaneously. An example of this would be a primary respiratory alkalosis occurring concurrently with a primary anion gap metabolic acidosis. Such conditions include early sepsis and salicylate toxicity, in which the pH is alkalemic from respiratory alkalosis but a substantial anion gap acidosis also exists.

The Approach to Acute Kidney Injury or Acute Renal Failure

Acute renal failure is a condition of rapidly increasing azotemia, defined as:

- Rapid increase in blood urea nitrogen (BUN) or Cr over baseline.
- Decrease in GFR of over 50% within days to weeks. (Remember that the serum Cr is inversely related to the GFR, so a doubling of Cr (1.0 → 2.0) means that GFR is cut in half.)

Renal failure can be either prerenal, renal, or postrenal. Table 4-9A shows how to distinguish them by cause and mechanism.

Work-up

When the cause is unclear by history and exam, look at the panel 7, order a urinalysis (U/A), fractional excretion of sodium (FENa*), and urine osmolality, consider placement of a Foley catheter, and obtain a renal ultrasound looking for hydronephrosis. A trial of IV fluid is helpful if prerenal failure is suspected and volume overload is not a concern. Table 4-9B shows the diagnostic work-up and treatment.

Table 4-9A. Characteristics of Different Forms of Renal Failure

	Prerenal	Renal	Postrenal
Mechanism	Caused by poor perfusion to the kidney or a relatively low effective arterial blood volume (EABV) state.	Caused by direct damage to the renal parenchyma.	Occurs from an obstruction after renal filtration has already occurred.
Causes	1. Volume loss: hypovolemia from diuretics (most common), bleeding: GI loss: emesis and diarrhea; other insensible water losses. 2. Effective low-flow states: heart failure, liver failure with poor forward flow. 3. Shock/sepsis.	1. Acute tubular necrosis (ATN) from prolonged prerenal ischemia or the toxins of sepsis. 2. Acute interstitial nephritis (AIN) from direct toxicity or hypersensitivity to drugs (commonly amphotericin B, aminoglycosides, radiocontrast dyes, penicillin, sulfonamides, NSAIDs, and diuretics) or infectious pyelonephritis. 3. Vascular causes: hypertension, vasculitis, cholesterol embolism, TTP/HUS, thrombosis of the renal artery or vein. 4. Glomerular causes: postinfectious GN, SLE, IgA nephropathy, infiltrative disorders, rapidly progressive GN, Goodpasture's disease, and many other causes of intrinsic renal disease.	1. Obstruction secondary to benign prostatic hyperplasia (BPH) is the most common cause. 2. Renal calculi. 3. Bladder/pelvic tumors. 4. Neurogenic bladder/ chronic Foley obstruction.
Prevalence	50%–70% of acute renal failure cases.	25%–40% of acute renal failure cases.	5%–10% of acute renal failure cases.
SiSx	Patient looks hypovolemic. May have orthostatic hypotension, tachycardia, reduced JVP, dry mucous membranes, and/or decreased skin turgor on exam.	Quite variable, depending on the cause. One may see signs of volume overload with oliguria and arrhythmias such as those resulting from electrolyte imbalances. Otherwise, the patient may be asymptomatic.	Abdominal pain (from renal calculi), history of frequent urination in small amounts (BPH), prolonged period of decreased urine output. A full bladder may be percussed.

Table 4-9B.   Diagnosis and Treatment of Different Forms of Renal Failure

	Prerenal	Renal	Postrenal
BUN:Cr*	>20:1	<10:1 (Cr increased more than BUN)	>15:1
Urine Osmolality	High, >500 mOsm/kg	Low, <350 mOsm/kg	<350 mOsm/kg
Urine Na+	<20 mEq/L Low because kidney retains Na+ to increase total body water.	>20 mEq/L High because Na+ is not reabsorbed properly in the damaged kidney.	>40 mEq/L
FENa†	<1%	>1%	>4%
Urinalysis	Normal or some hyaline casts, as tubular and glomerular functions are still intact.	The following are almost pathognomonic: 1. ATN—muddy brown casts with tubular epithelial cells, granular casts. 2. AIN—white cell casts, lymphocytes, eosinophils. 3. GN—RBC casts. 4. Antibiotic/drug induced allergic interstitial nephritis-eosinophiluria.	Hematuria with stones or pyuria with bladder infection may be seen. Urinalysis shows a trace or no protein and possibly crystals with certain stones.
Renal Ultrasound	No abnormality.	No abnormality. (Though echogenic, small kidneys, if seen, hint at underlying intrinsic renal disease, which is useful in diagnosing a first-time patient whose baseline Cr level is unknown.)	Renal ultrasound may show hydronephrosis but is only 80–85% sensitive for this condition. False negatives occur with acute obstruction, for retroperitoneal fibrosis, and in patients with hypovolemia. Spiral CT can be used to rule out urolithiasis but cannot detect indinavir calculi. IVP may also be useful.
Treatment	Trial of IV fluid or volume resuscitation to see if Cr improves in appropriate cases. Treat the underlying cause (i.e., severe heart failure or sepsis will require pressors), if known.	IV fluid will not change the course of the condition unless there was some component of prolonged prerenal azotemia initially. Finding and treating the underlying cause is the only method.	Placement of a Foley catheter if no GU trauma is suspected may reveal a large amount of fluid in certain cases. A bladder scan can also be useful in patients who are oliguric. Postobstructive diuresis will occur after obstruction is relieved. Patients with infection and obstruction have a medical emergency, and a urologist should be consulted to prevent urosepsis. The chance for recovery is inversely related to the duration of obstruction.

*Beware of things that can change the BUN/Cr ratio:
Artificially low: increased Cr from rhabdomyolysis. Cimetidine or TMP-SMX inhibits renal creatinine excretion so value is higher in the serum. Malnutrition causes a negative nitrogen balance and therefore, decreased BUN. *Artificially high:* increased protein intake increases BUN. This is also seen with steroid use, malnutrition, and cachexia which are all associated with breakdown of protein and thereby increases BUN.
†FENa [$(U_{Na}/P_{Na})/(U_{Cr}/P_{Cr}) \times 100\%$] gives the fractional excretion of sodium and is a way to correct the urine sodium level based on using the excretion of Cr as a correction factor. Note that if the patient is receiving diuretics or has preexisting chronic kidney disease, the calculation will not be very accurate. In such cases, one can use values for urea, a nonidiogenic osmole, instead of sodium (though this is rarely done). Substitute the urine urea and plasma BUN in the equation above. Values less than 35% suggest a prerenal state.

DISEASES OF NEPHROLOGY

Disorders of Water and Electrolyte Balance

Hyponatremia

D—Serum [Na^+] <135 mEq/L; <120 mEq/L is considered severe. Acute onset is a decrease seen in less than 36 hours. This disorder is due to water homeostasis problems rather than sodium balance problems. Total body sodium can be high, low, or normal in cases of *hyponatremia*, a term that refers only to the serum concentration.

Epi—Hyponatremia is the most common electrolyte abnormality in hospitalized patients. There is markedly increased mortality when it is seen in heart failure patients and those with end-stage liver disease.

P—More than 95% of total body sodium is extracellular. Causes of sodium loss include (1) diuretics (thiazide more than loop diuretics); (2) CHF, nephrotic syndrome, or cirrhosis, all of which cause decreased GFR and, subsequently, reduced water excretion and increased proximal convoluted tubule (PCT) sodium resorption during renal hypoperfusion; and (3) CNS trauma or medications that cause the system of inappropriate antidiuretic hormone (SIADH; see below).

SiSx—Symptoms include a change in mental status (ΔMS), seizures (if the hyponatremia develops rapidly), obtundation, coma, and even death. Muscle twitching may occur. Cheyne-Stokes breathing can be seen in severe cases of hyponatremia, where there is an alternating rapid and shallow rate of breathing.

Dx—

1. First, establish the volume status (hypervolemic, euvolemic, hypovolemic) based on the exam. Then check serum osmolality [to rule out pseudohyponatremia, as seen in hyperlipidemia, hyperglycemia, mannitol, or intravenous immune globulin (IVIG) with concomitant renal failure]. A correction for sodium in hyperglycemia is 1.6 mEq/L added for every 100 mg/dL of glucose above 200 mg/dL.

2. Calculate the osmolar gap = [Measured Serum Osmolality] – [Calculated Serum Osmolality]. The calculated serum osmolality = 2[Na^+] + [Glucose]/18 + BUN/2.8. The osmolar gap should be no more than 10 mOsm/kg, as normal osmolality is

Table 4-10. Causes and Treatment of Hyponatremia by Volume Status

Hypovolemic		Euvolemic	Hypervolemic	
U_{Na}>20 mEq/L	U_{Na}<20 mEq/L	U_{Na}>20 mEq/L in almost all cases	U_{Na}>20 mEq/L	U_{Na}<20 mEq/L
Implies renal losses: RTA, diuretics, adrenal insufficiency, salt-losing nephropathy.	Implies extrarenal losses: vomiting, diarrhea, third spacing from some other cause.	SIADH, psychogenic polydipsia, hypothyroidism, pseudohyponatremia (high lipid/protein or isotonic infusions).	Implies inappropriate renal losses, as in acute renal failure or chronic kidney disease.	Cirrhosis, nephrotic syndrome, CHF. In these conditions, the kidney tries to retain Na^+.
*Volume replete.	*Volume replete.	Restrict water and/or use demeclocyline (ADH inhibitor). Correct lipid and protein levels.	Diuretics.	Diuretics, fluid restriction.

*For volume repletion, the amount of water to replete is (Normal Na^+ – Current Na^+) $\times$ TBW.
Rapid correction is indicated in a patient with CNS symptoms; otherwise, slower correction is recommended to avoid central pontine myelinosis, a demyelinating condition of the pons that can involve acute progressive quadriplegia, dysphagia, and dysarthria along with changes in mental status. A rate of no more than 0.5 mEq/L/hr up to 12 mEq/day has generally been accepted. Acute changes in sodium lead to less osmole depletion in the brain and can generally be correctly more quickly. Hypertonic saline should be used with caution. It is indicated for severe CNS symptoms and in case of severe SIADH and cerebral salt wasting (*renal salt-wasting syndrome*).

285–295 mOsm/kg. If the measured value is hyperosmotic and the gap is >10, there are extra osmoles that must be accounted for. These are usually due to hyperglycemia or hypertonic infusions.

3. The other causes of hyponatremia are generally hypoosmotic. Urinary sodium determination is important because it establishes whether the cause is renal (>20 mEq/L) or extrarenal (<20 mEq/L when the kidney is working and wants to retain sodium for the body).

Tx—Treatment depends on the cause. See Table 4-10.

Hypernatremia

D—Serum [Na^+] >145 mEq/L.

P—All forms are associated with hypertonicity. There is no such condition as pseudohypernatremia. Causes include decreased fluid intake; increased water loss (excess sweating, burns); GI losses such as diarrhea and vomiting; excess osmotic diuresis with mannitol, high blood sugar where water losses >Na^+ losses; diseases causing nephrogenic diabetes insipidus (NDI) or central diabetes insipidus (CDI). Of note, hypertonicity is the main cause of secretion of ADH; therefore, ADH levels will be high in most patients without CDI.

SiSx—Symptoms include CNS depression, obtundation, coma, and seizures mostly in the young and old. Shrinking of brain volume can cause hemorrhage. Either polyuria or decreased renal output may be seen, depending on the cause.

Dx—Assess the volume status and use the guidelines in Table 4-11. Water deprivation tests and measurement of serum ADH may be useful. Urine Na^+ is also a helpful determinant, as in hyponatremia, to distinguish renal from extrarenal causes.

Tx—Treatment depends on the etiology. See Table 4-11 and the discussion of individual diseases presented elsewhere in this chapter.

Hypokalemia

D—Serum [K^+] <3.5 mEq/L.

P—Causes can be divided into two categories:
Renal
    Drugs: K^+-wasting diuretics (loop and thiazide), penicillin, amphotericin B; trimethoprim-sulfamethoxazole (TMP-SMX).
    Acute tubular necrosis (ATN).

Table 4-11. Causes and Treatment of Hypernatremia by Volume Status

Hypovolemic (Loss of water exceeds Na^+ loss)		Euvolemic (Free water loss)		Hypervolemic (Gain of water and Na^+)
U_{Na} >20 mEq/L	U_{Na} <10 mEq/L	U_{Na} <20 mEq/L	U_{Na} >20 mEq/L	Na^+ gain is the cause. Urine Na^+ invariably is >20 mEq/L.
Implies renal losses: loop/osmotic diuretic, glycosuria, postobstructive diuresis, intrinsic renal disease.	Implies extrarenal losses: vomiting, diarrhea, burns, fistulas.	Implies a renal cause: NDI, CDI, hypodipsia.	Implies an extrarenal cause: insensible losses (skin or respiratory loss).	Hypertonic solution administration, NaCl tablets. Primary hyperaldosteronism, Cushing's disease, congenital adrenal hyperplasia. Hypertonic dialysis—HD or PD.
Treatment is to give saline and hypotonic solutions thereafter since it is necessary to replete water and total body sodium.		Treatment is to administer free water PO or IV to correct level of Na^+ no faster than 0.5 mEq/hr.		Treatment is diuresis and/or dialysis.

Hypomagnesemia.

Renal tubular acidoses (RTAs) or any type of mineralocorticoid excess.

Vomiting (renal loss due to negative charge from excess bicarbonate in the collecting tubule lumen, secondary intravascular volume depletion, and hyperaldosteronism).

Extrarenal

Cellular redistribution, as seen in acute metabolic alkalosis (extracellular potassium exchanges for intracellular hydrogen), insulin effect, β agonists, which all shift K^+ into cells.

Diarrhea (GI loss can be high).

Decreased dietary intake (rare).

SiSx—Many are asymptomatic. In those with symptoms you may see:

Neuromuscular—weakness, paralysis, hyporeflexia.

Gastrointestinal—ileus.

Renal—polyuria, polydipsia.

Cardiac—T wave flattening and inversion, presence of u wave after T wave, ST depression.

Dx—First, determine if the patient is hypertensive and if serum sodium is elevated, pointing possibly to mineralocorticoid excess. If not, consider GI or renal losses. Consider RTA if the patient is acidotic. If urine K^+ is <20 mEq/L, this suggests extrarenal losses; levels >30 mEq/L suggest renal loses. A renin aldo stimulation test can also be done to look for hyperaldosteronism. An elevated urine Cl^- suggests GI-related K^+ losses.

Tx—Giving K^+ is the mainstay if therapy while trying to correct the underlying cause. Attempt to correct the acidosis with sodium bicarbonate ($NaHCO_3$) if it is severe (pH <7.2). Give IV KCl if the patient cannot take anything by mouth. An oral dose of 10 mEq KCl increases the serum $[K^+]$ by 0.1 mEq/L if the patient has normal GFR. Also, be sure to replete Mg^{2+} along with K^+; otherwise, the hypokalemia will be difficult to correct (the mechanism of action is unclear). Care should be taken in treating patients with significant kidney disease, as they may quickly become hyperkalemic.

Hyperkalemia

D—Serum $[K^+]$ >5.0 mEq/L.

P—It is most commonly seen in the following circumstances:

1. Decreased excretion—K^+-sparing diuretics (spironolactone, amiloride, triamterene), RTA-type IV, chronic kidney disease, NSAIDs, ACE inhibitors, mineralocorticoid deficiency or resistance.

2. Redistribution—acute metabolic acidosis (intracellular K^+ exchanges for H^+ ions in the serum), insulin deficiency.

3. Release from inside dying cells—tissue necrosis or hemolysis, rhabdomyolysis, and burns.

4. Excessive potassium intake or replacement.

5. Pseudohyperkalemia—test tube hemolysis, blood draw from an ischemic area.

SiSx—

Neuromuscular—weakness is a common complaint; paresthesias occur.

Cardiac—Symptoms usually occur with K^+ >6 mEq/L. The ECG shows peaked T waves, a wide QRS, flattened P waves, and a long PR interval. Ventricular fibrillation, ventricular tachycardia, severe bradycardia, and even asystole are possible.

Dx—Eliminate pseudohyperkalemia as the cause due to lysis of cells or platelets. This is a common occurrence and can be evaluated just by looking at the blood sample in the tube, so be sure to ask the laboratory. Consider newly started medications as a cause, and check the acid-base status. If the cause is not clear, calculate the *transtubular potassium gradient* using the formula [Urine K^+ / Plasma K^+]/[Urine osms/Plasma osms]. If the ratio is <8, renal K^+ secretion is impaired.

Tx—Stop using the offending agent if one is found. Acutely, however, severe hyperkalemia needs to be treated. Always check the ECG if K^+ >6 mEq/L or the patient has an arrhythmia. If ECG changes are noted, then acutely give:

1. Calcium gluconate 1 amp or 10–30 mL of 10% solution. This is thought to perhaps prevent potential cardiac complications.

2. Five to ten units of regular insulin IV with 1 amp D50 to shift K^+ into cells.

3. β agonists, which shift K^+ into cells.
4. Also, possibly give 50 mEq HCO_3^-; this therapy is controversial, but it is useful if the patient is also acidotic (pH <7.2).
5. Dialysis, if necessary, and when K^+ needs to be lowered quickly, especially in a patient with renal failure.

Then, to keep the K^+ concentration low and prevent redistribution, give:

1. Give 15–30 g of sodium polystyrene sulfate (Kayexalate), which is necessary for long-term removal of K^+; otherwise, K^+ will reaccumulate.
2. Diuretics—furosemide or acetazolamide to further remove K^+ from the urine. Dialysis is a powerful tool to reduce serum and total body potassium and is most often used in patients with advanced kidney disease.

Hypocalcemia

D—An ionized calcium <4.65 mg/dL or <1.1 mmol/L. Total Ca^{2+} is influenced by the acid-base status and the protein concentration. But if these are normal, <8.5 mg/dL is indicative of hypocalcemia. The correction factor is a 0.8 mg/dL increase for each 1 g/dL decrease in serum albumin below 4 g/dL.

P—Causes include low parathyroid hormone (PTH); vitamin D deficiency; Mg^{2+} deficiency (prevents peripheral PTH action, as may be seen in alcoholics); pseudohypoparathyroidism; severe bone diseases; rhabdomyolysis, tumor lysis syndrome; calcium chelation; hypothyroidism; and sepsis.

SiSx—

Cardiac—hypotension, long QT interval, T wave inversion.

Pulmonary—bronchospasm.

CNS/musculoskeletal—weakness, muscle spasm/tetany, *Chvostek's sign* (tapping on the facial nerve area in front of the ear elicits a twitch) and *Trousseau's sign* (inflating a blood pressure cuff elicits twitching in the arm), hyperreflexia, anxiety, and depression.

Dx—Diagnosis is made by the laboratory values for ionized or total Ca^{2+} with correction for albumin and acid-base status.

Tx—Treatment consists of a Ca^{2+} gluconate IV bolus, oral supplementation, and correction of the underlying cause if found (e.g., Mg^{2+} or vitamin D supplementation if either is found to be deficient). Low calcium is common in advanced kidney disease. It should be treated carefully only after serum acid and phosphorus levels are evaluated.

Hypercalcemia

D—Ionized Ca^{2+} > 5.28 mg/dL or total Ca^{2+} > 10.5 mg/dL in men and >10.2 mg/dL in women if total protein and acid-base status are normal.

P—Hyperparathyroidism and malignancy are by far the most common causes. Causes can be remembered by the mnemonic in Table 4-12.

SiSx—Remember the classic mnemonic rhyme: problems with "bones" (fractures), "stones" (renal), abdominal "groans" (anorexia, vomiting, constipation), and "psychic overtones" (weakness, fatigue, altered mental status).

Dx—After diagnosis is made by laboratory test results, evaluation should include an ECG (classically, the patient will have a short QT interval), total/ionized Ca^{2+}, albumin, PTH, vitamin D, and thyroid stimulating hormone (TSH) if the cause is not clear.

Tx—For severe or acute onset of disease, the treatment is IV hydration followed by furosemide diuresis. Give calcitonin, pamidronate, and then dialysis in refractory cases. Avoid

---

Table 4-12. Causes of Hypercalcemia

C—Calcium supplementation
H—Hyperparathyroidism
I—Iatrogenic, immobilization
M—Milk-alkali syndrome: triad of hypercalcemia, metabolic alkalosis, renal failure from intake of large amounts of calcium and absorbable alkali
P—Paget's disease of bone
A—Addison's disease, acromegaly
N—Neoplasm, especially squamous cell cancer (via production of a PTH-related protein) and myeloma
Z—Zollinger-Ellison syndrome (MEN I) with accompanying hyperparathyroidism
E—Excess vitamin A
E—Excess vitamin D
S—Sarcoidosis and other granulomatous diseases (production of hydroxylase-like substance that increases vitamin D conversion to its active form)

thiazide diuretics (which increase resorption of Ca^{2+}). Bisphosphonates can be harmful if the patient is vitamin D deficient, since he or she will not be able to reabsorb lost calcium.

Hypophosphatemia

D—Serum $[PO_4]$ <2.5 mg/dL. The normal level is 2.5–4.5 mg/dL. Concentrations are higher in children.

P—The average diet takes in 1 g daily. Most of it is absorbed in the gut by passive and active transport. Renal resorption occurs at the proximal and distal tubules via Na-P cotransporters, regulated by PTH, which induces increased urinary losses.

Phosphate is required for cellular energy in ATP and is a major buffer in intracellular fluid. Eighty-five percent is stored in bone. Loss is through either redistribution (most common cause), renal losses, or GI losses.

1. Redistribution occurs in respiratory alkalosis (hyperventilated patients and those with pain, anxiety, or sepsis), recovery from malnutrition (with refeeding, there is increased intracellular uptake by new cells after prolonged cell breakdown), recovery from diabetic ketoacidosis (DKA), hungry bone syndrome, excess epinephrine, or any process that drives glycolysis (uses up inorganic phosphate).

2. Renal losses: excess PTH due to any cause, vitamin D deficiency, RTAs, acidosis, carbonic anhydrase inhibitors, alcohol abuse, renal tubular defects as seen in multiple myeloma or other malignancy, Wilson's disease, Fanconi's syndrome, heavy metal poisoning, and glycosuria since glucose and sugar compete for the same transporter.

3. Gastrointestinal: inadequate diet, antacid abuse, vitamin D deficiency, chronic diarrhea or steatorrhea.

SiSx—Patients are usually asymptomatic, but with severe disease, one may see proximal myopathy, dysphagia, ileus, and even rhabdomyolysis. Respiratory failure can occur with diaphragmatic weakness. Cardiac contractility can be impaired due to adenosine triphosphate (ATP) deficiency. Central nervous system symptoms with severe depletion include metabolic encephalopathy, coma, and seizures. Hemolysis, thrombocytopenia, and impaired phagocytosis are also related to decreased ATP. Acute bone disorders can be seen in chronic hypophosphatemia with abnormal mineralization. Alcoholic patients are at increased risk for hypophosphatemia-related complications and should be treated earlier.

Dx—A urine phosphate level >100 mg/dL strongly suggests renal wasting. A low urine PO_4 suggests other causes. Glucose infusion with secondary insulin release is the most common cause in hospitalized patients.

Tx—Correct the underlying condition. Supplement with oral phosphate, 1500–2000 mg/day. Sodium or potassium phosphate can be given. Acute excessive IV repletion can cause hypocalcemia from calcium phosphate precipitation and can lead to shock, acute renal failure, and death.

Hyperphosphatemia

D—Serum $[PO_4]$ >4.5 mg/dL (>6.3 mg/dL in children).

P—Causes include the following:

1. Renal—Common in advanced kidney disease, as the failing kidneys are no longer able to keep up with the normal dietary phosphorus loads. For levels that exceed 10 mg/dL, consider other sources such as cell turnover/lysis. This is associated with secondary hyperparathyroidism, in which the PTH elevations attempt to drive phosphaturia and maintain phosphorus balance.

2. Extrarenal—Rhabdomyolysis and tumor lysis syndromes (can be >25 mg/dL), exogenous phosphate administration, hypoparathyroidism, tumoral calcinosis, growth hormone (GH) excess, hyperthyroidism, hemolysis of any sort, bowel infarction, and malignant hyperthermia.

SiSx—Signs of concomitant hypocalcemia may be seen; hypotension and acute renal failure or chronic kidney disease occur in many cases. The patient may be asymptomatic otherwise.

Dx—Diagnosis is made directly by the laboratory test values. Remember that in the absence of renal insufficiency, hyperphosphatemia is likely due to hypoparathyroidism, cell lysis, or tumoral calcinosis.

Tx—Acutely, if the patient is symptomatic, give IV fluids and acetazolamide; otherwise, patients with normal renal function should excrete the excess phosphate eventually if there are no acute symptoms. Hemodialysis (HD) may be necessary in severe cases. Chronic treatment involves phosphate binders. There are a number of agents, including aluminum and calcium salts, inert polymers, and lanthanum, that are used in specific patients for different reasons.

Hypomagnesemia

D—Serum $[Mg^{2+}]$ <1.0 mg/dL in most cases; <2.0 mg/dL in patients with heart disease or cancer.

P—Total body Mg^{2+} is about 20 g; 50% is in bone and 1% is extracellular. About 100 mg is excreted daily in the urine. Most regulation occurs at the distal tubule. Regulation is via serum Mg^{2+} levels. It is needed in all reactions that require ATP and in every step of replication and transcription of DNA and translation of RNA. Homeostasis depends solely on GI absorption and renal excretion as magnesium does not have a separate hormone control. Magnesium is absorbed in the small intestine in an unregulated fashion. Usually hypomagnesemia is seen with concomitant hypocalcemia, as magnesium is used as a cofactor for sensing and regulation, and low levels can be associated with decreased glandular PTH secretion. Hypomagnesemia also impairs the peripheral response to PTH, especially with bone. Two methods of loss occur: GI and renal.

1. GI loss includes inadequate diet, malabsorption, nasogastric (NG) suction, acute and chronic diarrhea, steatorrhea, acute pancreatitis, decreased cellular uptake as in alcoholic withdrawal, and primary intestinal hypomagnesemia—a rare genetic disorder of inborn metabolism.

2. Renal causes are seen in primary tubular disorders, drug-induced tubular loses (i.e., aminoglycosides, amphotericin B), chronic IV fluid therapy, osmotic diuresis (DKA, mannitol), postobstructive diuresis, hyperaldosteronism, and use of loop and thiazide diuretics. Hypercalcemia can also be a cause, as magnesium and calcium compete for the same binding sites.

SiSx—Symptoms are usually nonspecific. There may be muscle twitching, weakness, and tremor. Respiratory muscle weakness is evident in severe cases. Arrhythmias (usually ventricular) can occur, especially in those with a history of myocardial ischemia. Symptoms are similar to those of hypocalcemia, which may be seen concomitantly. Hypomagnesemia has also been implicated as a cause of osteoporosis.

Dx—Diagnosis is made directly by laboratory values. The ECG may show a widened QRS, T wave inversions, and U waves.

Tx—Replete the patient with a normal diet or supplementation. As magnesium is largely intracellular and control is based on the ambient serum concentrations, losses often have to be repleted slowly and oral salts are preferred in nonacute situations. One-half of an administered dose is usually excreted in the urine, so repletion of total body stores occurs slowly. Different salts of magnesium can be used to replace stores, but for the IV route magnesium sulfate is most often utilized.

Hypermagnesemia

D—The exact level is unclear for definitional purposes but is generally serum $[Mg^{2+}] > 4$ mg/dL.

RF—Risk factors are renal failure and laxative abuse.

P—Pathophysiology is usually iatrogenic, as the kidneys can secrete several hundred mEq/day unless there is concomitant renal failure. Laxative or antacid abuse and magnesium sulfate ($MgSO_4$) given during premature labor are common drug causes.

SiSx—The degree of symptoms depends on the serum level. Many problems arise from its competition with calcium ion binding sites.

4 to 6 mEq/L—CNS effects such as lethargy, drowsiness, nausea, vomiting, and decreased deep tendon reflexes (DTRs).

6 to 10 mEq/L—increased somnolence, hypocalcemia, absent DTRs, hypotension, bradycardia, ECG changes such as increased PR internal, increased QRS duration, and increased QT interval.

>10 mEq/L—muscle paralysis, heart block, and possible cardiac arrest

Dx—Diagnosis is made directly by serum laboratory values.

Tx—Acutely, give IV calcium, which is a direct antagonist. Hemodialysis may also be required in severe cases.

Metabolic Acidosis

D—Decreasing serum pH with decreased plasma bicarbonate.

P—It is caused by processes that result in loss of bicarbonate or accumulation of any kind of acid (see below).

SiSx—Symptoms vary with the specific etiology. With pH <7.2, the patient can have myocardial depression, fatigue, Kussmaul respirations (long, deep, rhythmic breathing that increases minute ventilation and reduces CO_2) with an increased ventilatory rate, and hypotension.

Dx—Establish the diagnosis with ABG and/or laboratory test values. Ask yourself whether the kidney is responding appropriately to the acid load, and examine the anion gap. The steps below will help you make the diagnosis:

1. First, calculate the anion gap (AG) = $[Na^+]$ – $[Cl^-]$ – $[HCO_3^-]$, which normally is 12 ± 2 mEq/L. There is a correction in hypoalbuminemic patients that consists of subtracting 2.5 mEq for each 1 g/dL albumin less than 4 g/dL. Table 4-13 is useful for interpretation.

Table 4-13. Characteristics of Metabolic Acidosis Based on Anion Gap

Characteristic of the Anion Gap	Possible Causes	Diagnostic Hints
Anion Gap Present (>14) Mnemonic: MUDPILES	Methanol Uremia DKA/alcoholic ketoacidosis Paraldehyde Iron/INH excess Lactate production Ethylene glycol/ETOH Salicylates/starvation	For ethylene glycol, methanol, isopropyl alcohol, or ETOH, a large osmolal gap will be present. Isopropyl alcohol will produce an osmolal gap (measured osmolality > calculated olmolarity) *without* acidemia. Classically, one may see papilledema and blindness with methanol poisoning; urine calcium oxalate crystals with ethylene glycol, and serum ketones in DKA. Salicylates may also cause a central respiratory alkalosis. Otherwise, check drug levels or other appropriate laboratory values.
Non-Anion Gap Acidosis (< 12–14) Mnemonic: DURHAM	Diarrhea—via HCO_3 loss Ureteral diversion RTA Hyperalimentation/TPN Acetazolamide/Addison's disease/ammonium chloride Miscellaneous (chloridorrhea, amphotericin B, etc.)	To distinguish the most common two causes, diarrhea and RTAs (if you cannot be guided by the history), use the urine ion gap (UG) = $[UrNa^+]$ + $[UrK^+]$ – $[UrCl^-]$). If the value is negative, consider diarrhea the culprit since this means the kidney is working well in excreting NH_4^+ along with Cl^-. If UG is zero or positive, consider an RTA. With low serum K^+, more common causes are diuretics, RTA type I or II, diarrhea, and Fanconi's syndrome. With high serum K^+ consider Addison's disease, renal failure, RTA type IV, K^+-sparing diuretics like acetazolamide or spironolactone, total parenteral nutrition, or other forms of hyperalimentation. Give IV fluid and then address the underlying cause.
Low Anion Gap (in presence of excess anions)	Bromide ingestion Multiple myeloma Hyperalbuminemia	Check total protein (TP) and for a large protein gap (TP-albumin).

2. If an AG is present, calculate the corrected bicarbonate delta gap (Δ-gap) to search for a mixed metabolic disorder present. The Δ-gap = AG − 12 + HCO_3. It will be 24 if all the acidosis is from a decrease in the body's bicarbonate (HCO_3^-), which is the normal value. If other anions are involved, this will not be the case. If the Δ-gap is >31, there is also a metabolic alkalosis from another process, as HCO_3 will be higher than normal. If it is <21, a non-AG acidosis is also present because HCO_3 will be lower than expected. Basically, the Δ-gap indicates if the gap is due entirely to a change in other anions (namely, Cl^-), giving rise to an acidic pH, or if there is an intrinsic change in HCO_3 from another condition. One may also calculate the ratio of Δ-gap/ΔHCO_3 meaning [Calculated AG − Normal AG (which is 12)]/[Normal HCO_3 − Measured HCO_3]. If the ratio is >2, this implies a concomitant metabolic alkalosis. Lactic acidosis will have a ratio of Δ-gap/ΔHCO_3 of about 1.6, since most lactate remains extracellular.

3. Finally, determine if appropriate respiratory compensation has also occurred. Generally, the $PaCO_2$ will be low, along with the HCO_3^-, because of compensatory hyperventilation. Appropriate respiratory compensation can be assessed by Winter's formula [$PaCO_2$ = 1.5 (HCO_3^-) + 8]. The limit of respiratory compensation is to hyperventilate down to a CO_2 of 20 mmHg. Inappropriate compensation implies mixed metabolic and respiratory acidosis.

Tx—This depends on correcting the underlying cause. HCO_3^- administration is usually reserved for severe acidosis (pH <7.20) in select cases or in severe non gap acidoses due to loss of bicarbonate such as diarrhea. Dialysis is also used for refractory conditions.

Metabolic Alkalosis

D—Increasing serum pH with increased plasma bicarbonate.

P—A process that both initiates it and maintains it is necessary. Initiation is usually through gain of bicarbonate [sodium bicarbonate ($NaHCO_3$)] administration, citrate, lactate, acetate, or via a loss of acid (vomiting, NG suction, diuretics, hypermineralocorticoid states). This must be maintained by the kidney through either volume depletion (contraction alkalosis from $NaHCO_3$ retention) or hypermineralocorticoid states.

SiSx—Symptoms include hypoventilation and its consequences, such as ΔMS from decreased perfusion of the heart and brain due to vasoconstriction.

Dx—Diagnosis is established by ABG and/or laboratory test values. To determine the cause, determine if the condition is responsive to NaCl administration. One needs to check urine Cl^- to verify this (see Table 4.14).

1. If urine Cl^- is low (<10 mEq/L), then it is saline-responsive alkalosis and due to HCl loss; consider the cause to be vomiting, contraction alkalosis, diuretics, and posthypercapnea (in an intubated patient whose hypercapnea has been corrected).

2. If urine Cl^- is high (>10 mEq/L), then it is saline-resistant alkalosis. Therefore, check the blood pressure. If it is high, consider primary hyperaldosteronism, Cushing's disease, renal artery stenosis, or renal failure plus alkali administration. If the blood pressure is low, consider hypomagnesemia, severe hypokalemia, Bartter's syndrome, $NaHCO_3$ administration, or licorice ingestion (which inhibits degradation of cortisol).

3. Finally, check for appropriate compensation; generally, the $PaCO_2$ will be high along with the HCO_3^- because of compensatory hypoventilation. Appropriate respiratory compensation can be gauged by $PaCO_2$ = 0.9 (HCO_3^-) + 15. The limit of respiratory compensation is 55–60 mmHg. Inappropriate compensation implies mixed metabolic and respiratory alkalosis.

Tx—For saline-responsive etiologies, administer an infusion of NaCl. An H_2 receptor blocker is useful in gastric alkalosis. For saline-unresponsive causes, try to enhance HCO_3 elimination with KCl and spironolactone/acetazolamide. If a mineralocorticoid excess state exists, treat with spironolactone or adrenalectomy.

Table 4-14. Summary of the Causes of Metabolic Alkalosis

Saline Responsive ($Ur_{Cl} < 10$ mEq/L)	Saline Unresponsive ($Ur_{Cl} > 10$ mEq/L)	
Blood pressure is not a consideration. Vomiting, NG suction, congenital chloridorrhea, diuretics, posthypercapnic response.	Blood pressure is normal or low. $NaHCO_3$ administration, hypomagnesemia, severe hypokalemia, Bartter's and Gitelman's syndromes, licorice ingestion.	Blood pressure is high. Mineralocorticoid excess states (e.g., primary aldosteronism, Cushing's syndrome), pseudohyperaldosteronism, renin excess, renal artery stenosis, renal failure with alkali administration.

Respiratory Acidosis

D—Increased blood $PaCO_2$ and decreasing blood pH.

P—It is caused by processes that prevent the body from excreting enough CO_2. There are three broad categories:

1. Lung/airway disease—Pneumonia, pulmonary edema, bronchospasm/laryngospasm, COPD, mechanical obstruction (foreign body, tumor).
2. Central nervous system—Drugs causing sedation or respiratory center hypofunction.
3. Chest cavity—Neurologic disorder, neuromuscular disorder involving the diaphragms, severe kyphoscoliosis, pleural effusion, pneumothorax.

SiSx—Symptoms are those of generalized CNS depression, perhaps because of increased cerebrospinal fluid (CSF) pressure; myocardial depression with acidosis and decreased cardiac output.

Dx—Attempt to find the underlying disorder by the history and exam. A chest X-ray may help delineate the pulmonary problems listed above. In patients with weak diaphragms, lying down flat causes shortness of breath within 10–15 seconds. Determine whether the process is acute or chronic since it takes time for the kidney to compensate for the lung. Appropriate compensations are:

1. Acute—For every 10 mmHg increase in $PaCO_2$, HCO_3^- increases by 1 mEq/L and pH decreases 0.08.
2. Chronic—For every 10 mmHg increase in $PaCO_2$, HCO_3^- increases by 3–4 mEq/L and pH decreases 0.03.

The maximum metabolic compensation is a HCO_3^- of 45 mEq/L.

Tx—Correct the underlying disorder if possible and use assisted respiratory therapy in cases where PCO_2 is high (>60 mmHg).

Respiratory Alkalosis

D—Decreased blood PCO_2 and increasing blood pH.

P—It is due to processes that cause excessive CO_2 elimination via the lungs. There are three broad categories:

1. Systemic—Infection/sepsis (especially gram-negative), salicylates, liver failure (via a direct CNS effect), hyperthyroidism, pregnancy.
2. Central nervous system—Anxiety, ischemia/cerebrovascular accident (CVA), tumor, infection, pregnancy/progesterone.
3. Pulmonary—PE, asthma, restrictive lung disease, hypoxia (pneumonia, pulmonary edema).

SiSx—Symptoms include a fast breathing rate, CNS disorders, obtundation, and a tetany-like syndrome.

Dx—After ABG and laboratory test values are obtained, one must determine if the alkalosis is acute or chronic, as the kidney cannot compensate for lung disease as quickly as in the reciprocal situation. Appropriate compensations are:

1. Acute—For every 10 mmHg decrease in $PaCO_2$, HCO_3^- decreases by 2.5 mEq/L.
2. Chronic—For every 10 mmHg decrease in $PaCO_2$, HCO_3^- decreases by 5 mEq/L. The maximum metabolic compensation is a HCO_3^- of 15 mEq/L.

Tx—Primarily, one has to correct the underlying disorder. Supportive care may be necessary, such as controlled ventilation in severe cases.

Disorders of Water Balance

Diabetes Insipidus (DI)

D—Polyuric syndrome of excessive water secretion in urine. Central diabetes insipidus (CDI) is caused by decreased pituitary secretion of antidiuretic hormone (ADH, also known as vasopressin), which normally causes water retention in the kidney. Nephrogenic diabetes insipidus (NDI) is caused by failure of the kidney to respond to ADH.

P—

1. Central diabetes insipidus is either idiopathic (30% of cases) or acquired from head trauma, postpituitary infarct, granulomatous infection, hypothalamic tumor, CNS infection or other CNS disease. Primary disease of the pituitary is rarely the problem. If anterior pituitary dysfunction is also seen, then underlying hypothalamic disease is likely to exist.

2. Nephrogenic diabetes insipidus can be familial. Mutations of the V2-type ADH receptor are X-linked; aquaporin 2 channel mutations are autosomal. Acquired forms may be caused by diseases involving the renal interstitium (e.g., secondary to sickle cell anemia, pyelonephritis, or amyloidosis) or by drugs that impair the renal gradient (e.g., lithium can cause temporary or permanent forms).

SiSx—Symptoms include polyuria, the degree of which varies with the degree of ADH responsiveness. Complete lack of ADH responsiveness causes water loss of up to 16–18 L/day. Polydipsia and nocturia are also seen. Patients usually compensate with increased free water intake, so one can elicit a history of thirst.

Dx—Patients usually exhibit euvolemic hypernatremia. Urine specific gravity is low (<1.010 g/mL), as is urine osmolality (<200 mOsm/kg). Serum osmolality can be >300 mOsm/kg. For suspected CDI, head MRI is necessary to rule out a mass if the cause is unclear. Perform a water deprivation test if it is unclear if the condition is CDI or NDI: hold all water for a while and measure serum osmolality until it is 295 mOsm/kg. Check urine osmolality and give subcutaneous vasopressin. Measure urine osmolality 1 hour later. Normal subjects will increase their urine osmolality less than 10%, since ADH is already maximally stimulated. In CDI, urine osmolality will increase by greater than 10%. In NDI, there is no change in urine osmolality (still dilute).

Tx—Medical intervention is recommended in any patient with polyuria of >4 L/d. Synthetic 1-deamino(8-D-arginine) vasopressin (DDAVP) has increased ADH activity two- to fourfold over endogenous forms. DDAVP nasal spray can be used for CDI. Patients should increase water intake and restrict salt intake. There is no good treatment for NDI, mostly volume contraction with thiazide diuretics to decrease the GFR.

Syndrome of Inappropriate ADH Secretion (SIADH)

D—Increased ADH secretion resulting in hyponatremia with an inappropriately concentrated urine.

Epi—This is a very common cause of inpatient hyponatremia.

P—It can be caused by CNS disease of any type or ectopic secretion by tumors [e.g., squamous cell cancer (SCC)]. It is rarely seen in pulmonary disease (pneumonia, tuberculosis), adrenal insufficiency, severe hypothyroidism, and by the use of certain drugs.

SiSx—Generally, the patient is not edematous or volume overloaded in appearance. If edema is seen, consider an additional condition as well. Otherwise, patients may be asymptomatic.

Dx—The individual should have euvolemic hyponatremia, however SIADH can sometimes occur with another entity so it is important to rule out other causes. One should see concentrated urine with urine osmolality >300 mOsm/kg and urine Na^+ >20 mEq/L to make the diagnosis. These values will be less in the context of volume contraction and low BUN and uric acid.

Tx—The condition resolves over time, with fluid restriction to 1 L/day, correcting the Na$^+$ by 5 mEq/day. Treat the underlying cause, if known. Otherwise, correct with the use of salt tabs and/or loop diuretics (which removes excess free water). In acutely symptomatic cases, consider hypertonic saline. Normal saline will not work with SIADH as urine osmolality (>300 mOsm/kg) is higher than that of NS, so giving this is in fact like giving patients back some free water and will lower sodium further. Hence, one needs to give a hypertonic saline concentration which has a higher osmolality concentration than the urine in order to remove free water. Demeclocyline (a tetracycline that inhibits ADH) can also be used in resistant cases.

Chronic Renal Insufficiency

Chronic Kidney Disease (CKD) and End-Stage Renal Disease (ESRD)

D—Decrease in renal function over at least 3 to 6 months from progressive and irreversible nephron damage. It is always associated with azotemia of renal origin. There are three forms of chronic kidney disease: (1) diminished renal reserve, (2) azotemia, and (3) uremic syndrome (occurs when GFR <20%). Classification by stage is shown in Table 4-15.

Epi—In the United States, 200,000 patients have ESRD. Common causes, in order of incidence in the United States, are diabetes (33%), hypertension (24%), glomerulonephri-

tis (GN, 17%), and polycystic kidney disease (PKD, 5%).

RF—Risk factors include a family history, older age, African American race, diabetes, and hypertension. Many cases have multifactorial etiologies.

SiSx—

Neuromuscular—Dementia, convulsions, coma.

Gastrointestinal—Anorexia, nausea/vomiting, unpleasant taste in the mouth, GI ulcers.

Cardiovascular—CHF, pericarditis, hypertension, hypervolemia.

Hematologic—Bleeding from platelet dysfunction, anemia.

Dermatologic—Yellow-brown macules, uremic frost (crystals from sweat), pruritis.

Bone—Diffuse osteopenia (a late finding).

Dx—Diagnosis is based not on absolute Cr or BUN values but on increasing BUN and Cr values over a period of time, that is, not during an episode of acute renal failure. The sequelae of poor kidney function are:

1. Acidemia from accumulation of sulfates, phosphates, and other organic acids.
2. Hyperkalemia since the patient cannot excrete K$^+$.
3. Volume dysregulation from aberrations in concentrating and diluting capabilities.
4. Hypocalcemia from lack of vitamin D action.
5. Anemia of chronic disease from lack of erythropoietin production.
6. Hypertension from an activated renin-angiotensin axis.

Ultrasound shows small (<9 cm), echogenic kidneys. Calculate the GFR to make sure, using the Cockroft-Gault equation:

$$GFR = (140 - Age \times Lean\ Body\ Weight\ in\ kg)/(Plasma\ creatinine_r \times 72)$$

- Multiply by 0.85 for women.
- Normal GFR is >90 mL/min/1.73m^2 of body surface area. The measurement is valid for GFR or Cr clearance *only in the steady state*, not during an episode of acute renal failure, as only during the steady state is a constant amount of Cr produced in relation to muscle mass. Also note that

Table 4-15.   Classification of CKD

Stage	GFR (mL/min/1.73m^2)
0	>90
1	90*
2	60–89
3	30–59
4	15–29
5	<15 or on dialysis

*Need an additional abnormality (e.g., abnormal sediment or proteinuria), blood tests, or an imaging study.

for a malnourished person with very little muscle, a Cr of 1.0 mg/dL can be very abnormal and GFR can be 30 or 40. In these cases, a complicated equation (called the MDRD equation) that includes albumin is more useful; it is readily available as an online calculator.

Tx—Correct any reversible factors, maintain electrolytes with supplementation, and institute dietary restriction of potassium, sodium, phosphates, and fluids. Supplementation with erythropoietin, calcium and vitamin D, and phosphate binders is usually done when the intact parathyroid hormone (iPTH) level is >200 pg/mL. Bicarbonate may be used to correct acidosis. Dialysis is commonly started when the GFR is <20 mL/min/1.73m² or when it is <10 or <15 mL/min/1.73m² in diabetics. Renal consultation for long-term dialysis or even transplantation should be started early.

Hepatorenal Syndrome

D—Acute renal failure seen in advanced liver disease as a result of decreased renal perfusion from increasingly severe hepatic injury. Diagnostic criteria are Cr >1.5 mg/dL in days to weeks, with severe acute/chronic liver disease and portal hypertension and no other causes found for renal disease. There are two types:

Type I—More serious; >50% decrease in CrCl, in <2 weeks, or twofold increase in Cr to >2.5 mg/dL.

Type II—Less serious; manifests as ascites resistant to diuretics; occurs over more than two weeks.

P—Chronic splanchnic vasodilation causes decreasing renal perfusion and decreasing GFR, with decreasing Na⁺ excretion as a result.

RF—The onset of renal failure in a patient with liver disease can be precipitated by spontaneous bacterial peritonitis (SBP), GI bleed (GIB), other infections, and rapid diuresis.

SiSx—Symptoms are those of known liver failure with new onset of renal failure. Specific symptoms of renal failure may be hard to detect but one may see increased volume overload with ascites and uremia.

Dx—The condition otherwise resembles prerenal failure. [Urine Na⁺] is <10 mEq/L (without diuretics). There may be oliguria with benign sediment, a slow rise in plasma Cr, and low Na⁺ excretion (cirrhosis). There is no improvement with volume expansion. It is hard to estimate the extent of renal failure because urea and Cr are both decreased in liver disease.

Tx—In early stages, try to decrease sympathetic tone and renovascular resistance. Use of subcutaneous octreotide along with midodrine may help decrease splenic vasodilation. Ultimately, one needs to reverse the liver disease (i.e., liver transplant to prevent ongoing disease). Otherwise, in patients who are not transplant candidates or whose liver disease is not reversible, it is futile to start HD or continuous venovenous hemodialysis (CVVHD) since there is no proven mortality benefit.

Renal Tubular Diseases

Renal Tubular Acidoses (RTAs)

D—Conditions with diminished net renal tubular acid secretion leading to non-anion gap metabolic acidosis from hyperchloremia as a result of retention of hydrochloric acid (HCL) or ammonium chloride (NH₄Cl) (which are equivalent) or a net loss of NaHCO₃ or equivalent. There are several forms (types I, II, and IV; type III doesn't exist for historical reasons).

P—Drugs are the most common cause, followed by primary diseases (see below).

SiSx—Symptoms depends on the etiology. Many patients are asymptomatic unless they have an underlying disease causing this problem.

Dx—Nongap acidosis is seen in patients without other causes. Distinguishing between RTAs is done using the characteristics listed in Table 4-16.

Renal Stones or Nephrolithiasis

D—Presence of calculi in the urinary system.

Epi—Calcium oxalate is the most common type, followed by struvite stones.

Table 4-16. Distinguishing Characteristics of Renal Tubular Acidoses

	RTA Type I (Distal RTA)	RTA Type II (Proximal RTA)	RTA Type IV (Hyperkalemic RTA)
Mechanism of Acidosis	Defect in H^+ ATPase pump at the collecting duct causing failure of acid secretion and inability to acidify the urine.	Failure to reabsorb HCO_3^- in the PCT.	Decreased aldosterone secretion or effect. Hyporeninemic hypoaldosteronism is the most common cause.
Urine pH	>5.5	>5.5 initially, then below	< 5.5
Serum [HCO_3^-]	<10 mEq/L (because it is lost in urine)	12–20 mEq/L (wasting only when the amount is above the absolute threshold downstream near the DCT).	>17 mEq/L
Serum [K^+]	Low, but corrects with alkali therapy	Low	High
Pathogenesis	Familial forms are mainly (but not exclusively) autosomal dominant. Acquired forms are seen in sickle cell disease, glue sniffing, lithium, Sjögren's syndrome, hypercalcemia, RA, hypergammaglobulinemia, amphotericin B toxicity, cirrhosis, SLE, and renal transplant patients.	Most common cause is from excessive light chains in multiple myeloma. It can also be seen in Fanconi's syndrome. Medications such as carbonic anhydrase inhibitors, ifosfamide, cyclophosphamide, and tetracycline are associated with this condition as is lead poisoning.	Primary hypoaldosteronism, NSAIDS, ACE inhibitors, K^+-sparing diuretics, diabetes, heparin, interstitial nephritis, and cyclosporine use are associated.
Complications	Nephrocalcinosis or urolithiasis	Osteomalacia	Hyperkalemia
Tx	Oral bicarbonate, K^+, perhaps protein restriction.	Give bicarbonate, K^+, and a thiazide. Children should be treated to prevent growth retardation.	Give fludrocortisones and K^+ bicarbonate; restrict K^+.

RF—Risk factors include extreme urine pH levels, medullary sponge kidney, polycystic kidney disease, and chronic obstruction.

SiSx—The symptom is sharp, intense, colicky pain that may radiate to the lower abdomen, testes, or labia. The condition can result in hydronephrosis or progressive dilation of the renal pelvis. Features include occult passage of asymptomatic stones and hematuria, which almost always occurs with stone movement and can be microscopic or visible, with or without pain. Urinary frequency and dysuria are common. Abdominal pain and tenesmus also occur. Infection can complicate the picture by producing back or flank pain as well as fevers and chills, especially in the presence of obstruction.

Dx—All efforts should be made to capture stones for analysis, which is the only means of definitive treatment. Cystoscopy is indicated for bladder calculi and for ureteral stones near the ureterovesical junction. Plain films identify most stones that are radiopaque. An intravenous pyelogram (IVP) is necessary to evaluate radiolucent stones. Ultrasound and CT may also be helpful.

Tx—Treatment depends on the type of stone. See Table 4-17.

Table 4-17. Treatment and Causes of Common Types of Renal Stones

Type	Characteristics	Causes	Tx
Calcium Oxalate (with pyrophosphate) (80–85%)	Radiopaque	Idiopathic hypercalciuria and other hypercalciuric states, hypouricosuria, hyperoxaluria.	Diet adjustments. Medications include potassium citrate for hypocitrauria, neutral phosphates for idiopathic calcium urolithiasis, thiazides for hypercalciuria (with concomitant sodium restriction), and allopurinol for hyperuricosuria. Primary hyperparathyroidism requires resection of parathyroid adenoma. If the stone is obstructive, depending on its size and position, percutaneous stone extraction (PERC) or extracorporeal shock wave lithotripsy (ESWL) or laser therapy may be indicated.
Ammonium Magnesium Phosphate [struvite stones] (10–15%)	Radiopaque	From alkaline urine, most often due to urease from *Proteus, Staphylococcus saphrophiticus,* UTIs. Can form large *staghorn calculi* in the renal pelvis and calices.	Give antibiotics for UTI and remove stone material surgically by PERC or possibly with ESWL.
Uric Acid (6%)	Radiolucent	Hyperuricemia (e.g., gout or increased cell turnover in, e.g., leukemia). Note, however, that more than half of all patients have neither hyperuricemia nor increased uric acid in urine.	Administer oral sodium bicarbonate to maintain alkaline urine. Consider allopurinol too. If the stone cannot be dissolved or is obstructive, ESWL is indicated.
Cystine (1–2%)	Cystine crystalluria seen in routine urine test. Also, positive nitroprusside test.	Autosomal recessive defects in amino acid (including cystine) reabsorption.	Urinary alkalization, cysteine chelators (e.g., D-penicillamine), high fluid intake. If the stone cannot be dissolved or is obstructive, PERC is indicated.

Diseases Associated with Proteinuria

Normal urinary protein excretion is <150 mg/day, the majority of which is small molecular weight proteins. Albumin excretion is <25 mg/day. Any amount in excess of this is proteinuria.

There are two main processes involved in proteinuria:

1. Tubulointerstitial nephritis—tubular proteins like Tamm-Horsfall protein and β_2-microglobulin are excreted. This is seen in drug-induced disease or chronic inflammatory disease.
2. Glomerulonephritis—proteinuria, specifically albuminuria, is common. The defect is in the filtering mechanism of the kidney.

There are also several types of proteinuria:

1. Glomerular proteinuria—From leakage of plasma proteins through a perturbed barrier.
2. Tubular proteinuria—From failure of resorption of low molecular weight proteins

that are normally filtered, resorbed, and metabolized by the tubular epithelium. It virtually never exceeds 2 g/24hr and therefore cannot cause nephrotic syndrome.

3. Overflow proteinuria—From filtration of proteins (usually light chains) that are present in excess.

Nephrotic Syndrome

- By definition, characterized by (1) urine protein >3.0–3.5 g/day, (2) hypoalbuminemia, (3) hyperlipidemia + lipiduria, and (4) generalized edema. There can be a variable amount of hypertension (mediated, at least in part, by sodium retention) and occasionally a tendency toward hypercoagulability if the proteinuria is severe (especially in membranous disease).
- Proteinuria is caused by disruption of the filtration barrier. This disruption can be mediated by decreased charge selectivity, decreased size selectivity, deposits into one of the layers of the glomerular basement membrane, or occasionally by abnormal permeability caused by circulating factors. Hypoalbuminemia is related in part to renal losses of protein and in part to decreased hepatic synthesis of albumin. Changes in hepatic synthesis of lipids account for the nearly universal feature of hyperlipidemia (and occasionally hyperlipiduria). The salt retention that leads to edema is incompletely understood but probably, in part, represents a primary renal defect in sodium handling and in part may reflect the response to disruption in effective arterial blood pressure. Hypercoagulability has been attributed to heavy urinary losses of antithrombin III, altered levels of proteins C and S, and hyperfibrinogenemia. The most common causes of nephrotic syndrome are shown in Table 4-18.

Nephritic Syndrome

This is a renal condition characterized by the following four criteria: (1) hematuria, (2) abnormal proteinuria, (3) renal insufficiency, and (4) hypertension. The presence of glomerulonephritis (GN) is common, and is characterized by an increase in cellularity either from hyperproliferation or from inflammation. Red blood cell casts are pathognomonic. The most common types of acute nephritic syndrome are listed in Table 4-19. Membranoproliferative glomerulonephritis, IgA nephropathy, Henoch-Schönlein purpura, systemic lupus erythematosus, mixed cryoglobulinemia, Goodpasture's syndrome, and Wegener's granulomatosis are all noninfectious causes of acute nephritic syndrome. Acute nephritic syndrome that develops into rapidly progressive GN most often results from conditions that involve an abnormal immune reaction.

Rhabdomyolysis

D—A disease of muscle necrosis with release of intramuscular substances into the circulation, sometimes causing acute renal failure and electrolyte abnormalities.

RF—Risk factors include trauma, postsurgical status, a comatose/postictal state, and extreme physical exertion. Drugs can cause this condition as well, such as cocaine overdose, as well as carbon monoxide and other myotoxins. Other risk factors include malignant hyperthermia and neuroleptic malignant syndrome, infections such as bacterial pyomyositis, and acute viral infections in some cases.

SiSx—Pigmenturia is seen in some cases (it may not be seen in cases where the filtered load of myoglobin is too low). Muscle pain may be present. Acute oliguric renal failure can be seen, along with signs of hyperkalemia and hyperphosphatemia from muscle breakdown and hypocalcemia from decreased bone responsiveness to PTH. Metabolic acidosis and severe hyperuricemia are also possible, depending on the severity of the condition.

Dx—A high degree of clinical suspicion combined with an elevated CK (sometimes over 100,000 units/L), renal failure, and electrolyte abnormalities can usually make the diagnosis.

Tx—Treat the underlying cause if known, in addition to using aggressive IV fluid to maintain a high urine output, using diuretics if the patient developed CHF. Alkalination of the

Table 4-18. Common Causes of the Nephrotic Syndrome

	Minimal Change Disease	Focal Segmental Glomerulosclerosis (FSGS)	Membranous Glomerulonephritis (MGN)	Diabetic Nephropathy
D	Nephrotic syndrome characterized by normal light microscopic findings.	Nephrotic syndrome characterized by focal pathologic lesion of parts (segmental) of the glomeruli involving sclerosis and hyalinosis.	Idiopathic nephrotic syndrome with a characteristic lesion involving the formation of new basement membrane.	Renal involvement in patients with diabetes mellitus characterized along a spectrum ranging from glomerular hypertension to ESRD.
Epi	Most common cause of nephrotic syndrome in young children. Peak incidence at 6–8 years.	Occurs in children and adults with refractory hypertension; cause of one-third of cases of nephrotic syndrome in adults and one-half of cases in African Americans.	Most common (30–40%) primary cause of nephrotic syndrome in white middle-aged adults.	The most common cause of ESRD in the United States. Complicates at least 30% of type I diabetes and 20% of type II diabetes.
P	Loss of the protein barrier via damage to the epithelial polyanions, possibly on an immunologic basis.	A nonselective proteinuria via destruction and hyalinosis of just part of the glomeruli. A collapsing variant can be seen, most commonly in HIV patients; most have a fulminant course. >50% of nephrons must be lost for secondary FSGS to develop.	A disease of idiopathic immune complex deposition. Seen with chronic inflammatory conditions.	Quite varied. May start with hypertension and microalbuminuria with early damage. By the time nephritic-range proteinuria occurs ESRD is not far off
RF	Majority of cases are idiopathic. Rare secondary causes associated with • Hodgkin's disease/ other lymphoproliferative malignancies • HIV infection • Interstitial nephritis from NSAIDs, rifampin, interferon-alpha.	Idiopathic primary disease seen in about one-third of cases. Secondary causes occur in the setting of: • HIV nephropathy. • Heroin addiction nephropathy. • Sickle cell disease nephropathy. • Massive obesity. • Other forms of focal GN (e.g., IgA nephropathy). • Advanced states of reflux nephropathy. • Unilateral renal agenesis.	Secondary causes can arise from: • Infections from entities such as HBV, HCV, syphilis, and malaria. • Malignancies (e.g., Lung and colon cancer as well as melanoma). • SLE. • Metabolic disorders (e.g., Diabetes and thyroiditis). • Use of drugs such as gold salts or penicillamine.	Poorly controlled diabetes.

SiSx	Hypertension or renal failure is rare. There is a benign urinary sediment.	Hypertension, mild renal insufficiency, urine sediment with RBCs and WBCs. One-third of patients present with subnephrotic-range proteinuria.	Nonselective proteinuria. Microscopic hematuria in 50% of cases, but RBC casts, macrohematuria, and WBCs are very rare.	First sign may be hypertension. Microalbuminuria is seen after about 5 years, defined as <30–150 mg/day of excretion. Nephrotic levels typically develop 5–10 years thereafter.
Dx	Usually by the history. Biopsy is rarely necessary. Light microscopy (LM)—normal glomerulus. Electron microscopy (EM)—epithelial foot process effusion and diffuse effacement. Immunofluorescence—no findings. Microscopic hematuria in 30%. Selective proteinuria: mainly albumin is seen on dipstick.	By renal biopsy LM—glomerular sclerosis that is focal and segmental. Loss of capillary loops. Immunofluorescence—IgM and C3. (In the collapsing variant, there is extensive foot process effacement and epithelial injury. Visceral epithelial cells appear to have reabsorption droplets.)	By renal biopsy LM—diffuse thickening of glomerular basement membrane (GBM) on the periodic acid–Schiff (PAS) test with capillary loops without inflammation or cell proliferation. EM—5–10 times thicker basement membrane. Spike (basement membrane) and dome (immune complex) deposits on subepithelial surface. Immunofluorescence—IgG and C3.	A history of diabetes and its severity are most suggestive, especially with progressive renal failure. Renal biopsy shows: LM—diabetes types I and II have the same pathology in the kidney. Increased basement membrane thickness and mesangial matrix, *Kimmelstiel-Wilson bodies*, capsular drops, and arteriolar hyaline change. Immunofluorescence—nonspecific albumin, IgG
Tx	Responds usually to steroid therapy. If not, other immunosuppressants are used. Has a very good prognosis. Adults respond more slowly and nonalbumin proteinuria is less likely to respond. Patients have a 95% 10-year survival.	Steroids are first-line therapy, with a 70% response in 16–24 weeks. Possible use of cytotoxic drugs later. ACE inhibitor use and plasmapheresis, if initiated early, may help. Recurrence occurs in 40% after treatment.	Remits spontaneously in 40%. From 30% to 40% have slowly progressive, relapsing, and remitting disease with no real response to steroids.	Blood pressure control and tight glycemic control with oral medication and insulin along with ACE inhibitors, when appropriate, can slow progress of disease. Renal transplantation with or without pancreatic transplantation is considered in candidates with ESRD who have few other comorbidities.

Note: Nephrotic syndrome is also seen in lupus nephritis, Henoch-Schonlein purpura HSP, and Membranoproliferative GN (MPGN), as described elsewhere in this chapter.

Table 4-19. Common Causes of the Nephritic Syndrome

	Acute Postinfectious GN (PIGN)	IgA Nephropathy (Buerger's Disease)	Membranoproliferative GN (MPGN)	Rapidly Progressive (Crescentic) GN (RPGN)
D	GN following an infectious process involving immune complex deposition in the kidneys.	GN secondary to deposition of IgA in the kidney.	GN characterized by thickening of the GBM and cellular proliferation.	A syndrome of GN that rapidly progresses to ESRD and is considered a medical emergency. A number of the types of GN including SLE, IgA nephropathy, Wegener's granulomatosis, and anti-GBM disease can lead to this condition if they are severe. Prognosis depends on degree of kidney failure at presentation.
Epi	A small number of patients progress to ESRD; otherwise, full recovery occurs spontaneously.	Most common worldwide cause of idiopathic GN. Uncommon in African Americans. From 40% to 50% progress to ESRD in 20 years.	Relatively uncommon. Most progress to ESRD. High rate of recurrence after renal transplants.	Crescents are nonspecific and are present in postinfectious GN, lupus nephritis, IgA nephropathy, MPGN, Henoch-Schönlein purpura (HSP), Wegener's granulomatosis, and microscopic polyarteritis nodosa.
P	From immune complex deposition 1–2 weeks after group A β-hemolytic streptococcus (*Streptococcus pyogenes*) infection. However, it can follow any type of bacterial or viral infection and is also seen with endocarditis.	Cause is unclear. Due to an abnormality in IgA regulation, perhaps from a chronically exposed antigen that caused an exaggerated mucosal response. Seen in association with conditions that increase circulating IgA levels, such as cirrhosis, gluten enteropathy, MPN, and HIV.	Two types exist: Type I (two-thirds of cases): deposition of immune complexes in the glomerulus with activation of classic and alternative complement pathways. Type II (one-third of cases): activation of alternative complement pathway only. Secondary causes are associated with chronic inflammatory conditions such as SLE, HBV, HCV, endocarditis, HIV lipodystrophy, α₁-antitrypsin deficiency, malignancies (CLL, lymphoma, melanoma), and hereditary complement deficiency states.	There are three types: Type I: anti-GBM antibodies occur with linear deposits of IgG and often with C3 along the renal basement membrane. Sometimes anti-GBM antibodies cross-react with pulmonary alveolar basement membrane to produce *Goodpasture syndrome*. Type II: immune complex mediated. Type III: pauci-immune or ANCA associated and can be a sequela of Wegener's granulomatosis or another polyangiitis.

SiSx	Classically, patients have smokey, cocoa-colored urine following a URI. If they have no signs of systemic infection, they may be asymptomatic.	One-half of patients have gross hematuria, which usually presents concurrently or within few days of a URI. Proteinuria can be up to the nephrotic range (which carries a worse prognosis). One-third of patients have microscopic hematuria on routine exam. Less than 10% have an acute GN that appears to be associated with HSP or may be a limited form of it.	Usually presents with a mixture of nephritic and nephrotic syndromes. Serum complement is usually low.	Progression from normal renal function to renal failure in days to weeks. Goodpasture's syndrome and Wegener's granulomatosis may also present with hemoptysis.
Dx	Urine RBC casts, azotemia, low C3, and positive serum ASO for streptococcal infection can make the diagnosis. If pathologic exams were done: LM—large, hypercellular swollen glomeruli, mesangial proliferation with PMNs and monocytes. EM—subepithelial "humps" of IgG and C3. Immunofluorescence—coarse granular pattern of IgG or C3 deposits along the basement membrane.	By renal biopsy. LM—mesangioproliferative and focal proliferative. Rarely, overt crescentic. Immunofluorescence—mesangial immune complexes of IgA and usually C3. C1q is absent (because of activation of the alternative pathway). EM—deposits in the mesangium.	By renal biopsy. LM—types I and II are indistinguishable. Mesangial proliferation, leukocyte infiltration, and thickened GBM. PAS shows a "double-contour" or "train-track" appearance due to mesangial and monocyte interposition. EM—type I has subendothelial electron-dense deposits. Type II has a deposition of unknown dense material in lamina densa of GBM. Immunofluorescence—type I has a granular pattern of C3. IgG, C1q, and C4 are also present. Type II has C3 on either side of the GBM. Type III (rare) has features of both types I and II.	By renal biopsy. LM—crescents seen between Bowman's capsule and glomerular tuft from depositing of fibrin, epithelial cell proliferation. EM—rupture in GBM. Immunofluorescence—linear IgG and C3 in Goodpasture's syndrome. One should attempt to find the underlying condition, with additional serology for Goodpasture's syndrome, Wegener's granulomatosis, or microscopic polyangiitis.
Tx	Typically, patient recovers fully with conservative treatment aimed at maintaining sodium and water balance.	ACE inhibitor in most cases and steroids in severe cases, which may be more beneficial in a certain subset. Cytotoxic agents are used in severe disease. ESRD develops in 15% at 10 years and in 20% at 20 years. Otherwise, there is a relapsing-remitting course.	Few remissions. Disease follows a slowly progressive but unremitting course. There is no effective treatment. There may be some role for antiplatelet agents, though this remains controversial. Patients with non nephrotic proteinuria have a more benign outcome.	Steroids and cytotoxic agents aim to prevent progression to ESRD but are not always successful.

urine may help solubilize myoglobin casts, although the data for this procedure are limited. Compartment syndrome is a potential complication if there is enough muscle breakdown.

Renal Disease Associated with Monoclonal Gammopathies

Renal Amyloidosis

D—Deposition of amyloid, a nondistinct pathologic proteinaceous substance in the kidney. It can be either primary or secondary from a reaction to a long-standing inflammatory disease. There are many different component of amyloid, depending on the disease process. The most common are as follows:

AL—from monoclonal immunoglobulin light chains, as in primary amyloidosis.

AA—a reactive secondary amyloidosis from an inflammatory condition.

β_2-microglobulin—long-term HD-related amyloidosis.

There is also a hereditary amyloidosis that is autosomal dominant.

P—

Pathophysiology includes the following:

Primary amyloid (AL)—usually derived from variable regions of λ light chains and forms fibrin tangles.

Secondary amyloid (AA) or reactive amyloidosis—associated with increased hepatocyte production of the acute phase reactant serum amyloid (SAA) protein, perhaps stimulated by interleukin-1 (IL-1) from chronic inflammation. The product is degraded by macrophages into smaller amyloid fragments that are deposited as fibrillin in tissues.

In secondary amyloid, RA accounts for up to 40% of cases in the United States. Others causing include ankylosing spondylitis, psoriatic arthritis, chronic pyogenic infections, inflammatory bowel disease (IBD), cystic fibrosis, renal cell carcinoma, Hodgkin's disease, and familial Mediterranean fever (FMF). It is rare in SLE.

SiSx—Symptoms depend on the site of involvement:

Glomerular involvement—Nephrotic range proteinuria with edema. Seventy-five percent of primary amyloidoses present with proteinuria. Urine sediment is typified by lack of inflammation at first. End-stage renal disease develops in 20% cases. Patients do not necessarily present with highly elevated Cr.

Vascular and tubular deposits—Narrowing of vascular lumens. Proteinuria and nephrotic syndrome with renal insufficiency are common in secondary amyloid. Degree of disease may be due to the size of the amyloid fragment. Less common is tubular dysfunction leading to type I RTA or NDI.

Crescentic GN—Rare complication superimposed on amyloidosis. Almost all cases are secondary amyloidosis due to RA. Consider this possibility when a patient has renal amyloidosis with acute renal failure and active urine sediment.

Dx—Renal biopsy is necessary. Amyloid has an antiparallel, β-pleated sheet secondary structure, which binds Congo red and is green birefringent under polarized light. Additionally, thioflavin-T turns the substance yellow-green. There is usually codeposition of serum amyloid P, glycosaminoglycans, and apolipoproteins. The different types of amyloid are indistinguishable by light microscopy (LM) and electron microscopy (EM). On LM, biopsy of the kidney shows diffuse glomerular deposition of hyaline material, first in the mesangium and then in the capillary. Immunofluorescence is negative for immunoglobulin (Ig) and complement in secondary amyloidosis but positive for monoclonal λ or κ light chains in the primary form. Alternatively, bone marrow biopsy can be useful as can liver/kidney biopsy, which is positive in 90% of cases. Abdominal fat pad testing is positive in 60–80% of cases.

Tx—In primary amyloid, there is no proven response to treatment. There is a 20% response rate with melphalan and prednisone. Autologous stem cell transplant allows higher doses of chemotherapy. Secondary amyloid can lead to ESRD, especially in patients with high SAA. It is best to treat the underlying inflammatory process in order to stabilize renal function and protein excretion. Colchicine has been tried and is most successful in FMF. Survival in patients with cardiac, renal, or hepatic failure is <18 months. These are the major causes of death. While associated with proliferation of single clones of plasma cells (thereby monoclonal), most patients with primary amyloidosis do not develop malignant characteristics of multiple myeloma (MM). Conversely, people with MM and light chain overproduction do not necessarily develop amyloidosis.

Light Chain Deposition Disease (LCDD)

D—Systemic disease caused by a monoclonal gammopathy with accumulation of monoclonal light chains in the kidney. Deposits have a fine granular structure (unlike amyloid, which has a fibrillar structure) and do not stain with Congo red or thioflavin T. They are more often κ (not λ, as in AL). Also, there are usually deposits in the glomeruli and in tubular basement membrane.

P—Instead of the variable portion of Ig (as in amyloid), the constant region of the light chain is deposited.

Epi—Most patients are <45 years old; 60% have MM. Others have Waldenströms macroglobulinemia or lymphoma. Sixty percent show nodular glomerulosclerosis similar to that found in diabetes. However, the features will not be brought out on silver stain.

SiSx—Nephrotic range proteinuria is seen in 50% of patients, along with renal insufficiency. Symptoms of malignancy may be present as well. Cardiac involvement, similar to that in amyloidosis, can also be seen.

Dx—On LM, biopsy shows a nodular sclerosing pattern with mesangial nodules of acellular eosinophilia that resemble those seen in diabetic glomerulosclerosis. Complement staining is negative.

Tx—The prognosis is poor, with death from cardiac or infectious complications. Melphalan and prednisone (as in amyloid) are generally not successful in patients with Cr > 4. Recurrence in renal transplants is reported.

Waldenstrom's Macroglobulinemia (See Chapter 10)

Renovascular Disease

Renal Artery Stenosis (RAS)

D—Stenosis of the main renal artery or its branches.

P—It is caused by (1) atherosclerotic plaques and (2) fibromuscular dysplasia, a disease producing structural abnormalities in the arterial wall. Decreased blood flow to the juxtaglomerular apparatus leads to renin activation and increased aldosterone production.

Epi—The disease accounts for 2–5% of cases of hypertension. Fibromuscular dysplasia is classically seen in young women.

RF—It is more common in patients with atherosclerotic disease.

SiSx—Symptoms include hypertension developing in a previously normotensive individual >50 or <30 years old or in a person who suddenly has very difficult-to-control blood pressure (BP). Classically, a high-pitched epigastric bruit is heard. Other features include hypokalemia secondary to hyperaldosteronism and metabolic alkalosis.

Dx—The best initial screen is ultrasound, which may show unilateral hypertrophy but normal echogenicity. Absence of contralateral hypertrophy should make one consider bilateral RAS. The captopril test has a sensitivity and specificity of >95%. (Oral captopril induces increased rennin production, which is more marked in RAS than in essential hypertension.) The gold standard is angiography, but magnetic resonance angiography (MRA) can also be done.

Tx—Definitive treatment involves surgery versus angioplasty to restore flow to the kidney. In the meantime, control of BP is important. Medical therapy alone is not an option. Angioplasty of the renal arteries can cure >50% of patients with fibromuscular dysplasia.

Renal Vein Thrombosis (RVT)

D—Thrombosis of one or both main renal veins.

RF—Risk factors include hypercoagulable states, nephrotic syndrome, trauma, extrinsic compressions (e.g., aortic aneurysm, tumor, lymph nodes), invasion by renal cell carcinoma, dehydration in infants, pregnancy, and use of oral contraceptives (OCPs).

SiSx—Symptoms depend on the abruptness of onset and the patient's age.

Children—Fever, chills, lumbar tenderness (with kidney enlargement), leukocytosis, hematuria, loss of renal function.

Young adults—Acute deterioration of renal function, exacerbation of proteinuria and hematuria.

Elderly individuals—Gradual thrombosis manifesting as recurrent PE or development of hypertension. Fanconi-like syndrome and RTA type II are also possible.

Dx—Renal venography provides definitive diagnosis. Magnetic resonance venography (MRV) may also provide definitive evidence.

Tx—Anticoagulation is necessary (to prevent PE). Consider using streptokinase and thrombectomy. Nephrectomy may be indicated in infants with life-threatening renal infarction.

Thrombotic Microangiopathies

In these conditions there is swelling of the basement membrane; detachment of epithelial cells; accumulation of fluid, fibrin, and cell debris; and partial or complete occlusion of the vessels such that there is trauma to circulating RBCs resulting in a microangiopathic hemolytic anemia. Associated diseases are thrombotic thrombocytopenic purpura (TTP), hemolytic-uremic syndrome (HUS), scleroderma, malignant hypertension, and antiphospholipid antibody syndrome. For a discussion of HUS/TTP and antiphospholipid antibody syndrome, see Chapter 9.

Hypertensive Nephrosclerosis

D—Sclerosis of the renal vasculature in response to sustained high systemic blood pressure leading to sustained glomerular capillary hydrostatic pressure. There are two forms: (1) benign nephrosclerosis, a disease of the media from chronic, nonspecific hypertension and (2) malignant nephrosclerosis in which there is a unique intimal lesion that can lead to renal ischemia and exacerbation of disease.

SiSx—Benign nephrosclerosis occurs in people with hypertension for 10–15 years. With malignant nephrosclerosis there can be sudden, abrupt increases in BP in those who previously only had moderately increased BP or who were normotensive. There may be associated acute renal failure, papilledema, hypertension encephalopathy, and an active urine sediment with hematuria and protein up to the nephrotic range.

Dx—Diagnosis is made primarily by the person's history and the clinical features. Renal biopsy shows the "onion skin" appearance of the renal vasculature.

Tx—The goal is to control BP. Without good control, benign nephrosclerosis can lead to ESRD. Malignant nephrosclerosis is considered a medical emergency and is approached aggressively.

Scleroderma Renal Crisis

D—Abrupt onset of renal failure accompanying scleroderma characterized by (1) acute renal failure, usually in the absence of significant renal disease, (2) abrupt onset of moderate to marked hypertension (although some patients are normotensive) due to ischemic activation of the renin-angiotensin system (hypertension is usually associated with grade III hypertensive retinopathy), and (3) a relatively benign urine sediment.

Epi—From 1% to 15% of patients with scleroderma develop this form of disease, although 60%–80% have some renal involvement.

RF—Risk factors include African American race, use of high-dose steroids, diffuse skin involvement (vs. limited cutaneous involvement) type of scleroderma, and cyclosporine use. The condition is also more common in cooler months, which raises the question of whether cold-induced vasospasm contributes to its pathogenesis.

P—The pathophysiology is renal ischemia and hypersecretion of renin leading to a hypertensive type of nephrosclerosis. On pathologic exam, one can see changes in the arcuate and interlobular arteries. Fibrin thrombi and fibrinoid necrosis are seen acutely. Upon healing, onion skin hypertrophy appears. It resembles the changes seen in malignant hypertension.

SiSx—Symptoms in addition to those in the definition include microangiopathic hemolytic anemia, pulmonary edema, headache, blurred vision, and hypertension encephalopathy with or without seizures. Nephrotic range proteinuria is unusual.

Dx—Renal biopsy does not establish the definitive diagnosis since the same changes can be seen in malignant hypertension, HUS, TTP, radiation nephritis, transplant rejection, and antiphospholipid antibody syndrome. The diagnosis is made therefore mainly by the patient history, exam and presentation.

Tx—If it is untreated, ESRD develops in 1–2 months. Control of BP is the mainstay of treatment. Aggressive treatment can save renal function before irreversible vascular injury occurs. Administer an ACE inhibitor to reverse the ATII-induced vasoconstriction. Captopril is the published agent of choice; it has a sulfhydryl group that may contribute to the effect. The goal is to reduce BP 10–15 mmHg/day until a diastolic pressure of 80–90 mmHg is reached. If BP reduction is too fast, it can precipitate acute tubular necrosis (ATN). Therefore, labetalol or nitroprusside should be avoided. Patients on an ACE inhibitors have been shown to progress to ESRD less quickly. If there is an inadequate response to the ACE inhibitor, calcium channel blockers can be used. Other alternatives include prostacyclin and epoprostenol. In the patient with scleroderma, the best approach is to screen the BP monthly, monitor the plasma Cr concentration, and monitor urine protein with a dipstick test every 3–6 months. Despite treatment, 20–50% of patients progress to ESRD. Renal transplantation has lower survival than for other indications and a 20% recurrence rate.

Sickle Cell Nephropathy

D—Decrease in renal function secondary to decreased renal capillary blood flow leading in many cases to papillary infarction.

SiSx—Volume depletion occurs, as there is an inability to concentrate urine after obliteration of the vasa recta and the concentrating system. Distal RTA (type IV) can also occur due to impaired function. Painless gross hematuria occurs in up to 50% of patients; this is seen in both sickle cell trait (Hb SA) or compound heterozygotes of sickle cell and hemoglobin C (Hb SC) (see Chapter 9). Papillary necrosis can be silent and progress to chronic renal insufficiency. Multiple urinary tract infections (UTIs) may occur. Nephrotic syndrome is seen in about 4% of cases.

Dx—In addition to a history of the above symptoms in a patient with documented sickle cell disease, one can demonstrate papillary infarction by biopsy, which otherwise shows membranoproliferative glomerulopathy with segmental and global sclerosis.

Tx—Treatment consists of volume repletion and treatment of acidosis, if present. Avoid K^+-sparing diuretics, NSAIDs, and potassium supplements.

Cystic Diseases of the Kidney

Autosomal Dominant Polycystic Kidney Disease (ADPKD)

D—A hereditary disease with a predisposition to cause development of large, cystic kidneys.

P—Ninety percent of cases are autosomal dominant, and 10% are sporadic. A defect in any one of three gene products of the polycistin gene complex is associated. Cysts have straw-colored fluid and can become hemorrhagic.

Epi—The prevalence is as high as 1:300. The disease accounts for 10% of ESRD cases in the United States.

RF—A family history is the main risk.

SiSx—Symptoms can present at any age but usually in the third to fourth decade. Gross and microscopic hematuria is common. Urolithiasis occurs in 15–20% of patients, with stones usually composed of calcium oxalate or uric acid. Seventy-five percent of adults will have hypertension due to intrarenal disruption of normal architecture; 50% have ESRD by 60 years of age. Extrarenal manifestations include hepatic cysts (in 50–70%) with normal LFTs. Also seen are cysts in the spleen, pancreas, and ovaries. Intracranial aneurysms are present in 5–10% of asymptomatic patients. Mitral valve prolapse (MVP) is found in 25%. Colonic diverticular disease is the most common extrarenal finding.

Dx—Ultrasound detects 100% of cysts in patients over 30 years old. Computed tomography may be more sensitive for small cysts. There is a greater chance for progression to ESRD in younger males with gross hematuria, hypertension, and increased renal size.

Tx—Treat hypertension and UTIs to slow the rate of progression. The most common causes events.

Simple Renal Cyst

D—A usually benign condition in which a cystic structure develops within or near the renal parenchyma.

Epi—It accounts for two-thirds of all renal masses.

P—Cysts are usually located at the outer cortex and are fluid-filled, with an ultrafiltrate of plasma.

Sx—Most cysts do not cause symptoms, but some can become infected and if they are large, they may cause flank pain.

Dx—Most cysts are found incidentally with ultrasound. The primary concern is to differentiate them from malignancy or an abscess. To be considered benign, they must be echo-free, smooth-walled, and easily demarcated and must have no calcifications or solid components with mixed echogenecity. They should be nonenhancing with contrast. If the diagnosis is in doubt, surgical exploration is needed.

Tx—Periodic reevaluation is the standard of care. Usually no treatment is needed.

Common Iatrogenic and Drug-Related Renal Toxicities

Aminoglycoside Renal Toxicity

D—Acute tubular necrosis secondary to aminoglycoside administration related to the preferential uptake and storage in the renal cortex, with subsequent damage to the (PCT) cells.

RF—It is due to concurrent renal failure from another cause.

SiSx—It can appear as late as 5–7 days after discontinuation of aminoglycosides because of the length of time aminoglycosides can be stored in the body. K^+ and Mg^{2+} wasting is sometimes apparent. Creatinine increases, but most patients are not oliguric. Note: Aminoglycoside renal toxicity differs by the specific antibiotic in the order of streptomycin > gentamycin > tobramycin from most toxic to least toxic.

Dx—The diagnosis usually involves a history of concurrent medication use and renal failure. Levels of aminoglycoside may be supratherapeutic.

Tx—The main therapy is supportive, with removal of offending nephrotoxins. The Cr level usually returns to normal within 3 weeks. Irreversible damage is uncommon.

NSAID Renal Toxicity

D—Renal failure from use of NSAIDs that can either be acute interstitial nephritis (AIN) or hemodynamically mediated by inhibiting prostaglandins in people with underlying renal disease. COX-2 inhibitors may also cause acute renal failure. Long-term use (>1 year) can lead to chronic renal disease.

P—The NSAIDs block production of vasodilatory prostaglandins, leading to decreased renal blood flow and acute renal failure.

SiSx—Acute interstitial nephritis may present with nephrotic syndrome due to minimal change disease or even membranous nephropathy. There may also be hyperkalemia, hyponatremia, and exacerbation of preexisting hypertension.

Dx—Diagnosis is usually made by a history of NSAID abuse/use.

Tx—Spontaneous recovery usually occurs within weeks unless chronic use has led to severe disease. In general, NSAIDs should be avoided or used as little as possible by anyone with any degree of renal disease or with concomitant comorbid conditions such as heart failure.

Contrast-Induced Nephropathy (CIN)

D—Acute renal failure following the administration of contrast dye, as used in cardiac catheterization or CT scans.

P—Contrast dye causes renal vasoconstriction, tubular obstruction, and direct tubular toxicity. These developments lead to decreased GFR.

RF—Diabetes and prior renal dysfunction can predispose to contrast-induced acute renal failure. The chance of CIN increases directly in proportion with the amount of iodine contrast that is used.

SiSx—Acute renal failure is seen by BUN and Cr testing, usually 24–48 hours after a dye load is given. Oliguria is a bad prognostic sign.

Dx—Diagnosis is usually made by the history and the absence of any other inciting cause. A low fraction excretion of sodium is usually found, as in prerenal acute renal failure.

Tx—Patients should recover within 1 week. Preventive measures for those who need a study with contrast include NS-forced diuresis before and afterward, low-ionic contrast agents, limiting the dose of the dye, and spacing repeated loads. Administration of N-acetylcysteine before and after the study, as well as the use of sodium bicarbonate infusions, have been shown in several studies (albeit equivocal) to perhaps help prevent worsening renal failure.

Radiation Nephritis

D—Renal dysfunction from radiation exposure (usually >23 Gy exposure within <5 weeks).

P—The pathophysiology is radiation-induced ischemia leading to tubulointerstitial damage.

SiSx—Symptoms include rapidly progressive renal failure, hypertension (may be malignant following unilateral renal irradiation), anemia, and proteinuria, which may reach the nephrotic range.

Dx—Diagnosis is made by a history of exposure and the absence of other causes.

Tx—Conservative management is used. Ipsilateral nephrectomy can be done in rare cases for unilateral renal irradiation.

CHAPTER 5

Gastroenterology

THE ABDOMINAL EXAM

Have the patient lay as flat as possible, with the arms at the sides.

1. Inspection
   - Get an overall sense of whether the patient is in any discomfort or pain before the exam.
   - Look at the overall shape of the abdomen (protuberant, flat, or scaphoid) and for asymmetry, scars, ecchymoses, striae (long red or purple stretch marks), and venous collaterals (if present, note the direction of blood flow).
   - Look for heavy use of abdominal muscles by patients in respiratory distress.
   - Look for peristaltic waves in patients with suspected intestinal obstruction.
2. Auscultation
   - Palpating before listening likely does not change the auscultatory findings, but auscultation should be performed next nonetheless.
   - The presence of bowel sounds usually means little, but their complete absence or a marked decrease from a prior exam is noteworthy, indicating possible obstruction or ileus.
   - High-pitched sounds may indicate obstruction.
   - Rarely, one may also hear venous hums that are benign or renal artery bruits indicative of renal artery stenosis. The latter are best heard just above and lateral to the umbilicus.
3. Percussion
   - Perform generalized percussion in all quadrants to determine a sense of dullness (bowel tissue, organs) or resonance (air).

- For the liver, start low down in the right lower quadrant (RLQ) and progress cephalad; otherwise, you will miss the difference in percussion if the liver is large.
- For the spleen, also start in the RLQ and progress diagonally up to the left costal margin. One can also percuss under the left costal margin while the patient takes large breaths (the spleen should move down on inspiration and hence will sound dull).

4. Palpation
   - Always note the patient's facial expression while palpating and start superficially, then deep. Be methodical, and examine any painful area last. If the patient's abdomen is rigid, bend both knees up all the way to relax the muscles.
   - Look for classic signs of peritoneal inflammation:
     1. Rebound tenderness (pain upon release of the hand rather than application of pressure, as muscles quickly resume their normal shape and move the peritoneum). Sometimes any quick movement of the abdomen can elicit this sign.
     2. Guarding is tensing of the abdominal muscles. Attempt to distinguish between voluntary and involuntary guarding.
        - In patients you suspect are feigning pain, while listening with the stethoscope, use it to press the area gently without giving advance warning.
        - Feeling for the liver and spleen is perhaps best done after percussion. To accentuate the findings, ask the patient to take a deep breath, and feel

both on inspiration and on expiration. An advanced trick for hepatomegaly is to listen with a stethoscope and simultaneously scratch the surface with a finger until there is a change in pitch at the liver border.

Specific findings on the physical exam can be found in the description of various diseases.

DIAGNOSTIC AND THERAPEUTIC MODALITIES

A number of noninvasive and invasive modalities exist to help evaluate many conditions affecting the GI tract. Choosing the appropriate study depends on the clinical question. Table 5-1 shows some of the more commonly used studies.

APPROACH TO COMMON PROBLEMS

Approach to Abdominal Pain

1. Major questions to always ask in order to help narrow the differential diagnosis:
   - **P**resentation/precipitating factors. Where is the pain (ask the patient to localize it with one finger if possible) and how did it come on (gradually or suddenly)?
   - **Q**uality. Is it sharp, like a jabbing knife, dull, or burning? Does it feel muscular or visceral? Remember, abdominal pain from bowel disease must be due to wall distention since this is the only place where pain receptors in the bowel are located.
   - **R**adiation. Does the pain go anywhere? Pain will always be poorly localized when the visceral surfaces are inflamed, but it becomes more localized when the parietal surfaces of organs are inflamed (as in appendicitis or cholecystitis). Referred pain for the right upper quadrant (RUQ) is to the right scapula and for the left upper quadrant (LUQ) is to the left scapula.
   - **S**everity/symptoms associated with the pain. How bad is it on a scale of 1 to 10? What brings it on and what relieves it, if anything (e.g., position, movement,

vomiting, defecation, or passage of flatus)? With relief obtained by vomiting or with a bowel movement, consider an obstructive process or ileus. With lack of a bowel movement or flatus, think of an obstructive process or ileus. With very severe pain, think of a perforation.
   - **T**iming. Does the pain come or go, or is it constant? How long does it last? For colicky pain (which comes and goes), consider an obstructive process in which temporary distention causes pain. For constant pain, think of an inflammatory process.
2. Make the differential diagnosis and decide on diagnostic procedure if necessary. Table 5-2 is useful for the quadrant approach to abdominal pain in generating differential diagnoses. Most likely causes of abdominal pain by area will vary, based on the patient's age and clinical circumstances.

Approach to Diarrhea

The following algorithm is useful:

1. First, determine if the patient really has diarrhea. Diarrhea is defined not just by an increased amount of stool but also by the weight (for adults it is usually >200 g) and consistency (i.e., one bout of watery loose stool per day may be considered diarrhea).
2. Distinguish between acute and chronic diarrhea. *Acute diarrhea* is roughly defined as that lasting for <3 weeks. It is most likely to be infectious in nature, and is the second most common cause of death worldwide and the leading cause of childhood death worldwide. *Chronic diarrhea* is defined as diarrhea persisting for >3 weeks. It is more common in developing nations, where it affects as much as 5% of the population. General complications of most types of diarrhea are metabolic alkalosis, hypokalemia, and dehydration.
3. Determine the type of diarrhea: secretory, osmotic, malabsorptive, or inflammatory. See Table 5-3.
4. Treat the underlying cause if possible. Depending on the situation, conservative management with rehydration (oral rehydra-

Table 5-1. Useful Radiologic and Endoscopic Techniques in Gastroenterology

Procedure	Description	Advantages	Disadvantages
Esophagogastroduodenoscopy (EGD)	Scope passed from oropharynx that in most cases can reach the second part of the duodenum.	Used to examine the mucosa for inflammation (e.g., esophagitis, gastritis, ulcers, strictures, and malignancies). Allows for biopsy, therapy of bleeding varices, and removal of foreign bodies.	IV conscious sedation is necessary in most cases.
Colonoscopy	Scope from below via the rectum where the cecum is reached in 95% of cases.	The gold standard for examining diseases of the colonic mucosa. Has greater sensitivity for polyps and malignancies than barium enema and allows for biopsy and therapy of arteriovenous malformations.	IV conscious sedation is necessary. Small risk of bowel perforation with insufflation. Requires significant bowel preparation beforehand to remove stool.
Flexible Sigmoidoscopy	Visualizes the rectum and a variable portion of the left colon, at most 60 cm from the anal verge.	Does not usually require conscious sedation.	Does not allow visualization of the whole colon in looking for pathology but is good for viewing left-sided colonic lesions.
Upper GI Series with or without Small Bowel Follow-Through (Also Called the Barium Swallow Study)	Barium is swallowed and then images of the bowel are taken under fluoroscopy, usually up to the last part of the duodenum. Small bowel follow-through to the cecum can be done with images later after the barium has traveled further.	Used primarily to look for structural abnormalities and to assess peristalsis.	Cannot demonstrate reflux disease and is insensitive to mild inflammation of the mucosa, so can identify only some ulcers. Radiographic reflux is seen in only 40% of patients with GERD and in 25% of normal patients.
Barium Enema	A non–water-soluble contrast material is passed into the rectum, and its shape is visualized under fluoroscopy. Air can also be injected to be used as a second contrast agent.	Best used to look for diverticula and strictures or to define anatomy.	If there is colonic perforation, barium will cause an intense inflammatory response. In such cases, the water-soluble alternative, gastrograffin, is preferred for enema.
Endoscopic Retrograde Cholangiopancreatography (ERCP)	An endoscope is passed from above down to the duodenum, after which a catheter is passed through the ampulla of Vater. This allows contrast material to be injected into both the biliary ducts and the pancreatic duct under fluoroscopy to view their shape.	Gives an accurate view of the biliary system. Can also be used for sphincterotomy (sphincter of Oddi), removal of stones from ducts, and dilation and stenting of strictured ducts.	Can cause pancreatitis in up to 5% of cases. Bile duct perforation is possible.
Endoscopic Ultrasound	Used to obtain images of the gut wall and adjacent organs.	Useful for staging esophageal, gastric, pancreatic, and rectal malignancies.	Cannot detect distant metastases.

Table 5-2. Causes of Abdominal Pain Based on Location

Area	Diffuse Periumbilical	Right Upper Quadrant	Right Lower Quadrant	Left Upper Quadrant	Left Lower Quadrant
Likely Causes of Disease	Prolonged constipation Pancreatitis Peptic ulcer disease Gastroenteritis Bowel obstruction Ingested toxins Pain related to diabetic ketoacidosis Pain related to narcotic withdrawal Aortic aneurysm Ischemic bowel Early appendicitis Rare: acute intermittent porphyria	Cholecystitis Biliary colic (cholelithiasis) Gastritis Peptic ulcer disease Right lower lobe pneumonia Hepatitis Liver abscess Pyelonephritis (more subcostal/flank)	Appendicitis Nephrolithiasis Inflammatory bowel disease Pelvic inflammatory disease Ectopic pregnancy Ovarian/testicular torsion Tubo-ovarian abscess	Splenic rupture Pyelonephritis Hiatal hernia Pancreatitis Bowel obstruction Ischemic bowel (watershed area) Left lower lobe pneumonia	Diverticulitis Nephrolithiasis Inflammatory bowel disease Sigmoid volvulus Pelvic inflammatory disease Ectopic pregnancy Ovarian/testicular torsion Tubo-ovarian abscess
Initial Test of Choice if Diagnosis Is Unclear	None or CT, depending on the history Abdominal X-ray might be useful if there is concern about obstruction: air-fluid levels will be seen	Typically ultrasound, then CT	CT and/or pelvic ultrasound	CT	CT and/or Pelvic ultrasound

Table 5-3. Distinguishing Characteristics of Types of Diarrhea

Type of Diarrhea	Secretory	Osmotic/Malabsorption	Inflammatory/Exudative
Mechanism	Anything causing increased secretion of electrolytes and water	Osmotic load in the gut draws water in, or there are intrinsic problems with absorption	Inflammatory process disrupts normal absorptive process and causes exudative shedding of GI tract
Classic Description	Watery diarrhea	Bulky, greasy, light-colored, floating stools	Bloody, filled with mucus
Causes	*Infectious* • Non invasive viral gastroenteritis, such as Norwalk virus, rotavirus, or adenovirus • Bacterial causes such as cholera or *Clostridium difficile* toxin. Parasitic infections as a cause are rare in the United States *Drugs* • Laxative abuse or procholinergic use *Tumor/neuroendocrine* • Carcinoid tumor (secretes serotonin) • Villous adenoma • Gastric acid increases with Zollinger-Ellison syndrome, vasoactive intestinal polypeptide-secreting tumor (VIPoma)	• Lactase deficiency • Bile salt malabsorption • Malabsorption syndromes (e.g., celiac sprue, pancreatic insufficiency of any cause, problems with bile production, mucosal atrophy) • Ingestion of sorbitol (a bulk sweetener in foods and a laxative) • Dumping syndrome (postsurgical) • Abuse of magnesium containing laxatives	• Association with chronic disease such as inflammatory bowel disease, irritable bowel syndrome, and connective tissue disease (e.g., scleroderma) • Radiation enteritis, ischemic colitis, and status postchemotherapy • Invasive microbials [CHESS mnemonic for organisms like *Campylobacter, H. pylori, E. coli* (enterohemorrhagic types O157:H7), *Salmonella,* and *Shigella*]. Also consider *Yersinia enterocolitica* and *Vibro parahemolyticus* in uncooked shellfish • Any motility disorder of bowel with bacterial overgrowth • Thyrotoxicosis, diabetes-associated enteropathy

Diagnostic Hints			
• Persists with fasting. Independent of food intake. Nonodorous • For infectious cases, consider S. aureus when symptoms occur <6 hours after eating; consider C. perfringens when symptoms occur 8–14 hours afterward and viral causes when they occur >14 hours after eating • If vomiting is a significant component, consider E. coli • Recent antibiotics use of any kind should make one consider C. difficile	• Improves with fasting. • Worse with food intake. • Malodorous • Can calculate the stool osmolar gap (Measured Stool $Osm - 2(Na^+_{stool} + K^+_{stool})$, which is usually >50 mEq/L, indicates osmotic diarrhea • Carbohydrate malabsorption involves acidic stool pH and intolerance of milk products. Urine D-xylose test is positive. (Xylose is an absorbable sugar that should be excreted in the urine. Less than 5 g in urine after administration is abnormal) • In fat malabsorption there are voluminous pale, fatty stools that can be screened for fat using a Sudan stain or confirmed with a 72-hour fecal fat test, wherein >8 g/day of fat in the stool after a special 100 g/day fat diet is abnormal • Protein malabsorption includes edema, muscle wasting, and hypoalbuminemia • In pancreatic insufficiency, bentiromide (normally cleaved by pancreatic chymotrypsin to PABA) administration will show a decreased amount of PABA in urine	• Generally independent of food intake • Patient may seem more toxic • Inflammatory cells seen in stool. Fecal leukocytes may be present, though sensitivity is debatable • Consider stool cultures for acute diarrhea for those who (1) are HIV positive, (2) have inflammatory bowel disease, or (3) have significant comorbidities. Culture identifies *Salmonella*, *Campylobacter*, and *Shigella* • Ova and parasite tests are ordered (1) if diarrhea is chronic, (2) if there is a high incidence of disease in the patient's location, or (3) if the patient is immunocompromised • Barium enema should be avoided in inflammatory colitis since it can exacerbate the condition • Perform sigmoidoscopy or colonoscopy if the cause still unclear	

tion in many cases) and alteration of diet is done. Depending on whether or not the patient is stable, antibiotics can be added; however, they are not helpful in *Staphylococcus aureus* toxin or *Bacillus cereus* infection. Antimotility agents like loperamide can be used in patients without fever or bloody stools.

Approach to GI Bleeding

The following is a useful diagnostic algorithm after the patient has been stabilized:

1. First, determine whether the source is an upper (UGIB) or lower GI bleed (LGIB). The boundary between the two is traditionally the ligament of Treitz (at the end of the duodenum). The presentation usually helps define this:

    Hematemesis—vomiting of blood. It is indicative of an UGIB. Bright red blood indicates vigorous bleeding, whereas "coffee ground"-colored emesis indicates that the blood has had time to mix with gastric acid and pepsin, which have degraded the hemoglobin.

    Melena—black tarry stool indicative of a UGIB above the ligament of Treitz or a slower LGIB. At least 75–100 mL is needed for bleeding to manifest.

Hematochezia—Bright red blood per rectum, usually from LGIB or extremely vigorous UGIB.

In some cases, it is not possible to distinguish a UGIB from an LGIB.

2. Generate a differential diagnosis based on the history. Common causes of GI bleeds are shown in Table 5-4.

3. Work-up and treatment of individual diseases are presented elsewhere. All patients must be stabilized hemodynamically and need two large-bore (at least 18-gauge) IV access sites, with a type and crossmatch for imminent blood transfusion. A Foley catheter will also be useful for determining the volume status. There is a 16% false-negative rate for nasogastric (NG) lavage, as one may not always see blood if the bleed is beyond a closed pylorus. If the fluid fails to clear after >500 cc of saline lavage, then consider more emergent need to find and treat the source by esophagogastroduodenoscopy (EGD). In patients with known varices, an NG tube is still indicated. Consider transfusing packed RBCs after a significant volume of normal saline (NS) has been given (usually 5 L) and transfusing platelets or fresh frozen plasma if multiple units of packed RBCs are given as these factors are being diluted out.

Table 5-4.   Common Causes of GI Bleeds

	Upper GI Bleed	Lower GI Bleed
Common Causes	1. Duodenal ulcer 2. Esophageal varices (one-third of patients with varices will also have other source of GI bleeds) 3. Gastric ulcer/gastritis 4. Mallory-Weiss tear 5. Erosive esophagitis 6. Arteriovenous malformation 7. Neoplasia	1. Diverticulosis—number one cause in patients >40 years old 2. Hemorrhoids and fissures 3. Neoplasia such as colon cancer (in patients >65, this is the diagnosis until proven otherwise) 4. Angiodysplasia or arteriovenous malformation 5. Vigorous UGIB (can mimic LGIB) 6. Ischemia 7. Inflammatory bowel disease
Signs and Symptoms	Hematemesis or coffee ground emesis, melena > hematochezia, orthostasis	Hematochezia > melena, but can be either
Management	Fluid resuscitate and stabilize. Place NG tube and perform lavage. Perform EGD if patient is stable and less than 150 cc blood returns via the NG tube. Otherwise, consider emergent EGD vs. performing surgery to stop refractory bleeding.	Fluid resuscitate and stabilize. Colonoscopy is the method of choice for diagnosis. Always rule out UGIB with NG tube and perform lavage. Radionuclide imaging may be useful to localize sources of active bleeding that are too small to see otherwise.

Approach to Dysphagia and/or Odynophagia

1. Determine if the patient has true dysphagia, which is characterized by a sensation of food arrest during swallowing because of difficulty in moving food through the oropharynx or the esophagus. Complaints of additional pain with swallowing (odynophagia) are thought to be a sign of underlying disease, especially in elderly individuals, and should be investigated.

2. Try to ascertain which type of dysphagia is present. There are two types: (1) *oropharyngeal dysphagia* (also called *transfer dysphagia*), which is caused by dysfunction of the muscles proximal to the esophagus and (2) *esophageal dysphagia*, which involves the rest of the esophagus more distally. Esophageal dysphagia can have mechanical or dysmotility causes. Patients without a known cause are said to have *functional dysphagia*. Some diagnostic clues are given in Table 5-5.

3. Patients with oropharyngeal dysphagia usually say that food gets stuck immediately on swallowing and point to the cervical region. Those with esophageal dysphagia have symptoms some time after swallowing and localize the area near the sternum. Those with webs or rings tend to have intermittent dysphagia.

4. Diagnostic techniques in cases where the etiology is unclear include video fluoroscopy, in which swallowing is studied on film under fluoroscopy. Otherwise, a barium swallow study is done, followed by endoscopy. Endoscopy usually is not done first, as it is unclear whether a stricture or another structural abnormality is present that may hinder the procedure.

5. Treatment, of course, depends on the underlying cause. Swallowing rehabilitation may be useful. Rings or webs can be cut endoscopically or surgically. Myomectomy or botulinum toxin can be used for sphincter dysfunction. Otherwise, treat the underlying disease.

Approach to Abnormal Liver Function Tests (LFTs)

It is important to remember that LFTs do not include just the transaminases [aspartate aminotransferase (AST), alanine aminotransferase (ALT)], alkaline phosphatase and bilirubin, but also measures of liver synthetic function such as the prothrombin time, which reflects clotting factors synthesis, and an albumin level, which reflects protein synthesis.

1. In generating a differential diagnosis, the history and physical exam should involve parts of the following:
   History
   General: Ask about known personal liver, biliary tract, or heart disease.

Table 5-5.   Diagnostic Clues for Dysphagia

Esophageal Dysphagia		Oropharyngeal Dysphagia
Dysphagia, Solids > Liquids	**Dysphagia, Solids and Liquids**	

• Think esophageal dysphagia with primarily a mechanical obstruction:
   • Carcinoma
   • Esophageal web or ring (more likely to cause intermittent symptoms)
   • Esophageal stricture from chronic reflux
 • Dysphagia lusoria (anomalous blood vessel crosses behind esophagus).
	• Think of dysmotility related issues
	 • Conditions include
	   • Achalasia
	   • Carcinoma in late stage
	   • Scleroderma
	   • Rare causes:
	     Diffuse esophageal spasm
	     Chagas Disease
		• Oropharyngeal dysphagia is more likely if a patient reports a feeling of food getting stuck up high, or if a patient has a cough after eating and/or aspirates easily.
		 • Usually due to a variety of neuromuscular disorders:
		   • Post stroke disease
		   • Polymyositis
		   • Myasthenia Gravis
		   • Parkinson's disease
		   • Myotonic dystrophy
		   • Sphincter dysfunction

Drugs: Ask about exposure to known hepatotoxins (both over-the-counter and herbal medications), as well as the alcohol history.

Infections: Investigate the possibility of viral hepatitis, looking at risk factors such as prior transfusion, a history of IVDU, and the patient's sexual activity. Consider rarer infectious causes [e.g., schistosomiasis, toxoplasmosis, tuberculosis, hepatitis A virus (HAV), cytomegalovirus].

Anatomic: Assess the body mass index (BMI) the presence of type II diabetes, and classic risk factors for gallstones, nonalcoholic steatohepatitis (NASH), and biliary tract disease.

Autoimmune: Ask about a personal history or family history of autoimmune diseases and inflammatory bowel disease. Consider autoimmune hepatitis, primary biliary cirrhosis (PBC), and primary sclerosing cholangitis (PSC).

Familial: Consider hemochromatosis, Wilson's disease, α1-antitrypsin deficiency, cystic fibrosis, and Gilbert's disease.

Malignancy: Ask about constitutional symptoms of weight loss, anorexia, and the presence of swollen glands.

Physical Signs of:

Chronic liver disease: muscle wasting, pruritis, jaundice, spider angiomata, palmar erythema, gynecomastia in men, testicular atrophy, xanthomas, and Dupuytren's contractures on the palms.

Cirrhosis: a small, nonpapable liver or a hard nodular liver.

Portal hypertension: ascites, abdominal venous collaterals including the umbilical caput medusae, splenomegaly, and presence of hemorrhoids.

Visceral malignancy: marked weight loss, an enlarged left supraclavicular node (Virchow's node), periumbilical nodes (Sister Mary Joseph's nodes), or a nodule on the digital rectal exam (Blumer's shelf).

Right-sided heart failure causing hepatic congestion: elevated JVP with an enlarged liver.

Hepatitis or gallbladder disease: RUQ pain, and positive Murphy's sign.

2. Next, look at the pattern of LFT abnormalities. If possible, try to distinguish acute from chronic abnormalities. Generally, hypoalbuminemia and a prolonged prothrombin time imply a subacute to chronic state of liver dysfunction, as the liver has a significant amount of functional reserve. Common patterns include:

a. *Hepatocellular pattern*: The AST and ALT are increased out of proportion to the alkaline phosphatase. This signifies a more destructive process affecting the hepatocytes themselves. In classic alcohol liver disease, the AST/ALT ratio is nearly 2:1. In viral hepatitis, ALT is usually greater than AST. Work-up in patients with an unclear history should include:

(1) Drug levels (e.g., acetaminophen)

(2) Hepatitis C virus (HCV) antibody, hepatitis B virus surface antigen, antibody (HBSAg), core antibody, HAV IgM (with or without IgG)

(3) Iron, total iron binding capacity (TIBC), ferritin studies for hemochromatosis

(4) Antinuclear antibody (ANA), serum protein electrophoresis (SPEP), anti–smooth muscle antibody (ASMA), anti–liver kidney muscle-1 (ALKM-1), and anti–liver cytosol antigen (ALC-1) (see Autoimmune Hepatitis section)

(5) Ceruloplasmin (if the patient is <40 years old) (see Wilson's Disease section)

b. *Cholestatic pattern*: The alkaline phosphatase and bilirubin are increased out of proportion to the ALT and AST. This may signify cholestasis or an obstructed biliary tract. Work-up includes an RUQ ultrasound to look for ductal dilation and the presence of stones. A CT or endoscopic retrograde cholangiopancreatography (ERCP) scan may be necessary to distinguish intra- and extrahepatic cholestasis. If biliary ducts are normal, check for an antimitochondrial antibody (AMA) to look for PBC or perform a liver biopsy. Also, check the level of gamma-glutamyl transpeptidase (GGT), which is more specific for cholestasis, or consider fractionating the alkaline phosphatase to make sure that the source of the problem is the liver and not bone or muscle.

c. *Isolated hyperbilirubinemia*

Direct—consider causes based on whether transaminases have a cholestatic or hepatocelluar pattern.

Indirect—consider work-up of hemolysis (check the hematocrit, lactic dehydrogenase, and haptoglobin), prolonged CHF, and Gilbert's syndrome.

3. If the etiology is still unclear, consider biopsy. Biopsy should almost always be done in patients who have persistently elevated transaminase levels more than two times normal with a negative or ambiguous work-up. Even when a diagnosis has been made, liver biopsy is sometimes used to assess the severity of the condition in order to modify the treatment. If the transaminase levels are less than twofold elevated and work-up for a chronic liver condition has been negative (no evidence of cirrhosis on ultrasound or CT and negative serologies), then clinical follow-up to see the progression or manifestation of disease may be more useful initially.

Diseases of the GI Tract

Esophageal Diseases

Anatomy

- Stratified squamous cells line the wall up to the gastroesophageal (GE) junction in normal patients. Metaplasia into other types of tissue, such as columnar cells, occurs in various diseases.
- The outside or serosal layer has many lymphatics in addition to arteries and veins, which provide easy access for tumor spread. The outer muscular layers are composed of skeletal muscle (upper one-third) and smooth muscle (lower two-thirds). See Figure 5-1.
- Esophageal veins drain into gastric veins and are therefore an important site of disease in portal hypertension.
- Peristalsis occurs through coordination of inner circular and outer longitudinal muscles. Primary peristalsis occurs along with a bolus of food, secondary peristalsis occurs in response to food that is not cleared, and tertiary peristalsis occurs during propulsive fibrillation and is always abnormal.
- Two areas of control exist: the upper esophageal sphincter (UES), which is useful in deglutition and consists primarily of the

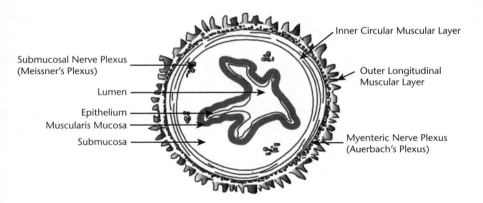

Figure 5-1. Esophageal Cross Section.
This cross section of the esophageal wall shows the major layers including, from inside to outside, the epithelium, muscularis mucosa, the submucosa, the inner circular muscle layer, and the outer longitudinal muscle layer and outer serosal layer. Areas of nerve innervation include Meissner's plexus (parasympathetic innervation) and Auerbach's plexus (parasympathetic and sympathetic innervation).

cricopharyngeus muscle, and the lower esophageal sphincter (LES), which acts to prevent reflux.

Inflammatory Lesions of the Esophagus

Gastroesophageal Reflux Disease (GERD) and Reflux Esophagitis

D—Gastroesophageal reflux is characterized by food moving retrograde in the GI tract and is a normal physiologic occurrence. Gastroesophageal reflux disease (GERD), however, occurs when gastroesophageal reflux leads to significant pathology or symptomatology and becomes problematic. Reflux esophagitis is a consequence of GERD, where acid reflux has caused an inflammatory response.

Epi—Up to 15% of people in the United States have gastroesophageal reflux symptoms once a week and 7% have daily symptoms.

RF—Risk factors include anything that causes delayed gastric emptying: drugs (e.g., high-dose steroids, β agonists, α antagonists, anticholinergics, calcium channel blockers, nitrates), the presence of a hiatal hernia, and pregnancy (progesterone inhibits the LES). One may also see it in scleroderma and after surgical vagotomy.

P—Transient LES relaxation is the most common primary etiology. This is due to decreased resting pressure, prolonged relaxation, or a transient increase in abdominal pressure.

SiSx

GI—Heartburn occurs usually 30–90 minutes after a meal and is described as substernal burning that worsens with reclining, with a concomitant sour taste in the mouth, regurgitation, and/or a feeling of dysphagia. Symptoms are usually worse at night. Hypersalivation (water brash) occurs in rare cases. Complications include strictures from healing esophagitis, esophageal ulceration, reflux-induced laryngitis, and ultimately Barrett's esophagus or cancer. A lump in the throat or odynophagia may signal an ulcer.

Non-GI—Anemia may be seen if bleeding occurs. Gastroesophageal reflux disease is a very common cause of chronic cough; asthma and laryngitis are also described as sequelae. Such symptoms are due in part to irritation from reflux of gastric contents into the proximal esophagus.

Dx—There are multiple modalities to investigate GERD and esophagitis:

1. For first-time complaints, symptomatic treatment with relief may be diagnostic.

2. The gold standard for diagnosis of GERD is 24-hour pH monitoring, in which a pH probe is placed at the GE junction for 24 hours and measures the pH while the patient records the timing of symptoms. One looks to determine if a pH <4 is associated with symptoms.

3. The Bernstein acid perfusion test (re-creation symptoms of GERD when 0.1 N HCl is placed in the midesophagus, reproducing heartburn twice, and is then relieved by saline). A negative Bernstein test, however, does not rule out GERD,

4. Barium swallow can evaluate abnormal anatomy or swallow dysfunction.

5. Esophageal manometry can evaluate for dysmotility. In this test, a tube with multiple pressure sensors tracks and measures peristalsis to see if it is coordinated and appropriate.

6. Esophagogastroduodenoscopy with biopsy should be done in patients with more long-standing GERD, refractory symptoms, ulcerations, Barrett's esophagus, or even malignancy.

Tx—Avoid drugs that exacerbate the condition and problematic substances such as spicy foods, chocolate, nicotine, caffeine, and peppermint for some patients. For reflux esophagitis, elevate the head of the patient's bed and use a proton pump inhibitor (PPI) or H_2 blocker, which is usually effective in many cases in decreasing acid production. To treat the underlying problem of reflux, drugs that increase LES tone and cause promotility (bethanechol, metoclopramide, or domperidone) are useful. Note that agents like carafate should not be used in combination with a PPI because PPIs need an acidic environment in which to work. In extreme cases refractory to therapy, antireflux surgery can be done—such as the Nissen fundoplication, in which the gastric fundus is wrapped around the esophagus to increase LES pressure.

Barrett's Esophagus

D—Complication of continued erosive reflux esophagitis in which the normal epithelium of the esophagus is replaced by intestinal epithelium. It is the most severe consequence of prolonged GERD and is considered to be a premalignant state.

Epi—It is more common in Caucasians and rare in African Americans. The mean age of diagnosis is 55 years, though the condition may even be seen in children. The overall risk is small, but it confers a 40-fold increased risk of adenocarcinoma.

P—Metaplasia occurs in which columnar epithelium replaces the stratified squamous epithelium of the esophagus after repeated insult and injury to the lining. This is a favorable adaptation to prevent further injury. There may be several types of columnar epithelium: gastric type with chief and parietal cells, specialized intestinal cells, or cells similar to those of the gastric cardia with mucus-secreting cells.

SiSx—The patient may have a history of heartburn, have overt GERD-like symptoms, or have esophagitis with odynophagia.

Dx—Esophagogastroduodenoscopy with biopsy is the only way to diagnose this condition. The test is only 80% sensitive, because short segments may be missed. Patients with more than 2–3 cm of metaplasia have a much higher risk of developing cancer.

Tx—Treat the same way as GERD, but perhaps be more aggressive. Also, surveillance EGD is needed to evaluate for progression to dysplasia or malignancy.

Infectious Esophagitis (See Chapter 8)

Esophageal Tears

Mallory-Weiss Syndrome

D—Longitudinal tears in the esophageal and/or gastric mucosa associated with forceful retching. These are not full-wall tears. Usually they do not produce significant life-threatening hematemesis, and surgical intervention is rarely required.

Epi—This condition accounts for 5% of UGI bleeding. A hiatal hernia is seen in many patients.

RF—Risk factors include alcoholism, older age, hiatal hernia, chronic prolonged vomiting, coughing, convulsions, hiccups under anesthesia, and closed chest massage.

P—Tears are usually due to a sudden increase in intra-abdominal pressure, as from retching. They can be single or multiple.

SiSx—The usual presentation is an acute UGIB associated with epigastric pain. Blood loss is typically small and self-limited but not always. Some cases can occur without bleeding and can be asymptomatic.

Dx—Esophagogastroduodenoscopy is the only way to diagnose the condition.

Tx—If the bleeding does not stop spontaneously, then control it during endoscopy with an injection of epinephrine. Nonbleeding lesions can be managed conservatively. From 40% to 70% of patients will require blood transfusions. An H_2 blocker or a PPI can be added to accelerate healing, but it does not affect the control of active bleeding.

Boerhaave's Syndrome

D—Spontaneous full-wall esophageal rupture, usually secondary to repeated vomiting. Most of the time, the tear occurs at the left posterolateral distal aspect of the esophagus. Cervical esophageal perforations can also occur.

RF—Risk factors include alcoholism and a history of peptic ulcer disease or Mallory-Weiss syndrome.

SiSx—Symptoms are retching and vomiting followed by excruciating substernal chest and upper abdominal pain. Because of contamination of the sterile mediastinum and surrounding structures with esophageal contents, dyspnea, sepsis, and shock can occur rapidly afterward.

Dx—The chest X-ray is usually abnormal and shows a widened mediastinum or free peritoneal air. Late manifestations can be pleural effusions, or subcutaneous emphysema in which there is air in the soft tissues of the chest. To confirm the diagnosis, gastrograffin (not barium, which can exacerbate inflammation) should be used as a contrast agent in a barium swallow study. Endoscopy has no role in diagnosis since it can extend the perforation and introduce more mediastinal air.

Tx—The condition is fatal in the absence of therapy. Surgery should be performed within 24 hours to repair the damage and debride the mediastinum. Until then, NG suction, IV antibiotics, and perhaps total parenteral nutrition (TPN) are necessary.

Structural and Motility Disorders of the Esophagus

Many of the more common and usually benign disorders are shown in Table 5-6.

Achalasia

D—Esophageal dysmotility characterized by the triad of (1) absence of normal peristalsis, (2) elevated LES pressure, and (3) incomplete relaxation of the LES.

Epi—The incidence is 1/100,000, and the condition occurs with equal frequency in males and females. The mean age at occurrence is 20–40 years.

P—It is due to decreased ganglion cell bodies with fibrosis and scarring of Auerbach's plexus via neuronal degeneration.

SiSx—There is dysphagia for *both* solids and liquids, weight loss in the great majority of patients, chest pain in 60%, and a nocturnal cough with or without recurrent pneumonia or bronchitis.

Dx—The gold standard is manometry testing, which shows the above triad. An upper GI series study shows absence of peristalsis. The esophagus may be very dilated, with a beak-like lower portion. Esophagogastroduodenoscopy is done to exclude malignancy, which is seen in a small number of patients.

Tx—Nitrates, anticholinergics, β agonists, and calcium channel blockers all work in less than 50% of patients. Forceful pneumatic dilation works in 70–90%. Endoscopic injection of botoxin or surgery (myotomy) are other options.

Table 5-6. Common Structural Disorders of the Esophagus and the Gastroesophageal Junction

Esophageal Webs	Webs are usually congenital abnormalities consisting of one or more horizontal fragile membranes found in the *upper and middle* esophagus. They usually protrude from the anterior wall and do not obstruct the entire lumen. 5% are asymptomatic. Usually they cause dysphagia for solids.
Esophageal Rings	Muscular structures that surround the entire wall of the esophagus. Usually found in the *distal* esophagus. A *Schatzki ring* is a mucosal ring seen in 6–14% of all patients undergoing EGD. Most are asymptomatic.
Esophageal Diverticulae	*Zenker's diverticulum*—a mucosal herniation (not true diverticulum) above the cricopharyngeal area. Also usually causes dysphagia for solids, halitosis, and regurgitation of undigested foods. *Traction diverticula*—in the middle and distal regions, secondary to an inflammatory process. *Epiphrenic diverticula*—in the distal esophagus, right above the LES, often asymptomatic.
Hiatal Hernias	Condition in which a portion of the stomach protudes up into the chest. Usually seen in pregnant women or people with chronically increased intra-abdominal pressure. Most cases are asymptomatic. Predisposes to GERD. *Type I*—"sliding." The GE junction is able to slide into the mediastinum. 95% of cases are asymptomatic. The few patients with reflux can usually be controlled with medications. The size of the lesion is unimportant. *Type II*—"rolling" or paraesophageal. The GE junction is normal and there is no reflux, so the patient is mostly asymptomatic. The fundus is prone to herniate into the mediastinum, which may lead to incarceration with strangulation requiring surgery. *Type III*—type I and type II together. A very large defect in the hiatus. Surgery is corrective.

Diffuse Esophageal Spasm

D—A dysmotility disease of nonperistaltic, large-amplitude esophageal contractions that cause chest pain.

P—It is due to a dysfunction of inhibitory nerves. Patchy neural degeneration of nerve processes (not cell bodies, as in achalasia) is seen on histologic exam. It may eventually progress to achalasia.

SiSx—It usually presents with chest pain and dysphagia. Chest pain occurs at rest but can be brought on with stress or swallowing. It can mimic cardiac chest pain with similar associated symptoms and radiation of pain to other parts of the body.

Dx—The condition is hard to distinguish clinically from other related motility disorders, but it is important to distinguish it from cardiac chest pain if nothing else leads one to think of this cause. The presence of dysphagia is perhaps the best clue. Barium swallow shows uncoordinated contractions that occur simultaneously, sometimes with large enough amplitude to obliterate the lumen. Manometry is the only way to make the diagnosis.

Tx—Anticholinergics are of limited value. Calcium channel blockers and other smooth muscle relaxants, such as sublingual nitroglycerin, are useful.

Plummer Vinson Syndrome

D—A triad of (1) esophageal webs, (2) iron deficiency anemia, and (3) dysphagia.

Epi—This uncommon disorder is seen mostly in elderly women. Patients are at increased risk of developing squamous carcinoma of the pharynx and esophagus.

P—The pathophysiology is unknown.

SiSx—One may also see spoon-shaped nails, as well as an atrophic tongue and oral mucosa, in addition to the defining characteristics of the disease.

Dx—Diagnosis is made by the clinical history and exam and specifically by demonstration of esophageal webs.

Tx—Correction of the iron deficiency can lead to resolution of the dysphagia and disappearance of the webs.

Eosinophilic Esophagitis (or Allergic Esophagitis)

D—A condition characterized by eosinophilic infiltration of the esophagus from an allergic or idiopathic cause.

Epi—It occurs in young or middle-aged adults, mostly men.

RF—Atopy, asthma, and allergies are associated conditions.

P—The etiology is unclear.

SiSx—Usually patients report a long history of dysphagia with or without food impaction. One may see it along with GERD that is unresponsive to PPIs, and it should always be part of the differential diagnosis.

Dx—Elevated IgE or eosinophilia on laboratory tests may be seen. The barium swallow may show a long, tapered, strictured esophagus with several concentric rings. The diagnosis is made by endoscopic biopsy showing many eosinophils in the mucosa. However, GERD can also cause this finding, especially in the distal esophagus, and must be excluded.

Tx—In children, a change in diet may cause improvement, as the esophagitis may be related in part to a food allergy. In adults, in addition to treating for any coexisting GERD, empiric topical steroids (swallowing inhaled steroids such as fluticasone) may help reduce symptoms, although relapse is common.

Gastric Disorders

Anatomy

The gross anatomy of the stomach is shown in Figure 5-2.

The fundus and body have parietal cells, which make HCl and intrinsic factor, and chief cells, which make pepsinogen. The antrum makes gastrin. Mucus-producing cells occur throughout. Gastrin, acetylcholine from vagal nerves, and histamine all act on receptors to cause acid secretion.

Acute Gastritis

D—Inflammation of the gastric mucosa, either diffuse or localized.

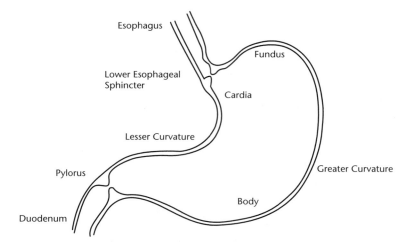

Figure 5-2. Gastric Anatomy.

P—The most common causes in the United States are drugs (primarily NSAIDs and alcohol), infection (*Helicobacter pylori*), and stress ulcers.

SiSx—Symptoms include epigastric burning pain, nausea/vomiting, and possibly a GI bleed.

Dx—Diagnosis consists of EGD with biopsy to show possible *H. pylori* or the presence of inflammation. Sometimes the diagnosis is based on the history and physical exam, and treatment is therefore empiric.

Tx—Once the condition is documented or suspected, remove the offending agents and treat with H_2 blockers or PPIs. Triple therapy is used for *H. pylori* (see the Peptic Ulcer Disease section).

Chronic Gastritis

D—Gastritis that is long-standing in nature. There are two well-characterized types, A and B. Type A is associated with autoimmune diseases; type B is associated with *H. pylori*.

P—There are superficial lymphocyte infiltrates in the lamina propria secondary to the same factors causing the acute form in most cases. "Fundal creep" occurs, which involves replacement of fundal tissue (parietal and chief cells) by antral mucosa (gastrin-producing cells). It is not precancerous, but it is common in older patients.

SiSx—Epigastric burning pain with nausea/vomiting and possible GI bleeding can be seen.

Dx—Esophagogastroduodenoscopy with biopsy is the classic way to determine the presence and chronicity of the condition. Table 5-7 presents some key differences between types A and B gastritis.

Tx—Treat the underlying conditions (e.g. *H. pylori*, autoimmune conditions), once documented.

Peptic Ulcer Disease

D—Condition in which there is breakdown of mucosal integrity of the stomach or duodenum with a localized defect or excavation.

Epi—There are 4 million new cases every year. Male patients outnumber females. Of these ulcers, 80% are duodenal and 20% are gastric. The mean age of occurrence is 40–50 years. Lifetime prevalence is 12% in men and 10% in women. The disease accounts for 15,000 deaths per year from complications. Duodenal ulcers are mostly (90%) within 3 cm of the pylorus. Gastric ulcers occur later in life and are more likely to be a harbinger of malignancy.

RF—Risk factors include smoking, use of drugs (NSAIDs, steroids, alcohol), a family history, COPD, *H. pylori* infection, multiple endocrine neoplasia (MEN) 1 syndrome, RA, atrophic gastritis, cirrhosis, and renal failure.

Table 5-7. Differentiation of Gastritis Types A and B

Type A	Type B
10% of cases	90% of cases
Involves the fundus and body, but the antrum is spared	Involves the antrum
Associated with parietal cell antibodies, pernicious anemia, high serum gastrin levels. Associated with other autoimmune diseases such as diabetes, hypothyroidism, and vitiligo	Associated with gastrin cell antibodies, *H. pylori* infections. Serum gastrin levels are normal or increased
Hypochlorhydria and achlorhydria will be seen	Patients have normal gastric acid levels
Increased risk of gastric polyps, gastric cancer, ulcers	Even higher risk of gastric cancer

P—Nonsteroidal anti-inflammatory drugs cause ulcers by inhibiting prostaglandin-mediated protection. In almost all cases not due to drugs, stress ulcers, or acid hypersecretion, there is overwhelming evidence that *H. pylori* is involved, especially in duodenal ulcers. *Helicobacter pylori* does not penetrate the gastric epithelia but allows acid to diffuse back and an ulcer to develop. It increases gastrin production by interfering with somatostatin release from D cells and releases ammonia via urease, which is toxic.

SiSx—Classically, one sees epigastric burning pain with eating if the ulcer is a gastric ulcer. Alternatively, pain is relieved with eating if a duodenal ulcer is present. However, 25% of patients may not have pain. A GI bleed is the most common complication and occurs in 15% of patients, either as coffee ground emesis or as melena. From 6% to 7% of patients have a perforation. Prolonged symptoms can cause weight loss. A scarred duodenal bulb can cause gastric outlet obstruction, which is seen in 1–3% of patients due to edema and inflammation. In this case, one may see repeated vomiting.

Dx—An upper GI series can miss an ulcer; therefore, EGD with biopsy is the test of choice. Multiple biopsies are usually done to rule out malignancy. In addition, EGD is useful in patients who are actively bleeding for localization and treatment. An upright film to assess for free air will help to rule out perforation. *H. pylori* culture or testing [via an enzyme-linked immunosorbent assay (ELISA), serum antibody test, or an EGD biopsy specimen that is specially stained] can also be done if there is little evidence to suspect other causes.

Tx—Remove known exacerbating factors. Intensive antacid therapy with H_2 blockers or PPIs is necessary to promote healing, which takes over 4 weeks in most patients. For *H. pylori* infection, triple-drug therapy is used to (1) protect the mucosa, (2) decrease acid production, and (3) eradicate *H. pylori*. There are multiple regimens, a common one being a PPI, amoxicillin, and clarithromycin. Surgery is rare nowadays but is needed for uncontrollable hemorrhage, perforation, obstruction, and intractability. The procedures done are usually a Bilroth I (vagotomy, antrectomy, gastroduodenostomy) or a Bilroth II (vagatomy, antrectomy, gastrojejunostomy). An oversew or patch repair can be done for simple perforation.

Stress Ulcer

D—Ulcer from severe stress in sick patients due to mucosal ischemia from hypotension, sepsis, hemorrhage, or hypovolemia. Usually it occurs in the fundus and body of the stomach, but it is also seen in the antrum, duodenum, and distal esophagus. Most ulcers tend to be superficial, but occasionally they can perforate. *Curling's ulcer* is specific to stress ulcers from a burn injury, *Cushing's ulcer* to patients with head trauma.

Epi—Stress ulcer is a common cause of GI bleeding in ICU patients. It is associated with a fivefold increase in mortality.

RF—Risk factors include shock, sepsis, hepatic failure, trauma, burns, organ transplant, a prior history of peptic ulcer disease, and UGIB.

P—Erosion begins within hours of the stressor. Some ulcers evolve after days and are usually deeper. Acid hypersecretion is seen in patients with head trauma. Defects in the glycoprotein mucous barrier are seen in critically ill patients, and ischemia is found in those with shock and sepsis.

SiSx—Massive UGIB is the usually finding. In the ICU, overt symptoms may be hard to distinguish. Abdominal pain may occur, depending on where the ulcer is located.

Dx—Diagnosis is made by a history of GI bleeding and EGD if needed. It may be diagnosed empirically.

Tx—Prophylaxis is key, either with a PPI, an H_2 blocker, sucralfate, or prostaglandin analogues. Treating the underlying condition is perhaps most important, but in severe cases one may need to perform endoscopic ligation, partial or total gastrectomy, or vagotomy to decrease acid secretion.

Gastroparesis

D—A disorder of gastric emptying that is not caused by obstruction, but rather by lack of normal peristaltic movement.

RF—Risk factors include diabetes for more than 10 years, the aftermath of viral infections, disorder of smooth muscle such as scleroderma or dermatomyositis, or idiopathic causes.

SiSx—Symptoms include nausea, vomiting, bloating or a frequent feeling of fullness with meals, and hard-to-control blood glucose. Diabetic patients may have other findings of autonomic nervous system dysfunction.

Dx—One can perform nuclear medicine gastric emptying studies of solids. Barium studies or EGD may be useful for cases in which mechanical causes of obstruction must be ruled out.

Tx—Prokinetics such as metoclopramide or cisapride are helpful, but not curative. Tight glycemic control in diabetics may improve symptoms.

Diseases of the Small and Large Intestines

Small Intestine Anatomy

The small intestine is composed of three sections:

1. Duodenum (25–30 cm)

Main processes are digestion and alkalinization via duodenal Brunner's gland secretions, pancreatic secretions, and bile. The duodenum is responsible for absorption of Ca^{2+}, iron, Mg^{2+}, folate, monosaccharides, and water-soluble vitamins.

There are four divisions:

First part—includes the duodenal bulb.

Second part—includes the ampulla of Vater, common bile duct, and pancreatic duct.

Third part—consists of the transverse segment.

Fourth part—consists of the ascending segment and ends at the ligament of Treitz, which defines the duodenal-jejunal border.

2. Jejunum (250 cm)

Major site of absorption for fatty acids, amino acids, monosaccharides, and water-soluble vitamins.

3. Ileum (350 cm)

Major site of absorption of fatty acids, amino acids, monosaccharides, bile salts, fat-soluble vitamins, and the vitamin B_{12}–(intrinsic factor) complex at the terminus.

The blood supply is via the gastroduodenal artery for the first part of the duodenum. Branches off the superior mesenteric artery (SMA) supply the rest of the small intestine.

Large Intestine Anatomy

Figure 5-3 shows the gross anatomy of the large intestine. The blood supply of the colon is via the SMA all the way to the splenic flexure. The inferior mesenteric artery (IMA) supplies from the splenic flexure to the superior rectal area. Finally, branches off the internal iliac supply the middle and inferior rectal areas.

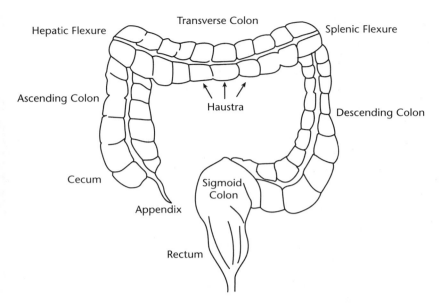

Figure 5-3. Anatomy of the Large Intestine.
Divisions of the large intestine are shown. The cecum is largest in diameter. The other sections vary with respect to their position along the peritoneum. The ascending and descending colons are retroperitoneal; the transverse and sigmoid colons are intraperitoneal; and the rectum is only partially retroperitoneal. Three thickened bands run along the colon (tinea coli) with perpendicular sacculations between them (haustra).

Disorders of Bowel Motility

Bowel Obstruction

D—Lack of passage of GI contents. It can be functional (e.g., paralytic ileus) or mechanical. For mechanical causes, one must distinguish between small and large bowel obstruction, as shown in Table 5-8.

Paralytic Ileus

D—Loss of peristalsis without structural obstruction.

RF—Risk factors include recent surgery/GI procedures, severe medical illness, hypothyroidism, diabetes, medications like anticholinergics and opioids, chemical or bacterial peritonitis, and severe intra-abdominal infection.

SiSx—Diffuse constant abdominal discomfort, nausea/vomiting, and abdominal distention can be seen, along with absence of flatulence, absence of bowel movements, and reduced or absent bowel sounds. There should be no peritoneal signs.

Dx—Diagnosis is based on distended air in bowels and air-fluid levels. Be sure to distinguish paralytic ileus from partial or pseudobowel obstruction, which improves with rest. Obtain supine and upright films to rule out perforation or obstruction.

Tx—Treat the underlying disease and decrease the use of narcotics when warranted. Initiate bowel rest with discontinuation of oral feeds. Perform NG suction and give IV fluids or, if necessary, TPN.

Volvulus

D—A rotation of the colon onto itself, tying itself into a knot, which may result in bowel obstruction. This condition usually occurs in the sigmoid colon (50–90% of cases) or cecum (10–40% of cases).

RF—Older patients (average age is the 50s), bedridden patients, newborns with malrotation, people with prior surgery, pregnant women, and patients with Hirschprung's disease are at risk.

Table 5-8. Comparison of Small and Large Bowel Obstruction

Type	Small Bowel Obstruction	Large Bowel Obstruction
Sx	Moderate to severe crampy abdominal pain, copious emesis *which relieves it.* Distention is worse the more distal the obstruction. Fever and signs of dehydration may be seen.	Constipation, obstipation, deep and cramping abdominal pain. Abdominal distention, nausea and less emesis but more commonly feculent.
Si	Exam shows abdominal distention (the more prominent the more distal the obstruction), tenderness, and visible peristaltic waves. Look for surgical scars and hernias; perform rectal exam. Listen for high-pitched bowel sounds (borborygmi), peristaltic rushes, or absence of bowel sounds.	Exam shows more abdominal distention, less acute onset, tenderness. Look for peritoneal irritation. May feel a palpable mass or see signs of shock or fever that may indicate perforation. Bowel sounds may be absent. Perform rectal exam.
P	Common causes are adhesions from postoperative care or inflammatory conditions, hernias, volvulus (in children), gallstone ileus, neoplasm, foreign body, intussusception, Crohn's disease, cystic fibrosis, stricture, hematoma.	Common causes are colon cancer, diverticulitis, volvulus, fecal impaction, and benign tumor. Assume that colon cancer exists until proven otherwise, especially in elderly people.
Dx	Obtain an abdominal X-ray. Consider contrast CT studies to determine if there is partial or complete obstruction. *Air-fluid levels are key* for partial or complete obstruction. A CT scan is useful to look for a transition zone of dilated proximal bowel and normal distal bowel to localize the area of obstruction.	Obtain an abdominal X-ray to look more for colonic pathology with air-fluid levels. Perform barium or water contrast enema (gastrograffin) if perforation is suspected.
Tx	Hospitalize the patient. Partial small bowel obstruction can be treated conservatively with NG decompression, but a complete small bowel obstruction usually is a more urgent indication for surgery. Make the patient NPO, give IV fluids, and use an NG tube for decompression. Consequences can be intraluminal volume loss, electrolyte disturbance, hypotension, sepsis, shock, and strangulation of bowel. There is a 25% chance of death for all those who present with this condition.	Hospitalize the patient. In some cases, the obstruction can be opened with a rectal tube, but surgery is the treatment of choice. Colon stenting is an emerging procedure as an alternative to surgery. Until then, make the patient NPO, give IV fluids, and decompress with an NG tube. A gangrenous colon requires colectomy. Treat any underlying cause if found. The condition is more emergent than small bowel obstruction, and the patient requires surgery without delay.

SiSx—Symptoms are similar to those of large bowel obstruction. They include colicky abdominal pain, nausea/vomiting, and obstipation.

Dx—An abdominal X-ray may show the "double bubble" sign with a pocket of air on either side of the obstruction. Diagnosis is usually made by barium or water-soluble contrast enema (with classic "birds beak" at the point of the volvulus) or CT. Do not perform barium enema in patients suspected of having intestinal gangrene or inflammation.

Tx—The main concern is to prevent the development of gangrene. Colonoscopic decompression is first-line therapy. Surgical resection may be indicated if colonoscopy fails or if volvulus recurs.

Ogilvie's Syndrome (Colonic Pseudo-obstruction)

D—Severe dilation of the cecum and right hemicolon in the absence of anatomic obstruction. Sometimes it may extend to the rectum.

Epi—Ninety-five percent of cases are associated with an underlying condition. The syndrome is seen mostly in elderly patients.

RF—Risk factors include trauma, infection, heart failure, recent abdominal surgery, neurologic conditions such as Parkinson's disease, the postoperative state, hypokalemia, hypomagnesemia, hypocalcemia, and opiate use.

P—The cause is unclear. It may have to do with impairment of the autonomic nervous system.

SiSx—Symptoms include nausea, vomiting, abdominal pain, constipation, and or diarrhea. Almost all patients have abdominal distention. Most have bowel sounds.

Dx—There is no diagnostic test. Exclude other causes of a dilated colon. Abdominal CT or a contrast enema can confirm the diagnosis by excluding a mechanical cause of obstruction or toxic megacolon.

Tx—Provide supportive care with removal of opiates, anticholinergics, and treatment of any underlying cause if found. Enemas may help, as may agents such as neostigmine. Colonoscopic decompression is used for patients who fail with conservative treatment, and surgery may be needed in those who have severe disease with peritoneal signs or who fail with all other therapy. Serial exams should be performed during observation to see if colonic dilation is improving.

Irritable Bowel Syndrome

D—Idiopathic disease of chronic bowel dysfunction described as abdominal pain with altered bowel motility, with either predominant constipation, diarrhea, or mixed symptoms.

Epi—This is the most common digestive disorder. The female/male ratio is 4:1. The condition is more common in Caucasians than in other racial groups. There is a possible association with past physical and sexual abuse and chronic pain syndromes. Half of the patients have comorbid psychiatric disorders. Most present at <45 years of age.

P—The cause is unclear. There may be a role for abnormal gut motor and sensory activity via the autonomic nervous system.

SiSx—Alternating constipation and diarrhea occur, along with abdominal pain. Symptoms are usually present for >3 months. Weight loss is not seen. Flatulence or belching is common.

Dx—Diagnosis is based on a normal physical exam and exclusion of other diseases. There are no diagnostic markers. It is a diagnosis of exclusion.

Tx—Most useful is a combination of emotional support, diet and fiber therapy, antispasmodics, antidiarrheals, and perhaps antidepressants, depending on the comorbid conditions.

Ulcerative and Inflammatory Diseases

Inflammatory Bowel Disease (Ulcerative Colitis and Crohn's Disease)

D—An idiopathic disease of chronic inflammation of the bowel that may have extraintestinal manifestations. There are two distinct entities, ulcerative colitis (UC) and Crohn's disease (CD).

Epi—The disease is more common in developed countries and especially in Caucasians, with the highest incidence in Ashkenazi Jews. The incidence in the United States is 7–11/100,000. The peak age of onset is 15–30 years, with a second smaller peak around 60–80 years. In UC, the number of male and female patients is equal. In CD, male patients outnumber females by 2:1.

RF—A family history is important. There is a 10% chance that a first-degree relative will be affected. There is a 67% concordance in monozygotic twins. Smoking causes a 1.7-fold increase. Use of OCPs is linked to CD.

P—The cause is unclear. Both environmental factors (viral or bacterial infections are associated) and a genetic predisposition (defective immune regulation) have been implicated. Ulcerative colitis and CD tend to have different anatomic distributions for unclear reasons (see Table 5-9).

SiSx

Intestinal Manifestations

UC—Tends to present with rectal bleeding, diarrhea, tenesmus (feeling of a frequent need to defecate with a sense of incomplete evacuation), and crampy abdominal pain. In children, both UC and CD may present solely with failure to thrive or to grow appropriately.

Table 5-9. Key Differences Between Crohn's Disease and Ulcerative Colitis

Feature	Crohn's Disease	Ulcerative Colitis
Symptoms	Bowel obstruction, fistulas, inflammatory mass, fever, diarrhea.	Rectal bleeding, diarrhea, tenesmus, crampy abdominal pain.
GI Tract Involvement	Any part of the GI tract from the mouth to the anus; usually spares the rectum. From 30% to 40% have small bowel disease alone; 20% have colitis alone. In those with any type of small bowel disease, 90% have terminal ileum involvement.	Colon only; usually all of the rectum. Twenty percent have full colonic involvement; 50% have rectosigmoid limited disease; 1–2% have backwash ileitis in the terminal ileum that is of no clinical significance.
Gross Inflammation	Skip lesions of ulceration that look like sausage links on films. Anal and GI tract strictures. So-called creeping mesenteric fat, seen with healing. There can be intra-abdominal abscesses and fistulas to bowel, skin, vagina, and perianal area.	Continuous inflammation and ulcerating lesions usually starting from the rectum and progressing proximally. No fistulas. Pseudopolyps may be seen with chronic reepithelization.
Histologic Characteristics	Transmural linear ulcers. Noncaseating granulomas seen in half of biopsies.	Mucosal or submucosal only; not full-thickness ulcers.
Complications		
Toxic Megacolon	Rare	More common
Carcinoma	Rare	More common

CD—Two classical patterns of presentation: as bowel obstruction with low-grade fever and crampy abdominal pain that is relieved with defecation or as a fistulizing form with enterocutaneous communications. Weight loss is common, and an inflammatory mass may be felt. More systemic signs are seen than in UC. Because of small bowel involvement, one can also see evidence of malabsorption and vitamin B_{12} deficiency in cases of terminal ileal involvement.

Extraintestinal Manifestations
Eyes—conjunctivitis, uveitis, episcleritis. The incidence is 1–10%. Findings may be seen even during remission.
Skin—erythema nodosum (10–15% of patients), pyoderma gangrenosum (1–12% of patients), vasculitis, and aphthous ulcers. *These conditions correlate with GI disease activity.* Perianal skin tags occur in CD. They may be seen even before overt GI activity.
Joints—arthralgias or arthritis that is usually asymmetric and polyarticular.

Exacerbations are correlated with GI disease activity. This is seen in 15–30% of patients. Ankylosing spondylitis and sacroilitis can also be found.
Hepatobiliary—primary sclerosing cholangitis (1–5% of cases, more common in UC), fatty liver, and cholelithiasis (more common in CD).
Urologic—nephrolithiasis is seen in CD, especially calcium oxalate stones from increased absorption of dietary oxalate.
Hematologic—increased clotting tendency because of changes in the activity of clotting factors/mediators. One may see DVT, PE, or even strokes.
Oncologic—greater risk for malignancy the longer one has the disease (more so in UC), with a small percent increase in risk per year.
Dx—Contrast films may be useful for study, such as an upper GI series with small bowel follow-up. However, if significant inflammation or perforation is a concern, one should avoid barium. Biopsy of a mucosal

lesion via EGD or colonoscopy that shows characteristic findings (see Table 5-9) and the anatomic location of disease along with the history is useful in most cases to make the diagnosis. But up to 15% of patients have indeterminant colitis, which will take longer to diagnose. In these patients, two antibodies can be used to help distinguish UC from CD: the perinuclear anti-neutrophil cytoplasmic antibody (p-ANCA) and the anti *Saccharomyces cerevisiae* antibody (ASCA). The p-ANCA is positive in 60–70% of UC patients and in 10–15% of CD patients, whereas ASCA is positive in 60–70% of CD patients and in 10–15% of UC patients. Some clinicians use elevated ESR or CRP to assess for disease activity, or to determine if symptoms are due to a flare or to another cause.

Tx—For both diseases, the mainstay of treatment is 5-aminosalicylic acid (5-ASA) and its derivatives. It is useful for acute therapy of a flare along with steroids. 6-Mercaptopurine (6-MP) and its prodrug, azathioprine, are now used significantly in inflammatory bowel disease as steroid-sparing agents for long-term maintenance of remission. However, the full effect takes 8–12 weeks. Antibiotics have no role in the treatment of active or quiescent UC, but ciprofloxacin plus metronidazole is useful in fistulous CD to prevent recurrence and is used for several months. Other agents for more severe disease refractory to steroids include methotrexate, cyclosporine, and infliximab (a TNF-α inhibitor). For refractory UC, colectomy is curative. Distinguishing characteristics of UC and CD are shown in Table 5-9.

Toxic Megacolon

D—Dilation of the colon that exceeds 6 cm in diameter. It occurs most commonly as a complication of severe inflammatory bowel disease from marked inflammation and mucosal destruction.

RF—Risk factors include inflammatory bowel disease, Hirschsprung's disease, heavy use of opiates and anticholinergics, and barium enema.

SiSx—It can result in sepsis, peritonitis or perforation and carries a high mortality rate.

Dx—Abdominal X-ray shows intraluminal gas along with a very dilated bowel. Usually the transverse colon is involved.

Tx—Surgical decompression is almost always necessary. In preparation, all patients have to be made NPO, given antibiotics and steroids, and have an NG tube placed. Rectal tube placement may also be necessary.

Microscopic Colitis

D—A syndrome of chronic secretory watery diarrhea with varying histology described by two forms: (1) collagenous colitis, which is characterized by a thickened subepithelial collagenous band in the colonic mucosa, and (2) lymphocytic colitis, which demonstrates subepithelial lymphocytic infiltration.

Epi—It is seen most commonly in middle-aged women.

P—The cause is unknown. It is unclear if the two diseases are related to each other, but this has been postulated. Causes range from abnormal collagen metabolism to the use of certain drugs such as NSAIDs. Diarrhea seems to be due to active chloride section.

SiSx—Symptoms include nonbloody, watery secretory diarrhea, weight loss, abdominal pain, and fatigue. They can be chronic and intermittent or continuous.

Dx—Laboratory findings are normal, though 50% of patients may have elevated ESR. Hypoalbuminemia and steatorrhea can be seen. Colon biopsy shows a thick layer of subepithelial collagen deposition. The diagnosis, as the name implies, is made by the histologic exam.

Tx—Antidiarrheal agents are used, as well as Bismuth, 5-ASA, and steroids.

Acute Mesenteric Ischemia and Ischemic Colitis

D—Insufficient arterial blood inflow or poor venous outflow from the gut. There are two major forms: (1) Mesenteric ischemia is from an acute occlusive event due to vascular occlusion via thrombolic or embolic disease that occurs predominantly in the SMA distribution in 80% of cases. (2) Ischemic colitis is a nonoc-clusive low-flow ischemic state seen in states of low cardiac output, with a greater tendency to occur at the watershed areas (splenic flexure, rectosigmoid junction) where vessels meet. Usually in ischemia, two of the three major visceral arteries must be affected because of extensive collaterals in the GI tract.

RF—Risk factors include increased age, atrial fibrillation, CAD, hypercoagulable states, endocarditis, CHF, shock, and rheumatic heart disease.

SiSx—Mesenteric ischemia presents with onset of severe diffuse abdominal pain that is out of proportion to that elicited by palpation on the physical exam. Pain is worse about 15–20 minutes after eating. However, 20–30% of patients may have no pain. Depending on the severity of the condition, one may find decreased/absent bowel sounds, occult blood to frankly bloody stool, and eventually hypo-tension, tachycardia, fever, and acidosis as transmural infarction/peritonitis develops. Ischemic colitis is more likely to present with bleeding in addition to pain. Chronic non-occlusive ischemia may present with malab-sorption and weight loss from avoidance of eating because of pain.

Dx—Flexible sigmoidoscopy or colonoscopy is used to demonstrate ischemic tissue in ischemic colitis. A CT scan may demonstrate colon wall thickening in classic locations. Mesenteric ischemia requires a high level of clinical suspicion. A CT scan may show a thickened small bowel. Diagnosis is made on the basis of angiographic findings (conven-tional or via CT/MRI).

Tx—Ischemic colitis is mainly self-limited, though attempt to reverse the low-flow state with fluid resuscitation or by increasing car-diac output, if possible, depending on the underlying cause. Immediate reestablishment of blood flow is key for mesenteric ischemia. This is done via angiography and embolec-tomy. Otherwise, necrotic areas must be removed by surgical resection. The distin-guishing features of these two entities are shown in Table 5-10.

Typhilitis

D—Poorly characterized inflammation typi-cally of the cecum (but can include the ileum and ascending colon) that occurs in neutro-penic patients. It is also called *neutropenic enterocolitis.*

RF—The risk factor is profound neutropenia (absolute neutrophil count < 500/µL).

P—The condition is not well understood. It is a combination of mucosal injury caused by cytotoxic chemotherapy, neutropenia, and an impaired host defense against microorgan-isms. The infection can lead to inflammation and necrosis of the cecal wall.

SiSx—Symptoms are fever and RLQ pain in a neutropenic patient. Abdominal distention, nausea, vomiting, and bloody diarrhea may

Table 5-10. Key Differences Between Acute Mesenteric Ischemia and Ischemic Colitis

Feature	Acute Mesenteric Ischemia	Ischemic Colitis
Patient age	Age varies, depending on the cause	Vast majority over age 60
Etiology	Thromboembolism usually into the SMA, from atrial fibrillation, hypercoagulable states, endocarditis or other causes	Low-flow state from low cardiac output (hypotension, dehydration, blood loss)
Symptoms	Severe pain out of proportion to exam / Rectal bleeding rare / Patient appears severely ill	Mild pain, mild tenderness / Rectal bleeding/bloody diarrhea typical / Patient does not appear severely ill
Diagnostic Test	Angiography (conventional, CT, MRI)	Colonoscopy
Treatment	Embolectomy / Surgical resection of necrotic small bowel	Conservative management; correct underlying cause of low blood flow (fluid resuscitation, transfusions, rate control of AF)

be present. Peritoneal signs and hypotension may indicate bowel perforation.

Dx—Diagnosis is based on characteristic findings of fluid-filled, thickened, dilated cecum on a CT scan. It is important to rule out *Clostridium difficile* colitis.

Tx—Conservative management includes broad-spectrum antibiotics, NG suction, and IV fluids. Surgical management may be needed if bowel perforation is present. Use of granulocyte-colony stimulating factor (G-CSF) may accelerate leukocyte recovery, possibly facilitating clinical recovery.

Diverticular Diseases

Diverticulosis

D—Presence of diverticuli in the small or large bowel. A diverticulum is either a congenital outpouching of the entire thickness of the wall of the GI tract, as in Meckel's diverticulum, or an acquired outpouching of the mucosa and submucosa through the muscular layer only of the intestinal wall, most commonly at the site of a nutrient artery. Diverticuli generally occur in the colon, but small bowel types are usually found in the proximal duodenum near the ampulla.

Epi—Diverticulosis is the most common cause of acute LGIB in patients >40 years of age. Diverticula are present in 50% of patients over 60 years old and in 20% of the population.

RF—Risk factors include a low-fiber, high-fat diet, old age, and connective tissue disorders.

SiSx—The condition is generally asymptomatic unless accompanied by rupture of a colonic vessel, in which case GI bleeding can occur. If it is symptomatic, it may present with left lower quadrant (LLQ) pain with eating and constipation.

Dx—Diverticuli are seen routinely on colonoscopy. A CT scan with oral contrast is the best noninvasive way to make the diagnosis.

Tx—Treatment involves a high-fiber diet. Diverticular bleeding stops spontaneously in 80% of cases. Consider surgery for recurrent GI bleeding or recurrent diverticulitis.

Diverticulitis

D—Obstruction of a diverticulum causing acute inflammation, perforation, or abscess. It occurs most commonly in the sigmoid colon.

Epi—It occurs in 10% of patients with diverticular disease.

P—Usually it is secondary to accumulation of undigested food and bacteria in the diverticulum leading to an inflammatory reaction and eventually to perforation because of increased intraluminal pressures.

SiSx—Symptoms include fever, constipation, LLQ pain, guarding, rebound tenderness, and occult rectal bleeding in 25% of cases, though diverticulosis is more likely to cause a massive GI bleed. With perforation, sepsis and shock can rarely occur.

Dx—Abdominal CT is the most useful way to make the diagnosis. Avoid colonoscopy unless the acute attack has resolved.

Tx—If there is no perforation, maintain bowel rest and give antibiotics for gram-negative bacteria and anaerobes. Abscesses can be drained percutaneously, but frank perforation warrants surgical resection.

Appendicitis

D—An obstruction of the appendiceal lumen from fecalith (35%), enlarged lymphoid follicles (60%), neoplasia, or a parasite.

Epi—There are 250,000 cases per year in the United States, with the highest incidence in 10- to 20-year-olds. Male patients slightly outnumber females. Perforations are highest at extremes of age.

P—Obstruction by fecalith is the most common mechanism of acute appendicitis in adults. In younger patients, lymphoid follicular hyperplasia is thought to be the main culprit following infection. In older patients, it is due to fibrosis, fecalith, or neoplasia. Once obstructed, the appendix distends, with resulting occlusion and/or thrombosis of the small vessels, and becomes ischemic and necrotic. Bacterial overgrowth occurs with anaerobic organisms first, then others including *Escherichia coli* and *Bacteriodes*.

Once perforation occurs, there can be localized abscess formation or diffuse peritonitis.

SiSx—Early signs are nonspecific, such as indigestion or flatulence. There may be poorly localized epigastric or periumbilical pain during the period of visceral inflammation, with eventual localization to the RLQ once parietal inflammation occurs. Anorexia and nausea/vomiting are concomitant once localization has occurred. Beware of abnormal appendix locations: in patients who are pregnant, it can be pushed up into the RUQ, and in those with malrotation, it is located in the LUQ. All signs of peritoneal tenderness at this point may be present, including rebound tenderness and involuntary guarding. Other characteristic signs are listed below. With perforation, the patient can become hypotensive and septic. The risk of perforation is 25% at 2 hours, 50% at 36 hours, and 75% at 72 hours.

Classic signs on physical exam are as follows:

Psoas—abdominal pain when the right hip and knee are fully extended.

Obturator—abdominal pain when the leg is internally rotated with the hip and knee flexed.

Rovsing—RLQ pain when the LLQ is palpated.

Tenderness at McBurney's point (one-third of the distance from the anterior superior iliac spine to the umbilicus).

Dx—A clinical diagnosis is made. Supporting evidence includes leukocytosis with a left shift and an abdominal X-ray showing loss of the psoas muscle shadow (indicating inflammation). In 10% of cases, one can see an appendicolith (a calcified deposit in the appendix). Free air on the abdominal X-ray/chest X-ray may suggest perforation. A CT scan with rectal or oral contrast is the best test in difficult-to-diagnose cases to show the appendix. It shows a thick wall, an appendicolith, a phlegmon, abscess, or free fluid. Sensitivity and specificity are about 90%, and CT will also help rule out an alternative diagnosis. Always perform a U/A to rule out UTI and a β-human chorionic gonadotropin (hCG) for women to rule out pregnancy.

Tx—Surgery is necessary for removal unless a retroperitoneal phlegmon has developed, in which case one should give IV fluids and antibiotics and perform elective appendectomy. The acceptable number of normal appendix removals varies from 10% to 20% in women with other pelvic processes that are harder to diagnose. Mortality is <1%. Initiate medical therapy in patients who have already developed an abscess or phlegmon that can be treated by nonemergent surgery.

Diseases of the Bowel Causing Malabsorption

Lactase Deficiency

D—GI intolerance to lactose-containing products, which are primarily dairy products.

RF—African Americans, Asians, Native Americans, Eskimos, and older people are among highest risk.

Epi—The prevalence of some degree of lactase deficiency is as high as 20% in Caucasians, but is higher among other groups, especially east Asians (95%), African Americans (70%) and Native Americans (80%)

P—It is due to either (1) genetically decreased small intestine brush border enzyme lactase, so that one cannot break down lactose in dairy products, or (2) mucosal injury leading to decreased activity of this enzyme. Osmotic diarrhea follows. In addition, bacteria in the colon break down some lactose into short chain fatty acids and hydrogen gas, leading to flatulence.

SiSx—Symptoms include osmotic diarrhea, abdominal pain, and flatulence after ingestion of milk or milk products.

Dx—Diagnosis is made by the history and by a trial of dairy products causing diarrhea. Cessation of diary product ingestion should eliminate the symptoms and also helps make the diagnosis. One can also do a breath hydrogen test to measure lactose nonabsorption or a lactose tolerance test in which, after an overnight fast, glucose levels are measured before and after a 50-g oral lactose load is given. A rise of <20 mg/dL over the baseline glucose level is abnormal. The sensitivity of the test is 75%, and the specificity is 96%.

Tx—Cessation of diary products is not necessary. Instead, patients can use lactaid products (where the lactose is already broken down into its components) or supplemental lactase enzyme pills. Make sure to supplement Ca^{2+} in patients who wish to avoid dairy products.

Celiac Sprue or Gluten-Sensitive Enteropathy

D—An intolerance to gluten, specifically to the gliadin component of gluten, which is found in wheat, barely, rye, and oats.

P—It is thought to be an autoimmune condition in which antibodies to gliadin lead to small intestine mucosal damage and subsequently to malabsorption.

RF—Risk factors include Caucasians race, a family history, and association with human leukocyte antigen (HLA)-DQ2.

Epi—It can become evident at any age throughout adulthood. There is increased risk of malignancy, particularly non-Hodgkin's lymphoma.

SiSx—Malabsorption with diarrhea may or may not be present initially, but it is usually seen. Sequelae include nutrient deficiencies, anemia, short stature, infertility, recurrent stomatitis, and dermatitis herpetiformis. Amenorrhea may be the first symptoms in girls, and there is failure to thrive in infants, with abnormal stools and bloating. One can see spontaneous remissions and exacerbations.

Dx—Duodenal biopsy via EGD is necessary for diagnosis; it shows blunted, flattened villi and an inflammatory infiltrate in the lamina propria. The response to a gluten-free diet is also helpful in making the diagnosis. Antibodies such as antigliadin, antiendomysial and antitissue transglutaminase (90–95% sensitivity and specificity) are frequently present. Antibodies should disappear once the gluten-free diet is started. The three antibodies, in order of increasing utility, are antigliadin, antiendomysial, and antitissue transglutaminase.

Tx—In most cases, a gluten-free diet can completely reverse the disease and cause the small bowel mucosa to return to normal. Steroids are given for refractory disease or to patients who are noncompliant. The most important complication is development of malignancy, which one should consider especially in those who are refractory to treatment.

Tropical Sprue

D—An acquired form of sprue that improves with antibiotic use. The etiology is unclear. Multiple nutrient deficiencies occur, such as deficiencies of vitamin B_{12} and folate.

RF—This is an acquired disorder found primarily in the Caribbean, South India, and Southeast Asia. It can affect up to 5–10% of people in some populations.

P—The role of bacteria in this disorder is not well understood. However, *E. coli*, *Klebsiella* and *Enterobacter* species are implicated in the pathogenesis.

SiSx—Symptoms include chronic diarrhea, steatorrhea, weight loss, and nutritional deficiencies.

Dx—Exclude other causes of diarrhea, such as cysts and parasites in patients from endemic areas. Diagnosis is made by intestinal biopsy showing a mononuclear infiltration in the lamina propria. A gluten-free diet does not help.

Tx—Tetracycline or other antibiotics should be given for up to 6 months with nutrient supplements.

Short Bowel Syndrome

D—Condition in which the total small bowel length of the small bowel is inadequate to support nutrition.

P—It is caused by massive intestinal resection (75%), mostly from complications of Crohn's disease, or in neonates from necrotizing enterocolitis, mesenteric occlusion, midgut volvulus, or disruption of superior mesenteric vessels with intestinal ischemia. While the small bowel adapts to its shortened length, sometimes this is not enough for adequate absorption. Patients without an ileocecal valve often have worse symptoms, as there is an increased flow of fluid into the colon.

SiSx—Diarrhea, electrolyte deficiency, and malnutrition are common. Findings such as gallstones, disruption of portal circulation, and hyperoxaluria-induced nephrolithiasis are also possible. Renal calcium oxalate crystals are seen due to increased absorption by the large bowel.

Tx—If there is >100 cm of jejunum of the small bowel, give calorie-dense foods (digested by colonic bacteria into fatty acids, which can then be absorbed), an oral rehydration solution, and antimotility agents. Total parenteral nutrition may be needed temporarily until small bowel adaption occurs. If <100 cm of small bowel and no colon remains, the patient requires IV fluids or TPN in addition to a modified diet.

Whipple's Disease

D—A rare systemic disorder that presents with fever, myalgias, and malabsorption. It affects many organs but mainly the small intestine.

RF—Middle-aged Caucasians men are most commonly affected.

P—It is caused by *Tropheryma whippelii,* a small gram positive bacillus.

SiSx—Symptoms include diarrhea, steatorrhea, weight loss, arthralgias, and CNS and cardiac problems. Dementia is a late symptom and has poor prognostic implications.

Dx—Jejunal biopsy is diagnostic. Periodic acid–Schiff-positive macrophages containing *T. whippelii* is the classic finding.

Tx—The disease is fatal if untreated. Antibiotics given for 1 year are curative. Trimethoprim-sulfamethoxazole (Bactrim) is usually used.

Protein-Losing Enteropathy

D—A group of GI and non-GI disorders in which there is hypoproteinemia without renal losses or known problems with protein synthesis. Hence, protein is lost mainly via the GI tract.

P—Normally, 10% of protein catabolism is via the GI tract. Common causes are heavy mucosal ulceration, celiac sprue or inflammatory bowel disease, lymphatic dysfunction,

and various types of congenital heart disease via unclear mechanisms.

Sx—Symptoms include generalized edema, a low serum protein level, and hence a tendency to develop a third space.

Dx—Diagnosis is made by the presence of peripheral edema, with not only low serum albumin but also low serum globulins in the absence of renal or hepatic disease.

Tx—Treat the underlying causes, if possible, and not just low albumin by direct replacement. Consider nutritional support with high-protein TPN or high-protein enteral feedings.

Radiation Enteritis

D—GI dysfunction after radiation treatment to the pelvis or abdomen.

RF—Risk factors include a total radiation dose >5000 cGy, previous abdominal operations, previous laparotomy, hypertension, diabetes, preexisting vascular disease and adjuvant chemotherapy (e.g., 5-fluorouracil, doxorubicin, actinomycin D, and methotrexate).

P—Radiation affects rapidly dividing cells of the small intestine epithelium and causes obliterative endarteritis of small vessels, leading to intestinal ulceration, strictures, and fistula formation. Associated intestinal bypass, bacterial overgrowth, or bile salt wasting may result in malabsorption.

SiSx—Symptoms range from diarrhea and abdominal cramping to bowel obstruction-like symptoms. Stricture or fistula formation can occur along with GI bleeding. All of these problems may occur even 20 years after radiation treatment.

Dx—Diagnosis is made by a history of radiation exposure and symptoms once other causes of diarrhea are ruled out.

Tx—There is no good treatment. One may try antimotility agents or cholestyramine. There is no indication for anti-inflammatory agents, as this is not an inflammatory disorder. Antibiotics can be given in cases of bacterial overgrowth. About 2–3% of patients will have obstruction, fistula formation, perforation, or bleeding and will require either surgical bypass or resection with reanastomosis.

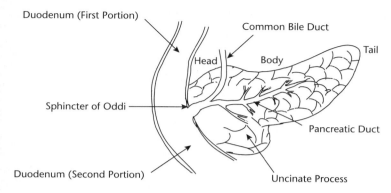

Figure 5-4. Pancreatic Anatomy.
The pancreas is a retroperitoneal structure composed of a tail, body, neck, head, and uncinate process. The pancreatic duct and common bile duct join together here before entering the duodenum.

Pancreatic Diseases

Anatomy

The gross anatomy of the pancreas is shown in Figure 5-4. On a microscopic level, the important features to note are the following:

- Endocrine cells of the pancreas are found in regions called the *islets of Langerhans*. They account for about 1–2% of the total pancreatic mass.
- The major endocrine cells include alpha cells, which make glucagon; beta cells, which make insulin and amylin; and delta cells, which make somatostatin.
- Exocrine cells include the acinar cells, which secrete digestive enzymes such as trypsin, chymotrypsin, pancreatic lipase, and amylase. The pancreas secretes 2 L of alkaline $NaHCO_3$-rich fluid a day full of these digestive enzymes.
- There is both sympathetic innervation (stimulates beta cell secretion) and parasympathetic innervation (simulates alpha cell secretion).
- The blood supply of the head is via the gastroduodenal artery and the inferior pancreaticodudenal artery off the superior mesenteric artery. The body and tail receive blood from the gastroepiploic and splenic arteries.
- At the first few weeks of gestation, the dorsal and ventral buds come together to form the pancreas, the main duct of Wirsung, and the minor duct of Santorini. Problems in fusion cause either *pancreatic divisum*, in which the pancreas is split into two separate halves, or an *annular pancreas*, in which the pancreas forms a ring around the second part of the duodenum and can constrict it.

Acute Pancreatitis

D—Leakage of pancreatic enzymes into pancreatic and peripancreatic tissue, causing inflammatory damage.

RF—This is most commonly due to gallstone disease (especially if the patient is >50 years old) or alcoholism. Other, less common causes are hypercalcemia, hypertriglyceridemia (usually >1000 mg/dL), trauma, viral infections, post ERCP procedure, and drug side effects (thiazides, sulfonamides, OCPs, and anti-HIV drugs most commonly).

SiSx—There is an abrupt, severe onset of non-crampy epigastric or diffuse abdominal pain that radiates to the back and may be relieved with sitting or standing. Nausea and vomiting usually are present, and shock can occur in advanced cases. Sympathetic pleural effusions secondary to peripancreatic inflammation can occur. If there is hemorrhagic pancreatitis, one may see flank discoloration (Grey-Turner's sign), periumbilical discoloration (Cullen's sign), or inguinal ligament discoloration (Fox's sign). In severe cases, the patient may have frank shock and develop ARDS.

Dx—Usually the clinical diagnosis is made by the symptoms and by increased amylase

Table 5-11.   Ranson's Criteria as Predictors of Mortality for Acute Pancreatitis

At Presentation	Within 48 Hours	(Number of Criteria)—Mortality
Age > 55 years	Serum Ca^{2+} < 6 mg/dL	(0–2)—5%
WBC > 16,000	Hematocrit decrease > 10%	(3–5)—15%
Glucose > 200 mg/dL	P_{O2} < 60 mmHg	(5–6)—40%
LDH > 350 IU/L	HCO_3 deficit > 4 mEq/L	(7–8)—100%
AST > 250 U/L	BUN increase > 5 mg/dL	
	Fluid sequestration > 6 L	

(more sensitive) and lipase (more specific) levels. A more definitive diagnosis can be made, however, if the ultrasound or CT scan shows an enlarged pancreas or the presence of an abscess or fluid collection around the pancreas. Additionally, on an abdominal X-ray, one may see the "sentinel loop" sign (dilated proximal small bowel) or the colon "cutoff sign" due to surrounding inflammation. Sympathetic pleural effusions may also be seen on a chest X-ray.

Tx—Remove offending agents and promote bowel rest with strict NPO orders. Perform NG suction and give analgesia. Meperidine may be better than morphine because it does not cause sphincter of Oddi contraction. Give IV fluids, and if NPO status is prolonged, consider nutritional support such as nasojejunal feeds (preferably) or TPN. From 85% to 90% of cases are mild and self-limited. The rest are severe and require monitoring in the ICU, where mortality is 50%. Long-term complications include pancreatic pseudocysts (which do not have a real epithelial lining), fistula formation, hypocalcemia, renal failure, chronic pleural effusions, and chronic pancreatitis. Pseudocysts are very common and usually resolve on their own. Persistent pseudocysts require either endoscopic or surgical drainage if they are symptomatic (causing pain, infection, or hemorrhage). They occur at least 1 week after a bout of pancreatitis, not sooner. People can function well with even less than 30% of the gland. If pancreatitis is due to gallstones, then remove them only after the pancreatitis has resolved. Indications for surgery include treatment of pancreatic abscesses, necrotizing pancreatitis, and correction of associated biliary tract disease. The prognosis

is classified by Ranson's criteria, shown in Table 5-11.

Chronic Pancreatitis

D—Irreversible parenchymal destruction from persistent inflammation leading to pancreatic dysfunction. It can be calcific, as from alcohol abuse, or obstructive because of scarring from multiple episodes of acute pancreatitis, papillary stenosis, pseudocysts, or tumors.

RF—Risk factors include alcoholism in 90% of patients, pancreatolithiasis, recurrent acute pancreatitis, hyperparathyroidism, and congenital malformation.

SiSx—Symptoms include persistent and recurrent epigastric pain with anorexia, nausea/vomiting, constipation, flatulence, and steatorrhea.

Dx—Increased amylase and lipase, glycosuria, pancreatic calcifications, and mild ileus are found on the abdominal X-ray and CT scan, the latter of which may show a dilated and strictured pancreatic duct.

Tx—It is necessary to maintain adequate pain control. Treat exocrine insufficiency by replacement of enzymes and urge the patient to completely discontinue alcohol use. Surgery may be indicated for intractable pain or structural causes. Methods include the Puestow procedure (attachment of the pancreas longitudinally to the bowel) and the DuVale procedure (distal pancreatectomy).

Diseases of the Gallbladder and Biliary Tract

Anatomy

The gallbladder is a thin-walled, contractile bag about 10 × 5 cm in size, sometimes

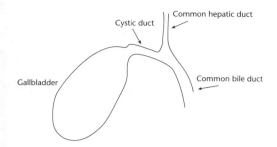

Figure 5-5. Gallbladder Anatomy.

covered completely by mesentery. It has a body, a neck, and an infundibulum with small ducts of Luschka that come off the wall opposed to the liver and go directly into it, as shown in Figure 5-5. The gallbladder empties directly into the cystic duct, which is lined by the spiral valves of Heister. This joins the common hepatic duct to make the common bile duct (CBD), which goes through the pancreas and joins the pancreatic duct to empty into the second portion of the duodenum at the ampulla of Vater through the sphincter of Oddi.

Cholelithiasis and Biliary Colic

D—Formation of stones in the gallbladder when solubilizing bile acids and lecithin are overwhelmed by increased cholesterol and bilirubin. *Choledocholithiasis* can also occur when stones pass into the CBD. There are three types of stones: (1) cholesterol stones (account for 75%), (2) pigment stones (account for 25%), and (3) mixed cholesterol and pigment stones.

RF—Classically, the characteristic patient fits the "4 Fs": fat, female, fertile, and around forty years old. Risk factors for cholesterol stones include Crohn's disease, cystic fibrosis, older age, fibrates, hyperlipidemia and hypercholesterolemia, estrogens, multiparity, radiation therapy, recent rapid weight loss, TPN use, and Native American origin. Those for pigment stones include conditions of chronic RBC hemolysis (black pigment stones develop), alcoholic cirrhosis, and biliary infection (brown pigment stones develop).

SiSx—There is postprandial abdominal pain in the RUQ that may radiate to the right subscapular region, associated with nausea/vomiting, fatty food intolerance, and dyspepsia. Pain has an abrupt onset, with gradual relief. "Biliary colic" pain is not really colicky but rather steady and severe, lasting for 1–4 hours. Stones cause no symptoms in up to 80% of patients.

Dx—Ultrasound of the RUQ is 95% sensitive for stones >3 mm and is the diagnostic test of choice. It allows one to see stones, the thickness of the gallbladder, dilation of the gallbladder tree, fluid, and other diseases. Consider an upper GI series to rule out ulcer and hernia.

Tx—Cholecystectomy is the definitive treatment in patients who are symptomatic. For asymptomatic patients, stone removal is necessary in those who have sickle cell disease, who have large stones (>3.5–4 cm), who are immunosuppressed, and who have porcelain gallbladder (repeated inflammation leading to a calcified, hard gallbladder). Dietary modification is helpful for those who are not surgical candidates. Pharmacologic dissolution of stones with bile salts can be done with or without extracorporeal shock wave lithotripsy, which is associated with a high recurrence rate. If the stones do not pass and end up stuck in the CBD (choledocholithiasis), then ERCP may be needed to remove them.

Acute Cholecystitis

D—Classical cholecystitis is caused by prolonged blockage of the cystic duct, usually from an impacted stone, resulting in postobstructive distention, inflammation, superinfection, and possibly even gangrene of the gallbladder. *Acalculous cholecystitis* occurs in the absence of a stone via biliary sludging from ischemia of the wall. *Emphysematous cholecystitis* results from infection of the gallbladder by gas-producing organisms such as anaerobes.

RF—The risk factors are the same as those for cholelithiasis. Acalculous cholecystitis is seen in patients who are chronically debilitated, in the ICU, on TPN, or have extensive burns.

SiSx—There is RUQ pain with nausea/vomiting, low-grade fever, and mild icterus. The pain is worse than that in biliary colic. There may be a positive Murphy's sign (inspiratory breathing arrest during deep palpation in the RUQ). The best sign is a "sonographic Murphy's sign," which is the same finding while pushing with the probe over the directly visualized gallbladder. Pain is poorly localized until the parietal surface of the gallbladder is inflamed. An enlarged gallbladder may be palpated in one-third of patients. Complications include empyema, hydrops (the obstructed gallbladder fills with a clear transudate secreted by the mucosa and can lead to perforation), gangrene, fistula, and gallstone ileus.

Dx—Laboratory tests may show a mild leukocytosis and elevated total and direct bilirubin. The diagnostic test of choice is a technetium hepatobiliary imino-diacetic acid (TcHIDA) scan, which shows stones and the anatomy; however, it can be a false positive in patients with TPN or active hepatitis. In a TcHIDA scan the patient is given cholecystokinin (CCK) to empty the gallbladder. Then, with labeled TC^{99}, one sees how the gallbladder fills 4 hours later; lack of gallbladder filling implies a blocked cystic duct, confirming the presence of cholecystitis. The test is 95% sensitive and specific. Ultrasound is also useful for diagnosis if the history is not classic. In emphysematous cholecystitis, one sees air in the wall of the gallbladder on an abdominal X-ray or CT scan. In acalculous cholecystitis, the diagnosis requires a high degree of suspicion. In many cases, TcHIDA shows a lack of response to CCK and ultrasound shows an increased amount of sludge. Ultrasound and CT are also useful for cholecystitis, showing an enlarged gallbladder and a thickened wall with pericholecystic fluid.

Tx—Either open or laparoscopic choleycystectomy, along with antibiotics to cover GI bacteria, is the treatment of choice and should be done within 48 hours. Sometimes if there is significant inflammation of the tissues and phlegmon develops, one can wait several weeks for this condition to subside before surgery. In acalculous cholecystitis the mortality is 50%. Treatment of choice for this entity is also cholecycstectomy once the patient is stable or percutaneous cholecystostomy if they are too unstable and are a high surgical risk.

Ascending Cholangitis

D—Infection of the biliary tract, either after obstruction by a stone or following a postoperative stricture.

P—High pressure from obstruction promotes migration of typical gut bacteria into the biliary tract and colonization. Common causes are *E. coli, Klebsiella, Proteus, Enterobacter, Pseudomonas, E. fecalis,* and *Clostridium.* Gallstones act as a nidus of infection, and obstruction favors migration of bacteria into systemic blood, causing sepsis.

RF—Risk factors include biliary obstruction and stasis from calculi or benign lesions, stricture, a prior procedure like ERCP, and a recent surgical procedure.

SiSx—Classically, the symptoms are Charcot's triad of sudden onset of RUQ pain (the patient can tell exactly when it begins), jaundice, and fever or Reynold's pentad of these three plus hypotension and a change in mental status (ΔMS), which causes immediate death in 15% of patients. One may also see dark urine from elevated levels of bilirubin pigments.

Dx—Ultrasound is a good first study to see if ducts are dilated and to look for the presence of stones. The TcHIDA test is not useful here. A CT scan is useful to determine the level at which the biliary tract is affected. Ultrasound is followed by ERCP to confirm the diagnosis and allows intervention with stone extraction sphincterotomy or stent insertion in the bile ducts. If there is high clinical suspicion, ERCP should be performed immediately.

Tx—Immediate relief of obstruction is essential via decompression by ERCP. Intravenous antibiotic therapy with ampicillin and gentamicin against enteric and gram-negative organisms is also important. Metronidazole can be added to cover anaerobes.

Gallstone Ileus

D—A condition in which a fistula forms between the gallbladder wall and a loop of small bowel through which a large stone passes, causing SB obstruction. The stone never passes via the bile duct. Classical impaction occurs at the ileocecal valve. Usually the stone is >2.5 cm.

Epi—This condition accounts for 1–3% of all cases of intestinal obstruction. It occurs in <0.5% of patients with gallstones and is much more common in females than in males. The mean age of occurrence is 70 years.

P—Fistula formation can occur between the gallbladder and duodenum or even between the gallbladder and colon secondary to pericholecystic inflammation that leads to adhesions after chronic episodes of cholecystitis. Pressure necrosis along the gall bladder wall occurs with larger stones. The stone becomes progressively larger as it moves down the bowel along with more sediment.

SiSx—The condition presents as subacute bowel obstruction with abdominal pain and vomiting, which may be relieved when the stone becomes disimpacted. Most patients are symptomatic.

Dx—Classically, air is seen in the biliary tree (via the fistula), either on abdominal X-ray or CT scan, which makes the diagnosis.

Tx—Removal of the stone and usually of the gallbladder is indicated after stabilizing the patient if necessary. The condition is associated with high morbidity and mortality.

Diseases of the Liver

Anatomy

- The liver is covered by the tough Glisson's capsule, which is rich in nerve endings. Its irritation is the source of RUQ pain in many liver diseases.
- All of the liver is covered by the visceral peritoneum except the so called "bare area" near the vena cava where it connects to the diaphragm.

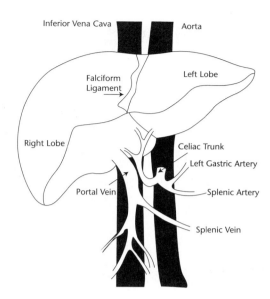

Figure 5-6. Liver Anatomy.

- The organ is divided into two lobes, as shown in Figure 5-6 by reflection of the peritoneum.
- The hepatic blood supply is from two sources: 30% is from the hepatic artery either off the celiac artery or replaced hepatic artery off the superior mesenteric artery (SMA), and 70% is from the portal vein.
- The liver makes 1L of bile per day, most of which is reabsorbed by the terminal ileum, with 5% escaping. It is recycled two to three times per day.
- Other functions of the liver include but are not limited to cholesterol storage and metabolism, fat metabolism and lipoprotein production, protein metabolism and synthesis, vitamin A, D, and B_{12} storage, iron storage, and drug and alcohol metabolism.

Disorders of Bilirubin Metabolism

These disorders are genetic conditions that focus on the formation and secretion of bilirubin. Figure 5-7 details the steps in this process, from degenerating RBCs to excretion in urine and feces. One very common disease process is considered here as many of the other conditions are quite rare.

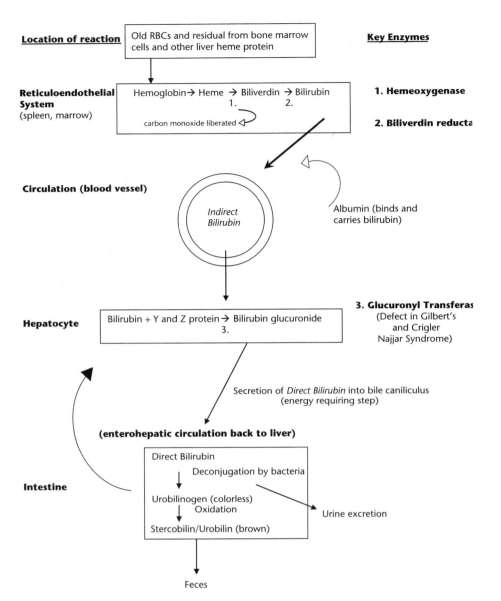

Figure 5-7. Metabolism of Bilirubin.

Bilirubin is formed from the breakdown of hemoglobin's heme moiety. It is the only reaction in the body that releases a molecule of carbon monoxide. Albumin is the main carrier of bilirubin in the circulation (called *indirect bilirubin*). In the liver, glucuronidation occurs where it is changed to *direct bilirubin* and thereafter occurs the major energy-requiring step in the entire process: secretion into bile. During many forms of liver disease, it is this energy-requiring step that is first impaired; hence, there is a backup and buildup of direct bilirubin in the blood. By contrast, hemolysis, involving excess breakdown of heme, causes an excess of indirect bilirubin.

Gilbert's Syndrome

D—A benign syndrome characterized by mild *unconjugated* hyperbilirubinemia in the absence of liver or biliary tract disease.

Epi—The overall prevalence is as high as 8%. The male/female ratio ranges from 1.5:1 to as high as 7:1 in some populations.

P—Genetic heterogeneity exists, but the predominant form in the United States and Europe appears to be autosomal dominant inheritance. There is a reduction in UDP-glucuronosyltransferase (UGT1A1) activity to 10–35% of normal, which reduces bilirubin clearance by a comparable amount. Genetic modifiers must exist, however, because substantial numbers of heterozygotes do not manifest disease. An associated disease is seen in infants and children called *Crigler Najjar-syndrome*, which is much more serious (type I is fatal) and is characterized by complete absence of UGT1A1 activity.

SiSx—Jaundice and scleral icterus are seen. Precipitating factors include stress, fatigue, reduced caloric intake, and illness.

Dx—Diagnosis is based on a family history of the disease with absence of known liver or biliary tract disease and chronically elevated unconjugated hyperbilirubinemia, usually <3 mg/dL (though it can be higher).

Tx—No intervention is necessary.

Systemic Diseases with Liver Involvement

Wilson's Disease

D—An autosomal recessive disease of systemic copper accumulation with sequelae involving the liver, CNS, eye, and kidney, among other organs.

Epi—The incidence is 1/30,000–1/100,000. The disease is rarely seen in patients <6 years or >30 years of age.

P—Mutations occur in the *ATP7B* gene, which encodes a transmembrane copper-transporting ATPase residing both on the hepatocyte canalicular membrane and in the perinuclear area. The defect causes lack of copper secretion into the bile (the main way to excrete copper); hence, there is buildup of free copper in the blood, which deposits in organs, causing pathology via free radical damage. Also, the defect does not allow production of ceruloplasmin (from apoceruloplasmin), and therefore, these levels are low. This latter condition has nothing to do with the disease, but it is used as a marker.

SiSx—Younger patients tend to present with liver disease ranging from acute to chronic cirrhotic liver disease to fulminant failure. One-half of these patients have Kayser-Fleischer rings, which are copper sulfate deposits in the Descemet's membrane of the cornea that do not affect vision. Older patients present with neuropsychiatric symptoms ranging from mild behavioral changes to depression and frank psychosis or a Parkinson-like syndrome with bradykinesia and tremor. Those with neuropsychiatric symptoms almost always have Kayser-Fleischer rings. Deposition in joints can cause arthritis, and deposition in the kidney can affect proximal tubule reabsorption. Sometimes an associated Coomb's negative hemolytic anemia exists due to free radical destruction of RBCs.

Dx—Liver failure in a young patient should make one suspect the diagnosis. Kayser-Fleischer rings are almost pathognomonic with other symptoms present. To establish the diagnosis, one must demonstrate decreased serum ceruloplasmin and elevated 24-hour urinary copper excretion. The diagnosis can be confirmed by the D-penicillamine provocative test of urinary excretion (which should increase excretion). If the results are ambiguous, perform liver biopsy and obtain quantification of copper (since cirrhosis can increase copper accumulation as well).

Tx—Remove excess copper stores and then prevent reaccumulation. Begin with dietary copper restriction (shellfish, liver, legumes, nuts). Administer D-penicillamine, a copper chelator, and oral zinc, which increases fecal excretion. Patients must always remain on a copper chelator to prevent reaccumulation. If they are noncompliant, it becomes much more difficult, if not impossible, to treat reaccumulation the second time. Transplant for those with cirrhosis and fulminant hepatic failure is curative.

Hemochromatosis

D—A disease characterized by excessive accumulation of body iron with toxic levels in the liver and pancreas. Two forms exist: familial and secondary hemochromatosis.

Epi—The incidence of the familial form is 1/220 among people of northern European origin. Male patients outnumber female ones by 5–7:1 (due to female physiologic iron loss in menstruation and pregnancy).

P—There exists no major pathway for iron excretion. In the familial form, there is a mutation of HLA-H, a HLA class I-like molecule involved in iron absorption (not fully characterized). The secondary form is due to iron overload, most commonly from multiple transfusions (e.g., in older hemophiliacs and in patients with thalassemias and sickle cell disease) and rarely from increased absorption (due to ineffective erythropoiesis) or increased intake (Bantu siderosis). Excessive iron results in (1) lipid peroxidation through iron-catalyzed free radicals, (2) stimulation of collagen formation, and (3) interactions with DNA, leading to cell death and predisposing to hepatocellular cancer.

SiSx—Elements of the classic triad of (1) hepatomegaly, (2) bronze skin pigmentation (from iron deposition and melanin), and (3) diabetes may be seen. Abdominal pain, restrictive cardiomyopathy, hypogonadism, and atypical arthritis are other features.

Dx—Transferrin saturation is elevated (>50%), and ferritin levels are elevated to around 1000–4000 ng/mL. Definitive diagnosis is made by liver biopsy, which shows iron deposits with Prussian blue stain.

Tx—Administer weekly phlebotomy for maintenance once serum iron levels decline. Iron chelators, such as desferoximine, can also be used.

Acute and Chronic Liver Failure

Acute Hepatic Failure

D—A clinical syndrome caused by the rapid development of liver synthetic dysfunction.

There are three classes of acute liver failure, depending on the interval between recognition of liver disease and development of hepatic encephalopathy: acute (<2 weeks), fulminant (2–8 weeks), and subfulminant (8–24 weeks). This entity may occur in patients who previously had normal liver function or well-compensated liver disease.

P—Causes include the following:

1. Massive hepatic necrosis: viruses (most commonly acute hepatitis B or A and rarely hepatitis C), drugs (e.g., acetaminophen, halothane, antituberculosis agents such as rifampin and isoniazid, and monoamine oxidase inhibitors), and industrial chemicals (e.g., carbon tetrachloride).

2. Dysfunction without necrosis: Reye syndrome, tetracycline toxicity, and acute fatty liver of pregnancy.

    Extrahepatic sequelae probably result from the liver's inability to detoxify enteric bacterial products in the blood.

3. Rare etiologies include autoimmune liver disease; infection with Epstein-Barr virus, herpes simplex virus, or cytomegalovirus; ischemic liver cell necrosis; *Budd-Chiari syndrome*; Wilson's disease; hyperthermia; primary graft nonfunction; and postsurgical partial hepatectomy.

SiSx—Direct manifestations of liver failure include jaundice and scleral icterus, coagulopathy, hypoglycemia, and metabolic acidosis. Systemic manifestations include rapid development of infection, peripheral vasodilatation with hypotension, pulmonary edema, renal failure, disseminated intravascular coagulation (DIC), and cerebral edema, which occurs when ICP > 30 mmHg (exhibited by systolic hypertension and increased muscle tone changing to decerebrate posturing). The latter complicates stages 3 and 4 of hepatic encephalopathy in 50%–85% of patients.

Dx—In addition to the symptoms described above, evidence of acute synthetic liver dysfunction includes prolonged clotting times, elevated direct bilirubin, low albumin, and elevated transaminases, perhaps with elevated ammonia (NH_3) that the liver cannot detoxify. Liver biopsy may be necessary to determine the exact cause if no noticeable drug history has been found. Biopsy must be carefully done in the face of a coagulopathy.

Tx—Liver regeneration may be possible with supportive care. Prevention of hepatic encephalopathy is essential with agents such as lactulose. Development of stage 2 or 3 hepatic encephalopathy (see the Hepatic Encephalopathy section), serious bleeding, sepsis, or recurrent bouts of hypoglycemia are indications for ICU admission. Patients with stage 3 or 4 hepatic encephalopathy may require endotracheal intubation to prevent aspiration. Coagulopathy should be treated with vitamin K. Definitive treatment for acute liver failure in which there is little recovery of function is orthotopic liver transplant.

Autoimmune Hepatitis

D—Syndrome of chronic hepatitis that may present as acute hepatic failure and is accompanied by a varying set of autoimmunologic abnormalities that ultimately leads to liver failure and cirrhosis. No other cause must be found for the underlying liver disease. Two types of autoimmune hepatitis exist, types I and II, which are different with respect to circulating antibodies.

Epi—Female patients outnumber males by 2:1. Type II more often affects young girls and women.

P—The condition is idiopathic but is thought to involve autoimmunity via a cell-mediated attack on hepatocytes triggered perhaps by environmental factors.

SiSx—The clinical picture fluctuates temporally as well as in severity from no symptoms to those of fulminant hepatic failure. Stigmata of chronic liver disease may also be present (see below). Sixty percent of patients also present with features of other autoimmune disease, including RA, thyroiditis, Sjögren's syndrome, and UC.

Dx—Marked increases in AST and ALT [up to several thousand international units/L (IU/L)] as well as increases in alkaline phosphatase and conjugated bilirubin are found.

Positive serum antibodies that may be found include ANA, anti-smooth muscle antibody (ASMA) in type I, and anti-liver kidney muscle-1 (ALKM-1) and anti-liver cytosol antigen (ALC-1) in type II.

Tx—Administer steroids acutely, using azathioprine or other immunomodulators for long-term maintenance therapy. Transplant is not often needed if patients are treated early. If the condition is untreated, 6-month mortality can be as high as 40%.

Alcoholic Hepatitis

D—Acute syndrome of liver disease that occurs in the setting of heavy alcohol consumption. Individuals with this usually condition consume, on average, at least 100 g/day of alcohol (30 oz of wine or about eight 12-oz cans of beer) for over a year.

SiSx—Fever, jaundice, and hepatomegaly with liver tenderness are seen. Ascites, encephalopathy, and varices occur after the onset of cirrhosis and portal hypertension. Ascites and encephalopathy can occur acutely without underlying cirrhosis and resolve as the acute alcoholic hepatitis resolves.

Dx—Elevated direct bilirubin, increased AST and ALT (usually below 300 U/L), and increased alkaline phosphatase are seen. Classically, AST exceeds ALT by a 2:1 ratio because of decreased pyridoxine intake. Viral hepatitis will produce the opposite ratio. Liver biopsy is diagnostic when the history is in doubt or when it is necessary to rule out other causes. Biopsy shows fatty liver with hyaline bodies (Mallory bodies) and hepatocyte necrosis.

Tx—Absolute abstinence from alcohol use is crucial. Administer B vitamins and folate supplements with a normal diet. Some improvement is seen with steroids or pentoxifylline.

Nonalcoholic Steatohepatitis (NASH)

D—Clinical entity in which there are symptoms of hepatitis in the absence of alcohol consumption, with findings otherwise indistinguishable from those of alcoholic hepatitis. No other cause, such as viral infection, can be found.

Epi—The incidence is 7–9% in all patients with liver biopsy but unclear in the greater population. The condition is found mostly in patients 40–60 years old.

RF—Risk factors are obesity, diabetes, IV hyperalimentation, and post-jejunoileal bypass surgery status.

P—The mechanism has yet to be elucidated. It is thought to involve insulin resistance leading to hepatic steatosis.

SiSx—Prolonged NASH can lead eventually to cirrhosis.

Dx—Modest increases in LFTs (two- to fourfold) are seen. Other causes of liver disease must be ruled out. Definitive diagnosis is made by liver biopsy. In addition to fatty liver, Mallory bodies are observed occasionally.

Tx—An obese patient should lose weight as a first step. There is no other proven treatment. Usually the disease has a stable course with no difference in life expectancy. In a small minority of patients, there is progression to end-stage liver disease (ESLD).

Budd-Chiari Syndrome (BCS)

D—Occlusion or diminished blood flow in the venous drainage of the liver due to a thromboembolic phenomenon. Clot occurs in the hepatic vein on the infrahepatic or suprahepatic inferior vena cava (IVC).

Epi—An underlying hypercoagulable state is found in the great majority of patients, with more than half of the cases caused by myeloproliferative disorders. Acute liver failure occurs most commonly in women.

RF—Risk factors include malignancy, OCP use, and other conditions leading to a hypercoagulable state.

SiSx—The presentation can vary from acute fulminant hepatic failure to subacute or even chronic liver failure. Patients typically have RUQ abdominal pain and hepatomegaly; jaundice and ascites develop rapidly soon afterward.

Dx—Transaminases (AST and ALT) are elevated (into the hundreds of IU/L) along with direct bilirubin. Doppler ultrasound can make the diagnosis by demonstrating abnormal flow of the hepatic veins or IVC as well as vessel wall thickening and dilation. A CT scan with IV contrast can also show filling defects or delayed filling of the hepatic veins. However, the gold standard is venography, which is more invasive and involves percutaneous assessment of hepatic vein and IVC pressures and flow. Liver biopsy has characteristic findings of congestion, necrosis, and hemorrhage and can be used to guide therapy based on the extent of damage and cirrhosis.

Tx—The goals of therapy depend on the severity of the clinical situation. First, one needs to prevent further clot via anticoagulation. Thrombolytics can be considered in the acute or subacute form of BCS (clot present for <4 weeks). Otherwise, decompression can be done by angioplasty or stenting, though reocclusion is common. Surgical thrombectomy usually is not feasible. For those with advanced liver disease, treatment of portal hypertension via shunting procedures can be done; ultimately, liver transplant should be considered.

Viral Hepatitis (see Chapter 8)

Acetaminophen Hepatotoxicity

D—Inability of the liver to detoxify acetaminophen, causing centrilobular necrosis. From 10 to 15 g of acetaminophen is enough to cause injury in someone with a healthy liver. Fulminant disease occurs with 25 g or more. In chronic alcoholics, the dose needed may be as low as 2 g.

P—Metabolism of acetaminophen involves phase I and phase II reactions in the liver. Phase I turns acetaminophen into a hepatotoxic metabolite called N-acetyl-p-benzoquinone imine (NAPQI), which is detoxified by binding to glutathione and then undergoes renal excretion. When glutathione is low, NAPQI binds hepatocytes and causes necrosis. Injury can be potentiated with alcohol or starvation, which reduces glutathione levels. Inhibitors of P450 can reduce the toxicity.

SiSx—Nausea, vomiting, diarrhea, abdominal pain, and shock can occur after 4–12 hours of overdose. After 24–48 hours, hepatic injury is more apparent. Symptoms are most apparent after 4–6 days.

Dx—Diagnosis is based on a history of acetaminophen ingestion and elevated blood levels. Elevations of AST and ALT up to 10,000 IU/L are not uncommon.

Tx—Treatment depends on the amount of time that has passed since the overdose. Within 30 minutes of an overdose, perform gastric lavage and give oral activated charcoal or cholestyramine to prevent absorption of any residual drug. After 30 minutes, activated charcoal will interfere with the antidote, N-acetylcysteine, which acts like glutathione in its reducing ability. Common nomograms are used to determine the probability of hepatotoxicity based on drug blood levels. Therapy with N-acetylcysteine is useful only in patient with levels above 200 μg/mL at 4 hours or 100 μg/mL after 8 hours. Otherwise, it is not necessary. The loading dose is 140 mg/kg, and then 70 mg/kg is given every 4 hours for a total of 15–20 doses. Survivors usually have no evidence of hepatic sequelae.

Primary Sclerosing Cholangitis

D—Inflammation, obliterative fibrosis, and segmental constriction of the medium-sized and large intrahepatic and extrahepatic bile ducts.

RF—The risk factor is inflammatory bowel disease, specifically UC.

Epi—Male patients outnumber females by 2:1. The prevalence is 5/100,000. The condition presents in the third to fifth decades of life; 50–75% of patients have inflammatory bowel disease. There is a 10–15% lifetime risk of developing cholangiocarcinoma and an increased risk of colon cancer.

P—The cause is idiopathic but is thought to involve autoimmunity.

SiSx—Symptoms are pruritis, jaundice, malaise, dark urine, light stools, and hepatosplenomegaly, with RUQ pain in 15% of patients.

Dx—Diagnosis is made when the characteristic multifocal stricturing and dilation of intrahepatic and/or extrahepatic bile ducts are seen on ERCP or MRCP. Other studies are supportive. Liver function tests show the cholestatic pattern. Serologic studies may show elevated IgM and hypergammaglobulinemia. Liver biopsy shows the characteristic onion skinning around bile ducts and is useful for prognostic purposes.

Tx—Cholestyramine or charcoal is used for pruritis, ursodeoxycholic acid to solubilize bile and facilitate bile flow, and fat-soluble vitamin replacements. Endoscopic retrograde cholangiopancreatography is used to remove stones and dilate ducts. Surgery is done for biliary drainage, and the patient is put on the liver transplantation list (third most common indication).

Primary Biliary Cirrhosis

D—A chronic, progressive, and sometimes fatal cholestatic liver disease characterized by destruction of intrahepatic bile ducts.

Epi—Over 90% of patients are women. Peak incidence occurs at 40–60 years of age. The condition is associated with RA, Sjögren's syndrome, sicca syndrome, scleroderma, CREST (calcinosis cutis, Raynaud's phenomenon, esophageal dysfunction, sclerodactyly, and telangiectasia), thyroiditis, membranous GN, and celiac disease in 75% of patients.

P—The condition is idiopathic but is thought to involve autoimmunity with inflammatory destruction of the small intraheptic biliary ducts. The damage gradually leads to cirrhosis and liver failure.

SiSx—Patients are asymptomatic early in the course, though they may have abnormal LFTs at that time. Insidious fatigue and extreme pruritis are the first symptoms, with jaundice developing months or years later. Hyperpigmentation, hirsutism, steatorrhea, weight loss, xanthomas (in 10%), and osteopenia (25%) are other features. There is an association with Sjögren's syndrome (in 75% of patients), antithyroid antibody in 25% of patients, RA, and the CREST syndrome (see Chapter 6).

Dx—Alkaline phosphatase is markedly elevated; AST and ALT are slightly elevated. Conjugated bilirubin increases with progression of disease and is a good prognostic indicator. One should rule out extrahepatic biliary obstruction with ultrasound. Serologic tests show IgM levels four to five times normal and positive antimitochondrial antibodies (AMA) in 90% of patients. Confirmatory liver biopsy should be performed and will show classic periductal granulomas, inflammatory destruction of the bile ducts with lymphocytic infiltration, and ultimately portal fibrosis.

Tx—Treatment must deal with both the disease and the sequelae of chronic cholestasis. For the former, steroids are ineffective. Ursodeoxycholic acid, colchicine, methotrexate, and various combinations thereof have been found to be of some value. For the latter, complications include pruritis, bone disease, hypercholesterolemia, malabsorption, vitamin deficiencies, and anemia, all of which must be addressed. Liver transplant can be successful in treating those with end stage liver disease from PBC.

Cirrhosis and Chronic Liver Failure

D—Cirrhosis is a late stage of progressive hepatic dysfunction characterized by distortion of the hepatic architecture with or without formation of regenerative nodules. There are two main types: (1) chronic sclerosis (cirrhosis with minimal regenerative activity of hepatocytes causing fibrosis without nodules) and (2) nodular cirrhosis (regenerative activity and numerous fine nodules with a large liver initially).

Epi—Most common causes include the following:
Toxins—alcohol and hepatotoxic drugs.
Infections—viral hepatitis (most commonly HCV), and schistosomiasis outside the United States.
Autoimmune—PSC, PBC, autoimmune hepatitis.
Vascular—cardiac cirrhosis (from longstanding right heart failure) and *Budd-Chiari syndrome*, involving thrombosis of the hepatic veins.
Hereditary—hemochromatosis, Wilson's disease, and α_1-antitrypsin deficiency.
Other—NASH and cryptogenic liver cirrhosis.

P—Most cases involve progressive fibrosis, in which hepatic stellate cells transform into myofibroblast-like cells and produce types I and III collagen in such a way that the portal vessels are directly connected to the terminal hepatic veins, bypassing the parenchyma.

SiSx—Many of the following symptoms may be present, some of which are discussed later in more detail:
General: anorexia, weight loss, weakness.
Skin: jaundice, pruritis, peripheral edema (from hypoalbuminemia), xanthomas, xanthelasmas (from an increase in lipids that are not metabolized), palmar erythema, and spider angiomas (blanchable vascular structures seen commonly on the chest). The last four result from hyperestrogenemia, which occurs due to lack of breakdown in the liver.
CNS: hepatic encephalopathy, asterixis (flapping of outstretched dorsiflexed hands).
GI: ascites, fetor hepaticus ("sweet and sour" body odor), evidence of portal hypertension such as splenomegaly, presence of extensive venous collaterals on the abdomen, hemorrhoids, and esophageal varices that predispose to UGIBs.
Renal: renal failure from hepatorenal syndrome.
GU: in males, hypogonadism and gynecomastia may also result from hyperestrogenism.
Heme: anemia and a tendency to bleed or bruise.
Bone: osteoporosis.

Dx—Liver biopsy is the gold standard to demonstrate cirrhosis. Besides obvious symptoms, evidence of liver synthetic dysfunction will be seen on laboratory tests, such as prolonged PT and hypoalbuminemia.

Tx—Liver transplant is the only definitive treatment for cirrhosis. Supportive therapy until then is necessary. Treatment of hepatic encephalopathy and relief of portal hypertension via shunts are discussed below. Treatment of the underlying condition may prevent the development of complications from portal hypertension/cirrhosis. Prevention of added insult to the liver includes HBV and HAV vaccination, as well as monitoring for hepatocellular cancer.

Classically, the prognosis for gauging the surgical outcome and 1-year survival was formerly determined by the Child-Pugh criteria, with classes A, B, and C. It incorporated many elements including albumin, the presence of ascites and bilirubin, the presence of encephalopathy and the PT. The currently used MELD (Model for End Stage Liver Disease) is an excellent predictor of mortality from cirrhosis and is used to rank patients on liver transplant wait lists. It is a complex formula based on (1) serum bilirubin, (2) creatinine, and (3) international normalized ratio (INR), with creatinine having the biggest impact on the overall score.

Ascites

D—Pathologic accumulation of fluid in the peritoneal cavity.

P—It can be the result of numerous causes. In cirrhosis, ascites results specifically from a consequence of increased back pressure from liver fibrosis into capillaries with portal hypertension, fluid overload from neurohormonal mechanisms, and decreased oncotic pressure from decreased albumin synthesis. It can also result from increased back pressure from thrombotic or venous occlusive disease, prolonged right heart failure, infectious causes, inflammatory causes such as pancreatitis, and malignancy (often ovarian cancer). With the increasing total extracellular splanchnic volume, there is decreased intravascular volume.

Therefore, the body increases renal sodium and water retention, primarily by elevating aldosterone. Lymphatic drainage of the peritoneum also decreases.

SiSx—Symptoms include increased abdominal girth with bulging flanks, umbilical herniation, pitting peripheral edema, pleural effusions, and SOB. Physical exam reveals shifting dullness. When you change the position of the patient from supine to side-lying, fluid always follow gravity, so dullness to percussion of the flank while the patient is supine will become resonant when the patient is lying with the opposite side down. A fluid wave shift may also be felt. Have someone press his or her arm down the middle of the abdomen to keep it taut and tap on one side. Pressure waves transmitted by the fluid may be felt on the other side of the abdomen.

Dx—It may be obvious by physical exam if more than 2 L of fluid is present, especially with a history of a rapidly increasing abdominal girth. Ultrasound is sensitive in detecting 100 mL of fluid. Paracentesis is the main way to characterize fluid and help determine the etiology. The test is sent for cell count, culture, chemistry with amylase and lipase, and cytology. One way to distinguish between transudative and exudative causes is to calculate the serum-ascites albumin gradient (SAAG), as shown in Table 5-12, which is the serum albumin minus the ascites albumin. Ascites signals an average of 2-year survival in patients with liver failure.

Tx—If possible, treat the underlying cause. In the case of liver disease, avoid alcohol in

Table 5-12. Serum-Ascites Albumin Gradient

If >1.1 mg/dL	If <1.1 mg/dL
Liver failure/cirrhosis with portal hypertension	Nephrotic syndrome
Heart failure	Peritoneal carcinomatosis
Massive liver metastases	Tuberculosis peritonitis
Fulminant hepatic failure	Serositis, as in rheumatic disease
Portal vein thrombosis	Pancreatitis-related ascites
Budd-Chiari syndrome	Bowel obstruction
Myxedema	Postoperative lymph leak

particular, restrict salt to 2 g/day, and use water restriction if hyponatremia is present but not if renal function is good. The diuretic mainstay in those with purely a liver etiology is spironolactone initially, with furosemide and spironolactone added later, depending on the patient's response. If necessary, large-volume paracenteses can be done, with albumin replacement (10 g for every 1 L) to maintain oncotic pressure. Weight loss should be slow, limited to 2 kg/day if possible. Transjugular intrahepatic portosystemic shunts and other forms of portovenous shunting (see below) can relieve some portal hypertension and thereby relieve ascites.

Hepatic Encephalopathy

D—Alteration in mental status with extrapyramidal and pyramidal symptoms due to hepatic failure. It may be acute and reversible or chronic and progressive.

RF—Precipitating factors for those with liver disease include (1) GI bleeding, (2) increased dietary protein, and (3) electrolyte disturbances (from diuretic-induced hypokalemic alkalosis, paracentesis, or vomiting), and (4) other infections.

P—The specific cause is unknown. It is thought that in the wake of hepatic failure, substances detoxified by the liver lead to abnormal neurotransmission in both the central and peripheral nervous systems. While NH_3 is perhaps the most widely followed substance found in excess, paradoxically the NH_3 level does not always correlate with the degree or severity of symptoms. Other incriminated substances include short chain fatty acids, phenol, and mercaptans, a group of sulfur-containing substances. There is usually a precipitating event in those with known otherwise stable cirrhosis.

SiSx—Stigmata of chronic liver disease are usually present. Disturbed consciousness is seen, ranging from minor changes in behavior to confusion to coma. Neurologic changes include asterixis (also seen in other forms of metabolic brain disease), rigidity, and hyperreflexia. Fetor hepaticus is a unique musty breath odor, also found in the urine, that is thought to be due to mercaptans. Clinical signs of cerebral edema occur when intracranial pressure (ICP) exceeds 30 mmHg.

Dx—Diagnosis involves demonstration of the four factors:

1. Acute or chronic liver disease.
2. Disturbances in awareness and mentation.
3. The aforementioned neurologic signs.
4. A characteristic (though nonspecific) symmetric, high-voltage, triphasic slow-wave pattern on the EEG.

The diagnosis is usually one of exclusion once other causes of mental status changes have been ruled out. Stage of encephalopathy is an important measure to follow in anticipation of a transplant (see Table 5-13). Note: the serum NH_3 level does not correlate with the stage.

Tx—Treatment usually consists of lowering the blood ammonia level by administering lactulose (acidifies intestinal contents and is cathartic, thereby decreasing NH_3 absorption). If the response is inadequate, neomycin or rifaximin is added to decrease bacterial overgrowth. Decreasing protein intake may help but also

Table 5-13.   Stages of Encephalopathy

Stage	Mental Status	Asterixis	EEG
I	Euphoria, depression, irritability, impaired handwriting, confusion, hypersomnia, sleep pattern inversion	None to minimal	Triphasic wave
II	Slurred speech, lethargy, amnesia, moderate confusion, hypoactive reflexes, loss of time	Present	Triphasic wave
III	Somnolence and marked confusion, incoherent speech, loss of place recognition, hyperactive reflexes, sleeping but arousable	Present	Triphasic wave
IV	Comatose; initially responsive to noxious stimuli, later unresponsive, dilated pupils, loss of self-awareness	Absent	Delta activity

can be harmful since the patient may already be hypoalbuminemic. In those with acute encephalopathy, the CNS symptoms are usually completely reversible with treatment.

Portal Hypertension

D—Condition in which the normally low portal pressure is more than 5 mmHg above the IVC pressure.

P—There are three sets of causes based on the relation to the hepatic sinusoids:

Prehepatic obstruction—portal vein obstruction.

Intrahepatic obstruction—cirrhosis or other causes of chronic liver disease.

Posthepatic obstruction—right-sided heart failure, constrictive pericarditis, hepatic vein obstruction (Budd-Chiari syndrome and veno-occlusive disease). Posthepatic obstruction causes the fastest rate of ascites accumulation, as both the portal and hepatic venous systems are obstructed.

In all cases, effective circulating blood volume is decreased as fluid is sequestered in the splanchnic circulation.

SiSx—Symptoms depends on the etiology. Often jaundice seen, with or without other signs of hepatic failure. Commonly, the signs of long-standing portal hypertension include ascites, evidence of venous collaterals such as hemorrhoids and esophageal varices, abdominal venous distention (called *caput medusa*, located around the umbilicus), splenomegaly, and hepatic encephalopathy

Classically four main sites of collaterals allow portal blood to return to the heart:

1. Esophageal varices—from left gastric vein to azygous vein drainage.
2. Hemorrhoids—from superior rectal to inferior rectal vein drainage.
3. Caput medusa (umbilical varices)—from periumbilical vein to inferior epigastric vein drainage.
4. Paravertebral and renal vein varices—from retroperitoneal vein communication.

Tx—Treatment depends on the underlying condition. Acute venous thrombosis may be reversible. Conditions in which there is chronic liver disease require transplant. Temporizing measures to relieve the major sites of compression include use of shunts, which allow better communication between portal and systemic circulations. Surgical shunts (such as a splenorenal or mesocaval shunt) are becoming increasingly rare; transjugular intrahepatic portosystemic shunt (TIPS) is the first-line shunt for the treatment of portal hypertension Shunting can worsening hepatic encephalopathy, as more blood becomes systemic and has not been detoxified by the liver.

Esophageal Varices

D—A manifestation of long-standing portal hypertension in which the venous collaterals in the esophagus become engorged, enlarged, and have tendency to bleed.

Epi—Up to 70% of patients with decompensated cirrhosis have varices at presentation. One third of those with compensated cirrhosis are thought to have varices. They account for about 10% of cases of upper GI bleeding.

RF—Risk factors include known chronic liver disease and alcohol use.

SiSx—The patient may be asymptomatic or present with UGIB.

Dx—Esophagogastroduodenoscopy is the only way to diagnose the condition. Varices are staged based on their size and the degree of obliteration of the lumen, with larger varices having a greater tendency to bleed. Other features noticed on endoscopy indicating a high likelihood of bleeding include cherry red spots, red wale marks (longitudinal red streaks), diffuse erythema, and a red color of the varix.

Tx—In the case of an acute bleed, after stabilizing the patient, sclerotherapy or rubber banding is indicated via EGD, which is successful in 80% of cases acutely. Short-term medical therapy includes octreotide to reduce splanchnic blood flow or vasopressin along with nitroglycerin. Long-term medical therapy includes use of β blockers to prevent bleeding. Eventually, release of pressure via a portosystemic shunt or, ultimately, liver transplant is indicated. β blockers are used to prevent bleeding of large varices and to prevent rebleeding.

Hemorrhoids

D—Painful swelling of the vascular cushions at the anal canal. They can be external and painful or internal and painless.

RF—Pregnancy, constipation, and portal hypertension are risk factors.

P—The primary cause is unknown, but the condition may be due to downward sliding of anal cushions associated with gravity, straining, and irregular bowel habits. Secondary causes include portal hypertension.

SiSx—Discomfort and pain with defecation are seen with external hemorrhoids. Internal hemorrhoids are painless and present with hematochezia or prolapse upon defecation. In this case, pain will occur only if there are fissures, abscesses, or external hemorrhoidal thromboses.

Dx—The history and physical exam (inspection during straining, digital rectal exam, and anoscopy) make the diagnosis. In some cases, it may be necessary to do colonoscopy or flexible sigmoidoscopy (to rule out inflammatory bowel disease or neoplasia).

Tx—For both internal and external hemorrhoids, dietary modifications, including consumption of fiber or bran and stool softeners, confer benefit in all situations, even after surgery. Over-the-counter suppositories have never been tested for efficacy. For external hemorrhoids, those that are thrombosed or symptomatic, yet refractory to conservative measures, require surgery.

CHAPTER 5 APPENDIX: DISEASES OF NUTRITION

Vitamins are small organic compounds that are required in small amounts. They cannot be made in sufficient quantity by the body and are therefore required in the diet. Fat-soluble vitamins are absorbed via the intestines. Water-soluble vitamins, in general, are not easily stored; hence, daily intake is needed. Tables 5-14 and 5-15 summarize conditions of vitamin deficiencies.

Trace elements are chemical substances that are needed in minute quantities to help maintain proper function. Common elements are shown in Table 5-16.

Table 5-14. The Fat-Soluble Vitamin Deficiencies

Vitamin	Function	Deficiency SiSx	Source
A	Component of photoreceptor pigments in retina and helps maintain normal epithelium.	Night blindness, conjunctival dryness, corneal keratinization. Dry skin. Severe deficiency therefore predisposes to infection, which occurs only after liver stores are depleted. Seen in fat malabsorption or severe liver disease.	Carrots and leafy green vegetables, egg yolk, cream, butter, liver, and fish oil
D (calciferol)	Calcium and phosphate absorption.	Rickets (children), osteomalacia (adults). Seen in a variety of circumstances that are not nutritional, such as chronic renal failure, liver disease, or malabsorption.	Made in skin exposed to sunlight. Also found in yeast, fish liver oils, egg yolks, and dairy products that are supplemented
E	Maintains cell membrane integrity by protecting lipids from oxidation (antioxidation).	Protein energy malnutrition, malabsorption, RBC hemolysis, and neurologic changes. Seen in cases of fat malabsorption.	Vegetable oils
K	Cofactor in clotting factor synthesis.	Problems with clotting because factors II, VII, IX, X, C, and S are vitamin K dependent in synthesis. Spontaneous bleeding, increase in PT >> PTT seen.	Leafy green vegetables, normal intestinal bacteria

Table 5-15. Water-Soluble Vitamin Deficiencies

Vitamin	Function	Deficiency SiSx	Source
B_1 (thiamine)	Cholesterol metabolism coenzyme	*Wernicke-Korsakoff syndrome* common in alcoholics with acute or chronic deficiency, with nystagmus, confusion, and confabulation. *Beriberi*—can be either the dry form, which is a bilateral symmetric peripheral neuropathy, or the wet form, which includes high-output cardiac failure. Increased need in pregnancy and hyperthyroidism.	Grains
B_2 (riboflavin)	A central component of 2 co-factors flavin adenine dinucleotide (FAD) and flavin mononucleotide (FMN) used in many metabolic processes.	Cheilosis (swollen, cracked, bright red lips) and angular stomatitis (fissuring at the angles of the mouth).	Milk or animal protein
B_3 (niacin)	Cholesterol metabolism coenzyme. A precursor for NAD and NADP	Seen in chronic diarrhea, cirrhosis, alcoholism, isoniazid use, carcinoid syndrome, and in people for whom milled corn is their staple diet. *Pellagra* is the result—diarrhea, dermatitis, dementia. Sequelae include symmetric cutaneous lesions, stomatitis, and glossitis (inflammation of the tongue).	Fruits, vegetables, and meat. Tryptophan is a precursor.
B_6 (pyridoxine)	Blood, skin, CNS metabolism	Seborrheic dermatosis, peripheral neuropathy, lymphopenia, anemia, cheilosis, glossitis, seizures in infants. Deficiency is rare.	Many different foods, including vegetables, meats, nuts, whole grains.
B_{12} (cyanocobalamin)	DNA synthesis and myelin formation	Pernicious anemia, neurologic disturbances, and ataxia	Meat and dairy products provide the only source.
Folate	DNA synthesis	Megaloblastic anemia without neurologic dysfunction	Most cereals are supplemented with this nutrient.
C (ascorbic acid)	Formation of collagen, maintenance of connective tissue, bone, and teeth.	Poor wound healing. Scurvy, which appears up to 1 year after deficiency state starts, is characterized by splinter hemorrhages, swollen and friable gums, myalgias, arthralgias, tooth loss, secondary infections, gangrene, and spontaneous hemorrhages.	Citrus fruits

Table 5-16. Trace Element Deficiencies

Element	Function	Deficiency SiSx	Source
Selenium	Required cofactor for protein and DNA synthesis. Has membrane-stabilizing activity.	Deficiency is very rare. Cardiomyopathy and skeletal muscle dysfunction may be seen. May be important in preventing cancer and heart disease.	Seafood, meat, eggs, whole grains, legumes, and Brazil nuts.
Zinc	Acts as a catalyst or cofactor for numerous enzymes in all organs. Absorbed mainly in the jejunum.	Impairs growth (can be severe if large deficiency); causes immune dysfunction, hypogonadism, poor wound healing, and vesiculobullous skin lesions. Causes *acrodermatitis enteropathica* which has characteristic GI and skin manifestations.	Oysters, red meat, poultry, beans, nuts, certain seafoods, whole grains, fortified breakfast cereals, and dairy products.
Chromium	Functions as a coenzyme or part of a metalloenzyme.	Glucose intolerance. Absorbed in the small intestine. Basically seen only in hospitalized patients with malnutrition.	Wheat germ and nuts
Iodide	Necessary for metabolism and homeostasis of thyroid gland function.	Goiter and ultimately hypothyroidism with all of its consequences. Developmental delay in children.	Most salts are supplemented
Copper	Ligand for a number of proteins and enzymes, such as monoamine oxidase (metabolized catecholamines).	Rare deficiency in premature infants on formula, those on chronic dialysis, and those with chronic diarrhea. Mimics iron deficiency anemia but does not resolve with iron supplementation.	Legumes, nuts, shellfish, and whole grains

CHAPTER 6

Rheumatology

THE BASIC JOINT EXAMINATION

In evaluating arthritis, one must determine whether or not there is inflammation. Typically, an inflamed joint will exhibit the cardinal signs of (1) redness, (2) warmth, (3) swelling, and (4) pain. Second, determine the location of the problem. Is it really in the joint, or is it in tendons (tendonitis), bursa (bursitis), or soft tissue areas (as in fibromyalgia)?

Any basic joint exam should therefore include the following:

1. Inspection
   Look for:
   - Joint redness and swelling around the joint indicating inflammation.
   - Asymmetry between similar joints on either side.
   - Muscle atrophy, which suggests lack of use, myositis or neurologic conditions.
   - Joint deformity, as chronic arthritis usually causes flexion deformities and misalignment of bones.
2. Palpation
   - Feel for warmth, joint swelling and tenderness, a sensitive but nonspecific sign of inflammation.
   - Compare both sides when possible. Assess the tension of any effusions.
   - Palpate areas to see if the pain can be reproduced.
   - Assess for warmth or a difference in temperature, which is best felt using the dorsum of the hand.
   - Crepitus, or a crackling sound or sensation as cartilage rubs together or bone rubs against bone.
3. Passive and active range-of-motion tests

- Test active (the patient moves the joint) and passive (the physician moves the joint, while the patient provides no effort) range of motion to assess limitations and pain.
- Depending on the joint, test various muscle groups and ligaments for injury (see below).

DIAGNOSTIC AND THERAPEUTIC MODALITIES

Arthrocentesis

In the presence of an inflammatory process, it is not uncommon for patients to develop joint effusions. Joint effusions are not specific to rheumatic diseases. When the etiology of an effusion is unclear, an arthrocentesis is performed, in which fluid is aspirated from the joint and sent for cell analysis, crystal analysis, culture, and Gram stain. Typical findings are shown in Table 6-1.

Note that:

- Crystals, as found in gout or pseudogout, can induce a high WBC count. A low WBC count does not necessarily rule out infectious causes, specifically in tuberculosis infection.
- The presence of crystals also does not rule out infectious causes. It is not uncommon to see blood in synovial fluid aspirates due to the vascularity of the synovium. However, synovium contaminated by blood should not clot in the tube, whereas pure blood is expected to clot in the tube.
- Bloody aspirates should make one consider coagulopathies such as hemophilia, synovial tumors, and tuberculosis if a traumatic tap is not suspected.

Table 6-1. Results of Synovial Fluid Analysis from Joint Tap

Condition	Cells	Color and Consistency		Example
Normal	0–200 WBCs	Pale yellow, clear, transparent	High viscosity	—
Noninflammatory	200–2000 WBCs	Yellow, transparent	High viscosity	Osteoarthritis, trauma
Inflammatory	2000–100,000 WBCs	Yellow, turbid, translucent to opaque	Low viscosity	Gout (crystals can cause an inflammatory reaction), RA
Septic	>50,000 WBCs with >75% PMNs	Purulent, opaque	Low viscosity	*Staphylococcus aureus*

Commonly Used Rheumatologic Serologies

Erythrocyte Sedimentation Rate (ESR)

The ESR, an *indirect* marker of active inflammation, measures the time required for RBCs to settle by gravity. When excess plasma proteins (e.g., acute phase reactants and immunoglobulins) are present, repellant forces between RBCs are decreased, allowing RBC clumping and thus a faster settling rate. A value of 0–20 mm/hour is textbook normal, but up to 40 mm/hr is normal for an 80-year-old person (a 4–6 mm/hr increase per decade occurs according to the formula age/2 + 10). An *ESR > 100 mm/hr* has a more narrow differential diagnosis that includes malignancy, vasculitis, osteomyelitis, endocarditis autoimmune disease, and severe systemic bacterial or mycobacterial infections. Noninflammatory conditions with excess immunoglobulin production or changes in RBC size or plasma viscosity also cause elevations in ESR (multiple myeloma, cryoglobulinemia, hepatitis, renal failure, anemia, and pregnancy). This test is commonly used as an adjunct to clinical information to determine whether an inflammatory process is occurring. In patients with known inflammatory disease, it can be helpful to monitor disease activity. While the ESR can be helpful in certain circumstances, remember that it is a nonspecific test and can be elevated in many nonrheumatologic conditions.

C-Reactive Protein (CRP)

This acute phase reactant, made by the liver in response to interleukin-1 (IL-1) and IL-6, is a useful test along with the ESR as a marker of inflammation. Unlike ESR, it is a *direct* inflammatory marker. Increases in CRP occur faster than in the ESR after the onset of an acute inflammatory process; therefore, CRP provides a more immediate picture of an inflammatory response. Normal values are 0–1 mg/dL, and levels >10 mg/dL are considered markedly elevated. Eighty percent of the time, such a high level is due to a bacterial infection. Mild elevations may be seen in obesity, hypertension, diabetes, and with tobacco use.

Rheumatoid Factor

Rheumatoid factor is an immunoglobulin, usually IgM (rarely also IgG or IgA), that is directed against the Fc portion of IgG molecules. Rheumatoid factor is nonspecific and, in addition to rheumatologic conditions, can be positive in subacute bacterial endocarditis (SBE), viral infections, and sarcoidosis. Eighty-five percent of those with RA will eventually become positive in the course of the disease, as will a fair number of Sjögren's syndrome and SLE patients.

Cyclic Citrullinated Peptides (CCP)

Testing for antibodies to CCP is a newer RA test that has lower sensitivity than rheumatoid factor, but high specificity for RA. Cyclic citrullinated peptides may be present in a third of

RA patients but up to 95% of patients who are CCP positive have RA. In addition, CCP may be present early in disease, even before clinical symptoms develop, and may help predict which patients may go on to develop RA. The presence of CCP is associated with a worse prognosis.

Antinuclear Antibody (ANA)

This general serologic test is used to detect autoantibodies to nuclear proteins. It is found in a multitude of rheumatic conditions. Antinuclear antibody has a high negative predictive value for SLE (if it is negative, the patient most likely does not have SLE). Laboratories differ on which titer is considered positive. In women, a titer of at least 1:160 is needed to be considered positive unless the history strongly suggests a connective tissue disease. Higher titers (>1:640) are more commonly seen in patients with SLE. The threshold is generally lower in men. Sometimes the fluorescent patterns of a positive ANA can suggest which specific antibody is present and direct further testing:

APPROACH TO COMMON PROBLEMS

General Approach to Joint Pain

The follow algorithm should be employed in any patient presenting with joint pain:

1. First, ascertain if the patient has true joint inflammation rather than joint pain without inflammation.
   - Arthritis is joint pain with inflammation, whereas arthralgia is joint pain without inflammation.
   - Signs of inflammation include warm, red, swollen, and painful joints.
   - Morning stiffness for >1 hour signifies an inflammatory condition, such as RA or SLE; stiffness for <1 hour is more common in osteoarthritis (OA).
   - "Gelling" is daytime stiffness after prolonged sitting or inactivity. It usually occurs for <30 minutes in OA and longer in RA.
2. Determine the number of joints involved (and modify the differential diagnosis accordingly).

   - A monoarthritis—consider trauma, infection (such as gonococcal infection in sexually active individuals or staphylococcal infections in IV drug users), or crystal deposition disease (commonly gout in the first metatarsolphalangeal [MTP] joint or pseudogout in the wrist or knee).
   - An oligoarthritis (two to four joints involved)—consider the seronegative spondyloarthropathies or crystalline disease.
   - A polyarthritis (more than four joints)—consider RA, SLE, or, rarely, polyarticular gout.
3. Determine which joint sites are involved.
   - The distal interphalangeals (DIPs) are involved—consider OA (common) or psoriatic arthritis.
   - The MCPs and wrists are involved—consider RA and SLE.
   - The first metatarsophalangeals are involved—consider gout, OA, and pseudogout (occasionally).
   - The knee alone—consider trauma, pseudogout, septic arthritis, OA, or gout.
4. Determine the pattern of joint involvement.
   - The axial skeleton is primarily involved—consider the seronegative spondyloarthropathies.
   - Peripheral joints are primarily involved—consider RA or SLE.
   - Symmetric joint involvement—consider RA or SLE.
   - Asymmetric joint involvement—consider psoriatic arthritis or reactive arthritis.
5. Decide if there is enthesopathy (inflammation of surrounding ligaments and tendons).
   - Enthesitis, which is inflammation of tendon insertions and can be seen in seronegative spondyloarthropathies.
   - Dactylitis, due to tendon sheath inflammation and appears as a "sausage-like" swelling of the digits.

The work-up of each of the following conditions is presented elsewhere in this chapter. Also, remember that most commonly, joint pain is not due to a rheumatologic condition but is the result of trauma or bursitis.

Approach to Knee Pain

Anatomy

See Figure 6-1 for the major ligaments and structures associated with the knee.

History

Be aware that hip problems can impact areas in and around the knee and vice versa. A history of intermittent locking while the knee is in extension indicates a loose ligament. Locking during flexion indicates a torn meniscus.

A feeling of the knee "buckling" or giving out during squatting indicates torn ligaments. Medial knee pain can be classic for medial compartment OA in the appropriate patient or indicates a medial meniscal tear. Patellofemoral syndrome, the most common cause of knee pain, is usually aggravated by descending stairs.

Exam

During gait, the knee should be extended only when the heel strikes the ground. At rest during standing, if one patella is higher than the other, there is asymmetry of muscle action.

When the knee is fully straightened, look for a swelling behind the knee in the popliteal fossa that may indicate a Baker's cyst—an abnormal communication with the bursa. Make sure to assess for effusions laterally and medially if they are not visible. Press firmly on the patella in patients who describe pain underneath. Also, assess surrounding soft tissue structures including the anserine bursa, which is just inferior to the medial joint line of the knee. Specific ligament tests are shown in Tables 6-2 and Figures 6-2 through 6-5.

To test passive and active range of motion:

- Extend the knee: 5° of hyperextension is normal. Painful active range-of-motion extension points to a quadraceps lesion. Weakness of extension suggests an L3 lesion. If flexion is painful, test the hip.

Flexion normally should occur such that the heel extends all the way to the buttock. Hyperflexion can be demonstrated by putting the hand in the popliteal fossa and flexing the knee.

The feel at the patient's end limit of passive range of motion is important. In arthritis, the resistance is very hard and in bursitis it is quite soft.

Table 6-2.   Specific Ligament Tests for the Knee

Structure	How to Test
Medial Collateral Ligament (MCL)	With the leg straight, push in against the lateral side of the knee with one hand while the other hand is holding the foot (valgus stress). Repeat at 30° of knee flexion. The knee should be stable and not give or cause pain. See Figure 6-2.
Lateral Collateral Ligament (LCL)	Same as above, but now push against the medial side of the knee away from the midline with one hand while the other is holding the foot (varus stress). See Figure 6-3.
Coronary Ligaments	These hold the menisci to the tibia. With the knee flexed, rotate the foot internally or externally. Medial (internal) foot rotation will strain the lateral coronary ligament. See Figure 6-4.
Anterior Cruciate Ligament (ACL) and Posterior Cruciate Ligament (PCL)	For the ACL, with the patient supine, the knee flexed at knee 90°, and the foot stabilized on the table, try to pull the tibia forward with a strong jerk. Normally, there should be only minimal outward movement of the tibia (*anterior drawer test*). One can repeat the test with the foot internally rotated (isolates the ACL). For the PCL, push the tibia posteriorly and observe the degree of backward movement (*posterior drawer test*). PCL tears are rare. See Figure 6-5.

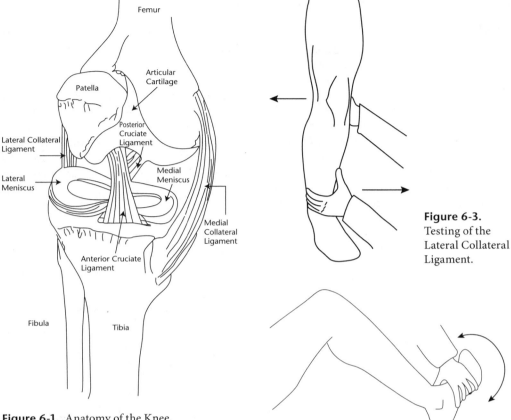

Figure 6-1. Anatomy of the Knee.

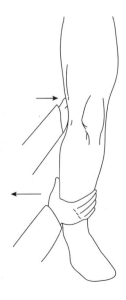

Figure 6-2. Testing of the Medial Collateral Ligament.

Figure 6-3. Testing of the Lateral Collateral Ligament.

Figure 6-4. Testing of the Coronary Ligaments.

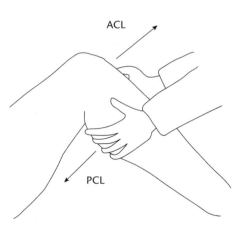

Figure 6-5. Testing of the Anterior and Posterior Cruciate Ligaments. ACL, anterior cruciate ligament; PCL, posterior cruciate ligament.

Approach to Shoulder Pain

Anatomy

See Figure 6-6 for the major ligaments and structures associated with the shoulder.

History

Rotator cuff tears present as limitations in shoulder function and pain with reaching, pushing, pulling, or lifting, especially with the arm above shoulder level. They typically occur with trauma such as falling onto an outstretched arm, repetitive subacromial impingement, direct blows to the shoulder, or rapid decelerating accidents.

When the joint capsule is involved, there is generally more significant limitation of lateral rotation. The normal shoulder can do 90° of abduction, 90° of medial rotation, and 90° of lateral rotation.

Exam

- Test abduction by holding the scapula with one hand and abducting the arm with the elbow flexed at 90°.
- Lateral rotation is tested with the elbow flexed at 90° and held in position against the patient's side. Pull the supinated wrist back away from the midline.

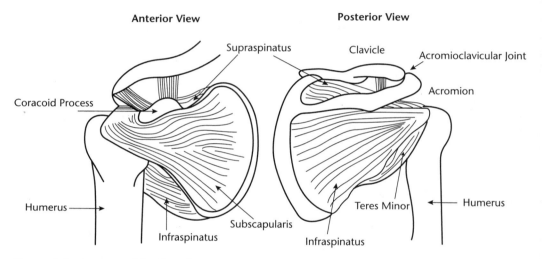

Figure 6-6. Anatomy of the Shoulder.

Table 6-3.   Testing Specific Rotator Cuff Muscles

Muscle	How to Test
Supraspinatus	Test resistance to abduction of the arm starting in midarc. If the elbow is bent, this is more of a test of the deltoid that is used in the initial movement of abduction. This is the muscle most commonly involved in rotator cuff tears. See Figure 6-7.
Subscapularis	With the elbow flexed at 90° and touching the flank, and with the forearm out to the side, see if there is resisted movement to moving the hand medially.
	The subscapularis is the rotator cuff muscle primarily responsible for internal rotation. Its strength can be assessed using the push-off, or Gerber's, test. This test is performed by having the patient place one hand behind the back and push posteriorly against resistance. See Figure 6-8.
Infraspinatus; Teres Minor	With the elbow at 90° and the palm of the hand on the abdomen, test resistance to external (outward) rotation. See Figure 6-9.
	The patient's arms are held at the sides, with the elbows flexed to 90°. The patient actively rotates externally against resistance. A positive test is indicated by weakness compared with the contralateral side and may be associated with infraspinatus or teres minor tendinopathy or tear. See Figure 6-9.

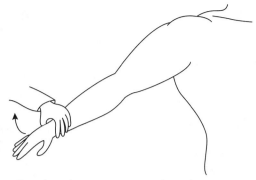

Have the patient move arm up against resistance

Figure 6-7. Testing of the Supraspinatus.

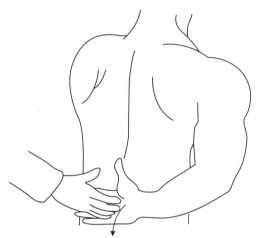

Have the patient push out against your hand

Figure 6-8. Testing of the Subscapularis.

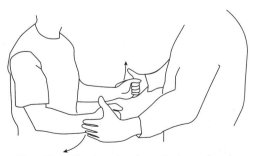

Have the patient push out against your hands

Figure 6-9. Testing of the Infraspinatus and Teres Minor.

- Internal rotation is tested with the elbow flexed at 90° and the arm behind the back. Starting with the hand in the small of the back, pull the hand back as far as possible and compare it with the other side. Specific rotator cuff muscle tests are shown in Table 6-3 and Figures 6-7 through 6-9.

Approach to Hip Pain

See Figure 6-10 for the major structures associated with the hip.

History

- When asked to point to the site of the pain, patients commonly indicate the area anteriorly at the groin, posteriorly at the buttock, or laterally.
  □ Lateral hip pain is usually not from the hip joint. If it is worse with direct pressure on the hip, this is a classic sign of trochanteric bursitis. If it is associated with paresthesia and hyperesthesia, this is a classic sign of lateral femoral cutaneous nerve entrapment (meralgia paresthetica) that is not influenced by direct pressure
  □ Anterior hip pain suggests involvement of the hip joint itself. If there is acute onset

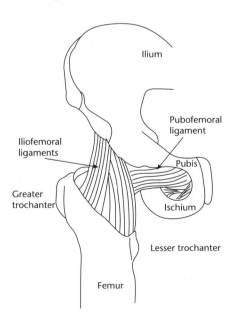

Figure 6-10. Anatomy of the Hip.

and worse with weight bearing, osteone-crosis, fracture, acute synovitis, or, less commonly, septic arthritis should be suspected. If it is not worse with pressure or flexion, an inguinal hernia may be present.

- ❑ Posterior hip pain is the least common and may be from sacroiliac joint disease, lumbar radiculopathy, zoster, or a rare presentation of a hip joint problem.

- Posterior hip pain may indicate greater trochanteric bursitis, which is a secondary condition to an underlying disorder that should be investigated. In some cases, a hip dislocation or displaced femoral neck fracture can be diagnosed just by inspection when the patient is supine. Posterior hip dislocation appears as a shortened limb that is internally rotated and adducted, whereas an anterior superior hip dislocation can present extended and externally rotated or inferior dislocations as flexed, abducted, and externally rotated.

Exam

Look at the gait. The foot on the affected side is sometimes in front of the other foot, and there is slight flexion and medial internal rotation of the affected side while the patient in standing. *Trendelenburg's sign* may also be present: when an asymptomatic person walks and stands unassisted on each leg in turn, the buttock of the weight-bearing leg should be lower since the other hip is lifted up to optimize the center of gravity for balance. If this is not the case, the test is positive for weakness in the hip girdle.

Range-of-Motion Tests

- With one knee at 90° flexion, check for hip flexion by asking the patient to place the knee of one leg on the chest. Stabilize the patient's pelvis and make sure that the other leg is straight by placing your other hand on that knee. During flexion, the contralateral knee begins to rise from the table when there is a limitation of hip flexion. Normally, a person can put the thigh on the trunk, but the last 45° of this movement is hip movement.

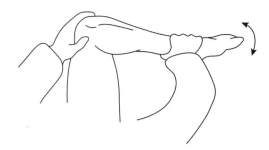

Figure 6-11. Hip Range-of-Motion Testing with the Knee Flexed.

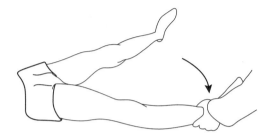

Figure 6-12. Hip Range-of-Motion Testing with the Knee Extended.

- Lateral and medial rotation of the hip is tested by flexing the knee to 90° and the hip to 90° and then moving the foot to and from the midline. Also, check abduction and adduction by moving the knee itself to and from the midline while the patient is in this position, as shown in Figure 6-11. Repeat with the knee extended, as shown in Figure 6-12. Normal hip abduction is about 45°.

- A subtle finding in arthritis is initial limitation in medial rotation of the hip, as seen by asymmetry between the right and left sides when the knees are flexed to 90° and the feet are pressed apart.

RHEUMATOLOGIC DISEASES AND SYNDROMES

Immune-Mediated Disorders

Rheumatoid Arthritis (RA)

D—An idiopathic, multisystem autoimmune disease characterized by chronic inflammation, proliferation, and hypertrophy of the synovial membrane lining peripheral joints. This leads to erosion of cartilage and bone, joint deformity, and dysfunction. A subset called *Felty's syndrome* is RA with splenomegaly and neutropenia.

Epi—As many as 1%–2% of adults are affected. Peak age at onset is 20–45 years. Female patients outnumber males by 3:1. A worse prognosis is associated with an increased number of joints affected, the presence of erosions, positive CCP, rheumatoid factor and rheumatoid nodules.

P—It appears to be due to autoimmune destruction of the joint space. What initiates this process is unclear, but immune-mediated vascular injury of the synovial lining occurs first, releasing many inflammatory mediators, such as tumor necrosis factor-α (TNF-α), IL-1, and IL-6. Synovial proliferation occurs with the accumulation of neutrophils and plasma cells that secrete rheumatoid factor. Complement activation also occurs, along with phagocytosis of collagen matrix and elastic tissues.

RF—Risk factors include a family history (30 times increase for monozygotic twins and 6 times increase for dizygotic twins) and human leukocyte antigen (HLA) DR4 and HLA-DR1 association (three to five times increased risk). In whites, these are markers for more severe RA.

SiSx

Articular manifestations

Rheumatoid arthritis commonly presents in 85% of patients as a symmetric synovitis of the MCP joints and proximal interphalangeal (PIP) joints and almost never of the DIP joints. Classically, patients have morning stiffness for >1 hour that subsides with activity. Associated fatigue, weight loss, fever, and subcutaneous nodules can occur, usually on bony prominences. Ulnar drift from tendon laxity and subluxation of the proximal phalanges may also be seen. Common deformities include the *swan neck deformity* and the *Boutonniere deformity* (see Figure 6-13). Rheumatoid

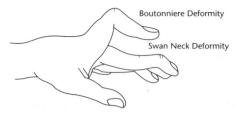

Figure 6-13. Hand Deformities in Rheumatoid Arthritis.

arthritis spares the thoracolumbar and sacroiliac joints. Cervical involvement can present paresthesias that radiate into the occiput or scalp. More severe involvement leading to atlantoaxial subluxation can cause cervical spinal cord compression leading to weakness of the limbs or sudden ataxia. Synovitis of knees can cause the formation of fluid-filled cysts (Baker's cysts) posteriorly in the popliteal space, with rupture causing thrombophlebitis.

Extra-articular manifestations—seen predominantly in patients with positive rheumatoid factor and longstanding erosive disease.

Cardiopulmonary—Exudative rheumatoid pleural and pericardial effusions (with characteristically low glucose), pleuritis, or pericarditis can be seen.

Eyes—Keratoconjunctivitis sicca or secondary Sjögren's syndrome, scleritis (RA is the most common systemic illness causing this condition), or episcleritis is seen.

Vascular—Small vessel vasculitis can be seen but is rare.

Neurologic—In rare cases, one may see mononeuritis multiplex, carpal tunnel syndrome, and mild peripheral sensory neuropathy.

Hematologic—Anemia develops with chronic disease; prolonged RA can lead to secondary amyloidosis.

Renal—Suspect secondary amyloidosis in any long-standing RA patient who presents with new proteinuria.

Other—Rheumatoid nodules (in 20–25% of patients) may be seen in areas of extensive trauma, such as the extensor surfaces, but may also be found in the lungs, heart, kidney, and dura mater.

Dx—The diagnosis is made if the patient meets at least four out of seven criteria (morning stiffness for >1 hour, three or more joint areas involved, hand arthritis, symmetry, nodules, positive rheumatoid factor, X-ray changes).[*]

The patient must also have had the peripheral polyarthritis for at least 6 weeks to make the clinical diagnosis. Rheumatoid factor is positive in 80% of cases but is not specific. Cyclic citrullinated peptide is present in one-third of RA patients, but as many as 95% of patients who are CCP positive have RA. Antinuclear antibody is positive in 15% of patients. On X-ray, one can see periarticular swelling, juxta-articular osteopenia, uniform joint space loss, or subluxations. Synovial fluid usually has >2000 WBCs, with polymorphonuclear leukocytes (PMNs) predominating.

Tx—Treatment includes several classes of drugs:

- Analgesics (acetaminophen, tramadol, capsaicin cream applied over joints and narcotics).
- NSAIDs—these are both analgesic and anti-inflammatory, but they do not alter the outcome of disease.
- Steroids—can be given orally, IV, or by intra-articular injection.
- DMARDs (disease-modifying antirheumatic drugs), which include methotrexate, leflunomide (Arava), azathioprine (Imuran), sulfasalazine, and hydroxychloroquine. Newer biologic DMARD therapies include (1) the TNF inhibitors: infliximab (Remicade), etanercept (Enbrel), adalimumab (Humira), and the IL-1 receptor antagonist anakinra (Kineret); (2) the B-cell depleter rituximab (Rituxan); and (3) the T-cell costimulatory blocker abatacept (Orencia).

---

[*] FC Arnett, SM Edworthy and DA Bloch, The American Rheumatism Association 1987 revised criteria for the classification of rheumatoid arthritis, Arthritis and Rheumatism 31 (1988), pp. 315–324.

Given the use of medications that can hamper the immune system, these patients are at risk for severe systemic infections. Overall in RA, one-third of patients will have destructive disease that is inadequately responsive to therapy, one-third will have an excellent response, and one-third will have an adequate response but will often need to take multiple drugs. Surgical arthroplasty or joint replacement is reserved for those who fail medical management, though it may not always improve function.

Juvenile Idiopathic Arthritis (JIA)

D—A chronic inflammatory arthritis that begins before 18 years of age. The lesions cannot be distinguished histologically from those of adult RA. This condition was formerly known as *juvenile rheumatoid arthritis* (JRA).

Epi—This is a rare condition with an incidence of 0.01% or lower. There are three different types: (1) Systemic onset JIA, also known as *Still's disease* (occurs in 10–20% of patients), is characterized by multiple extra-articular manifestations. The peak incidence is at 16–35 years of age. (2) Polyarticular arthritis (affecting 30–40% of patients) involves five or more joints. Systemic features do not predominate. (3) Pauciarticular arthritis (affecting 50% of patients) involves four or fewer joints. In all three forms of the disease, female patients outnumber males.

SiSx

1. Still's disease: There is a sore throat and sudden onset of high, spiking fever accompanied by a transitory, nonpruritic, erythematous, salmon-colored rash, which occurs mostly at night. Arthritis involves the PIPs, MCPs, wrists, knees, hips, and shoulders. Pericarditis is the most feared complication. In general, patients look quite ill and have weight loss and fatigue in addition to constitutional symptoms. Hepatosplenomegaly can be seen.

2. Polyarticular arthritis: The presentation is similar to that of RA. Individuals who are rheumatoid factor positive present

later in childhood. Those with rheumatoid factor positivity can and may have subcutaneous nodules, as in adult-onset RA.

3. Pauciarticular arthritis: Anterior uveitis (in 20%–40% of patients) may potentially lead to blindness and is unrelated to arthritis activity; it may be asymptomatic. Those with positive ANA are at the highest risk for this development. Axial skeleton oligoarthritis affecting mostly the sacroiliac joints in boys may be seen. Girls may initially present at any age with an oligoarthritis with prominent dactylitis and occasionally psoriasis as well.

Dx
1. Still's disease—a diagnosis of exclusion. Arthritis should be present in one or more joints for >6 weeks. In addition to the physical findings, one sees a very high ESR, anemia of chronic disease with microcytosis, and rare positive ANA or rheumatoid factor. Very elevated ferritin levels (usually in the 10,000 ng/mL range) can be highly suggestive of Still's disease in the right setting.
2. Polyarticular arthritis—a clinical diagnosis; rheumatoid factor and ANA are positive in only 20–40% of patients.
3. Pauciarticular arthritis—has few if any hematologic findings. Antinuclear antibody is positive in 60%, which indicates a higher risk of uveitis.

Tx—Still's disease—its course is one of disease-free intervals punctuated by flare-ups. A polyarticular arthritis is noticeable in the first 6 months. Fifty percent of patients recover completely with treatment.

Polyarticular and pauciarticular arthritis—treatment is the same as for RA, including the use of various cytotoxic medications. Other NSAIDs may be administered. Overall, 50%–75% of patients recover by adulthood; 10% develop severe functional abnormalities. All patients should be screened by an ophthalmologist given the consequences of uveitis. Intra-articular injections are important to help prevent premature closure of endplates.

Systemic Lupus Erythematosus (SLE)

D—A multisystem autoimmune disease of unknown etiology that may affect any and every organ system in the body. It is characterized by the production of autoantibodies. There are several variants. Drug-induced lupus, for instance, resolves when the medication is discontinued. Limited cutaneous forms do not have systemic involvement.

Epi—The incidence is 1/2000. The prevalence is 1 million in the United States. More than 80% of patients are young women. Most are between 14 and 45 years of age.

P—Genetic, environmental, and female hormonal factors are implicated in the development of autoantibodies, but there is no clearly understood cause. Damage is primarily due to antibodies by four mechanisms: (1) normal cells are removed by the reticuloendothelial system, (2) antibodies trigger immune complex formation with complement fixation that causes organ damage, (3) antibodies act directly against tissues to which they are directed, and (4) certain antibodies are thrombogenic and thereby cause organ damage.

RF—Risk factors include sun exposure and a family history, as there is a 1/40 chance of disease passing from mother to daughter and a 1/250 chance of its passing from mother to son. HLA-DR2 and HLA-DR3 are involved. African American race is also a risk factor (four times as many African Americans as whites are affected).

SiSx—
The presentation may vary from multiorgan to single-organ involvement, and the condition may be acute or chronic.
Cardiovascular/pulmonary—serositis of some kind (pleuritis, pleural effusions, and pericarditis) is seen in 50%.
GI—oral or nasal ulcers, GI vasculitis.
Joints—nonerosive, symmetrical polyarticular inflammatory arthritis that usually affects the small joints of the hands and feet.
Dermatologic:
Classically, a malar or butterfly rash on the face is a systemic sign of lupus in one-

third of patients. It rarely crosses the nasolabial folds but may affect the chin and forehead. Photosensitivity is quite common, resulting in a skin rash in sun-exposed areas.

Discoid lupus is associated with symmetric, well-circumscribed, erythematous patches on the neck, shoulders, back, and chest. They often scar, leaving behind hyper- and hypopigmented areas.

Subacute cutaneous lupus erythematosus produces extremely photosensitive annular lesions and few systemic features otherwise (usually Ro positive as well).

Other general skin findings include alopecia, Raynaud's phenomenon, livedo reticularis (a lace-like network of red and white discoloration on the skin), and signs of vasculitis (i.e., palpable purpura).

Neurologic—peripheral neuropathy, organic brain syndrome (a generalized decrease in mental functioning), CNS vasculitis, psychosis, and seizures.

Cardiovascular—pericarditis, Libmann-Sacks endocarditis. Coronary disease can also be seen, both as part of the disease and as a result of treatment.

Hematologic—hemolytic anemia, leukopenia, (usually lymphopenia) or thrombocytopenia, and possibly antiphospholipid syndrome with resulting thromboses.

Renal—many manifestations ranging from GN to nephrotic syndrome and ESRD. (See Chapter 4.)

Constitutional symptoms—fevers, weight loss, lymphadenopathy.

Other—Some have the sicca syndrome. *Neonatal lupus* is seen in infants of mothers with lupus. The entity is associated with congenital heart block due to maternal anti SS-A (Ro) antibodies. Transient rashes, thrombocytopenia, and hemolytic anemia are also characteristic.

Dx—The diagnosis is made when an individual meets 4 out of 11 of the criteria shown in Table 6-4. Antinuclear antibody is positive 95% of the time, and a negative test makes the diagnosis of SLE unlikely. Those who are

Table 6-4. American College of Rheumatology Criteria for Systemic Lupus Erythematosus

1. Malar rash
2. Discoid rash
3. Photosensitivity
4. Mouth ulcers
5. Arthritis
6. Serositis
7. Renal disease
8. Neurologic disease
9. Hematologic disorder
10. Immunologic abnormality (anti-dsDNA, anti-Sm, and/or antiphospholipid antibody)
11. Positive ANA

ANA negative, however, may have positive anti SS-A (Ro) or SS-B (La) antibodies. Anti-dsDNA and anti-Sm are the most specific antibodies for SLE, and the combination of hypocomplementemia and a positive anti-dsDNA is pathognomonic. Those with drug induced lupus have antibodies to histones, not to dsDNA or Sm, and seldom have hematologic abnormalities. Medications that can cause drug induced lupus include procainamide, hydralazine, isoniazid, methyldopa, quinidine, and chlorpromazine.

Tx—Sunscreens and avoidance of sun exposure can help avoid certain skin manifestations. In mild disease, hydroxychloroquine (Plaquenil) has been shown to prevent flares and is used in virtually all patients, including those with mild disease. Anti-inflammatory agents such as NSAIDs are also used for mild disease. For patients who are unresponsive to hydroxychloroquine or for those with visceral involvement, steroids are used along with a combination of other immunosuppressants such as methotrexate, azathioprine, mycophenolate mofetil, and cyclophosphamide. Rituximab, a B-cell depleter, is used in certain circumstances. Otherwise, treatment of complications both from the disease and from therapy is necessary. Overall, 10-year survival is 90%. Death is commonly due to infectious complications of immunosuppressive therapy, renal disease, and cardiovascular complications.

Table 6-5. Distinguishing Characteristics of Primary and Secondary Raynaud's Phenomenon

Primary Raynaud's	Secondary Raynaud's
Symmetric	Asymmetric
Frequent attacks	Infrequent attacks
No evidence of peripheral vascular disease	Ischemic signs or symptoms, digital ulceration
No tissue gangrene, digital pitting, tissue injury	Signs of a connective tissue disease (e.g. scleroderma,
Negative ANA and normal ESR	lupus)
Negative nailfold capillary exam	Positive nailfold capillary exam
More common in females, mostly with onset at menarche	More common over age 40; affects males and females alike

Raynaud's Phenomenon

D—A vasospastic disorder of small arterioles of the hands, toes, ears, and other body appendages. It can be primary or secondary if associated with a connective tissue disease.

Epi—Up to 5–10% of normal nonsmokers may have this condition. It is seen mostly in women.

RF—There is a higher incidence in patients with connective tissue diseases such as scleroderma and lupus and in smokers who develop Buerger's disease (see below). The condition is triggered by cold, stress, and drugs.

SiSx—There are three stages of vessel vasospasm that occurs most commonly in the fingers and toes:

1. Pallor stage—spasm decreases blood flow and results in numbness, paresthesias, and white-colored skin.
2. Cutaneous cyanosis—deoxygenated blood in the capillary bed causes blue discoloration of the skin.
3. Hyperemic phase—reopening of digital arteries causes blushing of the skin and a red color.

Complications include digital ulceration. Edema, periungual erythema, and livedo reticularis (lace-like network of red and white colors from changes in superficial circulation) may also be seen.

Dx—Diagnosis is made by the clinical exam and the history. If it is not associated with a connective tissue disease by other features, a positive ANA may suggest the development of a connective tissue disease in the future. A nailfold capillary exam with an ophthalmoscope can be helpful; blunting and enlargement of capillary loops suggest a connective tissue disease. Table 6-5 shows some features that distinguish primary from secondary Raynaud's phenomenon.

Tx—For primary Raynaud's phenomenon, avoid triggers such as cold weather or wear gloves. Ca^{2+} channel blockers, α blockers, and prostaglandin inhibitors may be administered. Avoid β blockers, which can make this condition worse (the mechanism is not entirely clear). Sildenafil can also be used in select cases. For secondary Raynaud's phenomenon, treat the underlying condition if found. Smoking cessation should also be advised.

Mixed Connective Tissue Disease (MCTD)

D—A rheumatic syndrome in which there is a high titer of anti-U_1RNP antibodies and a combination of clinical features from several connective tissue diseases such as scleroderma, SLE, and polymyositis.

Epi—It is seen in both children and the elderly worldwide and in all races. Female patients outnumber males by 16:1.

RF—Exposure to vinyl chloride and silica may be associated.

SiSx—Early symptoms are nonspecific, and it is unusual to see overlapping features of multiple connective tissue diseases at this time. However, almost any organ system can be involved, though several features may distinguish MCTD: usually there is absence of severe CNS or renal disease; in general, arthritis is more severe; and onset of insidious pulmonary hypertension is more common. Otherwise, Raynaud's phenomenon is the most common skin finding and may occur with hand edema with swollen digits. Myositis is the most common overlap feature with polymyositis, and is histologically identical. Esophageal dysmotility is the most common overlap feature with scleroderma and can be seen in up to 70% of patients. Finally, up to 25% of patients have CNS involvement. While 25% develop renal disease, diffuse nephritis is unusual and overall renal disease tends to be milder. Renal crisis, as in scleroderma, however, has been reported in some patients.

Dx—High titers of anti U$_1$-RNP antibody and features of multiple connective tissue diseases, which together are not sufficient to place the patient into a single disease category, make the diagnosis. Anemia of chronic disease is seen in the majority. Patients may have a positive Coombs' test but not necessarily hemolytic anemia. Hypergammaglobulinemia and positive rheumatoid factor are seen in 50%. Two-thirds of patients have clinically asymptomatic pulmonary involvement, as evidenced by decreased D$_L$CO (a measure of lung-diffusing capacity).

Tx—The majority of patients will have diagnostic criteria for one of the connective tissue diseases within 5 years. Until then, symptomatic treatment with anti-inflammatory or cytotoxic agents is given, depending on the severity of myositis, pulmonary disease, or vasculitis. The 10-year survival is 80%. Complications from pulmonary hypertension are the most common cause of death.

Diffuse and Limited Systemic Sclerosis (Scleroderma)

D—A disorder of connective tissue characterized by overproduction of collagen and matrix proteinases leading to small vessel obliteration and fibrosis of the skin and various internal organs. The limited form, so-called CREST, stands for calcinosis, Raynaud's phenomenon, esophageal dysmotility, sclerodactyly, and telangiectasia; it does not include involvement of internal organs except for the GI tract and lungs (pulmonary hypertension). Scleroderma may also exist in overlap forms, the most common of which is MCTD.

Epi—Female patients outnumber males by 3:1. There is a worldwide distribution, with all races affected. It is unusual in the young. The incidence is 75/100,000, and the peak incidence occurs at 30–50 years of age. The disorder is more severe in young black women.

P—The etiology is unclear, but generally, the process is one of vascular endothelial damage and fibrosis with intimal hyperplasia of small vessels and luminal narrowing, which leads to tissue ischemia.

RF—Coal miners are thought to be at higher risk.

SiSx

Skin—There is progressive thickening leading to decreased range of motion with different distributions in limited and diffuse forms (see Table 6-6). Raynaud's phenomenon occurs in 95% of patients. Subcutaneous calcifications and salt and pepper hyper/hypopigmentation of the skin can be seen. Microcapillary abnormalities, especially at the distal nail bed, where proliferation with dilatation and tortuosity of vessels are apparent under magnification, may be found. Skin ulcers may occur after infarction. Limited cutaneous forms, namely, *morphea* and *linear* scleroderma, exist.

Renal—Ten percent have renal crisis from malignant arterial hypertension with rapid kidney failure if not treated. (See Chapter 4.)

GI—GERD, esophageal dysmotility (75%), watermelon stomach (venous ectasia in the stomach can lead to a GI bleed), diminished peristalsis leading to bacterial overgrowth, malabsorption, large bowel involvement leading to "wide mouth diverticuli" and constipation.

Cardiopulmonary—Interstitial fibrosis and isolated pulmonary hypertension; cardiomyopathy.

Table 6-6. Summary of the Differences Between the Two Types of Scleroderma

Diffuse Scleroderma	Limited Scleroderma (CREST)
Skin involvement includes both proximal and distal extremities, trunk, and face.	Skin involvement usually includes just the distal extremities up to the elbows and the face.
Raynaud's phenomenon is seen within a year before skin changes.	Raynaud's phenomenon may precede skin disease by years.
Other systems involved are pulmonary, renal, cardiac, and GI.	Other systems involved are GI and pulmonary (especially pulmonary hypertension). Only <10% of patients have biliary cirrhosis.
ANA positive: nucleolar pattern. Anti SCL-70 positive (in 40%).	ANA positive: centromeric pattern.

Musculoskeletal—An inflammatory myopathy may occur and overlap with polymyositis. Fifty percent of patients develop joint and tendon swelling.

Dx—The diagnosis is based on the clinical and serologic findings. Antibodies help distinguish subsets of the disease. Ninety percent of patients are ANA positive. Finding ANAs in scleroderma is one of the few times when the pattern is helpful. Antinuclear antibodies in a *nucleolar* pattern are suggestive of systemic sclerosis, and ANAs in a *centromere* pattern are suggestive of CREST. Forty percent of those with the diffuse cutaneous form are anti-Scl-70 (an antibody against topoisomerase I) positive. The differences are highlighted in Table 6-6.

Tx—There is no real cure. Supportive care along with an ACE inhibitor to control hypertension may be helpful. This medication can be life saving in scleroderma renal crisis. Calcium channel blockers or other agents can be given for Raynaud's phenomenon. The pulmonary hypertension in this population is extremely difficult to treat, as it is refractory to vasodilatory therapy. Cytotoxic therapies (cyclophosphamide) may be beneficial in certain patients with interstitial lung disease. Drugs like steroids, methotrexate, and azathioprine can be used to treat arthritis and myositis. There is no good therapy for the skin condition, unfortunately. For GI symptoms, antibiotic are given for bacterial overgrowth and proton pump inhibitors (PPIs) for GERD. Promotility agents are used in certain circumstances.

Sjögren's Syndrome

D—A chronic, progressive autoimmune disease characterized by invasion of exocrine glands by lymphocytes and plasma cells with or without systemic involvement. The primary form (sicca syndrome) has a strong HLA-DR3 association with a broad attack on exocrine glands. Secondary Sjörgren's syndrome occurs in the setting of another rheumatic disease—mostly RA, SLE, and scleroderma—and has an increased association with HLA-DR4.

Epi—It is the second most commonly recognized autoimmune disorder after RA. It occurs at any age but mainly >50 years. Female patients outnumber males by 9:1. Patients have up to a 44 fold increased incidence of non-Hodgkin's lymphoma.

SiSx

1. Glandular symptoms—dryness and eventual ulceration of the eyes (keratoconjunctivitis) and mouth (xerostomia) from decreased lacrimal and salivary gland function, with or without concomitant lacrimal or salivary gland enlargement. There is a foreign body sensation in the eyes. Tooth decay may result from loss of protective saliva. Swallowing and talking are difficult due to dry mouth. Firm, nontender, bilaterally symmetric enlarged parotids are found in 67% of patients (only in primary Sjögren's syndrome), which are not painful.

2. Extraglandular symptoms—fatigue, malaise, myalgia, polyarthritis, lung involvement (primary Sjögren's syndrome may involve the entire respiratory tree), and peripheral neuropathy. Lymphadenopathy

may be seen and should be taken seriously, as lymphoma is seen in as many as 10%; these patients are at 40-fold increased risk.

Dx—A history of xerophthalmia (dry eyes), xerostomia (dry mouth), and large parotid glands, along with serologic evidence, makes the diagnosis. One should find positive ANA and positive anti SS-A (anti-Ro) in 70% positive anti SS-B (anti-La) in 40% of patients. Schirmer's test may be performed (filter paper in the eyes showing <5 mm tear wicking in 5 minutes) to confirm the presence of xerophthalmia. Rose Bengal staining of the eye may show keratitis. Salivary gland biopsy will show foci of mononuclear cells, and lip biopsy may show classic CD4 cell infiltration and destruction of minor salivary glands. Consider other associated autoimmune diseases as a primary cause. A sudden loss of autoantibodies may portend malignancy, commonly B-cell non-Hodgkin's lymphoma but also Waldenström's macroglobulinemia.

Tx—Symptomatic treatment first includes avoiding conditions and drugs (such as anticholinergics) that exacerbate the dryness of mucous membranes. Artificial tears and saliva benefit some patients. Parasympathetic agonists like pilocarpine and cevimeline can help the sicca symptoms. Cyclosporine eye drops may help decrease eye inflammation. Arthritis is one of the more common manifestations, and drugs similar to those used in lupus can be employed. For severe disease or in the presence of concomitant vasculitis, steroids and cytotoxic agents are used.

Inflammatory Myopathies

Polymyositis and Dermatomyositis

D—Idiopathic inflammatory muscle disease associated with prominent proximal muscle weakness.

Epi—This is a rare disease with an incidence of 1/100,000, peaking during childhood and late adulthood. Female patients outnumber males by 2:1. Dermatomyositis is much more common than polymyositis in children. Furthermore, patients with dermatomyositis have an increased incidence of various malignancies (i.e., ovarian, breast, and colon cancer as well as melanoma).

P—The condition is idiopathic, though it is thought to be related to viral infection. Inflammatory infiltrates are seen in muscle fibers, which appear shoddy from necrosis and degeneration. $CD8^+$ cells predominate in polymyositis.

SiSx

Skin—Findings are most prominent in dermatomyositis. There are erythematous patches over the face, neck, and upper chest in addition to extensor surfaces. Pathognomonic findings are heliotrope lids (violet discoloration and swelling of the eyelids); *Gottron's sign* (heaped-up, erythematous papules over the MCP or PIPs); "mechanic's hands" (roughened, erythematous skin and hypertrophic changes of the palms and fingers); the *V sign* of erythema over the anterior chest; and the *shawl sign* of erythema over the neck and upper back. Most of these signs do not occur in polymyositis.

Lung—Dyspnea on exertion (DOE) from chronic interstitial lung disease (ILD), especially with positive antisynthetase antibodies can be seen.

Joints—Mild arthritis occurs uncommonly and is rarely destructive. Eighty percent of patients with this symptom have the Jo-1 antisynthetase antibody.

Neuromuscular—most patients have slowly progressive muscle failure. Others have a fulminant progression with respiratory failure and myoglobinuric renal failure. Generally, the pattern of muscle weakness is symmetric in the proximal upper and lower extremities. Patients have difficulty rising from chairs, sitting in beds, or combing their hair. Pharyngeal muscle involvement may lead to swallowing difficulties and dysphagia, resulting in the risk of aspiration pneumonia. Cardiac muscle involvement is uncommon. Only in late stages are fine motor controls affected. Patients may have difficulty holding up their head (neck drop). The diaphragm may also be affected. The weakness progresses over weeks to months.

Oncologic—Visceral malignancy is seen in 10–25% of dermatomyositis sufferers, especially in elderly individuals with late-onset myopathy.

Dx—In addition to the aforementioned history and clinical symptoms, one should see an elevation in CK and aldolase. Frequently AST and ALT are elevated in these patients; this is usually indicative of muscle damage rather than liver injury. Serum myoglobin is also elevated in most patients. From 80% to 90% of patients have nuclear autoantibodies of some sort. If ANA is positive (>50%), it is usually of the speckled pattern. Antibodies not exclusive to polymyositis and dermatomyositis are Ro, La, ScL-70, and Ku. Exclusive antibodies are (1) antisynthetase, of which anti Jo-1 (directed against the histidyl tRNA synthetase) is the most specific but is seen in only 20% of cases; (2) anti-SRP (signal recognition particle) antibody; and (3) anti-Mi-2 antibody. Electromyography (EMG), along with muscle biopsy, helps to make the diagnosis. Electromyography of one side (i.e., the right arm and leg) is done, followed by biopsy of the contralateral side (i.e., the left quad) to avoid errors in biopy from the needle damage used in the EMG test. Magnetic resonance imaging (MRI) has now emerged as a helpful tool, since muscle inflammation can be seen as muscle edema and can help guide subsequent muscle biopsy. Muscle biopsy is important to help exclude inclusion body myositis. Work-up for occult malignancy should be done, including chest, abdomen, and pelvis CT scans for malignancy, especially in patients over 50 years of age.

Tx—Anti-Scl antibody patients are less responsive to treatment and tend to have more cardiac involvement. The anti-Jo-1 and anti-Mi-2 subsets tend to have better responses to treatment. In those with malignancy, removal of the tumor generally resolves the muscle disease, but the prognosis for such patients is generally poor. Large doses of steroids with other immunosuppressives as tolerated seem to be effective in controlling the disease in a majority of patients. Steroid-sparing agents such as mycophenolate mofetil (Cellcept), azathioprine (Imuran), and methotrexate are very important to help limit steroid exposure, as prolonged exposure can lead to steroid myopathy, thus confusing the picture. Intravenous immunoglobulin (IVIG) may be beneficial for steroid-resistant patients, but plasmapheresis, in general, is not. Hydroxychloroquine may help the rash of dermatomyositis. Physical therapy may ameliorate muscle weakness somewhat.

Inclusion Body Myositis

D—A subset of inflammatory myopathies that differs from dermatomyositis and polymyositis in that both distal and proximal muscle groups become weak.

Epi—Older males are more likely to be affected. It is the most common inflammatory myopathy in patients >50 years of age.

P—Cellular autoimmunity is implicated in which CD8+ cytotoxic T cells are directed against muscle fibers.

SiSx—Unlike other inflammatory myopathies, muscle weakness occurs in distal as well as proximal groups, especially foot extensors and deep finger flexors. Symmetry of weakness is almost the rule and is seen in 90% of cases. Falling is common because of early quadraceps involvement. Fine motor skills such as those required in knitting and writing are affected early on. Ocular muscles are always spared, so one should consider other diseases, such as mysathenia gravis, if these muscles are involved. Facial muscles may be affected. Dysphagia is seen in 60% of patients.

Dx—Creatine kinase elevation and characteristic myopathic changes are seen on EMGs. There is a typical absence of reactive autoantibodies. Muscle biopsy shows vacuolar changes under light microscopy (LM) and other characteristic abnormalities on electron microscopy (EM). Usually the diagnosis is made in retrospect after a patient with polymyositis does not respond to treatment.

Tx—The response to immunosuppressive therapy, as used in other inflammatory myopathies, is typically poor. However, the survival rate is generally high because of slow progression of the disease.

The Vasculitides

These diseases are defined by inflammatory conditions of blood vessels. All involve necrosis and inflammation of the vessel walls and can exist as a primary disease or as the secondary manifestations of infections, malignancies, or connective tissue diseases. They may affect arteries, veins, and even capillaries, and many patients have systemic or multiorgan involvement. They are primarily categorized by the sizes of the vessels affected, as shown in Table 6-7.

Small Vessel Vasculitis

Mixed Essential Cryoglobulinemia

D—Disorder in which there is deposition of immunoglobulins, which reversibly precipitate at cold temperatures. The result is vaso-occlusive and inflammatory injury of the vessels. There are three types of cryoglobulins. Vessel injury occurs most commonly in type II. Cryoglobulins may be found in otherwise healthy individuals with no disease.

Epi—The incidence is 1/100,000, and the mean age of occurrence is 40–50 years. Female patients outnumber males by 3:2. The frequency of type I is 25%; type II, 25%; type III, 50%.

P—

Type I is due to a specific monoclonal IgG in high concentration. A hyperviscosity syndrome may develop, which may lead to gangrene in extremities where blood pools. It is associated with multiple myeloma, Waldenström's macroglobulinemia, and lymphoproliferative disorders. The IgG does not activate complement efficiently, so destruction of tissues is not as substantial as in type II and III.

Type II is due to both a monoclonal IgM and polyclonal IgG, which bind the Fc site of other immunoglobulins. Thus, they are considered to be rheumatoid factors. They activate complement efficiently, cause the formation of immune complexes, and can result in vessel necrosis. Their formation may be primary or secondary to chronic infections such as HCV, autoimmune disorder, or lymphoma.

Type III is due to polyclonal IgM and polyclonal IgG. These are also rheumatoid factors but they do not occur in high enough concentration to cause necrosis. Their formation is correlated with hepatitis C virus (HCV) infection.

SiSx

Type I—often asymptomatic but may present with headaches, nosebleeds, and visual changes—all of which are related to hyperviscosity.

Type II—typically present as a nonsystemic small vessel vasculitis with palpable

Table 6-7. Classification of the Vasculitides

Small Vessel Vasculitis	Medium Vessel Vasculitis	Large Vessel Vasculitis

• The hypersensitivity vasculitides (also called leukocytoclastic or cutaneous vasculitides)
  • Mixed essential cryoglobulinemia
  • Henoch-Shönlein purpura
  • Serum sickness
  • Urticarial vasculitis
• Wegener's granulomatosis
• Churg-Strauss syndrome or allergic angiitis
• Microscopic polyangiitis
• Connective tissue disease–related vasculitis
	• Polyarteritis nodosa (PAN) (also has some small vessel involvement)
	• Isolated CNS vasculitis
	• Kawasaki's disease or mucocutaneous lymph node syndrome
		• Giant cell (temporal) arteritis
		• Takayasu's arteritis (also called aortic arch syndrome)
		• Behçet's syndrome

purpura, urticaria, and cutaneous ulcerations. Patients will have findings consistent with hepatosplenomegaly, pneumonitis, pulmonary hemorrhage, GN, serositis, and thyroiditis. Arthralgia, arthritis, and peripheral neuropathy are common.

Type III—symptoms of arthralgia and arthritis in 70% of patients. Polyneuropathy occurs in the majority. Palpable purpura may be seen. Renal manifestations of GN are seen in 30% of patients, with 15% progressing to ESRD. Cardiovascular compromise may also be seen.

Dx—For cryoglobulin testing, it is important to draw blood into a heated syringe, which must be kept warm until it is transferred to a cryotube. In type I, IgG is usually found in high concentration (1–5 g/dL). In type II, monoclonal IgM and polyclonal IgG are present. They precipitate more slowly (may take up to 3 days) and are found in smaller quantities (50–500 mg/dL). Complement levels are usually low as well. Polyclonal IgG and IgM are found in type III. Tests for associated HCV should also be positive. Usually one considers these diseases in the differential diagnosis of an individual presenting with palpable purpura, hyperviscosity syndrome, or other signs of small vessel vasculitis. When one orders tests for cryoglobulins, rheumatoid factor should also be included in case cryoglobulin levels are borderline high.

Tx—Asymptomatic cryoglobulinemia does not require treatment. Nonsteroidal anti-inflammatory drugs may be administered to patients with symptoms limited to arthralgias. Immunosuppressive agents such as steroids, azathioprine, or cyclophosphamide should be used in those with significant organ involvement such as renal, CNS, or skin vasculitis. Antiviral therapy with IFN-α for treatment of HCV is used in all patients with symptomatic type II cryoglobulins who are HCV positive. Those with severe disease (such as renal involvement or neuropathy) generally start antiviral therapy after immunosuppressive treatment. Plasmapheresis may be beneficial in select patients with the type I and type II forms.

Henoch-Schönlein Purpura

D—A systemic small vessel vasculitis generally seen in children, usually after an upper respiratory infection (URI).

Epi—It occurs primarily in children, though it is seen occasionally in adults. Peak incidence is between 5 and 15 years of age.

P—It is characterized by IgA immune complex deposition and therefore, perhaps, has the same pathogenesis as IgA nephropathy. Because it commonly follows a URI, the initiating factor is thought to be infectious.

SiSx—Palpable purpura is found on the buttocks and legs in a symmetric pattern. Renal involvement presents as proteinuria or hematuria and is more likely to occur if the skin lesions encompass the abdomen as well. Crampy umbilical pain is reported. Polyarticular arthralgias and arthritis are found in the knees and ankles. A GI bleed may also occur if there is mesenteric involvement. The disease may be more severe in adults than in children.

Dx—Diagnosis is made by the biopsy if the classic symptoms of purpura, hematuria, arthralgias, and abdominal pain are all present. Biopsy of skin, kidney, or vascular lesions demonstrates distinctive IgA deposition on immunofluorescence staining.

Tx—Most cases resolve spontaneously over days to weeks. If renal or GI involvement is severe, steroid administration is indicated.

Serum Sickness

D—A small vessel cutaneous immune complex vasculitis that often follows a drug reaction or foreign protein exposure after 7–10 days.

Epi—The incidence is decreasing since foreign antigens are less commonly used in medicine.

P—The antigen or hapten causes an antibody response to develop. Subsequently, immune complexes form and are deposited in vessels. The complement cascade is activated and inflammatory cells secreting proinflammatory cytokines are recruited, causing a leukocytoclastic vasculitis.

RF—Administration of a new drug or foreign protein, such as anti-lymphocyte globulin or tetanus antitoxin, is a risk factor.

SiSx—Symptoms include headache, fever, myalgias, and GI upset including nausea and vomiting. Rash or urticaria, purpura, and arthritis or arthralgias may be present. Some patients have nephritis with immune complex GN.

Dx—Diagnosis is based primarily on the clinical picture with a history of new drug or foreign protein administration. C3 and C4 levels should be low, as hypocomplementemia is a hallmark of this immune complex disease. Resolution upon discontinuation of the offending agent confirms the diagnosis.

Tx—Recovery after removal of the offending agent may take 7 to 28 days. Anti-inflammatory drugs may be given if necessary for fever. Antihistamines or steroids may also confer benefit.

Hypocomplementemic Urticarial Vasculitis

D—A small vessel cutaneous vasculitis characterized by the appearance of urticaria-like lesions, which are not transitory, as with normal urticaria. This condition may be associated with another rheumatologic condition or with malignancy. Another form of urticarial vasculitis exists that is not hypocomplementemic and is less common.

Epi—Female patients outnumber males by 2:1. The mean age of incidence is 43 years (range, 15–90 years).

P—There are four major causes: (1) drugs (e.g., ACE inhibitors, PCN, and sulfa drugs), (2) other rheumatic disease (SLE and Sjögren's syndrome), (3) viral infections (e.g., HBV, HCV, EBV), and (4) and idiopathic causes. Subsequently, a type III hypersensitivity reaction occurs in which antigen-antibody complexes are deposited in the vessel walls, with resultant chemotaxis of PMN and complement activation. Released proteolytic enzymes destroy the vascular lumen.

SiSx—Urticarial skin lesions occur, sometimes with arthritis. Renal and GI involvement may occur as well, as in Henoch-Schönlein purpura.

Dx—A clinical history of urticarial lesions that are not transitory and last for >24 hours is key to the diagnosis. Hypocomplementemia is a consistent feature with antibodies against C1q. Perform a biopsy if necessary to demonstrate vasculitis and confirm the diagnosis. Patients may be ANA positive, but they do not fulfill criteria for SLE.

Tx—There is a relapsing and remitting course. Administer steroids for disabling symptoms.

Wegener's Granulomatosis

D—A granulomatous vasculitis of small vessels with multisystem involvement. Typically, the upper and lower respiratory tracts as well as the kidneys are affected. Thus, this condition falls into the category of a pulmonary renal syndrome.

Epi—It occurs most commonly in males 40–50 years of age. The incidence is <1/100,000.

SiSx—

The classic triad is:

1. Upper respiratory tract problems—apparent in 85% of patients on presentation. Specifically, persistent sinusitis, mastoid infections, and otitis may be found.
2. Lower respiratory tract problems—presenting as cough and chest pain, with hemoptysis occurring in 20% of patients.
3. Renal disease—hematuria. Fifty percent of patients have RBCs in the urine. This is a later finding and may not be present initially.

Other symptoms include:

Skin—50% have necrotizing lesions. Patients are less likely to have skin involvement than in other vasculitides.

Joints—70–90% have monoarthritis or polyarthritis.

Eye—scleritis, red eyes, orbital proptosis from granulomatous inflammation of the retroorbit.

Other—associated with subglottic tracheal stenosis from chondritis and a saddle-nose deformity due to a perforated septum.

Dx—Clinical symptoms of a pulmonary renal syndrome or the combination of upper and lower respiratory tract symptoms should make one consider this disease. A supporting serologic finding is c-ANCA (an antibody directed against proteinase 3, a serine protease), which is positive in 80% of cases, especially during active multiorgan disease. Antibody titers may correlate with disease activity in select patients. Rheumatoid factor may be positive, and ESR and CRP will be elevated as general markers of an inflammatory condition. Anemia of chronic disease may be detected; eosinophilia is rare. Urinalysis may show GN or RBC casts. Chest X-ray or CT may show bilateral nodular cavitary infiltrates or nodules in 20% of cases. To make the diagnosis, evidence of upper and lower respiratory tract disease and GN, as well as a biopsy demonstrating necrotizing granulomatous vasculitis, are required. With regard to the latter, pulmonary tissue offers the highest diagnostic yield. Sinus biopsies typically have a low yield unless a mass is present, as random sinus biopsies typically show nonspecific inflammation.

Tx—Administer prednisone and possibly cyclophosphamide and/or methotrexate as well. Oral cyclophosphamide is a current standard of care in renal and pulmonary Wegener's granulomatosis and has been shown to prevent death and relapses. However, in Wegener's granulomatosis in its limited form (typically involving sinuses), less strong immunosuppressants such as methotrexate can be effective. Most patients will remit with at least once even while being treated with cyclophosphamide. If untreated, this condition is fatal, with mean survival of 5 months and 95% mortality within a year.

Churg-Strauss Syndrome (Allergic Angiitis)

D—A granulomatous vasculitis of small and medium-sized arteries that occurs in patients with asthma. Veins and venules are also commonly involved.

Epi—The mean age of onset is 40 years, with a range of 15 to 70 years. Male patients slightly outnumber females.

SiSx—This is a triphasic disease. The further apart these phases occur, the milder the disease.
1. The prodrome lasts more than 1 year, with allergic manifestations of rhinitis, nasal polyps, and asthma.
2. Peripheral blood and tissue (mainly pulmonary) eosinophilia develops. *Loeffler's*

syndrome (an eosinophilic endocarditis) may be seen. Chronic eosinophilic pneumonia may remit and recur over the years.
3. Small or medium-sized vessel systemic vasculitis with constitutional symptoms develops. Complications include eosinophilic gastroenteritis, mononeuritis multiplex, polyarthritis, cardiomegaly, pleural effusions, and pulmonary infiltrates and nodules.

Dx—Several of the abnormalities in the third phase may be detected on chest X-ray. The diagnosis is made by the following criteria:
1. A history or current symptoms of asthma.
2. Peripheral eosinophila $>1.5 \times 10^9$/L.
3. Systemic vasculitis of two or more organs other than the lungs.

Biopsy of the lung or skin will help confirm the presence of vasculitis and shows eosinophilic necrotizing granulomas in addition to small vessel vasculitis. Furthermore, pANCA is typically present, with two-thirds of patients having antibodies to myeloperoxidase (MPO).

Tx—Administer steroids, along with cytotoxic therapy if necessary, especially for severe lung, GI, cardiac, or other organ involvement. Eosinophilia resolves rapidly with steroids.

Buerger's Disease (Thromboangiitis Obliterans)

D—A segmental vasculitis of small and medium-sized arteries, veins, and nerves of the extremities. It is considered more of a vasculopathy than a vasculitis since autoantibodies are not present.

Epi—It occurs almost exclusively in young adult smokers. Male patients outnumber females. It is more common in Asia, the Middle East, and Eastern Europe. The incidence is 13/100,000 in the United States.

RF—It is strongly associated with smoking.

SiSx—Symptoms consist of the triad of (1) claudication of an extremity (mainly calves and feet or forearms and hands), (2) Raynaud's phenomenon, and (3) migratory superficial vein thrombophlebitis. Ulceration and gangrene may develop at the tips of fingers.

Dx—In general, the diagnosis is made clinically. Buerger's disease is distinguished from other vasculitides because ESR, CRP, complement, cryoglobulin, and autoantibody tests are usually normal. On biopsy of an acute lesion, a highly cellular, inflammatory thrombus without vessel wall involvement is seen. Subacute lesions show thrombus organization. Chronic lesions show no inflammation but rather vascular fibrosis and are indistinguishable from those in other types of vascular disease. Make sure to rule out other causes of emboli such as valvular disease by performing ECHO.

Tx—Usually the disease arrests upon smoking cessation. Otherwise, treatment consists of controlling pain and removing necrotic tissue.

Microscopic Polyangiitis

D—A small vessel vasculitis associated with pANCA (which stains for myeloperoxidase) and can give a clinical picture similar to that of other ANCA-positive vasculitides, namely, pulmonary renal syndrome and neuropathies.

Epi—The incidence is 4/1,000,000. The condition is more common in whites in the United States. Male patients slightly outnumber females. The mean age at diagnosis is 50 years.

SiSx—Constitutional symptoms of fever, malaise, and weight loss occur. A rash is seen in one-half of patients as palpable purpura. Proteinuria is common; rarely, nephrotic syndrome develops. Urinalysis shows RBCs and casts characteristic of GN. Renal insufficiency is common at presentation. Gastrointestinal involvement in the form of GI bleeding may be present, as in Henoch-Schönlein purpura. Other aberrations include mononeuritis multiplex, arthralgias, hemoptysis, and URI-like symptoms.

Dx—Classically, it is seen as a pulmonary-renal-skin syndrome, so when two or more of these systems are involved, it should be included in the differential. The pANCA test is positive in 50–90% of individuals; C3 and C4 are normal. The chest X-ray may show alveolar infiltrates from pulmonary hemorrhage of alveolar capillaries. Skin biopsy (or lung or kidney biopsy, for that matter, depending on disease involvement) shows necrotizing arteritis.

Tx—The aim of therapy is to induce and maintain remission. This is accomplished with cytotoxic agents such as cyclophosphamide or azathioprine, in addition to prednisone. Renal failure and pulmonary disease are the most common causes of death.

Medium Vessel Vasculitis

Polyarteritis Nodosa (PAN)

D—A systemic necrotizing vasculitic syndrome of medium-sized muscular arteries. It can also involve small vessels, but this occurs less commonly. It can be primary or secondary to HBV and HCV infections.

Epi—The incidence is 1/100,000, peaking during the fourth and fifth decades (though it may occur at any age). Male patients outnumber females by 2:1. Twenty percent may have active HBV or, less commonly, HCV infection.

SiSx—

Most patients have multisystemic ischemic dysfunction that evolves subacutely over months. Generalized symptoms include constitutional complaints such as fever and weight loss.

Renal—hypertension is the most common renal manifestation. Glomerulonephritis can also occur, particularly in those with small vessel involvement.

Neurologic—peripheral nerve mononeuritis multiplex occurs in 50% of patients and is characterized by infarction of nerve trunks in unrelated nerve distributions that develop one at a time.

Skin—50% of patients have skin involvement with palpable purpura, ulcers, livedo reticularis, and nodules. The lesions usually present on the distal leg and are associated with a localized burning sensation.

Musculoskeletal—asymmetric polyarthritis.

Gastrointestinal—50% of patients have abdominal pain with or without ulcers. Mesenteric vasculitis may cause diffuse abdominal angina.

Cardiovascular—usually rare but can result in MI as well as dilated cardiomyopathy.

Genitourinary—testicular infarction is also seen.

Dx—Most patients present with multisystemic disease. Blood tests show an elevated ESR, normocytic/normochromic anemia, and thrombocytosis (50% of patients). Up to 10% can be pANCA positive. Diagnosis rests on the biopsy of any affected organ or on an angiogram showing microaneurysms. Changes seen on biopsy of medium-sized muscular arteries are marked fibrinoid necrosis and neutrophilic infiltration with destruction of elastic laminae. Other areas may appear normal or healed. This variegated presentation in the same vessels is unique to PAN.

Tx—Untreated, PAN is almost always fatal, most often from renal disease. Prednisone and immunosuppressives such as methotrexate, cyclophosphamide, or azathioprine are used for treatment. Hepatitis B virus-associated PAN is treated with pheresis and antivirals.

Kawasaki's Disease (Mucocutanous Lymph Node Syndrome)

D—A febrile illness of infants and young children characterized by conjunctival injection, diffuse maculopapular rash and edema, erythema and eventual desquamation of the hands and feet, cracked lips, strawberry tongue, and nonsuppurative cervical adenopathy.

Epi—This is one of the most common vasculitides of childhood. The incidence is 2/100,000. It is more common in Asians.

SiSx—In addition to the symptoms mentioned in the definition, cardiovascular complications may include CHF and arrhythmia. A coronary vasculitis develops in 25% of patients and leads to coronary aneurysms, MI, or sudden death.

Dx—Diagnostic criteria include fever, which lasts for ≥5 days and is not attributable to another cause, and four of the following changes: bilateral conjunctival injection, mucous membrane changes in the mouth (strawberry tongue, erythematous pharynx, fissured lips, and so forth), palmar or plantar erythema or edema, periungual desquamation, polymorphous rash, and cervical lymphadenopathy (one node at least >1.5 cm). Elevated ESR or CRP, leukocytosis, thrombocytosis, and anemia may also be seen.

Tx—Intravenous immunoglobulin and aspirin is the treatment of choice. Coronary artery abnormalities may be prevented when treatment is administered early in the course of the disease. The condition is unresponsive to antibiotics. Coronary artery vasculitis is seen in almost all fatal cases (2.8% of patients).

Isolated CNS Vasculitis

D—Uncommon entity characterized by vasculitis restricted to the CNS vessels without other systemic involvement. Vessels of any size can be affected.

Epi—The average age at presentation is 45 years.

P—The etiology is unclear, but the condition is associated with CMV, varicella-zoster virus (VZV), and bacterial infections as well as Hodgkin's disease.

SiSx—Headaches are common and are associated with nausea and vomiting. Changes in mental status and acute focal deficits may be present. Constitutional symptoms of fever, weight loss, and arthralgia are uncommon.

Dx—Biopsy of brain parenchyma is not usually possible. Therefore, the diagnosis is made by characteristic vessel abnormalities on arteriography and biopsy of the leptomeninges if needed. A spinal tap showing WBC or protein elevation can be helpful in making the diagnosis, as can neuroimaging. High WBC and protein levels are consistent with CSF inflammation and are typically seen in CNS vasculitis.

Tx—The prognosis is poor. However, the disease may remit spontaneously in some patients. Steroids and other cytotoxic agents may prove beneficial. Young patients who are diagnosed early with acute disease usually have a good prognosis if they are responsive to steroids. Generally, the disease has a chronic progressive course.

Large Vessel Vasculitis

Giant Cell Arteritis (GCA)

D—A systemic segmental granulomatous inflammatory disease of the carotid arteries and its branches. It may also involve any medium-sized to large artery, such as the branches off of the aorta, such as the vertebral arteries. Occasionally, even veins may be involved. The pathology is indistinguishable from that of Takayasu's arteritis.

Epi—Almost all patients are >50 years old. One-half of patients have polymyalgia rheumatica (PMR). Female patients outnumber males by 3:1. The condition is more common in northern Europeans.

SiSx—Classically, the patient presents with a temporal headache with scalp tenderness, claudication of the jaw and tongue, and constitutional symptoms such as fever, weight loss, fatigue, and anorexia. Symptoms of PMR may also be present (see below). Possible eye involvement leading to blindness from ischemic optic neuritis via involvement of the ophthalmic or posterior ciliary artery may occur. Therefore, any visual changes should be taken seriously. The superficial temporal artery is commonly involved but is usually clinically silent.

Dx—Diagnosis is made by biopsy of the temporal arteries, which will show a mononuclear cell infiltrate or granulomatous changes. The biopsy specimen should be at least 3 cm in length, because involvement may be patchy. Color duplex ultrasound may show haloes indicative of arterial edema. Additional findings that aid in the diagnosis are an elevated ESR (usually >100 mm/hr, at least >50 mm/hr, but not always) and a normochromic, normocytic anemia.

Tx—For acute cases, administer prednisone 40–60 mg/day for several weeks until the ESR returns to normal. Most symptoms will respond within 24 hours. Higher doses of steroids may be required in patients with visual problems. Intravenous methylprednisolone may be given before a biopsy is performed if the degree of clinical suspicion is sufficiently high. In 24 months, one-half of patients are able to discontinue steroid therapy. No effective steroid-sparing agent has been found in GCA, and treatment with steroids is therefore the mainstay.

Takayasu Arteritis (Aortic Arch Syndrome or Pulseless Disease)

D—A chronic vasculitis affecting the aortic arch and its primary branches.

Epi—Female patients outnumber males by 4:1. The disease most commonly appears between 20 and 40 years of age. The incidence is 2.6/1,000,000.

RF—Asian women have an increased risk.

SiSx—Low-grade fever, arthralgias, and diminished pulses occur initially. Features of large vessel ischemia develop later: claudication, ischemic ulcers, and neurologic deficits. Aortic involvement may cause angina and CHF. Pulmonary and mesenteric vessels may also be affected. Renovascular hypertension and pulmonary hypertension may complicate this condition.

Dx—Complete arteriography of the aorta should be performed for diagnosis and to elucidate the extent of the disease. Stenoses are seen is almost all patients; aneurysms occur in only one-fourth. Magnetic resonance angiography is increasingly being used since contrast is not needed. Perform a baseline ECHO to assess for structural heart disease. Blood work-up may show an elevated ESR, anemia, and increased levels of gamma globulins.

Tx—Prednisone early in the course of the illness is necessary. Arterial bypass grafting or balloon dilation is performed on poor medical responders. Methotrexate or cyclophosphamide is useful in refractory cases. Survival is 90% at 10 years. Most patients die from CVA or CAD.

Behçet's Syndrome

D—A vasculitis with the presence of recurrent oral and genital ulcers as well as ocular involvement.

Epi—The distribution is worldwide. It is highest in Turkey, Iran, Saudia Arabia, and Japan, where the incidence is up to 1/10,000. The incidence in the United States is 1/150,000.

The syndrome occurs most commonly in young adults. Male patients outnumber females in the Middle East. The pattern is reversed in the United States.

P—The etiology is unclear, but vasculitis is the primary lesion, with a tendency toward thrombus formation. Fifty percent of patients have antibodies to mucosal membranes.

SiSx—Recurrent painful aphthous oral and genital ulcers are the classic symptoms. Ocular involvement includes uveitis and retinal vasculitis, with blindness as a possible outcome. The skin may exhibit erythema nodosum and papulopustular lesions. Central nervous system involvement may or may not occur. Arthritis is not deforming and involves the knees. Superficial or deep venous thrombosis is seen in 25% of patients. Superior vena cava (SVC) syndrome is apparent occasionally.

Dx—Diagnosis is based on recurrent oral ulceration and two of the following features: recurrent genital ulceration, eye lesions, skin manifestations, and a positive pathergy test (International Study Group, 1990).

Tx—The severity of disease usually abates with time. Life expectancy is usually normal. Mucous membrane involvement may respond to topical steroids. Thalidomide may also be effective. Colchicine or interferon can be used for arthralgias. Central nervous system involvement requires oral steroids or cytotoxic agents, especially azathioprine.

Disorders of Joints and Tissues

Common Osteoarthritis (OA)

D—Condition in which joint pain results from wear and tear of cartilage and articular surfaces. It is also called *degenerative joint disease*. There are several types: (1) primary idiopathic OA, (2) erosive OA (an autosomal dominant disease more common in middle-aged women), and (3) secondary OA due to another underlying disease (e.g., hemachromatosis, acromegaly, and many others) or trauma.

Epi—It affects 30% of adults and is the most common rheumatologic disease overall.

P—It is thought to be primarily either a mechanical problem (and therefore not inflammatory) or a problem of cartilage repair. Loosening of type II collagen occurs with mechanical stress and defects in collagen cross-linking or decreased proteoglycan synthesis may predispose to the earlier development of disease. After progressive focal degeneration occurs, there is formation of new bone at the joint margins.

RF—Risk factors include age, a family history, trauma, obesity, metabolic disorders such as gout, and any neuromuscular disease that places inappropriate stress on the joints.

SiSx—Classically, pain and stiffness are worse with activity and better with rest, but pain may persist in affected joints. "Gelling" or renewed stiffening occurs with prolonged rest. Morning stiffness is brief (<30 minutes) compared to inflammatory joint disease (>1 hour). Joint involvement is typically bilateral and asymmetric and can involve almost all other joints. There may be bony enlargement with decreased range of motion at affected areas. Hand involvement classically includes enlarged DIPs (Heberden's nodes) and enlarged PIPs (Bouchard's nodes) in addition to the MCPs (see Figure 6-14). Crepitus, a crackling noise heard with joint motion, may also be heard with passive movement, especially at the knee. In the spine, C4–C6 involvement is most common, followed by involvement of T8 through L3. Other presentations include isolated hip or shoulder OA.

Dx—Diagnosis is generally made by the exam and the history. Radiographically, one can

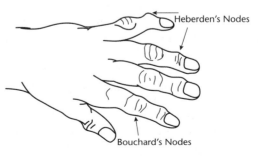

Figure 6-14. Common Deformities of the Hand in Osteoarthritis.

see nonuniform joint space loss, new sub-chondral bone formation, subchondral cysts, and osteophyte formation with normal mineralization. Usually the ESR and complete blood count (CBC) are is normal in primary disease. Antinuclear antibody and rheumatoid factor are unremarkable as well.

Tx—Advise patient to minimize joint overuse and repetitive trauma. Weight loss in areas of weight-bearing joints will also help. Arch supports, NSAIDs, acetaminophen, and other analgesics are also useful. Intra-articular steroids or hyaluronic acid injections (there are less data for the latter) can be used for intractable pain. For intractable pain or debility from advanced disease, joint replacement may be necessary. Oral steroids have no role in treatment.

Degenerative Disk Disease

D—Degeneration of the intervertebral discs of the spine, allowing impingement on spinal cord roots and thereby causing pain. It occurs most commonly in the lumbosacral and cervical regions. Nonspecifically, this condition may be called *spondylosis*.

P—Degenerative changes in the disk allow the inner nucleus pulposus to herniate out of the annular fibrosus capsule, causing impingement on the nerves. It occurs most commonly in the lumbosacral and cervical regions.

RF—Risk factors include OA, age, and trauma.

SiSx—Pain along the affected nerve root is elicited by activities such as rising from a seated or lying position, coughing, and laughing. Most commonly, L4 and L5 are involved. *Sciatica*, shooting pain down the leg in the L4–S1 distribution, involves the sciatic nerve. In addition to pain, there may be muscle weakness at the affected level. Urinary and bowel incontinence may indicate a large midline posterior herniation that compresses the cauda equina (the *cauda equina syndrome*). Cervical involvement most commonly causes pain at levels C4–C6 and may cause chronic suboccipital headache and local pain that radiates to the occiput, scapula, arm, or shoulder. An acute herniated disk may cause a cervical radiculopathy,

with pain and sensory abnormalities along the affected nerve root.

Dx—A passive straight leg lift (with the patient supine and both legs straight, lifting one leg up beyond 30°) will cause pain in lumbar disease. Neck flexion while supine or extension while standing may cause pain in cervical disease. A simple X-ray may show evidence of disk and/or spinal degeneration. A CT scan or myelography, in which contrast is injected into the subarachnoid space, can be used to show disk protrusion. Magnetic resonance imaging is also commonly used for diagnosis. Additionally, EMG tests can be done to assess nerve damage.

Tx—For mild symptoms, heat and anti-inflammatory agents such as NSAIDs can be used. Surgery may be needed for intractable pain or neurologic impairment.

Infectious Arthritis

D—Arthritis caused by an inflammatory response to infection. The most common types are due to disseminated gonococcal infection (DGI), nongonococcal bacterial infections, viral infection, and Lyme disease.

Epi—*Neisseria gonorrhoeae* is the most common cause in sexually active adults. In others, common agents include *Staphylococcus aureus* (60%), *Streptococcus* (15%), gram-negative rods (15%), and other bacteria. Disseminated gonococcal infection has a yearly incidence of 600,000 in the United States. One percent of patients have bacteremia.

RF—Risk factors include trauma, indwelling catheters, immunosuppression, and preexisting arthritis.

SiSx—The condition usually presents as a painful monoarthritis. The knee is involved in 50% of cases, but the wrists, ankles, and hips can also be affected. Twenty percent of cases are polyarticular. Most patients have fever and an associated infection such as cellulitis, URI, or UTI. Disseminated gonococcal infection can be initially a migratory arthritis and classically occurs with a pustular or vesiculopustular dermatitis. Pelvic inflammatory disease (PID)-like symptoms, including lower abdominal pain, and vaginal discharge may be present in women.

Dx—Aspiration of a septic joint shows >50,000 WBCs, >75% of which are PMNs. The WBC count is higher in nongonococcal bacterial infections and can be lower in patients already given antibiotics. Gram stain is positive in 50–75% of cases of acute bacterial arthritis. Synovial cultures will have a high yield (90%) for nongonococcal bacteria, whereas cultures from joints are often negative for gonococcus. In a sexually active individual, one can also check for gonococcus via the pelvic exam for women and a urethral swab for men. Gram stain, and cultures. X-ray may show joint space narrowing and erosion of the cortex after just 7–14 days.

Tx—A pus-filled joint is considered a relative medical emergency. Drain all purulent material from the involved joints and give antibiotics. For DGI, use IM or IV ceftriaxone followed by an oral regimen. Serial aspirates may be necessary, and surgery is required when needle aspiration is unsuccessful or inadequate.

Seronegative Spondyloarthropathies

These diseases have several common characteristics:

1. Patients are seronegative, meaning that they are rheumatoid factor and ANA negative.
2. The main effects are on the axial skeleton, particularly the sacroiliac joints. Appendicular skeleton involvement, if exhibited, is typically asymmetric and oligoarticular.
3. Patients may have enthesis or enthesopathy, which is inflammation of the bony insertions of tendons, ligaments, and fascia. Otherwise, this condition is seen only in sarcoidosis. It manifests as dactylitis, a "sausage-like" swelling of the entire finger or toe, which is different from the joint swelling seen in other arthropathies.
4. Extraskeletal features include uveitis, conjunctivitis, urethritis, inflammatory bowel disease, psoriasiform rashes, and aortitis.
5. Patients often harbor the HLA-B27 haplotype.

Ankylosing Spondylitis

D—The prototypical spondylarthropathy, characterized by chronic inflammation of the axial skeleton with variable ascension up the spine and to peripheral joints. The name literally means "fusion of spinal vertebrae."

Epi—There is an incidence of up to 1/1000 in Caucasians. Patients are usually <40 years of age. Male patients outnumber females by 9:1.

RF—There is a 90% HLA-B27 association in whites and 50% in African Americans/ Asians.

SiSx—There is insidious onset of lower back/ buttock stiffness and pain lasting for >3 months, as well as morning pain and stiffness, which are improved by exercise. The condition is associated with anterior uveitis (25%), aortitis (5%), aortic regurgitation, heart block, enthesopathy, and upper lobe pulmonary fibrosis. Eventually, patients may have difficulty taking deep breaths since chest expansion will be diminished. Pain is present in sacroiliac joints and/or peripheral arthritis of large joints, especially the hips and shoulders in more advanced, severe disease. On physical exam, decreased flexion may be measured by the Schober test, in which a 10-cm line measured vertically on the patient's back fails to increase to 15 cm with flexion. Chest expansion, as measured by the difference in the fourth intercostal space in males or below the breasts in females between maximal inspiration and forced expiration, is usually <5 cm. Additional direct compression over the sacroiliac joints causing pain may suggest sacroiliac involvement.

Dx—Radiographs show a straightened lumbar spine, bilateral sacroiliitis, and classically a "bamboo spine" in late disease with no subluxation or cysts.

Diagnostic criteria are as follows:

1. A history of inflammatory back pain.
2. Limitation of motion of the lumbar spine in both the sagittal and frontal planes.
3. Limited chest expansion relative to standard values for age and sex.

4. Definite radiographic sacroiliitis. Magnetic resonance imaging and CT can be used to detect early sacroiliitis that X-rays may not reveal.

Using these criteria, the presence of radiographic sacroiliitis plus any one of the other three criteria is sufficient to make the diagnosis.

Tx—Treatment involves NSAIDs and physical therapy. Anti-TNF agents are approved for the signs and symptoms and may help prevent disease progression. Only 6% of patients die from this disease. Fusion of the spine may take more than 10 years.

Reactive Arthritis

D—A reactive arthritis usually secondary to a complicating infection at another site, usually dysenteric or venereal. *Reiter's syndrome* was the old term for this condition.

Epi—Male patients outnumber females. The condition is seen mostly in young adults. It is the most common cause of chronic arthritis in young men.

RF—There is an 85% HLA-B27 association in males. Most commonly associated infections are *Yersinia, Salmonella, Shigella*, and *Campylobacter* in the GI tract and *Chlamydia* in the GU tract.

SiSx—Symptoms usually occur 2–6 weeks after initiation of infection. Classic symptoms are (1) asymmetric oligoarthritis of lower extremities that follows an episode of (2) urethritis or, in women, cervicitis and (3) bilateral conjunctivitis, uveitis, keratitis, or retinitis. Additionally, dermatologic manifestations may be found, including a painless mucocutaneous lesion on the glans penis (*circinate balanitis*) and mouth and hyperkeratotic lesions on the palms and soles (*keratoderma blennorrhagicum*). Aortitis or heart block is rarely seen.

Dx—Diagnosis is based mainly on clinical findings. An attempt to isolate the pathogen should be made in order to rule out other causes. Periosteal bone formation seen on X-ray near the Achilles tendon insertion is characteristic.

Tx—Consider joint immobilization and administration of NSAIDs. Topical corticosteroids may be used for skin lesions. Relapses occur at varying intervals. There is evidence that a course of antibiotic therapy, such as tetracycline for 3 months, may lessen the severity of the arthritis. Chronic disease is common in up to 60–80% of patients. Immunosuppressive agents are used for chronic disease.

Psoriatic Arthritis

D—A syndrome of cutaneous psoriasis and seronegative inflammatory arthropathy.

Epi—Most patients develop the disease in their late 30s to 40s.

RF—From 5% to 10% of people with psoriasis also have arthritis.

SiSx—Psoriasis usually precedes the arthritis. The arthritis involves the DIPs, often resulting in sausage digits (dactylitis) from the swelling. Nail pitting (onychodystrophy) is seen in 80%. Fifty percent of patients have peripheral symmetric oligoarthritis, 25% have symmetric RA-like disease, and 20% have spinal involvement. The PIPs, MCPs, and MTPs may be involved as well. Systemic manifestations are rare. In contrast to reactive arthritis, the arthritis tends to be located in the upper extremities.

Dx—All other causes of arthritis must be excluded. A biopsy-proven previous diagnosis of psoriasis is helpful. Otherwise, the diagnosis is purely clinical.

Tx—Treat the skin condition with topical preparations and administer anti-inflammatory drugs ranging from NSAIDs to cytotoxic agents such as methotrexate with or without etanercept, a TNF inhibitor.

Enteropathic Arthritis

D—An inflammatory arthritis induced or associated with inflammatory bowel disease as an extragastrointestinal manifestation. Spondylitis is associated with it in 50% of patients.

Epi—It afflicts 10% of patients with Crohn's disease (CD) and ulcerative colitis (UC).

RF—Whipple's disease (extremely rare) is a risk factor.

SiSx—Periarticular, transient, migratory arthritis is found. Arthralgia is the most common symptom, but synovitis with large joint effusions may also be seen. Lower extremities are more commonly affected. Joint pain does not correlate strictly with inflammatory bowel disease activity but does so more often in UC than in CD. Sacroiliitis develops in <20% of patients, most of whom are HLA-B27 positive. Attacks generally are worse during the first few years of bowel disease.

Dx—This is a clinical diagnosis in which extraintestinal manifestations are noted in a patient with known inflammatory bowel disease.

Tx—Treat the underlying inflammatory bowel disease (see Chapter 5).

Crystal-Induced Arthropathies

Gout

D—Disease of purine metabolism characterized by monosodium urate (MSU) crystals in and around the joints. Patients either overproduce (10%) or insufficiently clear (90%) the compound.

Epi—It is most common in men 30–60 years old and in postmenopausal women.

P—The defect causing MSU overproduction is from either a primary metabolic pathway problem or secondary to increased cell turnover associated with hematologic malignancies, hemolysis, or cancer chemotherapy. By contrast, decreased clearance is invariably due to drugs or renal disease. Immunoglobulin and WBCs become fixed to the crystals and evoke an inflammatory response.

RF—Risk factors include thiazide diuretics, trauma, alcohol, renal failure, and hyperuricemia (only 10% of patients, however, develop gout).

SiSx—Symptoms are divided into phases. (1) Asymptomatic hyperuricemia may extend 20–30 years. (2) The acute/interval gout phase is marked by sudden severe pain and inflammation in the first MTP (called *podagra*), midtarsal, or ankle (ordered by decreasing frequency) lasting for days to weeks. Fever is present in severe attacks. (3) Intercritical periods occur after the first attack and between subsequent flare-ups. Seven percent of patients will never have another attack, and most recurrent attacks occur within a year. (4) Chronic tophaceous gout occurs when tophi deposit in the pinna, at the site of chronically inflamed joints, on extensor surfaces of the arms, and at the infrapatellar and Achilles tendons. Usually a single joint (rarely a few) is affected. Tophi are large yellow- to cream-colored deposits that can ulcerate and exude chalky material.

Dx—Serum uric acid levels are not helpful acutely, since they may return to normal during an acute attack and then rise thereafter. The upper limit of normal is 7–8 mg/dL. Values >13 mg/dL and >10 mg/dL are considered elevated in men and women, respectively. Fluid aspiration is diagnostic if it shows classic urate crystals, which are needle-shaped and strongly negatively birefringent, that is, they are yellow under parallel and blue under perpendicularly oriented, polarized light.

Tx—The asymptomatic phase is generally not treated. Nonsteroidal anti-inflammatory drugs are the first line of therapy during acute gouty attacks. Oral colchicine may also be used in such situations because it inhibits neutrophil chemotaxis. Steroids are administered orally or by injection if the patient is nonresponsive or if there are contraindications to first-line agents. Injection of corticotrophin (ACTH) can also be used in acute gout. For prevention, modification of diet, allopurinol (a xanthine oxidase inhibitor), and/or probenecid (increases renal uric acid secretion) are prescribed.

These medications may prolong gouty attacks and should not be started until 2 weeks after an acute event resolves in those suffering recurrent episodes. Urate lowering therapy is typically reserved for those with frequent gout attacks and those with evidence of excessive urate burden (presence of tophi and/or history of urate nephrolithiasis).

Calcium Pyrophosphate Deposition Disease (CPPD) and Pseudogout

D—Gout-like arthritis that is caused by calcium pyrophosphate dehydrate. *Pseudogout* is the name for an acute inflammatory attack of CPPD.

Epi—It is half as common as gout and affects mainly the elderly.

P—The cause in most patients is unknown. A minority have a genetic form leading to metabolic aberrations. Other forms can occur as a result of severe OA or even result in severe OA.

RF—Risk factors include older age, OA, amyloidosis, hemochromatosis, hyperparathyroidism, hypothyroidism, gout, and Wilson's disease. Precipitation by a medical or surgical condition is common.

SiSx—Symptoms can range from acute attacks (25%) to chronic inflammation. In the acute situation the knee is most commonly affected, although any joint, including the first MTP, is susceptible. The clinical picture is similar to that of OA (50% of cases) or RA (5%). Twenty percent are asymptomatic, with incidental chondrocalcinosis on radiographs.

Dx—Synovial fluid crystals are short, cuboidal, and blue when parallel to polarized light (i.e., weakly positively birefringent). X-ray shows chondrocalcinosis (calcification of hyaline cartilage), though this finding may also be present in asymptomatic individuals who have never experienced an attack. Unlike MSU, CPP is radiopaque and may be visible in the clear space above bone atop cartilage.

Tx—Correction of the underlying metabolic disorder does not halt the progression of disease. Acute attacks are treated with aspiration of joint fluid, NSAIDs, and intra-articular steroid injections. Small oral doses of colchicine may be helpful in prevention.

Calcium Hydroxyapatite Deposition Disease

D—The typical form of calcium deposition in bone can also deposit in joint spaces, causing pathology.

Epi—One can find these crystals as commonly as CPPD during joint taps.

P—Mineral formation may be a result of abnormal cartilage metabolism.

SiSx—Episodes of acute inflammation occur. There may be discrete clumped bodies around shoulders, greater trochanters, wrists, elbows, digits, and other areas, which disintegrate within weeks after the acute attack. They may be associated with a chronic destructive arthropathy involving the knee and shoulder ("Milwaukee shoulder") in elderly patients

Dx—X-ray findings are nondiagnostic, showing calcifications around or in the joint space. Light microscopy material from tissue or synovial fluid shows brownish globules of crystals inside inclusion bodies of cells. Extracellular globules stain purple with Wright's stain and red with Alizarin red S. Ultimately, EM or IR is needed to make a definitive diagnosis.

Tx—Look for disorders of calcium and phosphate metabolism. Nonsteroidal anti-inflammatory drugs are used for acute episodes, or intra-articular steroid injections along with periodic aspirations may be given.

Periarticular Disorders of the Extremities

Bursitis

D—Inflammation of the bursa, the thin-walled sac lining synovial tissue where tendons and muscles overlap bony prominences. Subacromial bursitis is the most common type and accompanies rotator cuff injuries. Also common is trochanteric bursitis.

RF—Risk factors include excessive friction, trauma, connective tissue disease, gout, and infection.

SiSx—Trochanteric bursitis manifests as pain over the hip and upper thigh with tenderness over the greater trochanter. Subacromial bursitis presents as lateral and anterior shoulder pain.

Dx—It is primarily a clinical diagnosis after excluding other causes such as infection or crystalline disease.

Tx—Treatment consists of preventing additional irritation of the involved area. Immobilization, ice compresses, NSAIDs, bursal aspiration, or even local steroid injections may help relieve symptoms.

Adhesive Capsulitis (Frozen Shoulder)

D—Pain and restricted movement of the shoulder, usually without intrinsic shoulder disease. It may follow bursitis or tendinitis of the shoulder and may not be associated with systemic disorders.

Epi—Female patients outnumber males. The condition usually develops after 50 years of age.

RF—Prolonged immobility of the shoulder and reflex sympathetic dystrophy develop. The condition is very common in diabetics.

SiSx—Pain and stiffness develop gradually over several months. The shoulder is tender to palpation, with restriction of both active and passive movement.

Dx—The diagnosis is confirmed by arthrography with a small amount of contrast material.

Tx—In most patients, the condition improves spontaneously in 1 to 3 years, but some may have permanent restriction of movement, which can be prevented by early mobilization. Local steroids or NSAIDs may improve symptoms.

Lateral Epicondylitis (Tennis Elbow)

D—A painful condition of the lateral epicondyle thought to be due to small tears in the extensor aponeurosis from repeated resisted contractions of extensor muscles. It is usually due to repeated wrist extension and supination.

P—Most patients injure themselves by pulling weeds, carrying suitcases or briefcases, or using screwdrivers. The tennis injury occurs mostly when hitting a backhand with the elbow flexed.

SiSx—There is chronic pain at the lateral portion of the elbow that is worse with supination.

Dx—Diagnosis is made by the history and exam.

Tx—Use NSAIDs and ice. Avoid aggravating activities. Steroid injections may also help the pain. Occasional surgical release, if necessary, can be performed.

Medial Epicondylitis

D—A disorder similar to lateral epicondylitis thought to be due to repetitive wrist flexion and pronation, with microtears in forearm flexors.

Epi—It is most commonly due to work-related repetitive activity but is also seen in sports such as golf and basketball.

SiSx—Tenderness distal to the medial epicondyle with pain on resisting wrist flexion is found.

Dx—Diagnosis is made by the history and exam. Radiographs are normal.

Tx—Rest, NSAIDs, friction massage, icing, and steroid injections are useful. Occasional surgical release may be necessary.

Carpal Tunnel Syndrome (CTS)

D—A condition involving focal entrapment of the median nerve as it passes through the carpal bones and the transverse carpal ligament.

RF—Risk factors include pregnancy (the main cause), RA (a secondary cause), hypothyroidism, acromegaly, diabetes, mass lesions, edema, trauma, amyloidosis, and fracture.

SiSx—There is numbness in the distal arm and wrist in a median nerve distribution. Nocturnal pain is common. Pain may radiate to the shoulder, forearm, or upper arm. Physical exam findings include Tinel's sign (tapping over the median nerve on flexor surface causes a tingling sensation); positive Phalen's test [flexing the wrists 90° and holding them together for 1 minute causes numbness (see Figure 6-15)]; and positive carpal compression test (pressure over the carpal

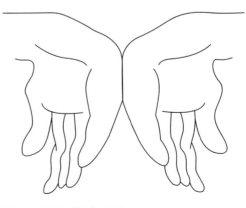

Figure 6-15. Phalen's Test.

tunnel with the thumb for 30 seconds causes symptoms). Late complications include atrophy of thenar muscles and permanent sensory loss.

Dx—This is a clinical diagnosis based on the signs described above, which can be confirmed first with a response to conservative treatment. Otherwise, nerve conduction studies ultimately make the diagnosis.

Tx—Minimize wrist movement with resting splints and use NSAIDs. Steroid injections resolve symptoms, but there is a high rate of recurrence. Surgical release should be performed if all else fails and symptoms persist. This relieves symptoms in 90% of patients.

Miscellaneous Rheumatologic Disorders

Polymyalgia Rheumatica (PMR)

D—An inflammatory condition characterized by pain and stiffness in the shoulders, pelvic girdle muscles, and torso.

Epi—Female patients outnumber males. Patients are usually >60 years old. Up to 15% have giant cell arteritis. The incidence is 1/200 cases over age 60.

P—The etiology is unknown. While closely linked to GCA, it is considered a separate disease process.

SiSx—Symmetric polymyalgias and arthralgias with a duration of >1 month are found. The most common symptoms are aching with stiffness of the neck, torso, shoulders, and arms. The hips, thighs and pelvic girdle are also commonly involved. Usually vague constitutional symptoms may be present, such as fatigue, sweats, and weight loss. Symptoms are worse in the morning and after prolonged sitting. Muscle strength is normal, and small joints are not involved.

Dx—This is a clinical diagnosis. An abnormal ESR is not necessary for the diagnosis, but it is usually elevated along with CRP. Work-up for GCA may be necessary, as is imaging of the great vessels. Rheumatoid factor and ANA tests are usually negative. An immediate response (within several days) to low-dose steroids is highly suggestive of PMR, and the absence of this response should make one question the diagnosis.

Tx—Prednisone 10–20 mg/day should relieve symptoms within 48 hours to 1 week; otherwise, another disease entity should be sought. Nonsteroidal anti-inflammatory drugs are also used.

Fibromyalgia

D—A disorder characterized by multiple complaints including, most commonly, musculoskeletal pain and stiffness, chronic general fatigue, difficulty sleeping, and multiple tender points on the body that are symmetrically distributed.

Epi—Female patients outnumber males by 8:1. The condition is seen in all races and all climates. The prevalence is as high as 3.5% in women and 0.5% in men, increasing with age >50. Many patients have associated psychiatric disorders such as depression or anxiety. Many may also have associated connective tissue diseases or chronic pain syndromes. Fibromyalgia is supposedly the second most common reason for lost work days after URIs.

P—The cause is unclear. Theories include decreased sleep or missed stage IV sleep, various medication exposures, and abnormal substance P or growth hormone levels. Symptoms may be triggered by emotional stress, trauma, and hypothyroidism.

SiSx—Generalized aching is the most common complaint, which first involves specific joints and then becomes diffuse over the entire body. Both muscle and skeletal pain are found. Stiffness occurs as well, especially in the morning. Patients also complain of exhaustion. Specific areas, called *fibromyalgia tender points*, can elicit intense pain when pressed with the finger tip using just mild pressure (enough pressure to blanch the finger nail of the examiner). These are symmetrically located on the body (see Figure 6-16). Psychiatric symptoms may also be manifest, including depression or anxiety. Sleep disturbance is very common and may contribute to the pathogenesis. Some patients have autonomic nervous system instability and may

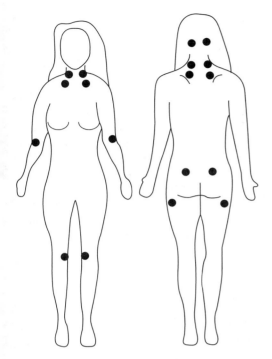

Figure 6-16. Fibromyalgia Tender Points.

fail tilt table tests, which are designed to test regulation of BP with changes in posture.

Dx—This is a clinical diagnosis. Demonstration of 11 of 18 tender points (see Figure 6-16), in addition to a history of pain, stiffness, and fatigue that cannot be attributed to another disease, is required.

Tx—The symptoms are variable, with some patients having a waxing and waning course and others having chronic features. Nonsteroidal anti-inflammatory drugs may be used but will be only partially helpful. Steroids and opiates should be avoided. Tricyclic antidepressants (TCAs) are useful in many patients when started at low doses initially. Treatment of associated connective tissue diseases or psychiatric conditions is also important. Regular aerobic exercise is recommended to reduce pain and stiffness.

Hypertrophic Osteoarthropathy (HOA)

D—A condition characterized by clubbing of the digits and enlargement of the extremities, with new periosteal bone formation and painful joints with synovial effusions. It can be primary (3–5% of cases) or secondary (the overwhelming majority) to other conditions such as intrathoracic malignancies (seen in 5–10% of these patients), suppurative lung disease or chronic lung conditions (e.g., CF), smoking, congenital heart disease, and GI disease such as inflammatory bowel disease.

Epi—It is more common in men than women

P—Primary HOA is autosomal dominant. The exact cause or final common pathway for multiple variants of the disease is unclear.

SiSx—Clubbing of the fingers is almost always a feature of HOA, but this can also occur with other disease entities. Skin changes are usually prominent, with thickening and coarsening. Deep skins folds develop. Joint effusions may be evident.

Dx—This is generally a clinical diagnosis. Evidence of effusions can be confirmed with an aspirate. New bone formation can be seen on radiographs.

Tx—Treat the underlying condition if one is found. In cases of neoplasia, removal of malignancy, when possible, usually leads to remission of the joint symptoms.

Relapsing Polychondritis

D— A rare inflammatory condition of unknown etiology that is characterized by episodic and progressive inflammation of cartilage of the ears, nose, and laryngotracheobronchial tree. It is also associated with systemic vasculitis, cardiac abnormalities, skin findings, GN, and scleritis.

Epi—Peak onset occurs at 40–50 years of age. Equal numbers of males and females are affected. Thirty percent of patients have another rheumatic disorder.

P—Immunologic mechanisms play a major role. There is deposition of immune complexes at sites of inflammation.

SiSx—Ear involvement is most common and classically is seen eventually in 85% of patients. Only the auricles (not the lobes) are affected since only they contain cartilage. Fifty percent of patients will eventually have nasal involvement; the bridge becomes red and swollen, with an eventual saddle nose deformity in severe cases. Arthritis is seen in 30% as the presenting problem, and is asymmetric and polyarticular. Eye manifestations, seen in 50% of patients, are inflammatory as well. Laryngotracheobronchial involvement is seen in 50%, with the possibility of life-threatening airway obstruction. Cardiac involvement is primarily valvular. Systemic vasculitis and other connective tissue diseases may be seen as well. The course of the disease is highly variable, with attacks lasting for days to weeks and subsiding spontaneously.

Dx—Major criteria include involvement of both auricles and the nose, accompanying arthritis, and involvement of the eye and the laryngotracheobronchial tree. Usually clinical symptoms are enough to make the diagnosis, but in unclear cases biopsy can be used.

Tx—Five-year survival is 75%. High-dose prednisone usually is effective, followed by cytotoxic agents for nonresponders.

Tietze Syndrome (Costochondritis)

D—Painful swelling of one or more of the costochondral articulations. Costochondritis may be used by some to refer to pain at these locations without swelling.

Epi—Onset occurs at around 40 years of age. Incidence is equal in males and females.

SiSx—Mostly only one articulation is affected, though sometimes several are. Most commonly, the third, fourth, and fifth articulations are the ones affected. Onset of pain can be gradual or sudden. Pain may radiate to the arms or shoulders and is aggravated by sneezing, coughing, deep inspirations, or twisting motions of the chest.

Dx—Diagnosis is made by the history and physical exam and after exclusion of other causes of chest pain. Replication of the pain with palpation is classic.

Tx—Give NSAIDs for pain. Avoid aggravating activities.

Chapter 6 Appendix

Many of the autoimmune conditions discussed in this chapter deal with serologic testing. Table 6-8 lists the conditions with which the most commonly used tests are associated.

Table 6-8. Summary of Common Autoantibody Tests

Condition	ANA	dsDNA	SM	His-tone	Ro	La	Scl-70	Cent-romere	RNP	Jo-1	RF
RA	30–60	0–5			5	2			30–40		85
SLE	**95–100**	**50–60**	**10–30**	70	20	15					20
Drug Induced Lupus				95							
Sjögren's Syndrome	40–70		70		**60–90**	**40–60**					75
Diffuse Scleroderma	80–95						**40**	10			25
CREST	60–80							**50–90**			25
MCTD			30						**100**		
PM	30–80							10		**25**	33

Note: Numbers represent the percentage of cases in which serology is positive. Values in boldface are more characteristic of the disease in question. RA, rheumatoid arthritis; MCTD, mixed connective tissue disease; PM, polymyositis; RF, rheumatoid factor.

CHAPTER 7

Endocrinology

APPROACH TO COMMON PROBLEMS

Approach to Inpatient Hyperglycemia

1. Focus on the following in taking the history and performing the physical exam:
   - History of diabetes or whether the patient meets the diagnostic criteria based on current sugar levels. Note the inpatient versus outpatient regimen and if the patient is insulin dependent.
   - Evidence of current infection.
   - Use of steroids now or in the past and any cushingoid features on exam.
   - Whether the patient is receiving excess sugar in IV fluids, TPN, or antibiotics.
   - Evidence of symptomatic hyperglycemia: hypovolemia, polyuria, polydipsia.
   - Evidence of other symptoms of glucose toxicity (ketosis or acidosis).
   - Food intake as an inpatient (compared to outpatient diet).
2. If sugar levels are highly elevated and the history and exam raise concern about diabetic ketoacidosis (DKA) or dehydration, check a panel 7 for electrolytes and the anion gap as well as serum ketone levels. If these are positive, treat the patient appropriately with IV fluids and IV insulin (see the Diabetic Ketoacidosis and Hyperosmolar Hyperglycemic State sections).
3. If the patient is otherwise stable but has evidence of diabetes, decide on an appropriate initial regimen or modify the current regimen. Most inpatient blood sugars are controlled with insulin. Starting an oral agent depends on the presence of comorbidities (see the Diabetes Mellitus section) and generally can be done on an outpatient basis after

conversion from insulin. Modifying the diet, altering the amount of dextrose or insulin in TPN, and treating underlying infections will all promote blood sugar control. In most cases, however, inpatient management of high sugar levels will involve insulin.

   a. *Starting a regimen*: Ultimately, all patients should be given both a basal, long-acting insulin to cover the body's background need for insulin (even in the fasting state) and a short-acting insulin to cover the insulin needed for meals. Figure 7-1 below shows both dose regimens. The glargine/short-acting insulin regimen is more physiologic, as there is a constant basal background insulin and the postprandial high sugar levels are treated at each meal with a very-short acting-insulin

   How do you determine how much insulin someone will need in a day (i.e., the *total daily dose*)? There are three methods:

   (1) For the first 24 hours, if sugar levels are not markedly elevated, one can use just a "correction dose" of short-acting insulin, formerly called a *sliding scale*. Here standard amounts of insulin are given for each cut-point of elevated sugar when checked several times a day. Then one counts all the short-acting insulin used.

   (2) If the patient is on an insulin drip, use the amount used in the last 24 hours.

   (3) Start from scratch and estimate how much insulin the patient may need based just on body weight. Use 0.5 units of insulin/kg. Divide it as 50% short acting insulin for meals and 50% basal long acting insulin. If the patient is NPO, all of the 24-hour total is converted to basal insulin.

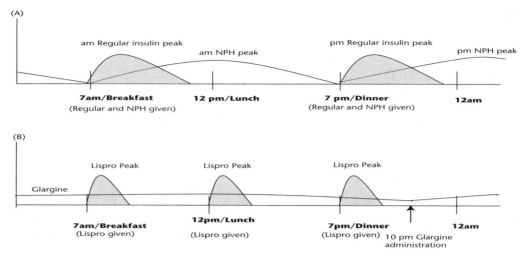

Figure 7-1. Inpatient Insulin Dosing Schemes Showing Insulin Levels (Y axis) Across Time (X axis). Shorting-acting insulins are shown in gray and long-acting insulins are clear.

Panel A: Older methods used a twice daily regular–NPH insulin combination. Postprandial lunch is not covered well in this scheme. Conversely, due to the peaking nature of NPH insulin, patients who are NPO may experience midday hypoglycemia.

Panel B: Newer methods use very-short-acting insulins, such as lispro, to cover elevated sugars after meals. The long-acting insulin, glargine, provides a 24-hour basal dose that doesn't have a major peak in its effect.

i. The older commonly used regimen was a mixture of neutral-protamine-Hagedorn (NPH) and regular insulin (see Figure 7-1, panel A). This is important to know for pathophysiologic reasons and because some patients are still taking these medications. Typically, the division is two-thirds of the total insulin with breakfast and one-third with dinner. The ratio of regular to NPH insulin varies, although the NPH dose is typically higher than regular insulin.

ii. Current guidelines use longer-acting basal insulin (i.e., glargine insulin, known as Lantus or detemir [Levemir] insulin) and shorter-acting bolus insulin (aspart, lispro, and glulisine; see Figure 7-1, panel B). In general, 80% of the calculated total daily dose is given this way (not 100% so that there is a safety margin), with 50% given as glargine and 50% as rapid-acting insulin spread across meals. Glargine is adjusted every 48–72 hours based on fasting morning sugar levels. Rapid-acting insulins are adjusted based on postprandial sugar levels. The fasting sugar goal is 90–130 mg/dL and the postprandial sugar goal is generally <180 mg/dL.

b. *If the patient is NPO and on insulin*: Hold the regular insulin and give one-half of the dose of the morning NPH; if the patient is on glargine, give the full dose the night before. Restart the prior formulation once the patient is eating. If the patient is not eating for an extended period of time and is normally on insulin, he or she will *still need some degree of basal insulin*, so do not hold it.

c. *Oral agents*: There are some noteworthy restrictions to the use of common oral agents in the inpatient:

1. Metformin is usually held in patients undergoing procedures with IV contrast because of the theoretical risk of lactic acidosis. It should also be held in any patient with acute renal failure.

2. Sulfonylureas should not be given to those with very poor oral intake because of the risk of hypoglycemia.

3. Thiazolidinediones are held in those with active congestive heart failure (CHF) or liver function test (LFT) abnormalities.

Approach to the Adrenal Incidentaloma

An incidentaloma is a mass found during radiologic screening for another condition (e.g., an abdominal CT scan for abdominal pain). Adrenal incidentalomas are seen in 3–5% of abdominal CT scans; most are nonfunctional adenomas.

Evaluation and treatment all depend on the answer to two questions:

1. Is the incidentaloma benign or malignant?
2. Is it functional?

The history and physical exam should focus on symptoms related to malignancy (weight loss, sweats, fevers, known history of cancer) and those indicating possible functional tumors (features of excessive cortisol on exam, symptoms of pheochromocytoma, hard-to-control hypertension, as seen with hyperaldosteronism). However, most individuals are asymptomatic. Ultimately, in these individuals, diagnosis relies on the characteristics of diagnostic imaging and functional testing.

1. *Benign or malignant*: Several characteristics on imaging help determine this status:
   - Size—The larger the mass, the more likely it is to be a malignant, whether metastatic or primary. The larger its size, the worse the prognosis. A unilateral mass >4 cm is very likely to be an adrenocortical carcinoma (a rare but aggressive adrenal cortex tumor portending poor survival).
   - Density on CT—If it is <10 Hounsfield units (i.e., the density of fat), it is extremely unlikely to be malignant.
   - Intravenous contrast washout on CT—Benign adenomas have very quick contrast washout (>50% is gone after 10 minutes); malignant ones do not.
   - Other imaging modalities—Positron emission tomography (PET) and MRI have questionable yield above and beyond abdominal CT except in cases of known malignancy (PET may be useful) or when pheochromocytoma is suspected (MRI may be useful).

   These distinguishing characteristics of common adrenal masses are summarized in Table 7-1.
2. *Functional or nonfunctional*: Most incidentalomas are nonfunctional, but many secrete subclinical levels of cortisol. Ten percent secrete cortisol, less then 5% are pheochromocytomas, and even fewer are aldosterone-secreting since many are diagnosed before they reach significant size on CT.

Work-up may include:

- Twenty-four-hour urine metanephrines and catecholamines and plasma metanephrines.
- Hypercortisol work-up with 24-hour urine cortisol especially if the incidentaloma is symptomatic or a 1-mg dexamethasone suppression test.
- Aldosterone and renin levels are useful if the individual is hypertensive.
- Androgen levels typically are not useful. Most patients will have signs or symptoms.

All incidentalomas larger than 4 cm should be resected, if possible, since many are likely adrenocortical cancers. For those that are not clearly benign or are considered malignant based on the above features, watchful waiting with repeat imaging is indicated. Fast-growing incidentalomas (>1 cm in 6–12 months) should be removed. Repeat hormonal testing can be done annually, although the data for this procedure are limited.

Approach to the Thyroid Nodule

1. *Important elements of the history and physical exam*
   - A history of head and neck radiation or a family history.
   - A rapidly growing, hard or firm lesion; lymphadenopathy.
   - Associated weight loss, sweats, fevers, bone pain.
   - Localized neck pain.
   - Signs of hyper- or hypothyroidism.
   - Age and gender: cancer is more common at extremes of age, and >5% of women may have thyroid nodules.
2. *Causes*

   Benign: multinodular goiter, Hashimoto's thyroiditis, cyst, follicular adenoma, Hürthle cell adenoma.

   Malignant: papillary, follicular, medullary, anaplastic, lymphoma, metastatic (breast, renal).
3. *Work-up*—See Figure 7-2.

Table 7-1. Characteristics of Common Adrenal Masses

Tumor Type	Benign Adenoma	Pheochromocytoma	Adrenocortical Carcinoma	Metastases
Appearance	Round, homogeneous, smooth margins	Variable shapes, cystic, hemorrhagic	Irregular shape Inhomogeneous, likely from central tumor necrosis Sometimes calcification is seen	Irregular and inhomogeneous
Size	Usually <4 cm	Variable size	Usually >4 cm	Variable size
Number	Unilateral	10% are bilateral	Unilateral	Usually bilateral
CT Characteristics	Rapid IV contrast washout Low attenuation <10 Hounsfield units	Delayed IV contrast washout	Delay IV contrast washout	Delayed IV contrast washout High attenuation (>20 Hounsfield units)
Other Features	Lipid-like characteristics on MRI	High T2 signal on MRI Usually highly vascular Do not biopsy (can precipitate hypertensive crisis)	High uptake on PET scan	PET useful if known metastasis Fine needle biopsy usually performed if there is known cancer

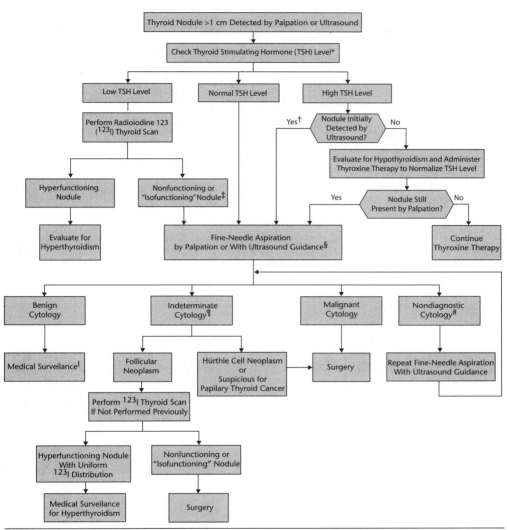

Figure 7-2 boxes:

Thyroid Nodule >1 cm Detected by Palpation or Ultrasound

Check Thyroid Stimulating Hormone (TSH) Level*

Low TSH Level

Normal TSH Level

High TSH Level

Perform Radioiodine 123 (^{123}I) Thyroid Scan

Nodule Initially Detected by Ultrasound?

Yes† No

Evaluate for Hypothyroidism and Administer Thyroxine Therapy to Normalize TSH Level

Hyperfunctioning Nodule

Nonfunctioning or "Isofunctioning" Nodule‡

Nodule Still Present by Palpation?

Yes   No

Evaluate for Hyperthyroidism

Fine-Needle Aspiration by Palpation or With Ultrasound Guidance§

Continue Thyroxine Therapy

Benign Cytology

Indeterminate Cytology¶

Malignant Cytology

Nondiagnostic Cytology$^#$

Medical Surveillance^l

Follicular Neoplasm

Hürthle Cell Neoplasm or Suspicious for Papilary Thyroid Cancer

Surgery

Repeat Fine-Needle Aspiration With Ultrasound Guidance

Perform ^{123}I Thyroid Scan If Not Performed Previously

Hyperfunctioning Nodule With Uniform ^{123}I Distribution

Nonfunctioning or "Isofunctioning" Nodule

Medical Surveilance for Hyperthyroidism

Surgery

*Cutpoints for low, normal, and high TSH levels vary according to laboratory.
†Evaluate for hypothyroidism.
‡Evaluate for hyperthyroidism.
§Indications for fine-needle aspiration guided by ultrasound include palpable nodule greater than 50% cystic, difficult to palpate or nonpalpable nodules, and nondiagnositc cytology on previous fine-needle aspiration.
lPerform diagnostic thyroid ultrasound if not previously performed.
¶Follicular neoplasm, Hürthle cell neoplasm, suspicious for papillary thyroid cancer.
$^#$Insufficient quantity of follicular thyroid cells.

Figure 7-2. Algorithmic Approach to the Thyroid Nodule.
JAMA December 1, 2004. 292(21):2632–264. Copyright © 2004 American Medical Association. All rights reserved.

231

Approach to the Hypercortisol State (Cushing's Syndrome)

1. *Suspected clues on history and physical exam*
   - New-onset hypertension, diabetes mellitus (DM), weight gain
   - New hirsutism, darker skin color [suggests corticotrophin (ACTH) hypersecretion], abdominal striae, new acne
   - Unusual fat distribution, "buffalo hump" over posterior neck, "moon faces," and supraclavicular fat pads are classic signs
   - History of poor wound healing
   - New-onset osteoporosis or unexplained fracture or avascular necrosis
   - Oligo/amenorrhea or impotence
   - Inability to concentrate, mood changes, psychosis
2. *Main causes*
   - Excess steroid use (oral, topical or inhaled, or progestin excess)
   - Cushing's disease (ACTH hypersecretion by pituitary adenoma)
   - Adrenal adenoma (excess cortisol secretion)
   - Ectopic ACTH (small cell lung cancer is the most classic symptom)
   - Unknown (15% of cases)
   - Pseudo-Cushing's syndrome—severe physical and psychological stress, severe bacterial infection, severe obesity or polycystic ovary syndrome, and, rarely, in those with chronic alcoholism.
3. *Work-up (inpatient or outpatient)*: Currently, there is no strict agreement on the proper algorithm.

1. *Screening tests*
   Overnight low-dose dexamethasone suppression test: 1 mg dexamethasone is given at 11 p.m. and at 8 a.m. cortisol and ACTH are measured. This low dose should reliably suppress ACTH in the normal pituitary gland, leading to cortisol suppression and reduced urinary excretion of cortisol as well. If the cortisol level is <5 µg/dL (fluorometric assay) or 2 µg/dL [high-performance liquid chromatography (HPLC) assay], this excludes Cushing's syndrome (98% negative predictive value). If the cortisol level is >14 µg/dL, the condition is probably Cushing's syndrome. Otherwise, the test result is equivocal.

   (*Note*: Drugs such as phenytoin, rifampin, primidone, and phenobarbitol increase dexamethasone metabolism and cause false-positive test results. Estrogens in oral contraceptives (OCPs) can prevent dexamethasone suppression. Therefore, check the 8 a.m. dexamethasone level if this is a concern; the ideal concentration is 2.0–6.5 ng/m.)

   Midnight serum cortisol/ACTH levels: These are checked at a time when the levels should be lowest. Typically, this is done three nights in a row. Cushing's syndrome is unlikely if the cortisol level is <5 µg/dL, but it may exist if the level is >7.5 µg/dL.

   Midnight salivary cortisol tests: Obtain samples on three consecutive evenings. Reference ranges differ widely, depending on the type of test. These tests are useful because they can be done on an outpatient basis, as the cortisol level is stable in the sample for hours.

2. *Confirmatory tests*
   Twenty-four-hour urine free cortisol: A ratio of >95 g cortisol per gram of Cr or more than three times the upper limit of normal for the assay confirms the presence of Cushing's syndrome. False positives occur with pregnancy, higher fluid intake, and use of carbamazepine and fenofibrate.

   Two-day low-dose dexamethasone suppression test: Dexamethasone 0.5 mg is given q6 hr x 48 hours. Six hours after the last dose, of cortisol/ACTH is drawn. Cutoffs are approximately the same. (This test is rarely done except on an inpatient basis, usually concomitantly with urinary testing.)

3. *Localization*
   If the above tests are positive and clinical suspicion is high, then localize the cause to either the adrenals, the pituitary, or an ectopic area.
   - If ACTH is low, with elevated cortisol, then this suggests an adrenal adenoma.

- If ACTH is high, with elevated cortisol, then this suggests Cushing's disease or ectopic ACTH.

The tests of choice are as follows:
- Pituitary MRI is performed, (adenoma is seen only in 50% of cases, however) followed by selective inferior petrosal venous sampling for ACTH, with corticotrophin releasing hormone (CRH) stimulation to confirm a pituitary source.
- An adrenal CT or MRI scan is done if ACTH is low and cortisol is elevated to look for an adrenal adenoma.
- A chest CT, MRI, or octreotide scan can be done for localization of ectopic sources of ACTH. Biopsy is done prior to resection in most cases.

[Note: Classically, the high-dose dexamethasone suppression test (8 mg overnight or for 2 days, similar to the low-dose protocol) was used to differentiate ectopic ACTH (which does not suppress) from pituitary ACTH adenoma (which does suppress); however, its utility has been questioned.]

Approach to the Patient with Amenorrhea

Amenorrhea is defined as the absence of menses, which can be primary (no menarche by age 16 with secondary sex characteristics or by age 12 with no secondary sex characteristics) or secondary (missing three cycles or 6 months in those who previously had menarche, which is the focus here.

1. Important elements of the history/physical exam
   - Recent stressors, weight loss, anorexia (hypothalamic amenorrhea).
   - Use of medications such as high-dose progestins, antipsychotics, or metoclopramide (increases prolactin levels).
   - Headaches/visual field deficits/galactorrhea (hyperprolactinemia).
   - Hirsutism, acne, irregular menses (hyperandrogenism).
   - Marked weight gain, striae, hypertension, DM (polycystic ovary syndrome, Cushing's syndrome).
   - Hot flashes, vaginal dryness, decreased libido (premature ovarian failure).
   - Recent obstetric procedures, endometritis or pelvic inflammatory disease (Asherman's syndrome).
   - Causes are shown in Table 7-2, and an algorithm for work-up is presented in Figure 7-3.

Table 7-2. Causes of Amenorrhea

1. Pregnancy
2. Hypothalamic hypogonadism leading to functional or hypothalamic amenorrhea as in eating disorder, excessive stress, or exercise and severe weight loss
3. Asherman's syndrome (scarring of the endometrial lining)
4. Ovarian failure
   Menopause
   Premature/gonadal dysgenesis (loss of oocytes/follicles)
   Medication related (chemotherapy)
   Infection (TB)
5. Hypothalamic-Pituitary-Adrenal axis dysfunction
   Hyperprolactinemia (prolactinoma/medications)
   Pituitary tumor
   Apoplexy
   Empty sella syndrome
   Cranial irradiation
6. Anatomic (usually primary amenorrhea)
   Absence of uterus, vagina, or cervix, müllerian agenesis
   Imperforate hymen/transverse vaginal septum
7. Thyroid disease (hyper- or hypothyroidism)
8. Exogenous androgens
9. Other (congenital adrenal hyperplasia, PCOS, androgen insensitivity)

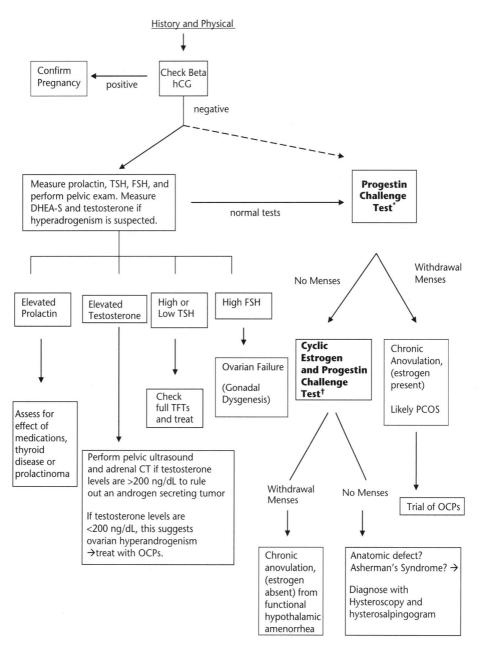

Figure 7-3. Diagnostic Approach to Amenorrhea.

*A progestin challenge is 10 mg of medroxyprogesterone acetate for 10 days.

†Commonly used regimens are oral conjugated estrogens for 35 days with medroxyprogesterone added (10 mg daily for the last 10 days).

DHEAS, dehydroepiandrosterone sulfate; FSH, follicle stimulating hormone; hCG, human chorionic gonadotropin; OCP, oral contraceptive pill; PCOS, polycystic ovary syndrome; TFTs, thyroid function tests; TSH, thyroid stimulating hormone.

Diseases in Endocrinology

The Thyroid Gland

Anatomy

- They thyroid gland is composed of two lobes connected by an isthmus (see Figure 7-4). The pyramidal lobe is a remnant.
- Abnormal development may present as (1) a *lingual thyroid* (a remnant posterior to the tongue) or as (2) *thyroglossal duct cysts* (parts left behind during migration).
- Innervation is via two recurrent laryngeal nerves and one superior laryngeal nerve branching off the vagus.

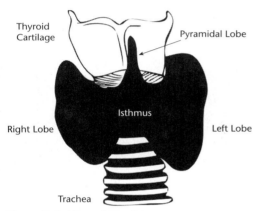

Figure 7-4. Thyroid Gland Anatomy.

Table 7-3. Differences Between T4 and T3

T4	T3
75% bound to TBG, albumin	99.6% bound to TBG, albumin
7-day half-life	1.5-day half-life
Secretion from thyroid only	20% from thyroid, 80% from conversion in liver, kidney, and pituitary
Converted in tissues to T3 (the active form to work on nuclear receptors)	Four times as potent as T4
Replacement medication = levothyroxine	Replacement medication = liothyronine

TBG, thyroid binding globulin.

Physiology

Two hormones are produced, triiodothyronine (T3) and thyroxine (T4) (see Table 7-3). Only the free forms are active. Their basic function is to stimulate protein synthesis, carbohydrate metabolism, fat turnover, increase cardiac contractility, and increase the number of β-adrenergic receptors, which are critical for brain and skeletal development.

Diagnostic Testing

Common tests used to evaluate thyroid function are shown in Table 7-4.

Diseases of the Thyroid Gland

Hyperthyroidism

D—A disease in which there is excess thyroxine hormone for normal homeostasis or the body somehow stimulates the release of excess thyroxine. There are multiple causes, as listed below.

Epi—Graves' disease is by far the most common cause, followed by nodular goiters, thyroiditis and adenomas. For Graves' disease, female patients outnumber males by 8:1.

P—Table 7-5 lists multiple causes of hyperthyroidism with their pathology.

SiSx

General—increased warmth, diaphoresis, weight loss, with normal or increased appetite, fevers, tremor, LAN.

Skin—dry skin, clubbing, phalangeal osteoarthropathy (*thyroid acropachy*), and pretibial myxedema (rare and the least common manifestation, usually not seen before exophthalmos develops) seen as a nonpitting thickening of the skin that is usually asymptomatic but can be painful.

Neck—pain is more common in subacute thyroiditis (de Quervain's disease) or suppurative thyroiditis and is not seen in Graves' disease or subacute lymphocytic thyroiditis. If there are palpable nodules, consider toxic multinodular goiter (TMG). Goiters may or may not be seen in Graves' disease.

Eyes—periorbital edema, proptosis, and lid lag can be seen (ask the patient to follow your fingers up and then down quickly; the

Table 7-4.   Diagnostic Tests of the Thyroid

TSH	The initial screening test for thyroid dysfunction. Most sensitive test of hyper- or hypothyroidism when the cause is not central (from anterior pituitary damage).
T4	Can be measured directly as free T4 (the active form of the hormone) or total T4 (protein bound). This total amount can fluctuate in states that alter TBG and albumin levels, such as pregnancy, oral contraceptive use, and liver disease.
T3 Resin Uptake	An indirect way to measure free T4. The patient's serum sample is mixed with radiolabeled T3 and resin to trap unbound T3. The test is used to distinguish changes in binding protein from true states of thyroid hormone over- or underproduction. The T3RU is inversely proportional to the amount of protein-bound T4. A free T4 index is used to calculate the free T4 level: take the T3 resin uptake divided by average normal T4 (which is 30%), then multiply by total T4.
T3	Useful when hyperthyroidism suspected in those with low TSH and T4 is normal. Occasionally, isolated T3 elevations are seen.
RAI Uptake	Radioactive iodine uptake test. I-123 is used for evaluation of thyroid function in hyperthyroid states. Scanning is done 24 hours after administration. I-123 is reduced in subacute thyroiditis, exogenous T4 production, and iodine-induced hyperthyroidism. Significant uptake is seen in Graves' disease (diffuse uptake) and large, functioning nodular goiters (patchy uptake) where the gland is iodine avid, with values >30%. Focally increased uptake is seen in solitary hyperfunctioning nodules. Prior use of IV contrast makes this test less reliable.
Pertecnetate Scanning	A nuclear medicine scan that does not employ iodine but can be used similarly to RAI to assess hyperthyroid states. Metabolically active thyroid tissues is compared to activity seen in the salivary glands. Takes less time than an RAI scan.
Serum Thyroglobulin (TG)	Made by the thyroid gland, used as tumor marker after thyroidectomy in cancer patients. Also used to differentiate hyperthyroidism from exogenous T4 (will be suppressed) vs. lymphocytic thyroiditis (will be elevated due to inflammation). An anti-TG antibody test is also performed, as these are common and can affect results as well.
Antibody Testing Antimicrosomal or Antiperodidase Antibody (anti-TPO)	Present in nearly all cases of Hashimoto's thyroiditis and 40–80% of cases of Graves' disease. But also seen commonly in type I DM (40%) and pregnancy.
Anti-TSH Receptor Stimulating Antibody	Up to 95% of Graves' disease patients will be positive. Occasionally seen in autoimmune thyroiditis. Helpful in predicting neonatal thyrotoxicosis in mothers with Graves' disease and conditions where RAI cannot be performed. Of note, not all antibodies are stimulatory. Some, as in autoimmune thyroiditis, block the binding of TSH and therefore can cause hypothyroidism.
Anti-TG Antibody	Up to 90% positive in autoimmune thyroiditis, but commonly seen in many other hyperthyroid states and in type I DM and pregnancy. This test is most useful when compared with TG levels.
Thyroid US	Useful for evaluating abnormalities in thyroid anatomy and for guidance in fine needle aspirates. Distinguishes solid from cystic masses and evaluates for abnormal lymph nodes in thyroid cancer.

Table 7-5. Different Causes and Pathogenesis of Hyperthyroidism

Causes of Hyperthyroidism	Definition	Pathogenesis	Diagnostic Clues
Graves' Disease	A syndrome of hyperthyroidism, goiter, ophthalmopathy/orbitopathy, and dermopathy.	Autoimmune condition from TSH receptor–activating antibodies and their sequelae, including activated T cells that increase the secretion of thyroid-specific autoantibodies from B cells.	Low TSH, elevated free T4 and/or T3 in the appropriate clinical setting. RAI is elevated, with uptake usually >30%. Thyroid is usually enlarged, with a bruit or thrill on exam. Two exam findings are specific to Graves' disease: infiltrating dermopathy (from dermal glycosaminoglycan accumulation) and orbitopathy causing exophthalmos (from extraocular muscle, fat, and connective tissue inflammation).
Toxic Adenoma	A single thyroid adenoma that produces excessive thyroid hormone, resulting in hyperthyroidism.	Somatic mutation of the TSH receptor, making it overactive.	RAI typically shows marked uptake that is focal and nonuniform.
Toxic Multi-nodular Goiter	Multiple autonomously functioning thyroid nodules producing T4 that results in hyperthyroidism.	A constitutively active mutation of the TSH receptor that can be present in up to 25% of cases.	RAI typically shows focal uptake, and patient has an enlarged thyroid nodule. Multiple hyperfunctioning nodules can be present, although one nodule may be dominant.
Subacute Granulomatous Thyroiditis (de Quervain's Thyroiditis)	A painful viral-mediated subacute inflammation of the thyroid gland that usually has a triphasic course of hyperthyroidism, hypothyroidism, and return to normal thyroid function.	Viral in origin, with significant inflammation. Many viruses, such as coxsackievirus, Epstein-Barr virus, adenovirus, echovirus, and influenza, have been associated, but viral inclusion bodies are not seen on histologic exam; hence, the immune response to the infection may also play a major role.	Can present as hyperthyroidism initially, which may be followed by hypothyroidism after all the TG and T4 are released. Neck pain is a prominent component and is very important in making the diagnosis. Diagnosis confirmed by low RAI uptake with high T4 and T3 in serum. RAI uptake is low because follicular cells are injured and unable to readily take up iodine.
Suppurative Thyroiditis	A painful thyroiditis usually due to nonviral infections.	Secondary to a bacterial infection; may be related to IVDU in adults.	Patient appears to be quite ill and the neck is painful. Fever and evidence of infection are usually apparent.

continued

Table 7-5. (*continued*)

Causes of Hyperthyroidism	Definition	Pathogenesis	Diagnostic Clues
Subacute Lymphocytic Thyroiditis	A painless thyroiditis due to an autoimmune process.	Cell-mediated autoimmune process similar to that in Hashimoto's thyroiditis; perhaps cytokines mediated in response to some other subclinical injury.	A hyperthyroid state but, importantly, painless. Usually there is no thyroid enlargement or a small goiter. RAI typically shows lower than normal uptake. TSH may be higher than expected as well. TG concentrations are low.
Postpartum Thyroiditis	A painless, self-limiting thyroiditis that usually resolves 2–6 months after delivery and that typically started with hyperthyroidism followed by hypothyroidism.	Very similar to subacute lymphocytic thyroiditis; also thought to be autoimmune related.	Can present as hyperthyroidism, hypothyroidism, or both. Seen even upto several months postpartum or postabortion. Painless and usually self limiting. A clinical diagnosis once distinguished from Graves' disease. Increases the risk of hypothyroidism later in life, however.
Amiodarone-Related	Derangement in thyroid hormone production and/or release due to amiodarone use.	Can cause both hyper- and hypothyroidism. Daily amiodarone 200 mg contains 20 times more iodine than a normal diet, and the incidence of hyperthyroidism is about 4% after the first year. Mechanisms include inhibition of conversion of T4 to T3 as well as T3 nuclear receptor binding (type I), resulting in increased T4 production. Alternatively, it can cause a destructive thyroiditis from the direct toxic effect (type II).	May be somewhat asymptomatic because of the AV nodal-blocking properties of amiodarone. The history is extremely important, as is exclusion of other causes. It is hard to distinguish between types I and II. RAI is results are difficult to interpret in making the diagnosis. In these patients, given their significant iodine exposure. Type I can often be treated with thionamides such propylthiouracil (PTU) and methimazole. Type II may require steroids in addition to stopping medication.
Exogenous Thyroxine Intake	Hyperthyroidism due to iatrogenic excessive administration of thyroid replacement.	Patient knowingly or unknowingly is taking excessive amounts of T3 or T4.	Mimics other types of hyperthyroidism in laboratory values and symptoms. RAI, if done, will be normal. Requires a high degree of suspicion if the patient is not forthcoming. Serum TG should be low, in contrast to that seen in Graves' disease or thyroiditis.

Table 7-5.   (continued)

Causes of Hyperthyroidism	Definition	Pathogenesis	Diagnostic Clues
Iodine-Induced Reaction	Hyperthyroidism from administration of iodine, sometimes called the *Jod-Basedow effect*.	Large doses of iodine via a contrast CT scan in cardiac catheterization usually given to a patient with abnormal sensitivity from underlying thyroid disease (e.g., with endemic goiter and iodide deficiency or nodular goiter containing autonomous nodules or Graves' disease) that causes significant overproduction of T4.	Clinical history.
Central Hyperthyroidism	Hyperthyroidism due to excessive TSH action on the thyroid gland causing overproduction of T4.	TSH-secreting pituitary tumor. This is quite rare, as are other TSH-secreting tumors.	Would expect to see an inappropriately normal or high TSH as well as high free T4 or T3.
hCG Tumor	Hyperthyroidism from overstimulation of the thyroid gland by a TSH-like substance that results in T4 overproduction.	The α subunit of hCG is similar to that of TSH. It may be seen in choriocarcinoma.	The hCG level will be markedly elevated. Consider this in the post- or peripartum setting.

hCG, human chorionic gonadotropin.

eyes follow but it takes a second for the lids to catch up, so you see a little more of the whites of the eyes). New exophthalmos is seen only with Graves' orbitopathy.

Cardiovascular—sinus tachycardia, atrial fibrillation, high-output cardiac failure (if prolonged), dyspnea on exertion (DOE).

Musculoskeletal—proximal muscle weakness

Bone—osteoporosis, hypercalcemia, irregular menses.

GI/GU—hyperdefecation.

(*Note*: older patients may have few symptoms except mild weakness instead, so-called apathetic hyperthyroidism.)

Dx—See above for specific findings. For most causes, the diagnosis is made by finding a low or undetectable thyroid stimulating hormone (TSH) combined with a high free T4, T3 resin uptake or T3. Thyroid stimulating hormone is the best initial screening test when used alone to rule out hyperthyroidism. It is most useful when central hyperthyroidism (pituitary disease) is not suspected, because in central hyperthyroidism TSH will be elevated along with thyroid function. Subsequently, if the diagnosis is not obvious by the history and exam, most patients will undergo thyroid scanning with radioactive iodine (RAI) or pertechnetate. In either study, one will not see significant uptake in subacute thyroiditis on exogenous T4 administration, but one will see increased uptake in Graves' disease and multinodular goiter (>30%). The RAI level is typically less than 1% in those with exogenous or ectopic hyperthyroidism from TSH suppression. Thyroglobulin (TG) is low in patients with exogenous T4 but high in those with subacute thyroiditis, iodine-induced hyperthyroidism, and struma ovarii (very rare condition of an ovarian tumor with functional thyroid tissue). Thyroglobulin levels are unreliable if anti-TG antibodies are present.

Tx—Treatment depends on the severity of the condition. With mild non-Graves' thyroiditis, a β blocker can be used until the thyroiditis resolves. In younger patients with Graves' disease, antithyroid medications are first-line therapy: methimazole (a daily drug and better for long-term therapy) or propylthiouracil (PTU, a three times a day drug that is preferred in pregnancy and used more often in acute situations since it has the added effect of blocking peripheral T4 to T3 conversion). These drugs may be used in conjunction with β blockers early on. Those who fail with such medication or older patients are more likely candidates for either radioiodine ablation or partial or full thyroidectomy as a last resort. Radioactive iodine ablates active tissue within weeks but can produce hypothyroidism requiring supplementation. For Graves' dermopathy (a late complication), one can try topical steroids, which may help lead to regression. For Graves' ophthalmopathy/orbitopathy in general, treatment of hyperthyroidism halts disease progression. Oral steroids can be used if symptoms are severe, as can decompressive surgery. Radioactive iodine may worsen Graves' eye disease. Finally, subacute thyroiditis is typically treated with NSAIDs, β blockers, and occasionally steroids. Less than 5% of patients have recurrence.

Thyroid Storm

D—An abrupt, severe exacerbation of thyrotoxicosis that is life-threatening.

RF—It is usually precipitated by a major stressor like infection, surgery, MI, or DKA in a patient with uncontrolled hyperthyroidism or one with an acute iodine load.

SiSx—High-grade fevers up to 104°–106°F are not uncommon. Marked anxiety/agitation, psychosis, hyperhidrosis, weakness, and tachyarrhythmias (typically at heart rates over 140 bpm are seen, along with CHF). Gastrointestinal symptoms such as nausea, vomiting, and diarrhea may be present, as well as fulminant liver failure.

Dx—Diagnostic criteria have been specified that include parameters such as the presence of CHF and liver dysfunction, as well as temperature, heart rate, and mental status. Typically, this is a clinical diagnosis in a patient with known or discovered hyperthyroidism that requires immediate attention.

Tx—Assess for and treat sepsis or any insulting factor. Otherwise, treatment is based on covering all physiologic mechanisms through which an overactive thyroid gland acts.

1. Thionamides (methimazole or propylthiouracil) are given initially at high doses to block the formation of new thyroid hormone.

2. This is followed by iodine (at least 1 hour following thionamide administration, usually as a saturated potassium iodide solution) to block the release of preformed thyroid hormone.

3. High-dose glucocorticoids can also be used to block the conversion of T4 to T3.

4. β blockers (very cautiously if the patient has florid CHF) such as propranolol or esmolol IV are typically used as well initially.

5. Finally, iodinated radiocontrast agents may provide a quick iodine load, but this treatment is not commonly used in the United States.

Subclinical Hyperthyroidism

D—Condition in which TSH is suppressed, while T4 and T3 levels are normal

P—It can be a precursor to Graves' disease, autonomous nodules, multinodular goiter, or following the use of antithyroid drugs/RAI after treatment for hyperthyroidism. Hospitalized patients, and those taking high-dose steroids and dopamine, are associated with this condition. It progresses to overt hyperthyroidism at the rate of 5% per year.

SiSx—All of the symptoms commonly associated with hyperthyroidism can be seen, including osteoporosis and cardiovascular effects. Alternatively, they may be relatively asymptomatic.

Dx—Diagnosis is made by the thyroid function tests mentioned above. Repeat tests may be needed, however, to confirm the diagnosis. Also, consider using 24-hour RAI uptake to rule out silent thyroiditis versus Graves' disease versus TMG.

Tx—Consider treatment with antithyroid drugs if the patient is older, TSH is <0.1 mU/L, or if the patient has evidence of osteoporosis or is very symptomatic.

Hypothyroidism

D—Thyroid hormone deficiency.

Epi—It is found in up to 15% of people >65 years old.

P—The most common cause is Hashimoto's thyroiditis, followed by iatrogenic disease (postradioablative or postsurgical) as a sequela of treatment for hyperthyroidism. Other causes include sequelae of subacute thyroiditis or postpartum thyroiditis (after the hyperthyroid phase), antithyroid drug excess (methimazole or PTU), specific drugs (lithium or amiodarone), iodine excess (inhibits organification of T 4 and T3) or deficiency (escape organification occurs when the thyroid is intrinsically abnormal), central hypothyroidism (reduced pituitary TSH), and Riedel's struma (replacement by fibrous connective tissue).

SiSx

General—fatigue, weight gain, cold intolerance, muscle cramps.

Cardiovascular/pulmonary—pleural or pericardial effusions, DOE, sleep apnea.

Eyes—periorbital edema.

Neck—goiter.

Hematologic—macrocytic anemia.

CNS—impaired memory, depression, carpal tunnel syndrome, decreased deep tendon reflexes (DTRs)

GI/GU—constipation, ileus, oligo- or amenorrhea, hypermenorrhea, or mennorhagia.

Skin—nonpitting edema, dry hair, thinning of brows, decreased sweating.

Dx—Diagnosis is made on the basis of elevated TSH and low T4 in primary hypothyroidism and low TSH and low T4 and T3 in central

hypothyroidism. Electrolytes should be checked since hyponatremia is common via the syndrome of inappropriate antidiuretic hormone (SIADH), which can occur with hypothyroidism. Hashimoto's thyroiditis is usually differentiated from the other causes of hypothyroidism on clinical grounds after eliciting a good history. Radionuclide scanning is not necessary to make the diagnosis.

Tx—T4 replacement is standard care, started at a lower dose in elderly patients, usually 25 µg, and is increased slowly. Thyroid stimulating hormone should be measured 6 weeks after dose adjustment. In central hypothyroidism, testing for panhypopituitarism is indicated. In this case, hydrocortisone is typically given before starting T4 because of the possibility of adrenal insufficiency. Note that there are drugs that affect thyroid hormone replacement, and patients should be instructed about these interaction if they take such drugs:

Decreased absorption: cholestyramine, sucralfate, iron or Ca^{2+} preparations.

Increased metabolism: antiseizure medications, rifampin.

Changes in thyroid binding globlin (TBG): estrogens increase TBG and therefore lower unbound T4 levels. As a result, higher doses are often required for patients with high estrogen levels—those taking OCPs or hormone replacement therapy (HRT) and pregnant patients. Conversely, TBG can be lowered by androgens, nephrotic syndrome, or cirrhosis.

Subclinical Hypothyroidism

D—Condition in which there is normal T4 with elevated TSH.

P—It can be a forerunner of primary hypothyroidism in the setting of high-titer antithyroid peroxidase TPO antibodies Many patients eventually develop hypothyroidism (estimated at a rate of 4% a year). Other causes include status post ablative therapy for Graves' disease and insufficient T4 replacement for hypothyroidism.

SiSx—Some patients may be asymptomatic; others may have symptoms consistent with mild hypothyroidism.

Dx—The TSH level is slightly but not markedly elevated (up to the 20 mU/L at most); however, free and total T4 will be normal, as will T3. In some cases (if the patient is markedly symptomatic), checking for anti-TPO antibodies may be useful.

Tx—The decision to treat is controversial. Currently, replacement with T4 is recommended for patients with subclinical hypothyroidism and a TSH level >10 mU/L.

Euthyroid Sick Syndrome

D—Abnormalities in the thyroid function test in the setting of a significant non thyroid illness but in the absence of underlying thyroid disease.

P—It is thought to be due to the release of cytokines such as tumor necrosis factor-α (TNFα), interleukin (IL)-6, and IL-1. There may be a deficiency of certain cofactors needed by the type I deiodinase enzyme (e.g., NADPH or glutathione) in the setting of severe illness.

RF—Risk factors include sepsis, renal failure, MI, starvation, burn/trauma, bone marrow transplant (BMT), and malignancy.

SiSx—Patients usually present with a significant underlying illness (e.g., infection, trauma, shock) and not with thyroid related symptoms.

Dx—The diagnosis is clinical. A variety of thyroid function test (TFT) abnormalities can be seen. The most common pattern of TFTs is low total/unbound T3 with a normal T4 and TSH. If checked, the reverse T3 (rT3) will be found to be elevated. Severely ill patients will also have a low T4 from altered binding to TBG. The TSH values are variable but are >0.05 µIU/mL. Ten percent of patients will have low TSH values.

Tx—Abnormalities are usually reversible after recovery from illness. Therefore, treating the underlying medical condition is indicated.

Myxedema Coma

D—A condition in which severe hypothyroidism leads to life-threatening complications.

Epi—It is now less common due to early recognition of hypothyroidism. It is seen mostly in elderly women.

P—It is usually precipitated by an acute event in the setting of long-standing hypothyroidism.

RF—Risk factors include sepsis, cold weather, use of CNS depressants, trauma, and surgery.

SiSx—Patients exhibit profound lethargy with a spectrum ranging from change in mental status to coma. Also seen are hypothermia, bradycardia, hypotension, hypoventilation, hypoglycemia delayed DTRs, and areflexia. Usually multiorgan system failure ensues.

Dx—This is mainly a clinical diagnosis, as treatment is urgent. Just before initiating therapy, TFTs should be performed in addition to checking the cortisol level (looking for concomitant adrenal insufficiency or panhypopituitarism). Checking electrolytes is also important since many patients also have concomitant low sodium levels.

Tx—Treatment should occur based on clinical suspicions without waiting for confirmatory results. Either T3 or T4 or both should be given in IV form (GI absorption may be impaired). Typically, a loading dose is given followed by daily maintenance dosing. Stress doses of steroids are given until adrenal insufficiency is ruled out. The rest is supportive care, which may include IV hydration, ventilatory support, and hypothermia correction with warming blankets. The mortality rate is 20–50%.

Thyroid Cancer

D—The most common endocrine malignancy. It is discussed here since it is managed primarily by endocrinologists rather than oncologists. Table 7-6 summarizes the most commonly encountered types.

Epi—Female patients outnumber males by 2:1 for most types. The total incidence is about 25,000 cases per year. Evidence of the papillary form of thyroid cancer is quite common at autopsy (up to 30%).

Tx—Postsurgical Treatment of Papillary Cancer: After thyroidectomy, there is almost always some degree of residual tissue left in the thyroid bed, which is seen on a postoperative radionuclide I-123 scan. Radioactive iodine (I-131) is used to ablate the remaining thyroid tissue after a period of thyroid hormone withdrawal. Thyroid hormone replacement is then reinitiated to induce TSH suppression. Thyroglobulin is a marker for recurrence and is monitored periodically along with

Table 7-6. Features of the Four Major Forms of Thyroid Cancer

Cancer Type	Papillary	Follicular	Medullary	Anaplastic
% of All Thyroid Cancer	60%–80%	10%	5%	<2%
Age	40 to 50s	All ages	50 to 60s unless MEN associated (20s–30s)	60 to 70s.
Mode of Spread	Lymphatic	Angioinvasion/hematogenous spread	Both lymphatic and hematogenous	Local spread, lymphatic and hematogenous
RF	Family history and neck irradiation	? Iodine deficiency Neck irradiation	Family history of MEN II or III. 80% of cases are otherwise sporadic	History of prior differentiated thyroid cancer
FNA or Biopsy Specimen	May see psammoma bodies (unencapsulated remnants of infarcted tumor papillae) in addition to the papillary structure overall and the presence of coffee bean nuclei.	Monotonous, uniform microfollicles resembling the normal microscopic pattern of the thyroid but with anaplastic-appearing cells.	Amyloid may be seen on histologic exam. Medullary thyroid carcinoma (MTC) is a neuroendocrine cell tumor.	Giant spindle cells. Usually develops from other differentiated tumors.
SiSx	Solitary thyroid nodule	Painless subclinical thyroid mass or nodule in many cases. Ten percent of patients have metastases at diagnosis with metastases to bone and lung and may present with a pathologic fracture.	Solitary thyroid nodule that occurs more commonly in the upper portion of thyroid, where most of the C cells are located.	Presents with a rapidly enlarging thyroid mass. Ninety percent have local spread at the time of diagnosis. Up to 50% have metastases at diagnosis which may involve lymph nodes, the larynx, trachea, esophagus, tonsil, and lungs. Patients will have a hard nodular neck mass that may be painful, sometimes with focal necrosis. compression can cause dysphagia, dyspnea, cough, and hemoptysis.

continued

Table 7-6. (*continued*)

Cancer Type	Papillary	Follicular	Medullary	Anaplastic
Dx	FNA Multiple forms exist: follicular variant (most common), tall cell variant (more aggressive), insular, columnar, Hürthle, clear cell, diffuse sclerosing. U/S is useful to look for lymph node enlargement due to possible spread.	FNA	FNA Immunohistochemistry may increase the diagnosis yield. Occasionally, paraneoplastic ACTH secretion is possible. Serum calcium to assess for hyperparathyroidism should be done preoperatively.	FNA
Serum Tumor Markers	Thyroglobulin from thyroid tissue.	—	Calcitonin from C cells	—
Poor Prognostic Factors	Age over 45, >5 cm size, and metastases to lungs and bones	Age >45, metastases	Age at the time of diagnosis >40	—
Tx	If >1 cm: total thyroidectomy,* <1 cm: total vs. hemi-thyroidectomy, postoperative radioiodine ablation† T4 suppression.	Total thyroidectomy* with or without radioactive iodine with surveillance.	Total thyroidectomy* with central neck dissection because the tumor is usually multicentric.	Usually fatal. Therapy is either thyroidectomy* for local disease or palliative treatment. Death is usually from upper airway obstruction and suffocation.
10-Year Survival	95%	60%–90%	50%	100% die at 2 years

*Postoperatively, one must monitor for hypocalcemia in the event of parathyroid injury.
†I-131 ablation doses are typically much higher (100–300 mCi) than those given for Graves' disease (10–15 mCi) and toxic adenomas (30 mCi).
FNA, fine needle aspiration.

thyroglobulin antibodies. Surveillance for recurrence also includes measurement of thyroglobulin after administration of recombinant TSH as well as surveillance I-123 scans.

The Pituitary Gland

Anatomy

- Figure 7-5 shows the various parts of the pituitary gland, which is divided into anterior and posterior sections. The pituitary blood supply is from superior and inferior hypophysial arteries. The former is a branch off the internal carotid, and forms a capillary plexus around the hypothalamus and drains into the hypophysial portal system.
- Hypothalamic hormones [growth hormone releasing hormone (GHRH), somatostatin, dopamine, thyroid releasing hormone (TRH), corticotropin releasing hormone (CRH), gonadotropin releasing hormone (GnRH)] are released by means of this portal system to the anterior pituitary.
- Vasopressin and oxytocin are sent directly via the nerve terminals to the posterior pituitary (see Figure 7-5).

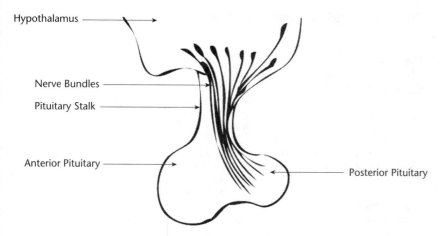

Figure 7-5. Pituitary Gland Anatomy.

Physiology

Secreted hormones and the conditions they cause in excess or deficiency are summarized in Table 7-7.

Pituitary Diseases

Pituitary Adenomas

D—A clonal neoplasm of the pituitary that can arise from any type of cell in anterior pituitary. Microadenomas are <1 cm in size; macroadenomas are >1 cm.

Epi—Asymptomatic adenomas are found in 15–20% of patients in imaging studies for other conditions.

P—Most common types are benign, nonfunctional, and nonsecreting tumors, followed by prolactinomas and then by growth hormone (GH)-, follicle stimulating hormone/luteinizing hormone (FSH/LH)-, and TSH-secreting tumors. Of note, pituitary hyperplasia occurs as a result of pregnancy or long-standing primary hypothyroidism/hypogonadism. Microadenomas <1 cm do not tend to compress surrounding structures. Symptoms are usually caused by localized effects or secretion of functional adenomas. The optic chasm is commonly compressed by large tumors, resulting in loss of superior visual fields followed by total bitemporal hemianopsia.

RF—A family history of multiple endocrine neoplasia 1 (MEN 1) syndrome (see Table 7-12) is a major risk factor.

SiSx—Most patients are asymptomatic. With compression, dull frontal headaches and visual changes are reported. With erosion through the floor of the cavernous sinus, injury to cranial nerves 2–6 are possible. Patients may have hypopituitarism (see below) from distortion of normal pituitary architecture or symptoms due to excess hormonal secretion.

Dx—Magnetic resonance imaging is the single best test for most sellar lesions. Evaluation of the hypothalamo-pituitary-adrenal (HPA) axis for hormonal hypersecretion [serum prolactin, insulin-like growth factor-1 (IGF-1), 24-hour urine cortisol, TFTs, FSH, and LH] is done when clinically indicated. In incidental adenomas measuring <10 mm, usually a prolactin test alone is appropriate and most cost effective. Hormonal deficiency is also possible, and work-up for hypopituitarism should relate to the clinical symptoms as well.

Tx—Treatment is dependent on the underlying cause. In asymptomatic cases after negative hormonal work-up, surveillance with MRI scans may be appropriate. For active or large LH/FSH-secreting tumors surgery is indicated, as medical therapy is ineffective. For TSH-secreting tumors, surgery is first-line therapy along with antithyroid drugs and/or octreotide.

Table 7-7. Hormones Secreted by the Pituitary Gland

	Excess	Deficiency	Tests
Anterior Pituitary Hormones			
GH	Acromegaly (in adulthood). Gigantism (congenital).	Growth failure in children. Few important features in adults except for an increase in adipose tissue and a decrease in muscle mass.	IGF-1 level Glucose tolerance test/GH
Prolactin	Galactorrhea, amenorrhea in females. Hypogonadism in males.	Postpartum failure of lactation in Sheehan's syndrome; otherwise, patients are asymptomatic.	Prolactin level. A level >200 µg/L is consistent with prolactinoma.
ACTH	Cushing's disease. Features of hypercortisolism with hypertension, hyperglycemia (e.g., weight gain, abnormal fat redistribution).	Adrenal insufficiency with symptoms of hypotension, nausea, weight loss, fatigue, and hypoglycemia.	A 24-hour urine cortisol test for excess along with an ACTH and cortisol level. For ACTH deficiency, a metyrapone test (for recent-onset or partial disease) and insulin-induced hypoglycemia test can be used.
FSH/LH	Neurologic symptoms due to mass effect. Rarely symptomatic (ovarian hyperstimulation, testicular enlargement, precocious puberty).	Amenorrhea, genital atrophy, loss of potency and libido.	FSH and LH levels, testosterone and estradiol.
TSH	Central hyperthyroidism (very rare).	Central hypothyroidism. Cretinism in children with marked mental retardation.	Thyroid function tests
Posterior Pituitary Hormones			
ADH	Syndrome of inappropriate ADH secretion (SIADH).	Central diabetes insipidus.	Urine and serum osmolality tests. Urine and serum Na for SIADH. Water deprivation test, ADH level and DDAVP stimulation test for diabetes insipidus.
Oxytocin	Pharmacologically used to induce labor.	—	—

ACTH, adrenocorticotropic hormone; ADH, antidiuretic hormone; FSH, follicle stimulating hormone; GH, growth hormone; LH, luteinizing hormone; TSH, thyroid stimulating hormone.

Prolactinoma, GH-secreting tumors, and hypopituitarism are discussed below.

Prolactinoma

D—A lactotroph tumor of the pituitary that secretes prolactin.

Epi—It accounts for 30–40% of pituitary adenomas. Female patients with microadenomas outnumber males. The condition is most common in the third and fourth decades. Mixed tumors secreting other substance in addition are also rarely seen.

P—Monoclonal expansion of a lactotroph is the primary cause. Many of the symptoms occur from prolactin itself and its disruption of the hypothalamic-pituitary-gonadal axis via effects on GnRH secretion Other causes of increased prolactin include:

Physiologic: pregnancy, breast feeding, post exercise, during sleep, the postprandial state, after seizure activity, and with hypothyroidism.

Pharmacologic: Antidopaminergic drugs (risperidone, haldol, metoclopramide) and estrogen.

Pathologic: Acromegaly (30–40% of GH tumors also secrete prolactin), renal failure, liver failure, hypothyroidism (decreased feedback), Craniopharyngioma (blocks suppressive dopamine transport from the hypothalamus), chest wall injury, or herpes simplex virus (HSV) that activates the circuitry responsible for suckling-induced prolactin secretion.

SiSx—Women may present with amenorrhea, infertility, galactorrhea, and virilization, and men may present with impotence, decreased libido, gynecomastia, and also galactorrhea. Osteopenia or osteomalacia can be seen. Signs of central CNS compression including headaches and visual defects are classical conditions causing bitemporal hemianopsia, but this not always present.

Dx—Check the prolactin level. If it is >200 µg/L, this is diagnostic and rarely exceeded in physiologic causes outside of pregnancy. If it is elevated and other causes are excluded, then MRI is the test of choice. Prolactin concentration varies with tumor size and a size >200 µg/L usually implies a macroadenoma, but patients with markedly elevated levels (>1000 µg/L) may give a falsely low value on testing because of the *high dose hook effect,* where significant excess of the antigen actually inhibits immune complex formation. The sample thus needs to be diluted and retested in highly suspicious cases.

Tx—Medical therapy is the first line of treatment even when visual symptoms are found, as therapy can ameliorate these symptoms, sometimes in a matter of hours. First-line treatment is dopamine agonist therapy, regardless of adenoma size (cabergoline or bromocriptine), which normalizes the prolactin level in 75–90% of cases and shrinks

the adenoma. Transsphenoidal surgical resection is the second line of therapy and is done for those who are nonresponsive to medical therapy with an uncontrollable mass effect. It can be complicated by panhypopituitarism and diabetes insipidus, however. Hyperprolactinemia resolves spontaneously in about 30% of cases of microadenoma, as microadenomas rarely progress to become macroadenomas. No treatment may be needed if fertility is not desired

Acromegaly

D—A condition resulting from prolonged GH hypersecretion in adults.

P—A pituitary somatotroph (GH-secreting) is the most common cause (95% of cases). Ectopic secretion is rare. Growth hormone stimulates hepatic insulin-like growth factor-I (IGF-I), which leads to many of the clinical manifestations of acromegaly.

Epi—The incidence is 7/100,000. Diagnosis is delayed because of slow progression of the disease. The mean age at diagnosis is 40–45 years.

RF—Secondary increases in GH occur in anorexia, malnutrition, DM, cirrhosis, stress, lung cancer, and breast cancer.

SiSx—Onset is slow and insidious, with an average interval of 12 years between symptom onset and diagnosis. Classic findings are enlarged jaw (macrognathia), enlarged hands and feet (increasing shoe, glove, and ring size), frontal bossing, enlarging space between teeth, and organomegaly. Associated conditions include carpal tunnel syndrome, DM, skin tags, galactorrhea (40% of patients also secrete prolactin), colonic polyps, sleep apnea, hypertrophic arthropathy, and valvular heart disease. Height is unchanged in adults.

Dx—Diagnosis is usually based on elevated IGF-1. Growth hormone is checked in patients with equivocal IGF-1 values, however GH levels have significant diurnal variation. Therefore, the glucose challenge test (measuring GH 1 hour after an oral load of 100 g glucose) can also be used (>10 ng/mL secures the diagnosis and <5 ng/mL excludes it). Serum prolactin should be checked as well for concomitant prolactin secretion, or from pituitary stalk compression which releases prolactin.

Tx—Transsphenoidal surgical resection is the first line of treatment. The second line of treatment consists of somatostatin analogues, such as octreotide, which normalize GH levels in two-thirds of patients and may shrink tumors. Dopamine agonists may be used as well in cosecreting tumors. Growth hormone receptor antagonists (e.g., pegvisomant) are third-line agents, and fourth-line therapy for refractory patients is radiation. The goal of therapy is to lower IGF-I concentrations to the normal range. Mortality usually results from cardiovascular diseases or cancer.

Hypopituitarism

D—Decreased secretion of one or many pituitary hormones due to either pituitary gland or hypothalamic diseases.

P—Causes include pituitary tumor-related conditions (the most common), congenital, trauma, radiation, infection, infarction (pituitary apoplexy or Sheenan's syndrome, involving infarction of the anterior pituitary during childbirth), infiltrative disorders such as sarcoidosis, amyloidosis, or hemochromatosis, empty sella syndrome, and extrapituitary tumors such as craniopharyngiomas, Typically, the first hormones lost are the least important for survival: first GH, followed by FSH/LH, TSH, and ACTH, in that order, in most cases of pituitary damage. Isolated TSH or ACTH deficiencies are very uncommon.

Sx—Symptoms include GH loss leading to fasting hypoglycemia, and delayed puberty, decreased muscle mass FSH/LH resulting in amenorrhea, gonadal atrophy, decreased hair, and decreased libido, TSH loss leading to hypothyroidism, and ACTH loss resulting in orthostasis, weakness, lethargy, coma, and even death.

Dx—Determine whether the defect is central or peripheral. Testing the different endocrine axes is necessary, including typically TFTs, morning cortisol and ACTH levels, IGF-1, prolactin, FSH and LH, testosterone, and estradiol. Remember to measure the target hormone level in addition to the pituitary hormone level.

Tx—Replace the missing hormone and/or or correct the underlying problem.

Empty Sella Syndrome

D—Extension of the subarachnoid into the sella turcica, filling it with fluid and causing compression of the pituitary.

Epi—It is found at autopsy in 5–20% of cases.

P—Primary empty sella is the most common cause. Secondary causes occur postpituitary surgery status, radiation, pituitary infarction, and hemorrhage of a pituitary tumor.

RF—Middle-aged, obese, hypertensive women are at risk.

SiSx—Headaches are reported. Cerebrospinal rhinorrhea and visual changes are quite rare. Associated hypopituitary symptoms may be present from compression.

Dx—An MRI scan is used to distinguish the syndrome from tumor or cyst. Pituitary function is typically normal. Endocrine function studies should be performed to exclude pituitary hormone insufficiency

Tx—Treatment for associated endocrine dysfunction is the mainstay of therapy, with surgery reserved for patients with progressive deterioration.

Cushing's Disease

D—Excess cortisol caused by an ACTH-secreting pituitary adenoma. It must be distinguished from Cushing's syndrome, which refers to any condition of steroid excess, endogenous or exogenous.

Epi—Female patients outnumber males by 3:1. The disease is most common in the 30s to 40s.

P—It usually results from a de novo pituitary adenoma or hypothalamic overproduction of CRH.

SiSx—Symptoms include proximal muscle weakness, osteoporosis, cutaneous striae, easy bruisability, fat redistribution (moon facies, buffalo hump truncal obesity), hypertension, emotional lability (ranging from depression to frank psychosis), hirsutism, and oligomenorrhea.

Dx—Biochemical diagnosis is based on either elevated urinary cortisol levels or elevated serum cortisol and ACTH levels after an overnight low-dose dexamethasone suppression test. Once the diagnosis has been confirmed, an MRI scan of the sella is used to locate the mass. If no mass is seen on MRI, high-dose dexamethasone suppression testing and inferior petrosal sinus sampling can be used to distinguish between an ectopic source of ACTH production and an ACTH-secreting pituitary adenoma.

Tx—Treatment consists of transsphenoidal resection of the pituitary and glucocorticoid replacement therapy. However, transsphenoidal surgery has a failure rate of about 10–20%. Those with recurrence can have bilateral adrenalectomy or stereotactic pituitary radiosurgery. Ketoconazole can be given to nonsurgical candidates.

Craniopharyngioma

D—An epithelial cell tumor that originate in the upper pituitary stalk, hypothalamus, or ventricles.

Epi—It accounts for 1–3% of intracranial tumors. Peaks occur in infancy and childhood and between 55 and 65 years of age.

P—It is due to remnants of cells from Rathke's pouch and is usually located above the sella turcica. Tumor size varies. Tumors can invade the sella turcica or displace cerebral structures.

SiSx—Pituitary hypofunction, visual difficulties, and severe headaches develop in children. Growth failure associated with either hypothyroidism or GH deficiency is the most common presentation in children, while hypogonadism is most common in adults. Men have erectile dysfunction, and most women have amenorrhea. Signs of hypofunction, such as hypothyroidism, are seen in 40% of patients and adrenal insufficiency in 25%. Severe headaches and visual dysfunction are also not uncommon.

Dx—Diagnosis is made by CT or MRI. Magnetic resonance imaging reveals a solid or cystic mass that may contain areas of suprasellar calcification(seen in 80%).

Tx—Treatment consists of surgery with craniotomy and/or radiotherapy.

Posterior Pituitary Syndromes

Diabetes insipidus and SIADH are discussed in Chapter 4.

The Adrenal Glands

Anatomy

The adrenal cortex has three layers of cells, each with a different function:

Zona glomerulosa (outer)—mineralocorticoids (aldosterone).

Zona fasiculata (middle)—androgens [dehydroepiandrosterone sulfate (DHEAS), dehydroepiandrosterone (DHEA), testosterone, and androstenedione)].

Zone reticularis (inner)—glucocorticoids (cortisol).

The center of the adrenal gland, the medulla, makes norepinephrine and epinephrine.

Disease of the Adrenal Gland

Adrenal Insufficiency (AI)

D—Deficiency of adrenocortical hormones.

P—Primary AI, also known as *Addison's disease*, results from impaired function of the adrenal gland. Causes of primary AI include the following:

Autoimmune—may be part of polyglandular autoimmune syndrome type I or II (see Chapter 7 appendix)

Infectious—CMV, cryptococcus, TB, atypical mycobacterial infection, fungal infection (histoplasmosis)

Metastatic (especially from lung and breast cancer or lymphoma)

Infiltrative (hemochromatosis, amyloidosis)

Congenital adrenal hyperplasia/adrenoleukodystrophy

Drugs—ketoconazole (inhibits the P450 system, which is essential for cortisol biosynthesis), rifampin, megestrol

Adrenal hemorrhage—as in adrenal vein thrombosis, heparin-induced thrombocytopenia (HIT) or antiphospholipid antibody syndrome.

Secondary AI results from deficient pituitary ACTH secretion. Steroid therapy with ACTH suppression is the most common cause of secondary AI. This condition can also be seen in the setting of panhypopituitarism.

SiSx—Symptoms vary quite widely. There may be weakness, fatigue, anorexia, nausea and vomiting, weight loss, and orthostasis. In secondary AI, there may be hyperpigmentation [due to increased secretion of pro-opiomelanocortin (POMC), the precursor of ACTH], especially in palmar folds, scars, and oral mucosa. Women may have decreased pubic and axillary hair. A craving for salt may be reported. The patient may also have features of hypothyroidism and hypogonadism if other hormonal deficiencies exist. Cortisol deficiency results in hypotension and hypoglycemia. Hyponatremia (sodium wasting leads to volume depletion) and hyperkalemia are caused by decreased aldosterone. This will not be seen in secondary AI, where mineralocorticoid (aldosterone) levels are normal since the renin-angiotensin II-aldosterone system remains intact.

Dx—Tests include the morning cortisol level and the ACTH stimulation test (either high-dose or low-dose). Random serum cortisol measurement in general is not helpful.

1. *Morning cortisol test.* This is performed at around 8 a.m., when cortisol levels are highest.
   If the level is <5 µg/dL, AI is very likely.
   If the level is >15 µg/dL, AI is unlikely.

2. *High-dose ACTH stimulation test.* Give 250 µg IV of ACTH (cosyntropin). Measure plasma cortisol levels at baseline and after 30 minutes and 60 minutes. If the peak cortisol value is >18–20 µg/dL, then adrenal insufficiency is unlikely. This test cannot rule out secondary or recent-onset AI.

3. *Low-dose ACTH stimulation test.* Give 1 µg cosyntropin IV and measure the cortisol level at baseline and after 30 minutes. Cortisol levels after 30 minutes of >18.5 µg/dL or an increase in cortisol by 7 µg/dL from baseline rule out the diagnosis. Some suggest that this is a better test for secondary AI. Simultaneous measurement of ACTH and cortisol levels can be used to distinguish between primary (elevated ACTH) and secondary AI (normal or low ACTH).

4. *Other tests*: The overnight metyrapone test and the insulin-induced hypoglycemia test (gold standard) can be used in the diagnosis of secondary AI. These tests are rarely used in the United States.

Electrolytes should be checked to assess for hyponatremia, hyperkalemia, and hypocalcemia. Other tests (e.g., tuberculin purified protein derivative for TB) or imaging for metastatic disease may be necessary to uncover the etiology.

Tx—Maintenance treatment consists of daily glucocorticoid (e.g., hydrocortisone) and mineralocorticoid (e.g., fludrocortisone) for those with primary AI. For those with secondary AI, maintenance consists of daily glucocorticoid only. Doses should be increased for illnesses or preoperatively to stave off adrenal crisis.

Adrenal Crisis

D—Acute life-threatening symptoms due to adrenal insufficiency in the setting of a medical stressor.

RF—Risk factors include anticoagulant treatment, bleeding diathesis, DIC, HIV, AIDS, sepsis, or following high-dose glucocorticoid treatment in the last 12 months.

P—Causes are the same as those of adrenal insufficiency in general. Here, however, there is a stressor requiring more than the normal amount of glucocorticoids and mineralocorticoids, (i.e., above the usual replacement doses). Causes include the following:

1. Acute stress (e.g., infection) precipitates the crisis in a patient with chronic adrenocortical insufficiency or on maintenance corticosteroid therapy.

2. Abrupt cessation of exogenous corticosteroid treatment.

3. Massive adrenal hemorrhage due to anticoagulant treatment, postsurgical DIC, or *Neisseria meningitidis* septicemia (Waterhouse-Friderichsen syndrome).

Note that other organisms may be responsible in the last condition. It is also seen in antiphospholipid antibody syndrome and in severe inflammatory disease.

Because cortisol maintains vascular tone and has inotropic affects, hypotension ensues.

SiSx—Symptoms include shock, fever, nonspecific GI complains, nausea, vomiting, abdominal pain, diarrhea or constipation, and postural dizziness or syncope. Hypoglycemia is a rare presenting symptom.

Dx and Tx—A clinical diagnosis is made initially, due to the urgent need for treatment, before a biochemical diagnosis can be confirmed.

1. Draw blood for measurement of cortisol (and of ACTH if the diagnosis is not clear).
2. Give normal saline (NS) with and 5% dextrose to reverse hypovolemia.
3. Give 4 mg dexamethasone IV immediately (does not confound tests).
4. Perform the low- or high-dose cosyntropin test as described above.
5. Give a bolus of hydrocortisone 100 mg every 6 hours. This is sufficient to cover both glucocorticoid and mineralocorticoid requirements.

When the patient is stable, switch to oral replacement treatment, including a combination of glucocorticoid and mineralocorticoid. Perform appropriate tests to uncover the underlying cause of the condition.

Primary Hyperaldosteronism

D—A condition of mineralocorticoid excess secondary to either an aldosterone-secreting adrenal adenoma (Conn's syndrome) or bilateral adrenal hyperplasia.

Epi—It accounts for as many as 5–15% of cases of hypertension. Female patients outnumber males.

P—Seventy-five percent of cases are due to unilateral adrenocortical adenomas (Conn's syndrome) and 25% to bilateral adenomas. Aldosterone increases sodium reabsorption, as well as urinary potassium and acid secretion. The fall in K^+ is accompanied by a metabolic alkalosis because of the hydrogen potassium ion exchanger in cells.

SiSx—The classic triad is (1) hypertension, (2) hypokalemia, and (3) metabolic alkalosis. However, few patients actually have hypokalemia. Hypokalemia may present as muscle weakness or cramps. Some patients have only diastolic hypertension; malignant hypertension is rare. Edema is rarely seen in the primary form due to an initial natriuresis.

Dx –Screening is recommended in those who have Joint National Committee (JNC) stage 2 or 3 hypertension (see Chapter 2) or drug-resistant hypertension, hypertension and hypokalemia, hypertension with adrenal incidentaloma, and early-onset hypertension, as well as in first-degree relatives of those diagnosed with primary hyperaldosteronism.

Mineralocorticoid receptor antagonists (spironolactone, eplereone) need to be discontinued prior to screening. Angiotensin converting enzyme inhibitors and angiotensin receptor blockers (ARBs) can raise plasma renin activity and make test results difficult to interpret. However, suppressed plasma renin activity while taking these drugs makes a diagnosis of hyperaldosteronism more likely. Morning measurement of the plasma aldosterone/renin ratio can be performed. A ratio of >20 or a plasma aldosterone concentration >15 should prompt further evaluation. Confirmation of the diagnosis is made by measuring urine aldosterone excretion and the plasma aldosterone concentration after salt loading. If biochemical testing implicates an adrenal aldosterone-secreting adenoma, a thin-section CT scan of the adrenals is obtained. A discrete adrenal adenoma (>1 cm in diameter with a normal contralateral adrenal) is found in 60–80% of such patients. However, about 20% of such "adenomas" are found to be hyperplasia at surgery. Therefore, it is often prudent to supplement CT localization with adrenal vein catheterization for aldosterone.

Tx—Laparoscopic adrenalectomy is performed for Conn's syndrome in most cases. If the patient is not a surgical candidate, suppression with aldosterone antagonists such as spironolactone can be used; this is also the treatment of choice for bilateral adrenal hyperplasia. Additional antihypertensive agents may also be necessary. Only 2% of aldosterone-secreting adrenal tumors are malignant.

Pheochromocytoma

D—An adrenal medullary tumor that secretes catecholamines, leading to hypertensive episodes that can be fatal.

Epi—Eighty percent of these tumors in adults are unilateral and solitary. Classically, they follow the rule of 10s: 10% are bilateral, 10% are extra-adrenal, and 10% are malignant. Most extra-adrenal tumors (paragangliomas) are located in the abdomen, though 10% are found in the thorax. In 5% of cases they are associated with MEN syndromes. Most occur in middle-aged adults.

P—The tumors are highly vascular and consist of chromaffin cells. Epinephrine, norepinephrine, and dopamine can be produced by these tumors. In familial syndromes, the *ret* proto-oncogene on chromosome 10 has been identified as a cause.

SiSx—Classically, there are episodic crises characterized by hypertension, anxiety attacks, headaches, excessive sweating, palpitations, and a sense of impending doom. In one-half of patients hypertension is sustained, though in others it occurs only in paroxysms. Hypertension is usually malignant and is resistant to multiple-drug regimens. Attacks can last for minutes to hours. Arrhythmias have been noted as well. Fatal paroxysms have been induced by medications including opiates, which can release catecholamines from the tumor.

Dx—There is no single best test. Initial tests may include measuring 24-hour fractionated urinary metanephrine and catecholamines which show markedly elevated levels. False positives can seen in patients on labetalol and α-methyldopa. Metabolites such as urinary vanillylmandelic acid (VMA), may also be elevated as well as plasma free metanephrine levels. This latter test has high sensitivity but low specificity. Imaging via MRI or by a nuclear scan with 123-I-metaiodobenzylguanidine (MIBG, a compound which is taken up by adrenergic tissue) can help to localize the lesion.

Tx—Initially, α blockers such as phenoxybenzamine are used over several weeks prior to surgical removal. Use of β blockers can produce an unopposed α-agonist effect leading to a paradoxical increase in BP. They are used only after α blockers have been started and usually when tachycardia has developed. In surgical candidates, metyrosine can be used. It inhibits tyrosine hydroxylase and decreases catecholamine production by the tumor. For patients with nonmalignant tumors, 5-year survival is >95%. Hypertension is cured in 75% of patients.

The Pancreas

Diseases of the Pancreas

Diabetes Mellitus

D—A group of metabolic disorders that are manifested by hyperglycemia.

P—These disorders are broadly categorized into type I and type II (see below). Other conditions include gestational diabetes, secondary diabetes from β-cell destruction (as in severe acute or chronic pancreatitis), maturity-onset diabetes of youth (MODY: an autosomal dominant defect in insulin secretion), drug-induced (steroids), and lipodystrophy related, among many others.

Epi—Type II has a recently increased prevalence and is seen in 25% of individuals >60 (and in 8% of all Americans). It is suspected that many more individuals have prediabetes, which has increased in parallel with the rise in obesity. The condition is most common in African Americans, Hispanic Americans, and Native Americans. Type I has the highest incidence in Scandinavia and the lowest in China and Japan. It is intermediate in the United States.

SiSx—Acutely, patients may present with signs of hyperglycemia: polydipsia, polyuria, polyphagia, dehydration, and visual and mental status changes. Otherwise, they may be asymptomatic, and diagnosis is made on routine screening. Chronic complications are many and include the following:

Diabetic retinopathy and macular edema leading to visual impairment/loss.

Diabetic neuropathy (sensor and motor/auto-nomic) leading to alteration/loss of sensation and orthostasis.

Diabetic vasculopathy [coronary artery disease (CAD), peripheral vascular disease (PVD), cardiovascular accident (CVA)].

Diabetic nephropathy leading to proteinuria, and renal insufficiency, or ESRD.

Gastroparesis.

Impotence and sexual dysfunction.

Cataracts/glaucoma.

Skin—diabetic ulcers from poor wound healing, diabetic dermopathy (an erythematous area evolving into circular hyperpigmentation), necrobiosis lipoidica diabeticorum (pretibial erythematous areas or papules that enlarge, with atrophic centers and central ulceration), and acanthosis nigricans (hyperpigmented dark areas on the neck, axilla, or extensor surfaces).

Patients are also at increased risk of infections.

Dx

1. Symptoms of diabetes (polyuria, polydipsia, weight loss) plus random BS >200 mg/dL or
2. Fasting plasma glucose level >126 mg/dL on more than one occasion (<100 mg/dL is normal, 100–126 mg/dL is impaired fasting glucose) or
3. Two-hour post–oral glucose tolerance test (OGTT) level >200 mg/dL (<140 mg/dL is normal, 140–200 mg/dL is impaired glucose tolerance) or
4. Hemoglobin A1c > 6.5%.

Screening is recommended in patients with a family history, obesity, a history of gestational DM, vascular disease of any sort, hypertension. hyperlipidemia, polycystic ovary syndrome (PCOS), high-risk ethnicity, or every 3 years in patients >45 years old. Hemoglobin A1c is not currently used to screen for DM.

Distinguishing between type I and type II is important, as it determines the course of therapy. Some of the differences between these two types are shown in Table 7-8.

Tx

Blood Sugar Control

The goal is usually HbA1c <6.5 –7.0%, and morning glucose <120 mg/dL and 2-hour postprandial glucose <140 mg/dL. Achieving these targets has important beneficial effects on most microvascular complications in type I (per the Diabetes Control and Complications or DCCT Trial) and type II (per the United Kingdom Prospective Diabetes Study or UKPDS trial). Oral agents and insulin are used. The different types are summarized in Tables 7-9 and 7-10.

Most common regimens include:

1. Mono- or combination therapy with oral agents.
2. Insulin plus single or multiple oral agents.
3. Insulin alone:
a. Basal bolus therapy: This is the most physiologic regimen. It consists of glargine insulin daily plus rapid-acting insulin given with meals [BID glargine insulin is

Table 7-8.   Differences Between Type I and Type II Diabetes

Type I	Type II
Autoimmune destruction of pancreatic β cells.	Insulin resistant initially, followed by relative insulin deficiency later in disease course; excess hepatic glucose production.
Insulin dependent.	Treatment includes oral with or without insulin.
Usually childhood onset.	Usually adult onset, although a rising prevalence in obese children/adolescents.
Prone to DKA (insulin deficient).	Prone to hyperosmolar hyperglycemic state (HHS).
30–50% monozygotic concordance.	100% monozygotic concordance. More related to family history.
0.2–0.5% incidence; equal in males and females.	2–4% incidence; female patients outnumber males.
HLA DR3, DR4 association.	No HLA association.

Table 7-9. Oral Agents Used to Treat Diabetes

Agent	Mechanism	Comment on Use	Side Effects/ Contraindications
Biguanides Metformin (Glucophage)	Inhibits hepatic gluconeogenesis and improves insulin sensitivity (mechanism unknown). Effective only in the presence of insulin.	First-line agent for many patients. Promotes weight loss. Less likely to cause hypoglycemia.	GI side effects (nausea, vomiting, diarrhea) usually reversible after dose is lowered. Very rarely, may cause lactic acidosis and contraindication in CKD (Cr >1.5), CHF, sepsis, hypoxia. Held in hospitalized patients and those receiving IV contrast.
Sulfonylureas Glyburide (Diabeta, Micronase, Glynase) Glipizide (Glucotrol) Glimepiride (Amaryl)	Increase β-cell insulin secretion. Sulfonylurea binding leads to inhibition of ATP-dependent potassium channels on β cells, which alters the resting potential of the cell, leading to calcium influx and stimulation of insulin secretion.	Given with meals to control postprandial hyperglycemia. Associated with weight gain. The different sulfonylureas are equally effective in lowering blood glucose concentrations	Useful only in patients with ß-cell function. Hypoglycemia is the most common side effect. Nausea, skin reactions, and photosensitivity also occur. Use cautiously in patients with renal and hepatic impairment.
Meglitinides Repaglinide (Prandin) Nateglinide (Starlix)	Act by regulating ATP-dependent potassium channels in pancreatic ß cells, thereby increasing insulin secretion in a glucose-dependent fashion.	Given with each meal. Expensive.	Use cautiously in patients with renal and hepatic impairment.
Thiazolidinediones Pioglitazone (Actos) Rosiglitazone (Avandia)	Increase peripheral glucose uptake. Increase insulin sensitivity. Work via activation of peroxisome proliferator-activated receptor (PPAR) gamma receptors.	Weight gain is dose dependent.	Fluid retention and pulmonary edema. Not used in class III or IV CHF or with LFT abnormalities. LFT monitoring required. Concern about increased CV events with rosiglitazone.
Alpha glucoside inhibitors Acarbose (Precose) Miglitol (Glyset)	Inhibit upper GI enzymes (α-glucosidases) that convert carbohydrates into monosaccharides in a dose-dependent fashion.	May also have beneficial effects on serum lipid concentrations.	Flatulence that can be severe. Not for use in patients with underlying GI disease.
Exenatide (Byetta)	Dose- and glucose-dependent augmentation of insulin secretion via binding to the GLP-1 receptor. Slows gastric emptying, suppresses glucagon release and causes appetite suppression.	Can be used with other orals. Provides added benefit of weight loss.	Nausea that usually resolves. Very rare cases of pancreatitis. Hypoglycemia seen when given in combination with sulfonylureas.
Sitagliptin (Januvia) and saxagliptin (Onglyza)	Dipeptidyl peptidase-IV (DPP-IV) inhibitor that prevents inactivation of GLP-1 thereby increasing insulin secretion and inhibiting glucagon release.	Use often in combination with other oral agents. Can be given renally.	GI upset or nasopharyngitis. Hyperreactivity with anaphylaxis, angioedema, or Stevens-Johnson syndrome is reported but is quite rare

Table 7-10.   Insulin Formulations Used to Treat Diabetes

	Insulin Type (Brand Names)	Onset	Peak	Duration
Rapid-Acting	Lispro (Humalog)	5–15 minutes	1–2 hours	3–5 hours
	Aspart (Novolog)	5–15 minutes	1–2 hours	3–5 hours
	Glulisine (Apidra)	5–15 minutes	1–2 hours	3–4 hours
Short-Acting	Regular (R)	30 minutes to 1 hour	2–4 hours	6–8 hours
Intermediate-Acting	NPH (N)	1–2 hours	4–8 hours	10–20 hours
Long-Acting	Glargine (Lantus)	1–2 hours	No peak	24 hours
	Detemir (Levemir)	1–2 hours	No peak	Up to 24 hours
	70/30 (Humulin) Contains 70 of N and 30 of R	30 minutes	2–4 hours	Similar to NPH
Premixed	70/30 (Novolin) Contains 70 of N and 30 of R	30 minutes	2–4 hours	Similar to NPH
	70/30 (Novolog) Contains 70 of N and 30 of aspart	10–20 minutes	1–4 hours	Similar to NPH
	50/50 (Humulin) Contains 50 of N and 50 of R	30 minutes	2–5 hours	Similar to NPH
	75/25 (Humalog mix) Contains 75 of N and 25 of lispro	15 minutes	30 minutes–2½ hours	Similar to NPH

used occasionally if the patient has a very high insulin requirement (>100 units), which requires multiple injection sites].

   b. Premixed insulin BID.

   c. NPH/regular insulin BID.

   d. Insulin pump continuous infusion (requires a highly compliant patient).

   e. Premixed regimens are rarely used today as initial therapy.

Treatment of Complications

Retinopathy—laser photocoagulation can be used to preserve vision.

Nephropathy—prevention or limiting progression: only tight BS, hypertension and lipid control; use of ACE inhibitors and ARBs. Microalbuminuria should be screened for annually.

Gastroparesis—smaller, more frequent meals; promotility agents: dopamine agonists (metoclopramide).

Neuropathy—commonly used agents are tricyclic antidepressants (amitriptyline, desipramine, nortriptyline), gabapentin, NSAIDs, capsaicin cream and the recently approved pregabalin, a 3-substituted analogue of gamma-aminobutyric acid (GABA). Selective serotonin reuptake inhibitors (SSRIs) are also used.

Orthostatic hypotension from autonomic neuropathy—may require fludrocortisone or midodrine, in addition to increased salt intake or support hose for the legs.

Pancreas transplant or simultaneous pancreas kidney transplant are the only curative options. Islet cell transplantation is experimental.

Diabetic Ketoacidosis (DKA)

D—Acute complication of type I DM. The condition is due primarily to uncompensated ketoacid production in the setting of insulin deficiency and hyperglycemia.

Epi—It accounts for 50% of DM hospital admissions, and it may be the first presenting symptoms of DM. The incidence is 1/2000. Mortality is as high as 10% in some cases and is higher in whites, females, and children than in other groups.

P—Insulin deficiency and excess glucagon are both needed for DKA to develop. Increased free fatty acid (FFA) release occurs in response to clinical stressors. Normally, FFAs are converted primarily to triglycerides and very low density lipoprotein (VLDL) instead of ketoacids in the liver. However, this balance shifts, favoring more ketoacid production (acetoacetate and β-hydroxybutyrate) in the setting of elevated glucagon. With the depletion of bicarbonate, ketoacid accumulation occurs and metabolic acidosis eventually ensues. In addition, glucagon and catecholamine excess in the setting of low insulin promotes glycogenolysis and hyperglycemia, as there is impaired glucose uptake into skeletal muscle and fat. Hyperglycemia causes an osmotic diuresis typically producing a water deficit of up to 5–10 L. Total body stores of electrolytes are lowered in this setting as well: sodium, potassium, chloride, phosphorus, and magnesium. Potassium loss is also worsened as intracellular potassium is lost to act as a buffer for the acidosis (via an H^+-K^+ exchanger). Triglyceride and VLDL levels are also increased due to both overproduction and reduced clearance. Hypertriglyceridemia results and can be severe enough to cause pancreatitis.

RF—The condition is usually due to a precipitating event: infection (UTI and PNA are most common), insulin noncompliance, pancreatitis (seen in up to 10%), alcohol abuse and withdrawal, trauma, MI, dehydration, and CVA.

SiSx—Symptoms usually develop over 24 hours and include nausea, vomiting, and abdominal pain (associated with the severity of the metabolic acidosis). Classic symptoms include Kussmaul respirations (deep, slow breathing) and fruity breath odor (from increased acetone). Signs of dehydration such as poor skin turgor, dry membranes, and orthostasis are usually present. A history of recent polyuria and polydipsia can also be elicited. Depending on the precipitant, the patient can experience severe hemodynamic compromise.

Dx—Biochemically, DKA is defined as (1) increase in serum ketones >5 mEq/L, (2) a glucose level >200 mg/dL, and (3) pH <7.4 with an anion gap metabolic acidosis. The proper method of ketone testing is important. Serum ketones are favored over urine ketones, which are measured with nitroprusside. This agent only reacts with acetoacetate but not with β-hydroxybutyrate; the latter makes up 75–90% of the ketoacids present. Serum testing assesses for hydroxybutyrate more accurately.

Tx—Prompt treatment initiation is important, perhaps even before diagnostic confirmation is obtained. Patients usually need admission to an ICU or a facility where frequent monitoring of blood sugar levels can be performed. The mainstay of treatment is (1) intravenous insulin, (2) aggressive intravenous hydration, and (3) electrolyte repletion where appropriate.

For fluid resuscitation, 2–3 L of normal saline (NS) over the first 3 hours is recommended, followed by ½ NS at 150–300 mL/hr in order to replete free water. The degree of resuscitation varies based on the clinical scenario; however, D5½ NS is started when the blood sugar level falls below 250 mg/dL, *as the primary goal is not to reduce the sugar level but to close the anion gap.*

For insulin, a bolus of IV (0.1 unit/kg) is given initially, followed by initiation of an IV insulin drip at a rate of 0.1 unit/kg/hr. Finger stick blood sugars are checked every 1–2 hours and panel 7s every 4 hours x 24 hours. Insulin is increased 2- to 10-fold if there is no response. If the K^+ level is very low, it must be corrected immediately before giving insulin. After the anion gap is closed and the patient is able to eat, give a subcutaneous injection of a long-acting insulin (NPH or glargine). The dose will depend on the patient's weight and insulin requirements. Long-acting insulin should be administered 2 hours before discontinuing the insulin infusion.

Potassium is the most important electrolyte to replete. Most patients are severely deficient, although this is not reflected in the panel 7. Add K^+ to the fluids at a rate of 10 mEq/hr when K^+ is <5.5 and 40–80 mEq/hr when K <3.5. Prophylactic phosphate administration is not indicated, as most patients are asymptomatic and repletion usually causes more harm than good. On the other hand, magnesium should be repleted as needed.

Complications of treatment include cerebral edema (most common in children) that occurs within 24 hours of therapy, presenting as headache and later as marked neurologic dysfunction. The cause is unclear but is thought to be due in part to worsening hyponatremia with overaggressive free water repletion.

Finally, looking for and treating the underlying causes is quite important and depends on the specific clinical scenario.

Hyperosmolar Hyperglycemic State (HHS)

D—Markedly elevated sugar levels in the absence of ketoacid formation, causing volume depletion and neurologic abnormalities. Coma, however, is infrequent (<10% of cases).

Epi—The incidence is 18/100,000 cases in the United States. The condition is more common than DKA and more common in the elderly. Mortality is up to 10%.

P—Hyperglycemia/hyperosmolarity leads to osmotic diuresis. Ketoacidosis does not develop, as the presence of insulin prevents ketogenesis but not hyperglycemia. In practice, however, DKA and HHS exist along a continuum of hyperglycemia, with or without ketosis.

RF—As with DKA, an antecedent illness such as a cardiovascular event, infection, or dehydration is often a precipitant.

SiSx—Classically, polyphagia, polydipsia, and polyuria are seen. Central nervous system involvement can range from lethargy to frank obtundation or coma when the plasma osmolality become very high. Seizure, hemiparesis, and visual changes may also be seen. Signs of volume depletion may also be present, including orthostasis and hypotension.

Dx—This is a clinical diagnosis based on the presentation with high sugar levels, dehydration, and no evidence of marked ketosis on serum ketones or an anion gap due to the presence of ketoacids. Creatine kinase levels should be checked, as rhabdomyolysis can trigger HHS as can dehydration. Bicarbonate should be normal or only mildly reduced.

Tx—The mainstay of treatment includes fluids and insulin. Patients typically have a significantly greater volume deficit than those with DKA; hence, fluid resuscitation is most important. Treating the underlying cause is also important. With glucose normalization, insulin requirement decrease. Typically, an IV insulin infusion and/or drip may be needed. In select cases, rapid-acting subcutaneous insulin can be used.

The Parathyroid Glands

Diseases of the Parathyroid Glands and Bone Metabolism

Primary Hyperparathyroidism

D—Hypercalcemia caused by an autonomously functioning parathyroid adenoma or, less commonly, glandular hyperplasia.

Epi—The incidence is 25/100,000. This condition causes 90% of hypercalcemia cases. It occurs most frequently over age 45. Female patients outnumber males by 2:1.

P—Parathyroid hormone (PTH) induces Ca^{2+} reabsorption in bone, the kidney, and the GI tract. It also decreases urinary PO_4 absorption and increases conversion of 25-hydroxyvitamin D to 1–25 dihydroxyvitamin D. Excess calcium affects the calcium-sensing receptor on the parathyroid gland and inhibits PTH synthesis and release.

The causes of primary hyperparathyroidism are as follows:

1. Solitary parathyroid adenoma (85%).
2. Hyperplasia in multiglandular disease (MEN I, IIa, or IIb).
3. Parathyroid carcinoma (rare).

SiSx—"Painful bones, renal stones, abdominal groans, and psychic overtones"

1. Bones: osteoporosis and osteitis fibrosa cystica leading to fractures.
2. Stones: nephrolithiasis.
3. Groans: constipation, nausea, peptic ulcers, pancreatitis, and gallstones.

4. Psychic overtones: depression, lethargy, and seizures.

There may also be aortic and mitral valve calcifications.

Dx—Diagnosis is based on finding elevated serum-ionized calcium (or corrected total calcium) and elevated PTH. Localization is often performed preoperatively with a sestamibi scan to determine which gland is hyperfunctioning.

Tx—Severe symptoms or significantly elevated calcium levels are treated with aggressive IV hydration with NS infusion. If heart failure develops, administer furosemide but keep giving fluids with the goal of achieving 100 cc/hr of urine output. Bisphosphonates, which inhibits bone reabsorption, are also a key to acute treatment.

Common indications for parathyroidectomy include significantly elevated serum calcium, younger age (<50 years), renal insufficiency, renal stones and significantly low bone mineral density.

Secondary Hyperparathyroidism

D—Overactivity of all parathyroid glands due to chronic depression of Ca^{2+}.

P—Causes include the following:
1. Chronic renal failure.
2. Vitamin D loss via malabsorption or inadequate intake/production.
3. Inadequate calcium intake.

Chronic renal failure is by far the most common cause. In this setting, hypocalcemia and inadequate phosphate excretion result in hyperphosphatemia and increased parathyroid gland activity. Rarely, in this setting, *tertiary hyperparathyroidism* may occur, in which one of the parathyroid glands gain autonomy, leading to hypercalcemia. It presents similarly to primary hyperparathyroidism and requires parathyroidectomy.

SiSx—Bone abnormalities are less severe than those in primary hyperparathyroidism. Calciphylaxis, vascular calcification leading to ischemia, may occur.

Dx—Diagnosis is based on finding low ionized calcium levels with elevated PTH, usually in the setting of chronic renal failure or malabsorption.

Tx—If the condition is due to chronic renal failure, administer phosphate binders—calcium carbonate, calcium acetate, or cross-linked polyallylamine hydrochloride (sevelamer) qac. Calcium salts may also be taken on an empty stomach. Vitamin D may cause hypercalcemia, so caution is needed. In refractory cases, a subtotal parathyroidectomy is performed in which three and one half glands are removed, leaving half of a gland left Calcimimetics such as cinacalcet are also used on occasion to treat this condition.

Familial Hypocalciuric Hypercalcemia (FHH)

D—A benign autosomal dominant disorder with mild to moderate hypercalcemia due to a defect in the Ca^{2+}-sensing receptor.

P—The Ca^{2+}-sensing receptor is present in many tissues, including the parathyroids, kidneys, and bone. An inactivating mutation in this receptor has several effects. The parathyroid gland requires higher levels of Ca^2 to reduce PTH secretion. Hence, PTH is not suppressed in this condition. In the kidney, more Ca^{2+} and Mg are reabsorbed as well.

SiSx—Patients may be asymptomatic and present with high calcium levels in childhood. Complications of urinary calculi and renal failure usually do not occur; however, cases of pancreatitis and chondrocalcinosis have been reported.

Dx—Suspicion should be raised by a mildly elevated calcium level and normal to elevated PTH, though this is also seen in some cases of hyperparathyroidism. Clinically, the condition is characterized by absence of hypercalcemic symptoms. Patients may also report a family history of hypercalcemia. Measurement of a 24-hour urinary collection for Ca^{2+} and creatinine to calculate the fractional excretion of Ca^{2+} is essential to distinguish FHH from primary hyperparathyroidism. A fractional excretion of calcium (FeCa) <1% is consistent with FHH.

Tx—Usually the course is benign. Subtotal parathyroidectomy does not cure the disorder. Family screening is the only recommendation.

Osteoporosis

D—Condition of low bone mineral density (BMD) defined as >2.5 standard deviations below the peak bone mass, leading to an increased risk of fragility fracture.

Epi—One-third of women and one-sixth of men in extreme old age experience hip fracture related to osteoporosis. Secondary complications of hip fractures include PE and nosocomial infections leading to 15–20% mortality.

P—Osteoporosis occurs primarily in postmenopausal (PMP) females but can also occur secondary to an underlying condition (see Table 7-11). Bone loss is either from decreased pubertal BMD accumulation or accelerated adult bone loss. Bone acquisition is almost complete by 17 years of age in girls and by 20 years in boys, and peak bone mass occurs by age 30. In PMP women, estrogen deprivation promotes bone remodeling by releasing constraints on osteoblastic production of skeletally active cytokines, which, in turn, stimulate the proliferation of osteoclast precursors.

RF—Risk factors include older age, family history, female gender, white or Asian race, low body weight, early menopause, low calcium and vitamin D intake, estrogen deficiency, smoking, and medications (i.e., glucocorticoids).

SiSx—Osteoporosis most commonly presents as a fracture. Otherwise, it is discovered on routine screening. Vertebral bodies, the distal forearm, and the proximal femur are the most common sites, but ribs and long bones also fracture. Vertebral body fractures may be silent. Most commonly, they are diagnosed with loss of height or spinal deformity (kyphosis, lordosis). Vertebral compression fractures can occur with sneezing, bending, or lifting light objects and most commonly happen in the middle and lower thoracic and upper lumbar regions. Hip fractures are associated with falls, more commonly to the side, where there is less tissue to cushion the impact.

Dx—Diagnosis is made mainly by dual-energy x-ray absorptiometry (DEXA) of either the lumbar spine or the proximal femur. Scoring is as follows:

T-score: the number of standard deviations away from the peak BMD of young normal subjects.

Z-score: the number of standard deviations away from the BMD of age-matched normal subjects.

A T-score less than –2.5 indicates osteoporosis.

A T-score between –1 and –2.5 indicates osteopenia.

Low Z-scores should prompt a search for secondary causes.

Tx—For the acute phase of vertebral compression, administer analgesics, muscle relaxants, heat, massage, and/or rest. An orthopedic back brace, physical therapy, and modification of the home environment may also help. For chronic osteoporosis, a regimen of weight-bearing exercise and fracture prevention measures are indicated

Prevention:

Calcium
   1200–1500 mg for <18-year-olds
   1000 mg for men and women 18–50 years
   1200 mg for men and women >50-year-olds

Table 7-11. Secondary Causes of Osteoporosis

Drugs
   Alcohol
   Heparin (chronic)
   Glucocorticoids
   Thyroxine
   Anticonvulsants

Endocrine
   Hyperthyroidism
   Hyperparathyroidism
   Hyperprolactinemia
   Hypercortisolism
   GH deficiency
   Hypothalamic amenorrhea
   Hypogonadism

Gastrointestinal
   Subtotal gastrectomy
   Malabsorption syndromes
   Chronic obstructive jaundice
   Primary biliary cirrhosis

Other
   Bone marrow disorders
   Anorexia nervosa

Vitamin D
   200 IU for <18 years
   400 IU for 18- to 70-year-olds
   600 IU for >70-year-olds
   800 IU for those with little sunlight exposure

The National Osteoporosis Foundation recommends treatment of PMP women (and men ≥50 years old) with a history of hip or vertebral fracture or with osteoporosis based upon BMD measurement (T-score of –2.5 or less):

Alendronate or residronate daily or weekly, or ibandronate monthly or zoledronate intravenously once yearly. All of these agents increase bone density and decrease fracture.

Raloxifene 60 mg orally daily for early PMP women and for the treatment of osteoporotic women has been shown to increase BMD and reduce the risk of vertebral fractures.

Estrogens are not indicated for the treatment of osteoporosis alone. Calcitonin (nasal spray) is a second-line treatment that has a modest effect on BMD and has been shown to reduce the incidence of vertebral fracture.

Parathyroid hormone is given for anabolic treatment as appropriate (it builds bone when given intermittently, as opposed to causing bone loss, as seen with normal physiologic secretion).

Paget's Disease of Bone

D—A disorder of focal bone remodeling characterized by an imbalance between osteoblast bone formation and osteoclast bone reabsorption.

Epi—It has an increased incidence in northern Europeans. It is rare in Africans and Asians.

P—The cause is unknown. A family history is seen in some studies. Histopathologic examination shows very vascular bone and large, bizarre osteoclasts. Abnormal bone reabsorption is the initiating event, which is increased to 10- to 20-fold above normal.

SiSx—The most common sites of involvement are the spine, femur, skull, and pelvis. Patients may present with pain in these areas, fractures (vertebral fractures are most common), or deformities. Most patients are asymptomatic. Complications include hearing loss, osteoarthritis, malignancy, and even high-output cardiac failure in severe cases from markedly increased blood flow to bone.

Dx—Most cases are discovered incidentally on radiographs. The alkaline phosphatase is high. Early imaging shows an osteolytic lesion. Over the years, one sees a mixed pattern with thickened trabeculae, enlarged or bowed long bones, a thickened iliopectineal line or pelvic brim, osteoblastic lesions of the vertebral bodies, and joint space narrowing as in osteoarthritis. Bone scans are uniformly positive in active Paget's disease and are useful once a focus has been found to delineate other sites.

Tx—Treatment is usually conservative, with pain control measures such as NSAIDs initially. Calcitonin and bisphosphanates can also be used to inhibit osteoclast action.

Reproductive Endocrine

Diseases of the Reproductive Organs

Polycystic Ovarian Disease

D—A condition presenting with signs of androgen excess, insulin resistance, oligomenorrhea or amenorrhea, and occasionally bilaterally enlarged polycystic ovaries.

Epi—It is the most common endocrine obesity-related syndrome in females.

P—It can be primary (idiopathic or hereditary, as with insulin receptor mutations) or secondary (i.e., associated with acromegaly and congenital adrenal hyperplasia). Originally, it was thought to be characterized by enlarged, polycystic ovaries, but there are now known to be many different pathologic findings in the ovaries, and the finding of cystic ovaries is not necessary to make the diagnosis. Most common are sclerotic ovaries with a thickened capsule and multiple cysts in various stages of atrophy. The exact cause is not known.

RF—Risk factors include premature pubarche, premature breast development, and a family history.

SiSx—Most women present with either infertility or hirsutism. Signs of hyperandrogenism may be present on exam: hirsutism in a male pattern and acne. Most patients have menstrual irregularity; two-thirds are anovulatory. Obesity is commonly seen; in one-half of patients with polycystic ovary syndrome (PCOS), it is often the presenting complaint. Signs of insulin resistance and overt diabetes may also be present in up to 40%. Acanthosis nigricans can accompany these findings.

Patients should be monitored for other features of metabolic syndrome, including BP and lipid abnormalities.

Dx—The diagnosis is clinical, though rough criteria exist (two of the following three findings:
1. Presence of menstrual irregularity, ranging from oligomenorrhea to anovulation.
2. Evidence of hyperandrogenism (by clinical exam or by elevated levels of serum androgen such as testosterone or DHEA).
3. Polycystic ovaries demonstrated by ultrasound.

Of course, other causes (prolactinoma, Cushing's syndrome, adrenal androgen secretion) should be excluded as well. Cortisol and TFTs may also be useful in the evaluation.

Tx—For hirsutism and acne, estrogen-progestin therapy is used in the form of OCPs in women not desiring pregnancy. Spironolactone can also be used for hirsutism. For amenorrhea, endometrial hyperplasia (from unopposed estrogen stimulation) can be reversed with progestational agents such as medroxyprogesterone acetate. Metformin and thiazolidinediones can be used to address the problem of insulin resistance. For pregnancy, clomiphene (GnRH analogues) can help stimulate ovulation.

CHAPTER 7 APPENDIX

Multiple endocrine neoplasia (MEN) syndromes encompass a wide range of clinical features inclu ded in both benign and malignant tumors. They are all autosomal dominant disorders, and although they are rare, it is important to recognize them when taking a detailed family history, as they impact treatment. The classic conditions seen in each MEN syndrome are shown in Table 7-12.

Another set of rare conditions in certain endocrinopathies that can be found together are the autoimmune polyglandular syndromes, shown in Table 7-13.

Table 7-12. Multiple Endocrine Neoplasia Syndromes

MEN I (Wermer's Syndrome)	MEN IIa (Sipple's Syndrome)	MEN IIb/MEN III
Hyperparathyroidism	Hyperparathyroidism	Marfanoid habitus
Pancreatic cell hyperplasia	Pheochromocytoma	Pheochromocytoma
Glucagonoma	Medullary thyroid cancer	Medullary thyroid cancer
Insulinoma		Benign neuromas of the eyelids,
Gastrinoma		lips, tongue, buccal mucosa,
Somatostatinoma		intestines, bladder, and bronchi.
VIPoma		
Pituitary adenoma		
Menin mutation	Ret mutation	Ret mutation

Table 7-13. Autoimmune Polyglandular Syndromes

Type I	Type II
Mucocutaneous candidiasis	Autoimmune thyroid disease
Hypoparathyroidism	Type I DM
Adrenal insufficiency	Adrenal insufficiency (adult onset)
	Gonadal failure, alopecia
Presents in childhood	Presents in adulthood
Sporadic or familial inheritance	Polygenic, autosomal dominant

CHAPTER 8

Infectious Diseases

DIAGNOSTIC TESTING

Numerous diagnostic tests are used to determine the specific etiology of infectious conditions. While, for most bacteria, cultures in specialized media help determine the particular organism after several days, use of the Gram stain early on may help make or narrow down a diagnosis. Table 8-1 shows the diagnostic stains for different categories of organisms.

APPROACH TO COMMON PROBLEMS

Fever of Unknown Origin (FUO)

The current criterion for FUO is a fever >101°F for at least 3 weeks without diagnosis after three outpatient visits or, if an inpatient, after 3 days of hospitalization.

There are several additional types:

- *Nosocomial FUO* occurs in patients who have a fever after admission with negative work-up over 3 days.

- *Neutropenic FUO* is defined as a fever in patients with absolute neutrophil count (ANC) <500 who have negative cultures without diagnosis for >3 days. The initial fever is either >101°F or can be a temperature of >100.4°F for more than one hour.
- *Human immunodeficiency virus—associated FUO* occurs in HIV-positive patients with fever for >4 weeks as an outpatient or 3 days as an inpatient.

The duration of fever changes the differential diagnosis:

- For those with acute or subacute fever, infections and cancer account for >60% of cases, and autoimmune diseases account for about 15%.
- For those with fever for >6 months, most cases are related to granulomatous disease (40%), factitious fever (25%), and cancer and autoimmune disease (20%). From 10% to 15% of cases remain undiagnosed.

Different causes of FUO are shown in Table 8-2.

Table 8-1. Diagnostic Stains for Infectious Organisms

Stain	Organisms Visualized	Comment
Gram Stain	Bacteria	Four components are used: (1) crystal violet (primary stain), (2) iodine (mordant), (3) ethanol (decolorizer), (4) safranin (counterstain).
Acid-Fast Stain (also called *Ziehl-Neelsen stain*)	Mycobacteria Nocardia	Acid-fast bacteria stain red, the color of the initial stain, and resist decolorization with acid-alcohol.
Gomori's Methamine Silver (GMS) Stain	PCP and fungi	GMS can be easily used on tissue, sputum, or closeup/or fluid. It stains the cyst wall.
Wright's Stain	Malaria	A combination of red acid and blue basic dye. Used in blood smears, bone marrow aspirates, cytogenetics. For WBCs in stool wet mount.
Tzank Stain	HSV	The vesicle is unroofed, the base scraped and treated with methylene blue. One looks for multinucleated giant cells.
Warthin Starry Stain	Spirochetes	This is a silver nitrate–based stain.

Table 8-2.   Causes of Fever of Unknown Origin FUO

	Causes	Comments
Infectious	Disseminated granulomatoses (TB, histoplasmosis, coccidiomycosis, blastomycosis, and sarcoidosis) Viral (EBV or CMV mononucleosis)	PPD is positive in less than 50% with TB patients who present with FUO.
	Abscess	Needs a high degree of clinical suspicion; obtain full body scan (chest, abdomen, pelvis) if one cannot localize the cause. Dental abscesses are frequently missed.
	Endocarditis	Difficult-to-culture organisms: • *Coxiella burnetii* (Q fever) and *Tropheryma whippelii* (cannot grow in cell-free media). *Brucella, Mycoplasma, Chlamydia, Histoplasma, Legionella,* and *Bartonella* require special media or methods. • HACEK group organisms (*Haemophilus* spp., *Actinobacillus, Cardiobacterium, Eikenella, Kingella*) require blood culture incubation for 7–21 days.
	Osteomyelitis	Vertebral and mandibular areas are common sites for FUO.
Neoplastic	Lymphoma (Hodgkin's and non-Hodgkin's), leukemia, renal cell carcinoma, hepatoma, atrial myxomas.	All suspicious lymph nodes should be excised for diagnosis or biopsied if appropriate.
Autoimmune	Lupus, Still's disease, mixed cryoglobulinemia, polyarteritis nodosum, temporal arteritis, Takayasu's arteritis, and Wegener's granulomatosis are the most common causes.	History is most useful to distinguish collagen vascular disease. Still's disease is a diagnosis of exclusion. ESR or CRP may be a helpful first test.
Drugs	Antibiotics, antihistamines, barbiturates, phenytoin, iodides, NSAIDs, hydralazine, methyldopa, quinidine, procainamide, antithyroid medication, and quinine (a contaminant of cocaine or heroin) are all possible culprits.	Eosinophilia presents in only 25% of cases. Stopping each medication is the only empiric way to assess this.
Other	Thromboembolic disease (PE), disordered heat homeostasis (hypothalamic dysfunction following stroke, hyperthyroidism), alcoholic hepatitis, hematomas, pheochromocytoma, and adrenal insufficiency.	Retroperitoneal, pelvic, or femoral hematomas may be hard to detect on exam.

In obtaining the history, one should focus on:

- Associated symptoms (chills, night sweats, cough, dysuria, pain, diarrhea, GI distress, itching)
- Risk factors for immunosuppression
- Sick contacts
- Travel
- Animal and insect exposure
- Drug and toxin history (including antibiotics, alcohol and illicits drug use)
- Immunizations
- Family history (cancer, autoimmune disease, familial Mediterranean fever, and so forth)

In addition to a complete physical exam, there are some subtle findings that may be noteworthy, as shown in Table 8-3.

Work-up: If the diagnosis is not clarified by the history and exam, then work-up should include:

- CBC with differential
- ESR and/or CRP
- Electrolytes
- LFTs
- LDH
- Urinalysis and microscopic examination
- Chest X-ray
- Blood cultures obtained three times while the patient is off antibiotics
- PPD
- HIV antibody assay
- antinuclear antibody (ANA)
- Rheumatoid Factor
- A heterophile antibody test (in children and young adults) for infectious mononucleosis.
- An Abdominal CT

Additional viral and fungal serologic tests may be obtained if the history suggests such an etiology. A tagged WBC scan may be obtained if the initial work-up is negative. If indicated, further work-up may include biopsy of the following sites: bone marrow, liver, lymph node, temporal artery, lung, pleural or pericardial fluid.

Treatment: Particular therapy should be delayed until the etiology of the fever has been identified. Febrile neutropenic patients or patients with nosocomial FUO who are severely ill, however, should receive empiric antibiotic coverage after cultures have been obtained.

Approach to the Patient with Sepsis

Sepsis is a systemic inflammatory process occurring in the presence of a documented infection that can lead to organ dysfunction, hypoperfusion (lactic acidosis, oliguria, or altered mental status), or hypotension and even shock. A related syndrome, the systemic inflammatory response syndrome (SIRS), occurs without the presence of a documented infection.

Table 8-3. Physical Exam Findings in Fever of Unknown Origin

Body Site	Physical Finding	Diagnoses to Consider
HEENT (head, ears, eyes, nose, and throat)	Tenderness around frontal and maxillary sinus	Sinusitis
	Nodules in the temporal arteries, reduced pulsations, jaw pain with repeated chewing motions	Temporal arteritis
Oropharynx	Aphthous ulcers	Lupus, Bechet's syndrome, disseminated histoplasmosis
	Tender tooth	Dental abscess
Fundi or Conjunctivae	Choroid tubercle or petechiae	Disseminated granulomatosis
	Roth's spot	Endocarditis
Thyroid	Enlargement, tenderness	Thyroiditis
Heart	New murmur or change in old murmur	Infective or marantic endocarditis
Abdomen	Enlarged iliac crest lymph nodes, splenomegaly	Lymphoma, endocarditis disseminated granulomatosis
Rectum	Perirectal fluctuance, tenderness	Rectal abscess
	Prostatic tenderness, fluctuance	Prostatitis
Genitalia	Testicular nodule	Periarteritis nodosum
	Epididymal nodule	Disseminated granulomatosis
Lower Extremities	Tenderness	Thrombosis or thrombophlebitis
Skin and Nails	Petechiae, splinter hemorrhages, subcutaneous nodules, clubbing, palpable purpura	Vasculitis Endocarditis

Frequent causes of sepsis are common infections that go uncontrolled such as:

- UTI/pyelonephritis
- Pneumonia
- Peritonitis
- Cholangitis
- Cellulitis
- Meningitis
- Abscess formation at any site

Microorganisms proliferate at these sites and may either invade the bloodstream or release their toxic components (e.g., Toxic shock syndrome toxin-1, or TSST-1, from staphylococci or lipopolysaccharide endotoxin from gram-negative bacteria) from the focal site of infection. These organism-derived products lead to release of inflammatory cytokines (TNF-α and IL-6) and in large amounts, they can produce profound physiologic effects on the vasculature (vasodilation and capillary leak) and organ systems.

Symptoms include fever (although 15% of patients present with hypothermia), tachycardia, tachypnea, and altered mental status. Hypotension and shock may occur in severe cases. Early sepsis can present with warm skin and extremities (warm shock: peripheral dilation) and may then progress to cool skin and extremities (cold shock: peripheral vasoconstriction). Petechiae or ecchymoses may suggest disseminated intravascular coagulation (DIC).

For the diagnosis, the patient should meet the SIRS criteria (see Table 8-4).

The following laboratory findings support the diagnosis of sepsis:

1. Neutropenia or neutrophilia with increased bands.

Table 8-4. The Systemic Inflammatory Response Syndrome Criteria

Temperature	≤36°C or ≥38°C
Heart Rate	≥90 bpm
Respiratory Rate	≥20 breaths/min **or** PaCO2 <32 mmHg
WBC Count	≥12,000 or ≤4000 cells/mL **or** >10% bands

2. Thrombocytopenia (in 50% of cases).
3. Positive blood cultures (in 40–60% of cases).
4. Increased BUN and creatinine levels [from acute tubular necrosis (ATN)].
5. Respiratory alkalosis may be noted initially secondary to hyperventilation, but may shift to metabolic acidosis with respiratory muscle fatigue and accumulation of lactate. This is one of the rare conditions in which there can be overcompensation for metabolic acidosis to create an alkaline pH.
6. Disseminated intravascular coagulation: prolongation of prothrombin time, decreased fibrinogen, and the presence of D-dimers.

Tx—Broad spectrum IV antibiotics are given empirically, and then later narrowed when culture data has returned. Early goal-directed therapy is used for resuscitation, which has become the standard of care at many institutions. It involves placement of a central venous catheter to monitor central venous pressure and mixed venous saturations to tailor resuscitation and pressors. Typically aggressive resuscitation with IV fluids is done first followed by the use of pressors if patients are still hypotensive. Removal of a focal source of infection and drainage (e.g., Foley catheter, infected line, abscess) is important. Patients with at least one acute organ dysfunction may be candidates for activated protein C (drotrecogin-α) which has shown some benefit in such patients. Other treatments include IV bicarbonate to correct acidosis and IV corticosteroids to treat relative adrenal insufficiency.

INFECTIOUS DISEASES BY PRIMARY SITE OF INFECTION

Head and Neck

Otitis Externa

D—Inflammation of the skin lining the ear canal and surrounding soft tissue. It is also known as *swimmer's ear*.

P—The outer ear is the cartilaginous portion that contains two-thirds of the ear canal up until the tympanic membrane. Inflammation is either infectious or, less commonly, allergic. Most common infectious agents are *Pseudomonas* and *Staphylococcus aureus*. Polymicrobial infections are seen in one-third of cases.

RF—Risk factors include excessive ear cleaning or itching of the ear with scratching (which removes the protective cerumen) and swimming (from excess moisture).

SiSx—Pain, pruritis, and a purulent discharge from the ear canal are common complaints. On exam, classically there is pain is elicited with movement of the pinna. An edematous and erythematous ear canal with a purulent discharge may be noted on exam.

Dx—This is purely a clinical diagnosis based on the symptoms and history.

Tx—Eardrops with polymyxin B, neomycin, and hydrocortisone can be used. Dicloxacillin is used for acute disease. Diabetics (in whom *Pseudomonas* is a chief etiology) and patients with severe infections should be treated with IV antibiotics due to their increased risk of developing malignant otitis externa and osteomyelitis of the skull base.

Otitis Media

D—An inner ear infection with concomitant fluid in the middle ear.

Epi—It is the most common diagnosis in sick children 6 months to 2 years old. Boys are affected more than girls.

P—The inner ear is the vestibule, semicircular canals, and cochlea. Infection usually follows an upper respiratory infection (URI) in which congestion of the nasopharynx and eustachian tube causes obstruction of the tube's isthmus. Middle ear secretions cannot leave and bacteria from the upper respiratory tract reflux there and grow, causing suppuration. The skin of the inner ear has no subcutaneous tissue and is in direct contact with the periosteum, allowing easier spread of infection. Most common bacterial agents are *Streptococcus pneumoniae, Haemophilus influenzae* (very few now due to type b), *Moraxella catarrhalis,* and viral causes (15%). Mycoplasma is associated with bullous myringitis. Tuberculous otitis media can be seen in developing countries.

RF—Risk factors include young age, immature anatomy, and attendance at a day care center.

SiSx—Symptoms include ear pain, vertigo, and even hearing loss. A discharge may indication perforation of the tympanic membrane. Fever, malaise, nausea and vomiting may accompany also occur.

Dx—Diagnosis is made by otoscopy, tympanometry, and the clinical history.

Tx—Most commonly, treatment involves amoxicillin to cover *Streptococcus pneumoniae*. Macrolides are useful for penicillin-allergic patients. Amoxicillin-clavulanate, cefuroxime, or ceftriaxone can be tried in those who fail amoxicillin. With recurrent disease, tympanostomy tubes can be placed to drain middle ear fluid. Poorly treated disease can result in hearing loss.

Acute and Chronic Sinusitis

D—Inflammation of the paranasal sinuses from a viral, bacterial, or fungal infection.

Epi—This is one of the top 10 common diagnoses in outpatient medicine and the fifth most common reason patients are given antibiotics.

P—The maxillary sinuses and sometimes the ethmoid sinuses are most commonly affected because they drain superficially against gravity. Frontal sinus infection is unusual and implies additional pathology. The most common causes of acute sinusitis (<1 month duration) are *Strep. pneumoniae, H. influenzae, M. catarrhalis*, and common cold-type viral infections, whereas chronic sinusitis (>3 months duration) is often due to obstruction of sinus drainage and ongoing anaerobic infections. Sphenoidal sinusitis is classically seen only with *Staph. aureus*. It occurs as a secondary infection after sinus obstruction or occurs after a URI which decreases mucociliary clearance of the sinuses, allowing infection to occur more easily.

RF—Risk factors include an immunocompromised state, allergic rhinitis, upper respiratory infection, asthma, nasal intubation, use of NG tubes, deviated septum, and nasal polyps.

SiSx—Symptoms include nasal congestion, nasal discharge, fever, headache, and facial pain near the affected sinus. Maxillary sinusitis causes pain over the cheeks and upper teeth; ethmoid sinusitis causes pain over the eyes or retroorbitally; frontal sinusitis causes pain over the eyebrows; and sphenoid sinusitis causes retroorbital pain with radiation to the occiput or upper face. Pain may be absent in chronic sinusitis, but nasal congestion, cough, and purulent drainage remain. Nasal examination reveals inflammation and pus.

Dx—This is a clinical diagnosis. Three symptoms—(1) unilateral facial pain or maxillary tooth pain, (2) a purulent drainage, and (3) the presence of symptoms for >7 days—are only about 30% sensitive for the condition but are enough to warrant treatment. A CT scan is rarely needed unless the condition does not respond to treatment, but it is more sensitive than X-rays. Special CT views of the head will show air-fluid levels or new opacification of a sinus. In chronic sinusitis that is unresponsive to treatment, sinus puncture (the gold standard for diagnosis) may be warranted.

Tx—Antibiotics may not be necessary, as there are little data to support their benefit over decongestants alone. Most cases, even bacterial ones, resolve without antibiotics. Antibiotics should be considered when symptoms last longer than a week. Usually amoxicillin, trimethoprim-sulfamethoxazole, or doxycycline is given for 10 days and symptomatic therapy (e.g., decongestants, steam inhalation, warm compresses) for treatment of acute sinusitis. For chronic sinusitis, antibiotics are given for 6–12 weeks with nasal steroids. Surgical drainage and correction of obstruction may be necessary if medical therapy fails.

Upper and Lower Respiratory Tract Infections

Acute Pharyngitis

D—An inflammatory condition of the oropharynx that may be infectious or noninfectious in origin.

Epi—It accounts for up to one-fifth of visits to outpatient physicians in the United States, the most for any infectious disease.

P—Noninfectious causes include a postnasal drip that irritates the lining of the throat. In such cases, the sore throat usually gets better during the day. Viral pharyngitis can cause sore throat by the same mechanism, eliciting a runny nose as well as a postnasal drip. Most cases are viral in origin. Of the bacterial causes, group A streptococcus accounts for 5–10% of all adult cases and is the only common cause that requires treatment to prevent complications such as rheumatic fever. Causative organisms are shown in Table 8-5.

RF—Risk factors include sick contacts and cold weather.

SiSx—Common symptoms of strep throat are sudden onset of sore throat, odynophagia, fever, headache, nausea/vomiting, and abdominal pain. Cough, hoarseness, and diarrhea are uncommon. Soft palate petechiae may also be present along with an exudate, though this can be seen with viral causes as well. Other symptoms include anterior cervical lymphadenopathy (anterior nodes drain the oropharynx), chills, myalgias, and malaise.

Dx—At the initial presentation in an otherwise healthy person, one needs to distinguish bacterial streptococcal infection from other causes. Clinical predictors of group A streptococcal infection are (1) fever >101°F, (2) lack of a cough, (3) tender anterior cervical lymphadenopathy, and (4) the presence

Table 8-5. Causative Agents in Upper Respiratory Tract Infections

Viral	*Common*: rhinovirus, coronavirus, adenovirus *Uncommon*: HSV (primary infection), influenza, parainfluenza, coxsackievirus (hand, foot, mouth disease), EBV (mononucleosis),CMV, HIV (seroconversion)
Bacterial	*Common*: group A and group B beta-hemolytic streptococcus *Uncommon*: Neisseria gonorrhoeae, diphtheria, *Arcanobacterium*, *Fusobacterium necrophorum* *Atypical*: Chlamydia, Mycoplasma

of exudates on the tonsils/oropharynx. If all four conditions are present, treatment is warranted without testing, although there is only a 35–55% chance of finding group A streptococcus on swab testing. If two or three conditions are present, clinical judgment should be used to decide whether or not to give antibiotics. If only one condition is present, group A streptococcal infection is unlikely and antibiotics maybe withheld. Other diagnostic studies used are the rapid streptococcal enzyme-linked immunosorbent assay (ELISA) test or throat culture, which takes 24 to 48 hours. Tests are done on a touch swab of both tonsils and the back of the pharynx.

Tx—Viral causes require supportive care only: antipyretics, fluids, and rest. If group A streptococcus is suspected or diagnosed, a 10-day course of oral penicillin or one IM shot is the treatment of choice (there is no significant resistance to penicillin). Azithromycin is given to penicillin-allergic patients. Cephalosporins can cause faster eradication rates (5 days instead of 10 days) and can also be used. If the patient is still symptomatic after several days, then work-up of the uncommon causes is in order.

Pneumonia

D—An inflammation of the alveoli/interstitium from infection by microorganisms. Different types are shown below and in Table 8-6.

Community-acquired pneumonia (CAP)— implies a normal or abnormal host with a common organism of high virulence, acquired outside of the hospital.

Atypical pneumonia—implies an infection by a less common organism.

Table 8-6.   Types and Causes of Pneumonia

Type of Acute Pneumonia	Most Common Organisms	Comments
Community-Acquired Pneumonia (CAP)	*Streptococcus pneumoniae* (50–75%) *Haemophilus influenzae* *Moraxella catarrhalis* *Klebsiella pneumoniae* Other enteric gram-negative bacteria	*Haemophilus influenzae* and *Moraxella* are also common in smokers. *Klebsiella* is classically seen in alcoholics and may present with "currant jelly"–colored sputum.
Atypical Pneumonia	*Mycoplasma pneumoniae,* *Legionella pneumophilia,* *Chlamydia pneumoniae* *Viral:* adenovirus, RSV, influenza, parainfluenza *Immunocompromised patients:* PCP or other fungal diseases such as histoplasmosis, coccidiomycosis, and blastomycosis	*Mycoplasma* is the so-called "walking pneumonia," more common in young adults who do not appear to be very sick. *Legionella* classically causes GI symptoms such as diarrhea and may present with, renal and hepatic dysfunction and/or ΔMS.
Nosocomial Pneumonias	Gram-negative bacilli (GNB): *Pseudomonas aeruginosa* (60%), *Escherichia coli, Enterobacter* Gram-positive cocci (GPC): *Staphylococcus aureus* (15%)	Double coverage for presumed *Pseudomonas* may be warranted unless cultures isolate other organisms.
Aspiration Pneumonia	Organisms of the mouth: *S. aureus,* group A streptococcus, anaerobes	*S. aureus* can form cavitations. Edentulous patients cannot develop such types of bacterial pneumonia, as they have no significant bacterial reservoirs. More common in such cases are viral or chemical pneumonias.

Nosocomial or hospital-acquired pneumonia—occurs by definition >48 hours after hospitalization or if the patient was recently discharged from a long hospitalization.

Aspiration pneumonia—implies oropharyngeal tracking of organisms into the lung, causing infection after an aspiration event.

Epi—Pneumonia is the number one cause of mortality from infectious diseases in the United States; 2–3 million cases occur every year. Up to 60% of cases do not yield a causative organism.

P—Different organisms have different virulence factors. For acute pneumonia, it is important to know the patient setting in order to identify the most common causes for appropriate antibiotic treatment. Chronic pneumonia is more likely to be due to mycobacteria (more suggestive if productive), fungi, parasites, and nocardia.

RF—There are many risk factors, including an immunocompromised state, chronic illness, cancer, COPD, asthma, cystic fibrosis, smoking, and influenza infection. Advanced age, impaired gag reflex, and decreased level of consciousness all predispose to aspiration pneumonia.

SiSx—Symptoms may include a productive cough (purulent yellow or green sputum or even hemoptysis), dyspnea, fevers/chills, night sweats, and pleuritic chest pain. Pneumonia due to atypical organisms may present with a more gradual onset, dry cough, headaches, myalgias, and pharyngitis. Physical signs vary and can include decreased or bronchial breath sounds, crackles, wheezing, dullness to percussion, egophany, and tactile fremitus. Elderly, diabetic, or COPD patients may have minimal findings on exam.

Dx—A clinical diagnosis of acute pneumonia can be made with a new onset of fever, productive cough, and focal crackles on exam. A chest X-ray may demonstrate lobar consolidation, as seen in most bacterial pneumonias, or patchy or diffuse infiltrates, as seen in atypical or viral pneumonia. Cavitations may also be seen with more virulent organisms such as *Staph. aureus*. A negative chest X-ray, however, does not always rule out pneumonia. Pleural effusions, if present, should be tapped and the fluid analyzed for evidence of infection. Parapneumonic effusions, if infected, need a chest tube. A CBC may reveal leukocytosis with increased neutrophils. Sputum Gram stain and culture may identify the organism, though the yield is generally quite poor, especially in patients who have already been started on antibiotics. If the patient appears to be very ill, obtain blood cultures to assess for sepsis and an ABG to demonstrate acid-base disturbance.

In those who fail therapy or have organisms (such as with *Pneumocystis jiroveci* pneumonia) that require diagnosis by other means, additional procedures can be performed. Flexible bronchoscopy with bronchoalveolar lavage has significant limitations for lower respiratory flora because it is easy to have contamination. This test is usually reserved for immunocompromised patients at high risk for TB or PCP in whom a diagnosis needs to be made. Open lung biopsy is reserved for severely ill non-immunocompromised patients who are not responding to therapy.

Tx—Antibiotics are the mainstay of therapy for acute pneumonia. Patients who are admitted to a hospital generally need IV antibiotics. Criteria for hospital admission have roughly been defined by the Pneumonia Outcomes Research Trial (PORT) Score, which includes a point system based on numerous factors including abnormal laboratory tests findings and vital signs, as well as comorbid lung, heart, liver, and kidney diseases. The PORT score, however, does not account for HIV-positive and otherwise immunocompromised patients and should not substitute for clinical judgment if the patient looks sick. Specific antibiotics or other treatment depends on the suspected organisms and the type of pneumonia (see Table 8-7). Admission to an ICU is indicated in those with severe respiratory distress with a high risk of becoming septic.

Table 8-7. Empiric Therapy for Pneumonia

Patient	Suspected Pathogens	Common Coverage Regimens
Outpatient <60 years of age	*Streptococcus pneumoniae, Mycoplasma pneumoniae, Chlamydia pneumoniae, Haemophilus influenzae*	Macrolides: clarithromycin or azithromycin Doxycycline
>60 or with comorbid disease	*S. pneumoniae, H. influenzae,* gram negatives (e.g., *Escherichia coli, Enterobacter, Klebsiella), Staphylococcus aureus, Legionella,* viruses	Second-generation cephalosporin or trimethoprim-sulfamethoxazole or amoxicillin. Add macrolide if atypical organisms are suspected.
CAP requiring hospitalization	*S. pneumoniae, H. influenzae,* anaerobes, gram negatives, *Legionella, Chlamydia*	Third-generation cephalosporin (such as ceftriaxone) + azithromycin clarithromycin or doxycycline Fluoroquinolone (note: ciprofloxacin has less coverage against *S. pneumoniae*)
Nosocomial pneumonia	Gram negatives including *Pseudomonas, S. aureus, Legionella,* and other mixed flora	Third-generation cephalosporin + azithromycin (or levofloxacin). If patient is at risk for *Pseudomonas*: piperacillin-tazobactam + azithromycin or cefepime + levofloxacin
Aspiration pneumonia	Anaerobes	Levofloxacin + clindamycin (or metronidazole) Piperacillin-tazobactam

Tuberculosis (TB)

D—A multisystemic disease with primarily pulmonary manifestations caused by *Mycobacterium tuberculosis* (Mtb) and characterized by a granulomatous response of tissue inflammation and damage.

Epi—This is the number one cause of infectious morbidity and mortality worldwide, with up to one-third of the worldwide population infected. There are 8–10 million new cases each year with 2–3 million deaths. The disease is most common in Southeast Asia, Latin America, and sub-Saharan Africa. In the United States, 10–15 million individuals have latent infection. The incidence of TB peaked in 1992 with acquired immunodeficiency syndrome (AIDS) and changes in immigration and has decreased since then.

P—*Mycobacterium tuberculosis* has no natural reservoir except for infected individuals. It is an obligate aerobe and a facultative intracellular parasite attacking tissue with high oxygen tension, with the ability to proliferate within mononuclear phagocytes. Cell walls contain mycolic acids that are resistant to decolorizing by acid-alcohol (hence they are called *acid-fast bacilli*). Transmission is mostly by aerosolization of respiratory secretions, which have to be small enough (1–5 μm) to reach the distal alveoli, where bronchial mucociliary clearance is more difficult. Such small particles can be generated mainly by forceful coughing and may remain suspended in the air for several hours. They are then taken up by macrophages, and a complex cell-mediated defense occurs that, in >90% of cases, is successful in containing the initial infection over a few weeks to months. During this time, the bacilli may disseminate to other pulmonary and extrapulmonary sites for potential reactivation later. Residua of primary infection may be seen in the lungs as hilar granulomas (called the Ghon focus) or apical fibronodular areas (called Simon foci) or as granulomas in other tissues.

RF—Risk factors include HIV, crowded living conditions, incarceration, homelessness, immunosuppression, alcoholism, diabetes, advanced age, immigration from developing nations, and contact with TB-positive individuals.

SiSx—Eighty-five percent of patients present with pulmonary disease; 15% present with extrapulmonary disease, increasing to 60–80% in immunocompromised patients, especially those with AIDS. Classic generalized symptoms include fevers, chills, profuse night sweats, and weight loss. Pulmonary symptoms include cough, which is almost universal. It is dry initially but then productive, with variable amounts of hemoptysis that can be heavy if there is cavitation into a nearby bronchial artery (*Rasmussen's aneurysm*). Malaise, weight loss, dyspnea, and nonpleuritic chest painare also common. Middle and lower lobe involvement is seen in primary infection, whereas reactivation of disease involves the upper lobes primarily. Areas of extrapulmonary TB are shown in Table 8-8.

Table 8-8. Sites of Extrapulmonary Tuberculosis

Location	Manifestations	Comments
Lymph Nodes	Usually unilateral and painless. Can cause massive lymphadenopathy.	More common in young adults. Responds slowly to medication. May need excision.
Pleura	Can occur in acute primary disease or from indolent condition. Pleural effusions may also occur. Pleuritic chest pain may be a sign of this. Elevated adenosine deaminase in the pleural fluid may aid in diagnosis.	Responds to medication. Drainage via thoracotomy generally is not done. Thought to be due to a delayed type hypersensitivity reaction. Burden of organisms is low and hard to obtain without pleural tissue.
GU	Kidneys, ureters, bladders, uterus, or fallopian tubes can be affected.	Can be a cause of obstructive uropathy. Cannot diagnose with an AFB on urine. Imaging may be suggestive, as is sterile pyuria and urine culture.
Bone/Joint	Potts disease is the most classic example and is more common in the elderly. It affects the lumbar and dorsal spine and weight-bearing joints.	Debriding and spine stabilization is needed. Diagnosis is made by CT-guided biopsy.
Disseminated Disease	This is more common in immunocompromised hosts. Adrenal involvement may lead to insufficiency.	Up to 50% are PPD negative; chest X-ray abnormalities may not be seen initially. Culture of multiple fluids, including gastric aspirates, can be done if a negative sputum smear. Liver biopsy has the highest yield of all tissue. Bone marrow biopsy may be positive only in those with pancytopenia.
CNS	Meningitis can present with cranial nerve palsies as TB affects the base of brain. Fever and headache may be seen early on; later, confusion, seizures, and coma can develop.	Lumbar puncture shows elevated levels of protein and white blood cells, decreased glucose, and high opening pressure. Steroids are needed in most cases. This is a hard condition to diagnose. PCR may be useful, though a negative result does not exclude the diagnosis.
GI	Ileal involvement can be mistaken for Crohn's disease.	Laparoscopic biopsy may be needed.
Pericardial Disease	Cough, dyspnea, and vague symptoms may be the presenting signs. Acute chest pain is quite rare.	Widened cardiac silhouette and left pleural effusion may be seen. Steroids may decrease the size of the effusion. Pericardiectomy may be needed for tamponade.

Dx

Sputum: Examination by acid-fast stain (Ziehl-Neelsen or Kinyoun) is a common method to assess for active TB. Obtaining three expectorated morning sputum samples on three consecutive days gives the best yield (up to 80–90% positive in cases where TB is later shown to also be positive by culture). Gastric aspirates in the morning can also be used and reflects swallowed sputum during the night, but this test is rarely performed. Induced sputum is not superior to expectorated sputum. Growth in culture is slow, and can take up to 5 weeks. If clinical suspicion is very high (i.e. suspicious imaging but negative or poor quality sputums), then bronchoscopy for bronchoalveolar lavage or lymph node biopsy to obtain additional material is necessary.

Skin testing: Tuberculin purified protein derivative (PPD) is the most commonly used method (see Table 8-9), though it is used mainly to test exposure and not to exclude or include active pulmonary TB, since for these purposes it is not sensitive or specific. In fact, the PPD can be falsely negative in 20–25% of patients with active TB, especially in immunocompromised, malnourished, or elderly patients. In such patients, an anergy panel may be helpful.

Imaging: Chest X-ray or CT may show apical fibronodular infiltrates with or without cavitations. Most common sites of reactivation are (1) the posterior and apical right upper lobe (RUL), (2) the apical-posterior left upper lobe (LUL), and (3) superior segments of the lower lobes. Lower zone disease is more common in diabetics and those with endobronchial involvement.

Tx—All cases should be reported to local and state health departments. All patients with suspected active TB requiring hospital admission require respiratory isolation. This is usually done before the diagnosis is made. Treatment depends on the stage of TB and the host factors. If the person is treated as an outpatient, he or she needs to wear a mask in the presence of others.

Latent, inactive TB: Preventive chemotherapy for reactivation is recommended, as it markedly reduces the chance of reactivation; it should be done in all high-risk populations. Typically, isoniazid (INH) with pyridoxine (to prevent peripheral neuritis from INH) is given as monotherapy for 9–12 months. Patients should abstain from alcohol and liver toxicity should be monitored. Patients >35 years old with a low risk of reactivation may choose to forgo INH prophylaxis, however, because of the risk of INH-induced liver toxicity, which increases with age. Daily rifampin for 4 months is used in those with INH-resistant but rifampin-sensitive TB. In HIV-positive individuals, rifampin can interact with highly active antiretroviral therapy (HAART) medication. In these patients, rifabutin may be a more appropriate choice.

Active TB: A multidrug regimen is necessary, as mutations are common; a four or five-drug regimen is used initially in many cases. This commonly includes pyrazinamide, ethambutol, isoniazid, rifampin, and sometimes streptomycin, among others. Directly observed therapy programs are useful to prevent resistance.

Actinomycosis

D—A chronic bacterial infection that can create both a suppurative and a granulomatous response. It is noteworthy for its ability to cross anatomic boundaries in its mode of spread, creating external sinuses in its path.

Table 8-9. Criteria for Positive Tuberculin Purified Protein Derivative Finding

A positive PPD is indicated by the size of the induration and the patient risk factors:	
>5 mm	HIV or risk factors, close TB contacts, and those with chest X-ray evidence of TB.
>10 mm	Homeless, from a developing nation, IVDU history, chronic illness, residents of health care or correctional facilities, health care workers.
>15 mm	None of the above risk factors.

Epi—It is a rare infection in the United States, given the improved dental hygiene. Mostly young and middle aged adults are affected.

P—The organism is a non-acid-fast, gram-positive coccobacillus with filamentous branches and require microaerophilic conditions for growth. Multiple species exist, but *Actinomyces israelii* is most common in human infection. *Actinomyces* is part of oral flora, adheres to dental plaques, and is also found in fecal flora as well as in the female reproductive tract. Unlike *Nocardia*, this is not an opportunistic infection and few systemic infections have been reported in immunodeficient patients.

RF—Risk factors include low socioeconomic status and poor dental hygiene.

SiSx—There are several well-recognized presentations:

Cervicofacial: In the setting of tooth decay and poor oral hygiene, tissue swelling or a suppurative inflammatory mass can develop, most commonly in the submandibular area. Symptoms of trismus (tonic contraction of jaw muscles) and a colorless exudate may be present. Infection can extend to the tongue, salivary glands, pharynx, and larynx. Cervical spine and cranial bone infection may lead to subdural empyema and invasion of the CNS with time.

Thoracic: In the setting of aspiration, infected oropharyngeal material. Pulmonary actinomycosis can spread commonly across lung fissures into the pleura and chest wall and can eventually destroy ribs as well. Some patients have a history of underlying lung disease.

Abdominal/pelvic: Usually this is a chronic localized process often preceded several weeks by abdominal surgery for an acute appendix or perforated colonic diverticula. The ileocecal region is most commonly involved, with formation of an inflammatory mass lesion. Persistent draining from sinus tracts can form. Pelvic inflammatory processes with actinomycosis have an association with intrauterine devices (IUDs) which have been left in for years.

Dx—The gold standard is anaerobic culture from fluid taken directly from a lesion or biopsy. It takes 3–10 days, however, to culture this organism. Other classic features that may help make the diagnosis are the presence of sulfur granules in drainage from a sinus tract or cultured fluid, though these granules are not universally present. The presence of non-acid-fast, gram-positive, filamentous branching organisms seen with microscopy is very suggestive.

Tx—Penicillin G is the treatment of choice. It is given in high doses over prolonged periods since infection has a tendency to recur. Usually 2–6 weeks of IV treatment is followed by oral therapy for months for deep-seated infection. Resistance is minimal. Tetracyclines, macrolides, or first-generation cephalosporins can also be used.

Nocardia

D—A subacute or chronic bacterial infection causing an intense suppurative response that involves the lung primarily and has the potential to seed to other areas, including the skin and CNS.

Epi—Three times as many males as females are affected. There are 500–1000 new cases per year in the United States.

P—Like *Actinomyces*, it is a gram-positive, filamentous, branching aerobic organism with bacillary and coccoid forms. However, it is weakly acid fast. Reservoirs include grass, soil, and rotting vegetations. *Nocardia asteroides* is the most common species infecting humans, usually as an opportunistic infection in immunocompromised, individuals; however, normal hosts can also be affected on occasion. The disease is thought to be acquired by inhaling airborne bacteria; thus, the lung is a primary site of infection in most cases. Virulence is due in part to production of a superoxide dismutase and catalase that block the phagolysosome action.

RF—An immunocompromised state is the major risk factor. Skin infection can be seen in immunocompetent individuals after inoculation.

SiSx—Pulmonary manifestations are the most common (75% of cases), presenting with fever, cough, dyspnea, pleuritic pain, and weight loss. The infection can disseminate to other organs in 20–40%, especially in post-transplant patients. Central nervous system involvement may present with headache and focal neurologic defects. Other sites include the liver, eye, kidney, lymph nodes, and skin.

Dx—Chest X-ray can show nodules, infiltrates, multiple abscesses, and cavitation in 20–50% of cases. Cultures of sputum, pleural fluid, bronchoalveolar lavage, or a lung aspirate or biopsy can help make the diagnosis. One should see filamentous branching rods that stain unevenly with crystal violet to give a beaded appearance and may be acid fast. Skin lesions should be also aspirated or biopsied, as they may reveal sulfa granules. The typical lesion seen on biopsy is one of liquefactive necrosis with abscess formation. Granuloma formation is infrequent and fibrosis is rare, unlike actinomycosis. Culture can take up to 14 days.

Tx—Trimethoprim-sulfamethoxazole, which also has good CNS penetration is a common first-line therapy. Most nocardia species are sensitive to this drug. Alternatives are imipenem or minocycline. Mortality in patients with CNS involvement can be as high as 40% and can be 15%-20% in those with pulmonary disease.

Other microorganisms involving the respiratory tract are discussed elsewhere in this chapter.

Central Nervous System Related Infections

Meningitis

D—Inflammation of the leptomeninges, usually from bacterial, viral (called *aseptic meningitis*), or fungal causes. Occasionally, malignancy and collagen vascular diseases can cause a similar inflammation.

RF—Risk factors include an immunocompromised state, recent sinopulmonary infections, and recent neurosurgical procedures.

SiSx—Patients classically present with fever, malaise, headache, neck stiffness, photophobia, altered mental status, and, rarely, seizures. Signs of meningeal irritation include Brudzinski's sign (neck flexion while the patient is supine causes hip flexion) or Kernig's sign (neck pain is elicited with extension of the knee while the hip is flexed, when the patient is supine and flat). Neurologic deficits are an ominous sign, especially if they involve cranial nerves, as seen in TB meningitis. In cases of gonococcal meningitis, a diffuse rash may be seen.

Dx—Bacterial meningitis initially should be a presumptive clinical diagnosis. In this case, empiric antibiotics should be given and lumbar pucture (LP) performed within 4 hours if papilledema or focal neurologic deficits are absent. Fever work-up including blood cultures should also be done. A CT scan of the head is required to rule out a mass effect in patients with a neurologic deficit, poor mental status, or known immunocompromised status, though this should not prevent early treatment. The LP is routinely sent for a cell count with differential (tubes 1 and 4), protein and glucose (tube 2), and other studies such as polymerase chain reaction (PCR) or culture (tube 3) of various bacterial, viral, or fungal etiologies. The LP can be done with the patient in a fetal position (opening pressure should always be measured in this position) or sitting with a hunched-over posture. Classic findings are shown in Table 8-10.

Tx—Treat bacterial meningitis with an immediate dose of empiric antibiotics and supportive care (see Table 8-11). Do not wait for LP or CT scan results to treat given the high mortality rate. Ideally and LP or CT should be done within 30 minutes of antibiotics administration to provide a good diagnostic yield. A CT scan is done before LP if the patient has a focal neurologic deficit or is immunocompromised given the chance that a mass lesion or abscess is present, whereby an LP may cause brain herniation. Viral meningitis can be treated with supportive care alone, except for herpes meningoencephalitis, which is treated with acyclovir. All contacts of patients with meningococcal meningitis should receive rifampin prophylaxis.

Table 8-10. Cerebrospinal Fluid Findings in Meningitis

Organism	Opening Pressure	WBC*	Protein	Glucose
Normal	5–15 mmHg or 65–195 mmH$_2$O	<10 mononuclear cells /mm^3 and < 1 polymorphonuclear cells/mm^3	15–45 mg/dL	CSF/blood glucose ratio >0.6
Bacterial	↑	↑ polymorphonuclear cells	↑↑	↓
Viral	normal/↑	↑ mononuclear cells	normal/↑	normal
TB/Fungal	↑↑	↑ mononuclear cells	↑↑↑	↓

Note: viral meningitis can have predominance of neutrophils early on, in which case glucose, protein levels, and the clinical picture are critical. HSV may present with a significant number of RBCs.
*A rough correction of WBCs for a bloody/traumatic tap is to subtract 1 WBC for every 1000 RBCs.

Table 8-11. Empiric Therapy for Bacterial Meningitis

Age	Organism	Antibiotics
<1 month	Group B streptococci, *Escherichia coli*, *Listeria*	Cefotaxime + ampicillin
1–3 months	Pneumococci, meningococci, *Haemophilus influenzae*	Cefotaxime + vancomycin
3 months–adult	Pneumococci, meningococci	Ceftriaxone + vancomycin
>60 years/alcoholism/ chronic illness, pregnancy	Pneumococci, gram-negative bacilli, *Listeria*	Ceftriaxone + vancomycin + ampicillin
Immunocompromised	Pneumococci, meningococci, *H. influenzae*, gram-negative bacilli, *Listeria*	Cefepime + vancomycin + ampicillin

Encephalitis

D—Inflammation of the brain parenchyma, usually characterized by the presence of cognitive or neurologic defects.

Epi—Several thousand cases are reported to the Centers for Disease Control (CDC) each year. The exact incidence is unknown, but the number of cases due to herpes simplex virus (HSV) is estimated at 0.2/100,000 per year.

P—Disease is due either to direct injury from the virus itself, which invades neuronal cells, or to postinfectious encephalitis injury, in which the virus may not cause direct tissue damage but inflammation/demyelination probably results from an autoimmune cause. Postinfectious encephalitis is most commonly seen with measles (known as *subacute sclerosing panencephalitis*) but also occurs with varicella-zoster virus (VZV), rubella, and influenza. Common causes of encephalitis are listed in Table 8-12.

RF—Risk factors include extremes of age and an immunocompromised status.

SiSx—Symptoms can be nonspecific but generally include headache, fever, nausea, and vomiting. Meningeal signs are usually absent, though nuchal rigidity can be seen. Neurologic derangements are present and range from a change in mental status or focal neurologic deficits to full obtundation. Classic presentations for HSV are strange behavior, aphasia, or olfactory hallucinations (the disease has a penchant for the inferior frontal and medial temporal lobes). West Nile virus more classically is characterized by diffuse paralysis and peripheral neuropathy. Toxoplasma encephalopathy presents in up to 40% of HIV-positive patients with headache, encephalopathy, and focal neurologic complaints or frank seizures.

Table 8-12. Viral Causes of Encephalitis in the United States

Causes	Comment
Enteroviruses	Aseptic meningitis; rarely leads to encephalitis
Coxsackievirus	More common in the fall and summer
Echovirus	
Poliovirus	
Arboviruses	Geographic variation noteworthy
California encephalitis	California (misnomer) virus found in the northern Midwest and the East
St. Louis virus	St. Louis virus is found in urban areas around Mississippi
West Nile virus	West Nile virus is found in the northeastern and southeastern United States
Western equine virus	Western equine type is found just west of Mississippi
Eastern equine virus	Eastern equine type is found in New England
Powassan virus	Powassan virus is the only one transmitted by ticks
Herpesviruses	CMV, EBV are the most common
	HSV-1 greatly exceeds HSV-2 as a cause
	VZV is rare except in immunocompromised patients
Other	Diagnosis can usually be made by other historical clues
HIV	
Rabies virus	
Influenza virus	

The syndrome of inappropriate antidiuretic hormone (SIADH) and its sequelae occur in 25% of patients with St. Louis encephalitis. Overall, seizures are more common with encephalitis than with meningitis.

Dx—The initial CSF exam is usually nondiagnostic, showing inflammation, as in aseptic meningitis. Elevated levels of RBCs in the CSF, when nontraumatic, may suggest HSV. Viral cultures are important, depending on the clinical scenario, with the highest yield for coxsackievirus and echovirus and the lowest yield for Epstein-Barr virus and CMV. The polymerase chain reaction (PCR) test on CSF should be done for HSV (>95% sensitive and specific, but less so into the second week of illness), West Nile virus, and enteroviruses (the yield is up to 75%). Neuroimaging studies are an important adjunct, as is EEG in cases where the diagnosis is not certain. Classically, HSV has increased signal intensity in the frontotemporal, cingulate, or insular regions on T2 MRI and/or low-amplitude or "flattened" activity on EEG. Ten percent of cases of PCR-positive HSV encephalitis will have a normal MRI, however. Brain biopsy is reserved for patients with nondiagnostic PCR studies, focal MRI abnormalities, and worsening clinical progress despite treatment.

Tx—Varicella-zoster virus and HSV are the only treatable causes; acyclovir is used. Untreated, the mortality of HSV encephalitis is high (>50%), with morbidity in survivors of long-term deficits. Varicella-zoster virus encephalitis can easily be fatal in immunocompromised patients. Japanese encephalitis and eastern equine encephalitis are just as severe. Subacute sclerosing panencephalitis (SSPE) from immune-resistant measles virus can be fatal. Many other causes are usually benign in the immunocompetent patient and require only supportive care, but they can be lethal in immunocompromised hosts.

Creutzfeldt-Jakob Disease (CJD)

D—A uniformly fatal condition with rapidly progressive dementia resulting from an infectious proteinaceous particle known as a *prion*.

Epi—This is the most common human prion disease but it remains quite rare, with an incidence of 1/1 million cases per year.

P—Sporadic (90%) forms, familial forms, variant forms, and iatrogenic forms are all recognized. Iatrogenic sources are from human pituitary hormone administration and dural graft transplants, among others. The incubation time is thought to be about 10 years on average. The prion protein is thought to induce conformational changes in normally expressed CNS proteins, disrupting normal cellular function. Familial cases are associated with a mutated protein expressed in normal neurons. In sporadic cases, the abnormal prion protein is thought to have a different form of secondary folding that acts as the etiologic agent. Other human prions cause Kuru, a dementing disease in certain New Guinea tribes spread by cannibalism, and fatal insomnia, characterized by insomnia and autonomic dysfunction. They are also found in animals. New-variant CJD, also known as *bovine spongiform encephalopathy* ("mad cow disease"), has an earlier onset (at 30 years of age) and a longer course (>1 year) and is thought to be transmitted to humans by eating brain or spinal cord of infected animals.

SiSx—Rapidly progressive mental deterioration, ataxia, and stimulus-induced myoclonus are the hallmark symptoms of sporadic CJD. New-variant CJD may have other features affecting vision and cerebellar or thalamic function. Changes in behavior, memory, judgment, and mood are early signs. Dementia becomes the most prominent finding and advances quickly. Myoclonus that can be induced by startling the patient is seen in many cases at some point during presentation. Hyperreflexia, primitive reflexes, and increased spasticity may also be seen.

Dx—An MRI scan in sporadic CJD may show hyperintensity of the cortical ribbon on MRI diffuse weighted imaging (DWI) or T2 hyperintensity in the caudate and putamen. With disease progression, prominent neuroimaging findings are generalized atrophy and ventricular dilation. In new-variant CJD, MRI may show hyperintensity of the pulvinar (caudal most nucleus of the thalamus) on DWI. An EEG may show classic periodic synchronous bi- or triphasic sharp wave complexes at some point during the course. Elevated CSF protein without pleocytosis is usually seen. The 14–3–3 protein, a neuronal signaling protein that is released into the CSF after neuronal death, is elevated in 85–95% of patients with sporadic CJD. The positive predictive value of this test is dependent on high clinical suspicion. Brain biopsy is the gold standard diagnostic test, demonstrating spongiform changes (numerous vacuoles) with neuronal loss and accumulation of the prion protein seen by immunohistochemistry. The histopathologies of sporadic and new-variant CJD are different.

Tx—Supportive care is the mainstay of treatment. Currently, there is no effective therapy and the condition is fatal.

Gastrointestinal Infections

Pseudomembranous Colitis

D—A condition of inflammatory exudative plaques or pseudomembranes of the colonic mucosa, most commonly due to overgrowth of *Clostridium difficile* and, in most cases, presenting with diarrhea and usually associated with antibiotic use.

Epi—It is one of the most common nosocomial infections.

P—*Clostridium difficile* is part of the normal GI flora, but overgrowth and disease occur most commonly as a complication of antibiotic or cancer-related chemotherapy. It produces two exotoxins. Toxin A is an enterotoxin that affects the intestinal mucosa. Toxin B, which is 1000 times more potent is less commonly diagnosed. In fact, 75% of isolates produce both toxins. Disease occurs when enough of either toxin binds to the brush border cell receptors to cause loss of actin filaments and shedding of cells into the lumen, creating ulceration. The presence of inflammatory exudates result in appearance of pseudomembranes. Persistent carriers are thought to have IgG against toxin A that prevents them from developing diarrhea and colitis.

RF—The most common antibiotics associated with this condition are penicillins, clindamycin, quinolones, and cephalosporins but virtually all antibiotics are implicated, even those used in treatment, such as metronidazole and vancomycin, as these can also disturb the balance of normal GI flora.

SiSx—Symptoms range from none (in carriers) to toxic megacolon. Acute watery diarrhea with abdominal pain is the most common presentation. Fever and leukocytosis are commonly seen. Bloody diarrhea is rare. Many hospitalized patients are asymptomatic carriers. Symptoms can occur even up to several weeks after an antibiotic has been discontinued.

Dx—Usually toxin testing is performed with separate samples at least 8–12 hours apart. Newer assays may require less repeat testing. In highly suspicious cases, toxin B studies are performed. Endoscopy will show the classic pseudomembranes and may be done in those with persistent diarrhea and negative toxin studies. A CT scan may show a thickened colonic wall.

Tx—Treatment depends on the severity of the disease. In mild cases, withdrawal of the offending antibiotic can result in resolution. Until a diagnosis is made, antidiarrheal agents such as loperamide should be withheld, as they increase the risk of toxic megacolon. The treatment of choice once a diagnosis is made is metronidazole. In the case of treatment failure, metronidazole can be repeated for a longer course. Refractory or severe cases can be treated with oral vancomycin. Additional treatments include replacement of colonic flora using the probiotic lactobacillus.

Viral Hepatitis

A condition caused mainly by one of five unrelated viruses. All of them can produce similar clinical pictures and have four phases:

1. *Incubation period* (2–20 weeks, depending on the virus and the amount of exposure): The virus becomes detectable in blood. Bilirubin, AST, and ALT are normal. Specific antiviral immunoglobulins are not yet detectable.
2. *Preicteric phase* (3–10 days): The viral antigen titers peak. The patient begins to suffer from fatigue, nausea, poor appetite, and vague RUQ pain. Virus-specific immunoglobulins, and AST and ALT begin to rise.
3. *Icteric phase* (1–3 weeks): Viral levels decrease. Dark urine appears along with jaundice. Pruritis, light-colored stools, anorexia, and weight loss are accompanying symptoms. Exam reveals hepatic tenderness and possibly hepatosplenomegaly. Bilirubin (both total and direct), AST, and ALT peak.
4. *Convalescent phase*: Virus is cleared. Bilirubin, AST, and ALT, return to normal levels.

Table 8-13 highlights main points of the various forms of viral hepatitis.

Table 8-13.　Summary of Types of Viral Hepatitis

Etiology	Transmission	Acute/Chronic	Dx
Hepatitis A (picornavirus)*	Fecal-oral (contaminated food, water, shellfish)	Acute hepatitis only. Does not cause chronic hepatitis.	Positive HAV IgM antibody makes diagnosis. IgG antibody indicates exposure and immunity.
Hepatitis B (DNA hepadnavirus)*	Blood and other body fluids, including saliva	Causes both acute and chronic hepatitis in 5–10%; 1% suffer fulminant or fatal acute hepatitis. Cause of hepato-cellular carcinoma (HCC).	Based on: HbsAg Anti-HBs Anti-HBc HBeAg and Anti-HBe
Hepatitis C (similar to a flavivirus)	Blood—formerly a major cause of post-transfusion hepatitis	Causes acute but mostly chronic hepatitis. Major cause of cirrhosis and ultimately HCC.	Anti-HCV antibody
Hepatitis D (Delta agent)	Blood	Causes acute or chronic disease only in association with HBV.	Anti-HDV Ig with positive HBV as well
Hepatitis E (unclassified RNA virus)	Fecal-oral (especially water-borne)	Acute hepatitis that can be severe or fatal in pregnant women (its main association).	Anti-HEV IgM

*Vaccine available.

Hepatitis A Virus (HAV)

D—An RNA virus of the family Picornaviridae.

Epi—Affects 1.4 million people per year worldwide, including 30,000 in the United States. It accounts for 20–40% of the viral hepatitis in the United States. Seroprevalance may be as high as 40%.

P—The virus is a positive-strand RNA picornavirus of 7.5 kb. A single serotype exists. Humans are the only known reservoir. Spread is fecal-oral. The incubation period is 15–45 days. Outbreaks can be sporadic or epidemic. Liver damage is from the body's immune response, specifically from CD8+ T cells and NK cells.

RF—Risk factors include travel to endemic areas, consumption of shellfish from contaminated waterways or raw fish, low socioeconomic status, lack of sanitation and poor hygiene, and anal sex. Day care centers are common places of outbreak.

SiSx—Usually this is an acute, self-limited illness and may be subclinical in children. Symptoms include fatigue, malaise, nausea/vomiting, RUQ pain, and, after a week, jaundice, pruritis, light stools, and dark urine. Hepatomegaly can be seen in up to 80%; splenomegaly and lymphadenopathy are less common. Fulminant hepatic failure can occur very rarely; it is seen more commonly in those with concomitant chronic HCV or another underlying liver disease. There is also a rare association with a relapsing or cholestatic clinical illness that can trigger an autoimmune hepatitis in some cases. Rare extrahepatic manifestations described include vasculitis, arthritis, aplastic anemia, and transverse myelitis seen in prolonged illnesses.

Dx—Transaminases are usually high (several thousand), with ALT levels exceeding AST levels and increased direct bilirubin and alkaline phosphatase. Diagnosis is made by the anti-HAV IgM antibody, which is the gold standard for acute illness. Antibodies are positive during the onset of symptoms and remains so for 4–6 months. Immunoglobulin G remains detectable for years. Anti-HAV IgG appears early in the infection. Anti-HAV IgM wanes after 4–12 months.

Tx—Treatment is usually supportive, as the condition is self-limited. Hospitalization is rare except for those with complications or significant comorbidities. Bilirubin should normalize in most patients by 3 months. Prevention via improved sanitation and hand washing is important in appropriate environments. The most commonly used HAV vaccine is inactivated; a live attenuated form also exists. Vaccination is appropriate for travelers to endemic areas and for those at higher risk of complications from HAV infection (HIV- and HCV-positive individuals or those with any chronic liver disease). Postexposure prophylaxis is given to those with recent exposure to HAV in the form of a single dose vaccine within 2 weeks of the last exposure.

Hepatitis B Virus (HBV)

D—A DNA virus of the family Hepadnaviridae.

Epi—From 400 to 500 million individuals are infected worldwide.

P—Spread is by the parenteral or sexual route. The incubation period is 30–150 days, during which time certain components rise: hepatitis B surface antigen (HBsAg), hepatitis B early antigen (HBeAg), and HBV DNA. By the preicteric period, antibodies to the core antigen (anti-HBc) appear. At this time, HBV DNA and HBeAg begin to fall. Eventually, the convalescent period is marked by the development of antibodies to the hepatitis B surface antigen (anti-HBs).

RF—Risk factors include immigration from endemic areas (Southeast Asia, China, Micronesia, sub-Saharan Africa, India, and the Middle East), travel to and high-risk behavior in endemic regions, IVDU, multiple sexual partners, anal sex, transfusion (less common), and heath care work.

SiSx—Beyond nonspecific symptoms of generalized acute or chronic hepatitis, extrahepatic manifestations of hepatitis B include vasculitis, glomerulonephritis, and polyarteritis nodosa. Disease course is variable. From 5% to 10% of patients go on to develop chronic HBV and over decades may develop cirrhosis. Others have clinical remission but may have relapses. Rarely (<1%), patients have fulminant hepatic liver failure, in which case liver transplant should be contemplated

Dx—Diagnosis is made by serologic testing, as shown in Tables 8-14 and 8-15. Acute HBV is diagnosed by the presence of positive HBsAg, HBc IgM and no anti-HBs. If HBV DNA and/ or HBeAg is positive this suggests a time of high infectivity and replication. In the period of acute hepatitis known as the "window period," there will be positive IgM anti-HBc but negative HBsAg and negative anti-HBs. Hence, it is always important to check the core antibody. In previous HBV infection, there will be positive anti-HBs and positive IgG anti-HBc. Persistant HBsAg suggests chronic hepatitis B infection.

Table 8-14. Clinical Utility of Hepatitis B Tests

Hepatitis B surface antigen (HBsAg)	Appears 1–10 weeks after exposure. Seen before ALT elevation. Becomes undetectable in the serum after 4–6 months. If it persists longer, then infection is considered chronic and may take longer to clear, sometimes many years.
Antibody to the hepatitis B surface antigen (Anti-HBs)	This antibody forms causing disappearance of HbsAg (except in cases of chronic hepatitis B). Persists for life, conferring long-term immunity. May not be detectable even though HBsAg disappeared several weeks to months earlier (the so-called window period). Here IgM core must be used. If both HBsAg and Anti-HBs are seen, then the antibody is unable to neutralize the Ag. These people are carriers.
Hepatitis B core antigen (HBAg)	An intracellular antigen called the *core antigen,* which is found only in infected hepatocytes. It is not detectable in serum and therefore is not measured.
Antibody to the hepatitis B core antigen (Anti-HBc)	IgM to the core antigen that forms during acute infection that then becomes IgG. The sole marker of infection during the window period. May be detectable years after infection as IgG, which indicates that there has been prior cleared infection in a noncarrier, as HbsAg will be negative. May increase in exacerbations of chronic HBV.
Hepatitis B early antigen (HBeAg)	A secretory protein that is marker of replication/infectivity. It is associated with high rates of transmission. If it persists, it indicates chronic infection.
Antibody to the hepatitis B early antigen (Anti-HBe)	Seroconversion to anti-HBe occurs faster than seroconversion of HBsAg to anti HBs, but can be delayed in chronic infection. During seroconversion HBV DNA usually disappears. Seroconversion can be delayed in chronic infection.
HBV DNA by PCR	Disappears during recovery. Used to assess replication and, if the patient is suitable for antiviral therapy in chronic disease.

Table 8-15. Common Serologic Patterns in Hepatitis B Infection

HbsAg	Anti-HBs	Anti-HBc	HBeAg	Anti-HBe	Interpretation
+	–	IgM	+	–	Acute HBV
–	–	IgM	+/–	–	Acute HBV, window period
+	–	IgG	+	–	Chronic HBV with active viral replication
+	–	IgG	–	+	Chronic HBV with low viral replication
+	+	IgG	+/–	+/–	Chronic HBV with so called "heterotypic anti-HBs" (10% of cases), hence HbsAg is still detected
–	+	IgG	–	+/–	Recovery from HBV (immunity)
–	+	–	–	–	Vaccination (immunity)

Tx—For patients with established chronic infection, interferon alpha or peginterferon is used for treatment. Patients without AST and ALT elevations usually do not respond to treatment. Side effects of interferon treatment include fatigue, myalgia, fever, and depression. More serious but rare side effects include psychosis, renal and cardiac failure, bacterial infection, and autoimmune disease. A rise in ALT after 2–3 months of treatment is normal.

Oral antivirals, often used in combination, such as lamivudine, adefovir, tenofovir, entecavir, and telbivudine, are alternatives to interferon with fewer side effects. Indications include intolerance to interferon. Treatment can be discontinued if HBeAg falls with a rise in anti-HBe IgG; this, however, rarely occurs. Treatment with lamivudine alone beyond a year to achieve complete resolution, but leads to drug resistance in 20–25%.

Vaccination to prevent hepatic B is recommended for all newborns and children, and is given as three shots at 0, 1, and 6 months of age. Adults with the risk factors listed above should also receive vaccination. In addition, household and sexual contacts of patients should be immunized. Postexposure prophylaxis with hepatitis B immune globulin (HBIG) is warranted for newborns and patients with parenteral exposures to an HBV-infected individual, though this is controversial.

Acute Hepatitis C Virus Infection

D—RNA virus of the family Flaviviridae.

Epi—There are approximately 36,000 new cases per year in the United States.

P—Spread is by IVDU (60%), sexual exposure (15–20%), maternal–fetal transmission, and needle stick accidents. The incubation period varies considerably from 15 to 120 days. Hepatitis C virus RNA can be detected 1–3 weeks after exposure and anti-HCV Ig develops some time after onset of symptoms and ALT and AST elevations. Serum HCV RNA disappears if the disease is self-limited, but chronic disease develops in 70% of patients. Fulminant disease is rare. Chronic infection occurs >75% of the time after acute infection even when transaminase levels are normal.

RF—Major risk factors include older age, male sex, alcoholism, IVDU, coinfection with another hepatitis virus, and HIV-positive status.

SiSx—Most patients are asymptomatic and are identified by testing after review of risk factors. Disease progression is usually slow, with cirrhosis occurring many years after infection. Malaise, joint pain, fatigue, URI symptoms, nausea, vomiting, and/or changes in bowel habits followed by jaundice and fatigue are possible symptoms. On exam, jaundice, scleral icterus, tender hepatomegaly, possible splenomegaly, and lymphadenopathy may be noted. Patients at a late stage of disease can present with progressive liver failure and also have an increased risk of developing hepatocellular carcinoma (HCC).

Dx—Test for anti-HCV Ig. Since it may appear weeks or months after symptoms develop, testing for anti-HCV Ig repeatedly or for HCV RNA may be necessary. Quantitation of the RNA does not correlate with disease severity.

Tx—Wait 2–4 months after the onset of symptoms to ascertain whether the disease is self-limited. No preventive treatment is currently recommended for needle stick exposures.

Chronic Hepatitis C Virus Infection

D—Condition in which the body is unable to clear the initial hepatitis C viral infection and low-grade infection persists.

Epi—This is the rule for most HCV infections rather than the exception. Most of these infections are newly diagnosed after an initial infection many years earlier from blood transfusions or other causes.

P—Marked genetic heterogeneity, termed *quasispecies diversity*, may account for the proclivity toward chronicity. Genetic differences of 1–5% may be found among HCV isolates from a single individual alone. Hepatitis C is classified into 6 genotypes and 90 subtypes. The most common genotypes in the United States are 1a and 1b (75%), 2a and 2b (15%), and 3a (7%). Different genotypes give the same clinical presentation but differ in susceptibility to treatment. Progression to chronic hepatitis is more common with genotype 1b. After the acute episode, AST and ALT levels vary widely. Usually patients are diagnosed with chronic hepatitis C 10–20 years after the initial viral exposure. One-third progress to cirrhosis with development of ESRD or HCC.

SiSx—In addition to findings associated with cirrhosis (see Chapter 4), look for extrahepatic manifestations including signs and symptoms consistent with cryoglobulinemia, glomerulonephritis, mucocutaneous vasculitis, sicca syndrome, non-Hodgkin's B-cell lymphoma, porphyria cutanea tarda, and lichen planus.

Dx—Anti-HCV antibodies make the diagnosis and should be done in patient with unexplained elevated ALT and AST levels or risk factors for HCV infection. Most patients should also have a liver biopsy at some point to stage the degree of liver inflammation and fibrosis or cirrhosis that is present.

Tx—Patients with genotype 1 are less amenable to therapy. Those with genotype 2 or 3 usually have a better response. Indications for treatment with peginterferon-ribavirin include raised ALT and AST levels and at least moderately severe chronic hepatitis on liver biopsy. Contraindications to peginterferon-ribavirin treatment include decompensated liver disease, renal failure, immunosuppression, cytopenia, severe psychiatric disease, active substance abuse, or lack of any bridging or portal fibrosis on biopsy in genotype 1 patients. Contraindications to ribavirin treatment are hemolysis, anemia, significant CAD, or renal insufficiency. Due to ribavirin's teratogenicity, both men and women should practice contraception during treatment and for 6 months afterward. Side effects of interferon and ribavirin may limit therapy. Finally, alcohol abstinence and HAV and HBV vaccination of the patient are warranted.

Routine HCC screening is important for patients with chronic hepatitis C and cirrhosis and includes a yearly RUQ U/S with serum AFP levels. If the patient is HIV positive, these tests are initially done every 6 months.

Hepatitis D Virus

D—Hepatitis D virus (HDV) is an RNA virus requiring HBV for replication. The RNA encodes a large and small delta antigen. The large antigen is involved in viral assembly and secretion and the small antigen in replication.

P—Spread is most common in HBV carriers with repeated parenteral exposure to HDV, known as *delta superinfection*. Clinically, the patient presents with acute hepatitis in addition to sequelae of <u>chronic</u> hepatitis B. *Delta coinfection* is the term for simultaneous <u>acute</u> HDV and HBV hepatitis. The clinical progression is similar to that of HBV infection, but a second elevation in AST and ALT levels may occur due to delta virus replication. Fulminant and chronic diseases are more common in co-infection than in acute hepatitis B alone.

SiSx—Symptoms are usually more severe than those of acute hepatitis B alone, but otherwise similar.

Dx—Superinfection is demonstrated by a positive HBsAg and anti-HDV Ig but negative anti-HBc IgM. Coinfection will give positive results for all three.

Tx—Currently, there is no specific treatment. Most cases of coinfection are self-limited. For HBV carriers, preventing parenteral exposures is key.

Hepatitis E Virus

D—Hepatitis E virus (HEV) is an RNA virus that is unclassified.

Epi—Large outbreaks have occurred in India, Pakistan, China, northern and central Africa, and Central America.

P—Spread is by the fecal-oral route, most commonly from swine or rats in the United States. The incubation period is 15–60 days. Hepatitis E virus virions and antigen are found in stool during the incubation period.

RF—Risk factors include travel to and residence in endemic areas. Pregnant patients are more susceptible to adverse events.

SiSx—Jaundice can be more severe than other acute viral hepatitis infections. Otherwise, hepatitis E manifests like acute HAV. The disease is much more severe in pregnancy.

Dx—A cholestatic (high bilirubin and alkaline phosphatase) as opposed to a hepatocellular pattern is more often seen on LFTs. Diagnosis is made if acute hepatitis occurs in the setting of recent travel to endemic areas, especially if the tests for other hepatitis viruses are negative. An anti-HEV IgM test and other HEV assays exist but are not standardized.

Tx—Currently, there is no specific treatment. Individuals should be cautioned against drinking water and eating uncooked foods in endemic areas. A vaccine is currently under development.

Food-Borne Illnesses

D—Illnesses resulting from ingestion of a wide variety of foods contaminated with pathogenic organisms or microbial toxins.

Epi—Up to 81 million food-borne illnesses occur annually in the United States.

SiSx—Common pathogens and their specific symptoms are presented in Table 8-16.

Table 8-16. Pathogens in Food-Borne Illness

Pathogen	Source	SiSx	Treatment
Bacillus cereus	Reheated fried rice Toxin mediated	Abrupt vomiting within 1–8 hours followed by watery diarrhea.	Self-limited.
Campylobacter jejuni	Poultry, raw milk	Fever, abdominal cramps, and *bloody* diarrhea within 16–48 hours.	Self-limited. Erythromycin, ciprofloxacin can be used if severe.
Clostridium perfringens	Rewarmed meat Toxin mediated	Abrupt, profuse, watery diarrhea within 8–16 hours.	Self-limited.
Clostridium botulinum	Home-canned food Honey (infants) Toxin mediated	Nausea, vomiting, and diarrhea followed by flaccid paralysis within 1–4 days. May occur in infants who are fed honey (ingest spores).	IV antitoxin.
Enterotoxigenic *Escherichia coli*	Uncooked foods, fecal contamination, fresh produce	Abrupt diarrhea. "Traveler's diarrhea."	Self-limited.
Enterohemorrhagic *E. coli* producing Shiga toxin. *E. coli* 0157:H7	Uncooked foods, fecal contamination, fresh produce	Fever, abdominal cramps, and bloody diarrhea within 3–8 days.	Associated with HUS; Symptoms can be severe.
Norwalk-like viruses	Shellfish, salads	Abdominal cramps, vomiting, headache, and watery diarrhea within 16–72 hours.	Self-limited.
Salmonella	Poultry, eggs, dairy products	Fever, abdominal cramps, bloody diarrhea, nausea and vomiting within 16–48 hours.	Self-limited. Antibiotics may prolong carrier state and increase relapse rate in patients with nontyphoid salmonellosis.
Shigella	Fecal contamination	Abrupt bloody diarrhea with mucus. Lower abdominal. cramps.	Ciprofloxacin if severe.
Staphylococcus aureus	Meats, dairy products (mayonnaise) Toxin mediated	Abrupt, intense vomiting and diarrhea within 1–8 hours.	Self-limited.
Vibrio cholerae	Shellfish, endemic areas (toxin mediated)	Severe, profuse "rice water" diarrhea within 16–72 hours.	Vigorous fluid and electrolyte replacement
Vibrio parahaemolyticus	Shellfish	Fever, abdominal cramps, and watery diarrhea within 16–72 hours.	Self-limited unless patient is immunocompromised.
Yersinia enterocolitica	Pork, milk, tofu	Fever, abdominal pain, inflammatory diarrhea. Can resemble acute appendicitis or right-sided colitis.	Ciprofloxacin if severe.

Dx—Diagnosis is based on positive stool culture or blood culture.

Tx—Replace fluid losses either orally or parentally. Antiemetics and antiperistaltic agents can be used for symptomatic relief, but antiperistaltic agents are contraindicated in patients with high fever, bloody diarrhea, or fecal leukocytes. See Table 8-16 for antibiotic use. Most illnesses are self-limited.

Infections of Skin and Bone

Cellulitis

D—An infection of the skin with extension into subcutaneous tissues. *Erysipelas* is a more superficial infection and does not affect subcutaneous tissues.

Epi—Males are affected more often than females; the lower extremities are most commonly involved.

P—After entrance, bacteria multiply and exotoxins evoke an inflammatory reaction that can spread subcutaneously. The most common cause is β-hemolytic streptococci followed by *Staph. aureus*. Other organisms to consider are *Pseudomonas aeruginosa* following puncture wounds, *Aeromonas hydrophilia* or *Vibrio vulnificus* after freshwater exposure, and *Pasteurella* after dog or cat bites. Diabetics are more likely to have polymicrobial disease.

RF—Risk factors include lymphedema, leg ulcer, trauma, intertrigo, venous insufficiency, leg edema, obesity, and tinea pedis.

SiSx—The symptoms most commonly seen are macular erythema, swelling, warmth, and tenderness. Red streaks on the skin moving upward (lymphangiectasia) are a sign of lymph involvement. Tender regional lymphadenopathy, lymphangitis, and abscess formation can also be seen. Sharp, well-demarcated margins are more commonly seen in erysipelas. Signs of systemic infection are fever, chills, and myalgias, which may occur in some cases. Lack of erythema, warmth, swelling, or local tenderness makes the diagnosis very unlikely. Crepitus may be heard and felt in patients with anaerobic organism infection such as *Clostridium perfringens*.

Dx—This is purely a clinical diagnosis. Establishment of microbiology is not necessary in most cases. Blood cultures are generally not necessary unless systemic infection is suspected, patients are not responding to therapy, or unusual exposure is noted.

Tx—Antibiotics are necessary. The decision to admit the patient to a hospital depends on whether IV antibiotics are needed. First-line empiric therapy is cefazolin for staphylococcus and streptococcus infections. Penicillin can be given to patients with erysipelas. Clindamycin or a quinolone can be given to penicillin-allergic patients. Vancomycin should be given if hospital-acquired methicillin-resistant *Staph. aureus* (MRSA) is suspected; otherwise, trimethoprim-sulfamethoxazole or clindamycin should be given for community-acquired MRSA. Diabetics require broader coverage for gram-negative infections with IV ampicillin sulbactam. For outpatients, trimethoprim-sulfamethoxazole with metronidazole, to cover patients for anaerobes, may be a reasonable option.

Lack of response to treatment should prompt a search for osteomyelitis or another organism (e.g., fungal infection or TB). Oral suppression therapy can be given to patients who have two or more episodes a year.

Osteomyelitis

D—Bone infection secondary to a soft tissue infection (80% of cases) or to hematogenous seeding (20% of cases). Hematogenous seeding usually occurs in children, affecting the metaphyses of the long bones, and in IV drug users, affecting vertebral bodies.

P—Different microorganisms are involved, depending on the host. These are shown in Table 8-17.

SiSx—Fever and localized bone pain are the most common presenting complaints. Localized warmth, erythema, tenderness, and limited motion of adjacent joints can be noted on exam.

Dx—Elevated WBC, ESR (>100 mm/hr), and CRP levels may be helpful but do not have to

Table 8-17. Causes and Features of Osteomyelitis.

Condition	Bones/Joints Affected	Pathogen
Healthy patient	Multiple bones	*Staphylococcus aureus*
Sickle cell disease	Multiple bones	*Salmonella, Streptococcus pneumoniae*
IVDU	Vertebral bodies, disc space	*S. aureus, Pseudomonas aeruginosa*
Penetrating foot injury	Foot bones	*P. aeruginosa*
Hemodialysis	Ribs, thoracic vertebrae	*S. aureus*
Ingestion of unpasteurized dairy products	Knee, hip, sacroiliac joint	*Brucella*
Rash and arthritis	Multiple	*Neisseria gonorrhoeae, N. meningitidis, Haemophilus influenzae, Moraxella osloenia, Streptobacillus moniliformis*
Diabetic foot ulcer	Site of ulcer	Streptococci, anaerobes, gram-negative bacilli
Foreign body	Site of ulcer	*Staphylococcus epidermidis*
Dog or cat bite	Site of trauma	*Pasteurella multocida*, anaerobes
Human bite	Site of trauma	*Eikenella corrodens*, anaerobes
Tick exposure	Large joints, especially knees	*Borrelia burgdorferi*

be elevated. Blood cultures may be positive. Radiographs may show periosteal elevation, but they are often negative until 10–14 days after the acute presentation. Bone scans are more sensitive but not specific. Indium-labeled leukocyte scanning is more specific. An MRI study will show increased signal in the bone marrow consistent with bone marrow edema and may also show associated soft tissue infection. It is the best imaging test. Definitive diagnosis is made with bone aspiration with Gram stain and culture.

Tx—Treat patients with IV antibiotics for 4–6 weeks. If *Staph. aureus* is suspected, consider oxacillin, nafcillin, vancomycin (in MRSA), or a quinolone plus rifampin. If gram-negative coverage is required, consider a third-generation cephalosporin, gentamicin, or quinolone. Surgical debridement may be required for necrotic bone. Left untreated, osteomyelitis may lead to systemic sepsis, chronic osteomyelitis, soft tissue infection, and/or septic arthritis.

Genitourinary Tract Infections

Urinary Tract Infections/Pyelonephritis

D—Infection of part of the urinary tract with significant bacteriuria in the presence of symptoms.

Epi—Females are affected more frequently than males.

P—The most common organisms are *Escherichia coli* (80% of cases), *Staphylococcus saphrophyticus*, *Klebsiella*, *Proteus*, and *Enterococcus*.

RF—Risk factors include Foley catheter or other urologic instrumentation, anatomic abnormalities [e.g., benign prostatic hyperplasia (BPH), vesicoureteral reflux], a history of previous UTIs or pyelonephritis, diabetes, recent antibiotic use, immunosuppression, and pregnancy. Occasionally, a UTI can develop from a simple inoculation of the lower urinary tract during sexual intercourse.

SiSx—Symptoms include urinary frequency, dysuria, burning, suprapubic pain, malodorous or cloudy urine, and urgency. With acute pyelonephritis, vomiting, fever, and flank pain may be the presenting complaints. Urosepsis must be considered in an elderly patient with altered mental status.

Dx—Urine dipstick may reveal increased leukocyte esterase, elevated nitrites, elevated urine pH (characteristic of *Proteus* infections), and/or hematuria (seen with cystitis). Microscopic analysis may reveal more than five leukocytes per hpf and a bacterial pathogen. White blood cell casts on urinalysis indicate acute pyelonephritis. Clean-catch urine culture with >10^5 bacteria per milliliter is the gold standard. Negative cultures but persistent evidence can suggest *Ureoplasma* or *Chlamydia*. Herpes simplex virus needs special culture media, as does *Neisseria gonorrhoeae*.

Tx—Antibiotic treatment depends on the patient, complications, and pathogen. Oral trimethoprim-sulfamethoxazole or ciprofloxacin for 3 days is the treatment of choice in healthy young females. Fluconazole can be used to treat *Candida albicans* in symptomatic patients. Patients with Foley catheters who are asymptomatic should have their catheter changed but do not need antibiotics. Elderly patients, patients with comorbid disease, or those with acute toxicity in the setting of acute pyelonephritis should be hospitalized and treated with IV antibiotics (ciprofloxacin or ampicillin and gentamicin to cover *Enterococcus*).

Herpes Simplex Infection

D—Viruses that affect primarily the oral (HSV-1) and genital areas (HSV-2). Primary disease and reactivation of disease exist as the virus finds a reservoir within the body, commonly the trigeminal nerve ganglia for HSV-1 and the sacral ganglia for HSV-2.

Epi—About 500,000 cases of genital HSV occur annually. The prevalence is currently about 30 million cases in the United States.

RF—Risk factors include, a prior sexually transmitted disease (STD), and an increased number of sexual partners.

SiSx

Mucocutaneous (more common with HSV-1)—Painful vesicles form and ulcerate after several days and are induced by stress, fever, infection, sunlight exposure, and chemotherapy. Pruritis is also a common finding, and regional lymphadenopathy may occur as well.

Extragenital—This may include, urinary retention due to sacral autonomic dysfunction (rare), and skin lesions elsewhere.

Ocular—Keratitis, keratoconjunctivitis, and blepharitis may be seen. This is usually unilateral.

Neurologic—Encephalitis and meningitis are the major disease processes. This is different from than other forms of aseptic meningitis in that behavioral and speech disturbances may also be seen. This is because HSV has a propensity for the temporal lobe.

Gastrointestinal—Esophagitis is usually seen in immunocompromised patients. Disseminated infection to numerous organs can also occur in the setting of a poor immune system. Reinfection is commonly unilateral and may not be vesicular. Lesions usually last for only 10 days instead of 2 weeks.

Dx—Diagnosis is usually clinical, but viral cultures of vesicular fluid or direct fluorescent antibody testing of scraped lesions can confirm the diagnosis. Polymerase chain reaction can identify the virus in the serum and in CSF. Lumbar puncture will show lymphocytosis and normal glucose. EEG, may show focal temporal slowing and periodic epileptiform discharges. Ocular HSV can be diagnosed with branching dendritic ulcers that stain positive with fluorescein dye.

Tx—Antivirals, usually acyclovir, are used, with IV treatment initially for encephalitis.

Sexually Transmitted Diseases

Syphilis

D—An infection caused by the *Treponema pallidum* bacterial spirochete.

Epi—About 6000 new cases occur each year, mostly in the southeastern United States. The incidence peaked in the early 1990s.

P—Transmission is usually from direct contact with an infectious lesion during sexual intercourse. Access is gained through disrupted epithelium, with transmission occurring in as many as one-third of patients who are exposed. The incubation period is up to 2–3 weeks.

RF—Risk factors include the presence of other sexually transmitted diseases (STDs), African American race (confers a 30-fold higher risk), and men who have sex with men.

SiSx—There are several stages that are categorized into early syphilis (primary, secondary,
and early latent) and late syphilis (late latent
and tertiary forms) as shown in Table 8-18.

Dx—*Treponema pallidum* cannot be cultured
in vitro. Several methods exist for diagnosis.
For primary syphilis, darkfield microscopy
allows spirochete visualization from primary
lesions. Serologic tests are likely to be negative at this time. Direct fluorescent antibody
testing (DFA-TP) or PCR can also be done.
For secondary syphilis, serologic testing is
best done using treponemal and nontreponemal tests, as shown in Table 8-19.

False-positive test results occur in a small
percentage of the population and are most
commonly due to collagen vascular diseases,
IVDU, chronic liver disease, and HIV infection. False-negative results occur when tests
are done prior to the development of antibodies or when a "prozone" reaction occurs
during a mismatch between concentrations
of antibody and antigen. Central nervous
system syphilis is best assessed with cerebral spinal fluid Venereal Disease Research
Laboratory test (CSF VDRL). Although this
test is specific, it is quite insensitive, so a
nonreactive CSF-VDRL does not rule out
neurosyphilis.

Tx—Early syphilis is a reportable infection. Treatment is prolonged since *T. pallidum* divides slowly. It is highly sensitive

Table 8-18. Stages of Syphilis

Primary syphilis: days to weeks	More than one chancre is rare. Usually it heals spontaneously in 3–6 weeks. Transmission rates are high and systemic spread of syphilis occurs during this phase.
Secondary syphilis: weeks to years	(1) Rashes (25% of patients): (a) a reddish brown symmetric maculopapular rash involving the entire trunk, the extremities, and especially the palms and soles. It is rarely pustular; (b) large gray-white lesion in warm, moist, membranous areas such as the mouth and perineum called *condyloma lata*. (2) Systemic symptoms—fevers, malaise, anorexia, headache, sore throat, myalgias, and weight loss. Diffuse, minimally tender lymphadenopathy involving, among other sites, the epitrochlear nodes. Patchy alopecia with a "moth-eaten" appearance may also be seen. (3) CNS—personality changes, depression, dementia.
Early latent: <1 year	Period during which there are no symptoms but infection is demonstrable by serologic testing. Patients are considered potentially infectious. Defined as a period of 1 year's duration from the initial infection if this can be documented.
Late latent: >1 year	Period during which transmission is thought to be much less likely. Requires a longer course of treatment.
Tertiary: up to 25–30 years	(1) Gummas—granulomatous lesions that can occur anywhere. On the skin, they may be ulcerated or serpiginated. In the GI tract, they may be mistaken for Crohn's disease, TB, or histoplasmosis. In the CNS, they can cause mass lesions. (2) Neurologic—called the *great imitator* because so many manifestations occur 1–25 years after the initial disease, causing a diagnostic dilemma. (a) Asymptomatic invasion of the CSF is common early on. Fifteen percent of primary infections and 40% of secondary infections have either protein or cellular abnormalities on CSF, which is the only way they might be diagnosed. (b) Acute meningitis 1–6 years after infection that presents as cranial nerve palsies, including eighth nerve palsy or hydrocephalus. (c) Meningovascular disease—presents as CVAs. It is more common than meningitis. An endarteritis can cause vascular occlusion in the area of the great cerebral vessels. Aphasia and hemiparesis are the most common symptoms, though symptoms depend on which arteries are involved. (d) *General paresis* is due to an infection of the meninges and cerebral cortex with changes in personality, depression, and eventually dementia. (e) *Tabes dorsalis*—rarely seen now. A disease of the posterior columns and dorsal roots with manifestations of diminished reflexes and loss of position and vibratory sense, paresthesias, and sharp pains in the extremities and trunk. *Argyll Robertson pupils* may be present as well—small, fixed pupils that do not react to light well but do react to convergence/accommodation. (3) Cardiovascular—classically, the ascending aorta can become dilated and result in aortic regurgitation. Coronary thrombosis and heart failure are possible.

Table 8-19. Tests for Syphilis

Nontreponemal Tests	Treponemal Tests
Rapid Plasma Reagin (RPR)	Fluorescent treponemal antibody absorption (FTA-ABS) test
Venereal Disease Research Laboratory (VDRL)	Microhemagglutination test for antibody to *Treponema pallidum* (MHA-TP)
Used as a screening test. Based on reactivity of serum to cardiolipin-cholesterol-lecithin antigens forming IgG and IgM antibodies. Positive tests are used to follow the response of treatment.	Used as confirmatory tests. Based on detection of antibody against treponemes

to penicillin. A single dose of penicillin G is sufficient for treatment of disease up to the early latent phase if one can present a nonreactive syphilis test in the last year or good documentation of the primary chancre within that time. For patients who do not respond, as seen by a decreased VDRL titer of at least fourfold over 6 to 12 months, reinfection have occurred, and retreating is necessary. Alternatives to penicillin because of allergy are a 14-day course of doxycycline, or macrolides for pregnant patients. Tertiary syphilis requires longer treatment: three weeks of IM shots penicillin or doxycycline for 1 month. Several weeks of frequent Intravenous penicillin dosing (every 4 hours or continuous infusion) is needed for neurosyphilis. Contrary to popular belief, treponemal tests do not always remain positive for life and reversion to a nonreactive status can occur in certain patients. This actually occurs with a greater tendency in those who are HIV positive.

Chlamydia

D—An STD caused by the organism *Chlamydia trachomatis*. It is usually more indolent than gonococcus.

Epi—It is the most common STD in the United States, with about 4 million cases per year. It accounts for up to 40% of cases of nongonococcal urethritis (NGU) in men. Coinfection with gonococcus occurs in 30% of cases.

P—Chlamydia lacks the ability to form adenosine triphosphate (ATP) and therefore is an obligate intracellular organism. It prefers columnar epithelial cells. The replication cycle involves extracellular elementary bodies that first attach to epithelial cells and are ingested via pinocytosis. After 48–72 hours of replication, they form reticulate bodes that eventually occupy almost all of the cytoplasmic space and are then released to infect new cells.

Vertical infections in the neonate (neonatal pneumonia and conjunctivitis), meaning they occur at the time of birth, are from serovars B and D–K. L serovars cause lymphogranuloma venereum (LGV; see below). Serovars A–C cause endemic trachoma, an ocular infection and a common cause of blindness in the developing world. Atypical URIs and pneumonias are also caused by serovar C.

RF—Risk factors include young age (the strongest predictor), African American race, multiple or new sexual partners, lack of barrier contraception, low socioeconomic status, and prior STDs.

SiSx—In general, chlamydia has fewer acute manifestations than gonococcus but more long-term ones. Many men are asymptomatic carriers. In those who are symptomatic, acute urethritis is common, which, compared to gonococcus, is usually less severe and is less purulent, with a thinner discharge. Dysuria is also less common, and no lymphadenopathy or systemic signs develop. Chlamydia also has a longer incubation period (up to 3 weeks vs. 1 week for gonococcus). Women, 50% of whom are asymptomatic, can present with cervicitis characterized by dysuria, vaginal discharge, and abdominal pain. On exam there is a mucopurulent cervical discharge, and the cervix appears friable and edematous. A major complications in women is pelvic inflammatory disease (PID), which develops in 30% of patients left untreated. It is associated with higher rates of infertility than pelvic inflammatory disease from gonococcus. Another complication is a perihepatitis called the *Fitz-Hugh–Curtis syndrome,* involving inflammation of the liver capsule. This can also be seen with gonococcus.

Dx—Culture remains the gold standard; however, it is rarely done. Direct fluorescent antibody, ELISA, and gene probe on cervical swab specimens have a sensitivity of 80–95% compared to culture. Polymerase chain reaction has a sensitivity and specificity of >95% in high prevalence populations and can be used on urine samples.

Tx—Chlamydia is susceptible to the tetracyclines and macrolides. Azithromycin 1 g po or doxycycline 100 po BID × 7 days are appropriate doses. Levofloxacin 500 mg po × 7 days is an appropriate alternative. All pregnant women should be screened for *Chlamydia* and should avoid treatment with doxycycline (contraindicated in pregnancy). Otherwise, screening is recommended in all sexually active women under age 25 and in those older than 25 with risk factors. One should also evaluate for the presence of other STDs at the same time.

Gonorrhea

D—An STD caused by transmission of the gram-negative diplococcus *N. gonorrhoeae,* also called *gonococcus,* which can have both local and systemic consequences.

Epi—It is the second most common STD in the United States after *Chlamydia.* There are about 300,000 cases annually.

P—Infection involves the four stages of attachment, local invasion, proliferation, and inflammatory response. Pili facilitate attachment. Opa (opacity-related proteins), which are also involved in attachment, undergo antigenic variation to avoid antibody formation. Local invasion occurs via various adhesion proteins and other Opa proteins that bind to heparin sulfate proteoglycan receptors. Gonococci are then are engulfed by mucosal cells and undergo intracellular replication. They can resist the destructive oxidative burst of the phagolysosome and can replicate within these organelles. Gonococcus is adaptive and can grow in both anaerobic and aerobic environments. Another virulence factor is the secretion of an IgA-1 protease.

RF—Risk factors include young adults, new or multiple sexual partners, single status, low socioeconomic status, substance abuse, and a prior history of STDs. It is more common in men who have sex with men.

SiSx—Symptoms can involve any part of the genital tract and oropharynx in both men and women. Disease may also become disseminated. The presentation differs in men and women, as shown in Table 8-20.

Table 8-20.   Differences in Presentation of Gonorrhea by Gender

Men	Women
Only 10% are asymptomatic	Up to 50% are asymptomatic
Most commonly causes urethritis. Presents with penile discharge and/or dysuria. Discharge may be spontaneous at the meatus and may be purulent in color. Acute unilateral epididymitis can be a complication but is more common in Chlamydia infection, which presents as unilateral testicular pain and swelling. Anorectal and pharyngeal infections are uncommon in heterosexual men and more common in men who have sex with men. Pharyngeal infections are usually asymptomatic, though they may cause cervical lymphadenopathy.	Most commonly causes a cervicitis. Symptomatic infection causes a vaginal pruritis and purulent discharge and/or dyspareunia. Abdominal pain signifies an upper GU tract infection. The exam may show a friable cervix. Anorectal infection may be asymptomatic. Oropharyngeal isolation usually represents colonization. Rarely, Bartholin's and Skene's glands become infected and are usually symptomatic. The most serious complication is pelvic inflammatory disease, which occurs in 10–40% and can lead to infertility, ectopic pregnancy, and chronic pelvic pain.

Dx—Culture on Thayer-Martin medium is the gold standard and takes up to 48 hours. It has high sensitivity in symptomatic women but lower sensitivity in those who are asymptomatic. Gram stain can also be used to look for gonococci as intracellular or extracellular diplococci. This test can make the diagnosis in about 60% of symptomatic women and 100% of symptomatic men. In men, the swab is taken 2 to 3 cm into the meatus. Electroimmunoassay can be done on a cervical swab or urine and is usually done only in patients from high-prevalence groups. Polymerase chain reaction tests are now more popular since they are less invasive and can be done on urine samples. Commercial kits use DNA probe technology that has the same sensitivity and specificity as culture. The decision to test for other STDs depends on the patient's sexual behavior. There is an increased risk of HIV transmission with gonococcus, as it is thought that the inflammatory response causes an increase in HIV shedding in vaginal secretions.

Tx—Treatment is the same for men and women. Ceftriaxone 1.25 g as an intramuscular injection and oral cefixime (400 mg once) are commonly used treatments. In populations with >20% prevalence of co-infection with chlamydia it is useful to treat the patient for chlamydia as well. Azithromycin 2 g will treat both chlamydia and gonococcus, but it may cause GI side effects and is not preferred due to the emergence of azithromycin resistance. Other regimens specifically for gonococcus are levofloxacin 250 mg orally once and ciprofloxacin 500 mg orally once, although quinolone resistance has also increased, making them less preferred agents.

Lymphogranuloma Venereum (LGV)

D—An STD causing genital ulcers due to specific strains of *C. trachomatis*: L1, L2, and L3.

Epi—It is most common in tropical areas. There are only several hundred cases in the United States per year.

P—It has a predilection for lymphoid tissue and causes a lymphoproliferative reaction. It also can cause lymphangitis and lymph node necrosis with abscess formation. The incubation period is up to 2 weeks.

SiSx

Primary infection—causes a genital ulcer that usually heals in a few days.

Secondary infection—2 to 6 weeks later there is direct local extension to regional lymph nodes that may form abscesses and rupture. Proctitis can also occur.

Late infection—fibrosis and strictures can occur anywhere along the anogenital tract.

Dx—Primary infection is typically missed. Lymph node aspiration can be used for culture in secondary infection. Diagnosis more commonly involves serologic tests such as complement fixation or microimmunofluorescence. A positive test is a titer >1:256, whereas a negative test is a titer of <1:32. Unfortunately, these tests cannot distinguish current from past infection; therefore, the clinical history and exam are quite important for diagnosis.

Tx—Antibiotics cure the infection and prevent further damage. Buboes may require needle aspiration or incision. Doxycycline for 21 days is the treatment of choice. Alternatives are the macrolides erythromycin or azithromycin.

Chancroid

D—An STD due to *Haemophilus ducreyi* which causes painful genital ulcers.

Epi—It is more common in developing countries and very rare in the United States, accounting for only several hundred cases per year. The incidence is probably highly underestimated.

P—*Haemophilus ducreyi* is a small gram-negative rod. Its virulence factors include lipopolysaccharide (LPS) with fibronectin and secretion of a cytotoxin that contributes to ulcer development. The incubation period ranges from 1 day to 1 month.

SiSx—The chancroid ulcer begins as a papule that changes to a pustule and then to an ulcer.

It can be as large as 2 cm and even larger in immunocompromised patients. It is characteristically very painful. The ulcer base has a yellow exudate when scraped and bleeds easily. Most commonly the ulcer occurs on the glans, prepuce, or corona in men and on the introitus, labia, and perianal areas in women. Inguinal lymphadenopathy may also be seen and can be painful.

Dx—The former standard method of diagnosis was culture on hemin plate medium on which gray to tan-colored colonies form. On Gram stain there is a classic "school of fish" appearance of long parallel strands from clumped organisms. Polymerase chain reaction is now the standard method for diagnosis.

Tx—Ciprofloxacin, azithromycin, or ceftriaxone are all appropriate treatments. Buboes may require drainage.

HIV and Associated Opportunistic Infections

HIV

D—A retroviral infection leading to immunodeficiency, which results in opportunistic infections and malignancies as well as a host of systemic conditions.

Epi—About 700,000 people in the United States and 10 million worldwide are presumed to be infected.

P—Human immunodeficiency virus is a retrovirus, meaning that it has a reverse transcriptase (RNA polymerase, which makes DNA) allowing it to replicate in host cells. It has three basic structural proteins: pol (polymerase), env (envelope), and gag (group antigens). Two types, HIV-1 and HIV-2 (seen mainly in West Africa), have been identified. The virus infects all types of cells that have the CD4 antigen (T cells, B cells, macrophages, oligodendrocytes), which allows it to attach to the cell. Entrance into the cell occurs via CCR5 and CXCR5 receptors. Patients with CCR5 deletions are less likely to become infected. Replication occurs with integration of the latent virus into the genome. As the viral load increases, the CD4 cell count falls. B cells are also affected, as are macrophages, which may help transmit the infection to other organs and can serve as a reservoir.

RF—Risk factors include sexual contact with infected individuals, transfusion of infected blood, needle sharing and IVDU, and perinatal exposure.

SiSx—Many patients are initially asymptomatic with seroconversion. However, some present with a flu-like illness at this stage (acute seroconversion) with pharyngitis, rash, and hepatitis. Otherwise, the presentation usually involves frequent infections or an opportunistic infection that ultimately leads to the diagnosis.

General—fever, night sweats, weight loss. Weight loss is seen in long-standing HIV infection, with disproportionate amount of muscle mass lost.

Pulmonary—frequent pneumonias, PCP presenting with slow-onset dyspnea and cough. TB reactivation can occur. Other presentations include fungal pneumonia, Kaposi's sarcoma with pulmonary involvement, nonspecific interstitial pneumonitis, and chronic sinusitis.

Neurologic—manifestations may include cerebral toxoplasmosis—the most common space-occupying lesion in HIV, presenting with headache, focal neurologic defects, or ΔMS. Multiple lesions are more typical. Central nervous system non-Hodgkin's lymphoma is the second most common lesion, usually occurring as a solitary lesion. Another development is AIDS dementia complex—usually slow and progressive. Cryptococcal meningitis may present with fever, persistent headache, and elevated intracranial pressure. Progressive multifocal leukoencephalopathy with focal neurologic deficits is also seen in advanced disease. Human immunodeficiency virus myelopathy with paraparesis and sensor ataxia is another recognized entity. In addition, HIV causes peripheral neuropathies. Retinitis, especially CMV also can be seen.

Table 8-21.   Prophylaxis Guidelines for HIV

CD4 Count	Condition	Agents
>500	None	None
<200	Candidiasis	Fluconazole
	PCP	Trimethoprim-sulfamethoxazole (alternatives include dapsone, atovaquone, and inhaled pentamidine)
<100	Toxoplasmosis	Azithromycin weekly
<50	CMV, MAC	Trimethoprim-sulfamethoxazole. C Test for IgG, consider ganciclovir

Gastrointestinal—Common manifestations include oral candidiasis (thrush) and candidal esophagitis (odynophagia in an HIV-positive patient is candidal esophagitis until proven otherwise); hairy leukoplakia on the lateral tongue (from EBV); acalculous cholecystitis; enterocolitis; mycobacterium avium complex (MAC), which can present with chronic loose stools; and AIDS enteropathy.

Endocrine—CMV infection of the adrenal gland with resultant adrenal insufficiency.

Skin—Commonly seen conditions are HSV and more severe zoster infections (i.e., distribution in multiple dermatomes); molluscum contagiosum, bullous impetigo, and folliculitis; bacillary angiomatosis from *Bartonella henselae* or *Bartonella quintana* infection; Norwegian scabies, psoriasis, xerosis, and seborrheic dermatitis (more severe).

Oncologic—Kaposi's sarcoma, primary CNS lymphoma (treated with radiation). non-Hodgkin's lymphoma (NHL)—mostly diffuse large B-cell infection; invasive cervical cancer or anal dysplasia and squamous cell cancer.

Gynecologic—vaginal candidiasis, cervical dysplasia, and cervical neoplasia (AIDS-defining illness in someone who is HIV positive).

Dx—The first diagnostic test is ELISA for antibody detection. If it is positive, confirm the diagnosis with a Western blot, which has 99.5% sensitivity and almost 100% specificity. A rapid diagnostic HIV test is also available now available with high sensitivity. Most patients develop antibodies within several months of infection; therefore, retesting is important in high-risk populations. Anemia, leukopenia, and thrombocytopenia may also be seen. The CD4 count provides important prognostic information. Acquired immunodeficiency syndrome itself has several definitions but mostly involves having an AIDS-defining condition: a CD4 count below 200 or a percentage below 14.

Tx—Routine care is given, including the following:

Check the CD4 count every 3–6 months with viral load (VL) testing.

PPD (a positive test is >5 mm), rapid plasma reagin (RPR), Venereal Disease Research Laboratory (VDRL) test.

Toxoplasma IgG and CMV IgG

Influenza and pneumococcal vaccine

Screen for HAV, HBV, and HCV

Pap smear every 6 months

Consider anal Pap smears for patients practicing receptive anal intercourse

Prophylaxis for certain conditions is based on clinical features and the CD4 count, as shown in Table 8-21.

Highly active antiretroviral therapy (*HAART*): Initiation of this therapy is patient dependent, but in general it may be started when the CD4 count is <300–350 or the VL count is >30,000 or in the presence of certain opportunistic infections. Compliance with the regimen is very important since resistance rates are quite high. Current drugs are shown in Table 8-22.

Table 8-22. Antivirals Currently in Use in the United States

Class	Example	Comment
Nucleoside Reverse Transcriptase Inhibitors (NRTIs)	Zidovudine (AZT)	First approved drug Thrombocytopenia Anemia
	Didanosine (ddI)	Neutropenia Pancreatitis Painful neuropathy (15%) Fulminant hepatic failure
	Stavudine (d4T)	Peripheral neuropathy Pancreatitis Hepatitis Lipoatrophy
	Lamivudine (3TC)	Few side effects Used with zidovudine or stavudine
	Abacavir	Hypersensitivity syndrome (5%) with flu-like syndrome
	Emtricitabine (FTC)	Diarrhea, nausea, rash, flatulence, renal toxicity
	Tenofovir (TDF)	Asthenia, diarrhea, nausea
	Zalcitabine (ddC)	Associated with neuropathy.
Nonnucleoside Reverse Transcriptase Inhibitors (NNRTIs)	Nevirapine	Rash (40%) that is treatable
	Efavirenz	CNS and psychological complaints
	Delaviridine	Least potent Rash
	Etravirine	Active against some viruses; resistant to others in the class
Protease Inhibitors (PIs)	Indinavir	Calculi in 40%; hydration important; rarely used now in the United States.
	Nelfinavir	Diarrhea
	Ritonavir	P450 inhibitor Increases bioavailability of most other protease inhibitors. Except for nelfinavir, all other protease inhibitors should ideally be given together with ritonavir.
	Saquinavir	GI side effects
	Lopinavir/ritonavir	Diarrhea
	Tipranavir (TPV)	Hepatitis, intracranial hemorrhage, diabetes
	Fosamprenavir (APV)	
	Atazanavir (ATV)	Avoid concomitant use with PPIs
	Darunavir	
Fusion Inhibitors	Enfuvirtide (T-20)	Blocks entry of HIV into cells
CCR5 Receptor Antagonists	Maraviroc	Test must be performed to evaluate if virus attaches via CCR5 receptor (*tropism* assay)
Integrase Inhibitors	Raltegravir	Does not cause dyslipidemia

Common HAART regimens: (1) two NRTI + NNRTI; (2) two NRTI + "boosted" PI (PI together with ritonavir).

Pneumocystis Jiroveci (Formerly carinii) Pneumonia (PCP)

D—A fungal infection causing pneumonia that manifests commonly in HIV-positive individuals and other immunocompromised hosts. New nomenclature now distinguishes *P. jiroveci* from *P. carinii,* which is found only in rats.

Epi—There is a worldwide distribution in animals and humans.

P—Transmission is airborne. The fungus is harmless in immunocompetent hosts. Normally, alveolar macrophages ingest and kill it.

RF—Risk factors include prior PCP infection, a CD4 count <200 (seen in 95% of patients), recurrent fever, thrush, and unexplained weight loss.

SiSx—Symptoms include fever, nonproductive cough with minimal sputum production, and dyspnea that is usually worse with exertion. Symptoms may be subtle and occur gradually over weeks in HIV patients or several weeks after long steroid tapers in non-HIV patients. In those previously given aerosolized pentamidine, there may be disseminated disease in lymph nodes, pericardium, spleen, liver, intestines, and bone marrow.

Dx—Classically, the chest X-ray shows diffuse bilateral interstitial infiltrates, although almost any chest X-ray finding can be seen, including cavitary lesions, pleural effusions, lobar pneumonia, or a "negative" film. Those receiving aerosolized pentamidine for prophylaxis may have more upper lobe disease, as seen in TB. An ABG may show an increased arterial-alveolar gradient. Obtaining the organism is the best way to make the diagnosis. Specimens by induced sputum or bronchoalveolar lavage (more sensitive) can be stained with methenamine silver, toluidine blue, or Wright's Giemsa, which selectively stain *P. jirovecii* cysts. Transbronchial biopsy or open lung biopsy is a last resort. Serum LDH can be helpful; if the LDH is low, the condition is unlikely to be PCP.

Tx—Empiric therapy is usually started first, especially in situations where the patient is hypoxic or needs hospitalization. Prognostic indicators are an increased arterial-alveolar gradient and a low PaO_2. Trimethoprim-sulfamethoxazole is the treatment of choice, and is given both for primary treatment (a 21-day course) and for prophylaxis. PCP prophylaxis should be considered in patients with CD4 counts <200 in those with other opportunistic infections such as oral candidiasis with HIV, or in immunocompromised patients such as those receiving a bone marrow transplant (BMT). Alternative regimens are dapsone, clindamycin and primaquine, or atovaquone. Intravenous pentamidine can also be used, but it is more toxic. Steroids should be given to those who are hypoxic with PaO_2 <70 mmHg or a significant A-a gradient. Patients get worse for a few days with treatment before they get better. Treatment before diagnostic bronchoscopy is fine with respect to the yield if bronchoscopy is done within several days.

Mycobacterium Avium Complex (MAC)

D—Infection caused by *M. avium* or *M. intracellulare*, two non-TB mycobacteria that occur in both HIV-infected and noninfected hosts.

Epi—Infection is also seen in non-HIV patients; however, the frequency is increased in those with HIV infections.

P—It usually presents as disseminated disease, although localized forms have become more common after the use of antiretroviral therapy. The organism is ubiquitous in the environment, with infection via inhalation or ingestion, not by reactivation.

RF—The risk increases most when the CD4 count is <50, as well as with consumption of raw fish/shellfish and the use of an indoor pool for swimming.

SiSx—Localized disease may present as fever and focal lymphadenopathy (cervical, abdominal, mediastinal). Disseminated infections are nonspecific, usually with fevers, sweats, weight loss, diarrhea, and cough.

Dx—Blood cultures are usually negative in localized infection but positive in disseminated infection. Isolation from lymph nodes after biopsy is the best way to diagnose localized disease. Bone marrow culture also has a higher yield, although it takes a while.

Tx—Prevention in appropriate patients involves weekly use of azithromycin. Established disease is associated with shortened survival in AIDS patients and is treated with multiple drugs. Drugs of choice may include ethambutol, rifabutin, and a macrolide such as clarithromycin or azithromycin. Streptomycin can be used for extensive cavitary disease.

Cytomegalovirus

D—A double-stranded herpes virus that causes a wide variety of disease in children and adults.

Epi—Seroprevalance increases with age. One percent of newborns in the United States are infected. Spread involves prolonged, repeated contact rather than casual contact. Transmission of CMV is usually sexually or by blood transfusion.

P—Viral replication is associated with the formation of large intranuclear inclusions and smaller cytoplasmic inclusions.

RF—Human immunodeficiency virus infection is a risk factor. Cytomegalovirus is also a major pathogen in transplant recipients from direct infection and reactivation.

SiSx—Most patients are asymptomatic. Acute infection is similar to that of infectious mononucleosis, though the development of pharyngeal symptoms is unusual. Cytomegalovirus has been associated with many of the following conditions, in advanced HIV: retinitis, esophagitis, gastritis, colitis, diffuse pulmonary infiltrates, encephalitis, myelitis, and radiculopathy, among others.

Dx—Diagnosis involves Tzank smear and tissue biopsy shows characteristic owl's eye appearance of CMV infected cells; they are enlarged and have intranuclear and intracytoplasmic inclusions. Cytomegalovirus antigenemia and PCR are helpful but do not definitively diagnose invasive disease.

Tx—Severe acute infections require IV ganciclovir. Other agents include valganciclovir, or foscarnet and cidofovir in specific situations such as ganciclovir-resistant disease.

Toxoplasmosis

D—Caused by a ubiquitous obligate intracellular protozoan.

Epi—There is a worldwide distribution, with hosts being humans and many species of animals and birds. The cat is considered the definitive host. The positive antibody prevalence in the United States is 15–30%.

P—It has several forms: trophozoites (rapid proliferation, causes acute disease), cysts (latent form, persists indefinitely, ingested via uncooked meat), and oocysts (passed in feces). The incubation period is 1–2 weeks.

RF—It is found in undercooked meat, contaminated food/water, cat litter, and soil-eating children. Reservoirs are rodents and birds eaten by cats.

SiSx—The primary infection is usually mild and resembles influenza or mononucleosis. There may be some generalized lymphadenopathy. Reactivated disease in the immunocompromised host is most relevant for HIV and can affect the brain, lungs, eye, skin, GI tract, and liver. Classically in HIV, encephalitis can develop, as well as focal neurologic deficits with cerebral toxoplasmosis. Myocarditis, which can also occur, is much less common.

Dx—The condition should be suspected in an HIV patient with new focal neurologic deficits. Diagnosis is based on either serologic tests of blood or CSF with ELISA for IgM and IgG antibodies or biopsy of tissue. Brain imaging studies may show the classic single or multiple ring enhancing lesions. In uncertain cases in which the brain MRI demonstrates characteristic findings, empiric treatment can be used for 2 weeks to assess for clinical and MRI improvement before proceeding to brain biopsy.

Tx—Either trimethoprim-sulfamethoxazole or dapsone/pyrimethamine is used for prophylaxis. Treatment requires pyrimethamine with sulfadiazine and folinic acid followed by pyrimethamine with clindamycin and folinic acid until clinical and radiographic resolution has been achieved.

IMPORTANT DISEASES BY ORGANISM CLASS OR RELATED CONDITIONS

Noteworthy Zoonoses

Tularemia

D—A zoonosis caused by the bacterium *Francisella tularensis.*

Epi—It affects individuals of all ages, all races, and both genders. More than 50% of U.S. cases occur in Arkansas, Oklahoma, and Missouri. Scandinavian countries also have an increased incidence.

P—It is mainly a disease of wild animals spread to humans incidentally via blood-sucking insects or by contact with animals. The organism can persist in animal carcasses, mud, and water. Ticks and wild rabbits are the classic carriers. Domestic dogs and cats and other animals, however, may also harbor the organism. Histologically, the disease resembles TB, forming noncaseating granulomas early on, but may later form into abscesses.

SiSx—Disease starts with a nonspecific viral prodrome. Classically, after 1–14 days of incubation, an ulcerative lesion forms at the site of inoculation. Lymphadenopathy occurs regionally with or without lymphadenitis. Systemic disease can then ensue, including tularemia pneumonia and typhoidal-stage tularemia involving severe bacteremia. Other manifestations are ocular, causing conjunctivitis, or GI, causing a membranous pharyngitis or mesenteric lymphadenopathy. Some diseases may present as a FUO.

Dx—Diagnosis is made by a smear of clinical specimens or via serologic testing with antibodies. Urine testing is currently not widely available. Culture of the organism is difficult.

Tx—Streptomycin is the drug of choice, given IM for 10 days. Gentamicin is another acceptable agent; tobramycin appears to be ineffective. If the disease is untreated, symptoms can last for up to 4 weeks. Typhoidal or tularemia pneumonia has a high morality if untreated (>30%). Vaccination is available in high-risk populations.

Rabies

D—A preventable zoonotic disease caused by a neurotropic RNA virus.

Epi—It has the highest case fatality rate of any infectious disease, causes up to 70,000 deaths a year, mostly in developing countries. Rare cases occur in the United States.

P—Virtually all transmission occurs via the bite of rabid animals, mainly dogs but also bats, raccoons, skunks, and foxes. Many strains of Rhabdoviridae, single-stranded RNA viruses, exist. The virus spreads from wound to dorsal root ganglion to brain; it is neurotropic and likes the brainstem, thalamus, basal ganglia, and spinal cord, where it replicates. The average incubation period is 1–3 months.

SiSx—Symptoms are divided into two classic forms:

1. Encephalitic—classically, involves hydrophobia, pharyngeal spasms, hyperreactivity, and encephalopathy (80%).
2. Paralytic—presents with quadriparesis with sphincter involvement and delayed cerebral involvement.

Nonclassical forms can present with neuropathic pain, sensory or motor deficits, cranial nerve palsies, and seizures. This pattern is more often seen with bat-associated rabies. Severe symptoms can be preceded by a flu-like prodrome followed by evidence of encephalitis or paralysis. Coma can eventually result.

Dx—Usually the diagnosis is based on a clinical history of a bite or recovery of the virus from a captured animal. Otherwise, antemortem testing may include sample collections for tests requiring saliva, as well as neck/skin biopsy with hair follicles, serum, and CSF fluid. Antibodies may not be present until after clinical signs of rabies appear. Cerebrospinal fluid chemical analysis does not distinguish rabies from other encephalopathies.

Tx—Treatment is usually supportive, since the disease is generally fatal unless the patient was previously vaccinated against it. Prevention includes giving the rabies vaccine for preexposure prophylaxis in high-risk groups.

Brucellosis

D—A zoonotic infection, also called *undulant fever* or *Malta fever*, caused by gram-negative intracellular coccobacilli.

Epi—It is most common in the midwestern United States and in endemic countries (Mexico, Spain, South and Central America).

RF—It is caused by ingestion of unpasteurized milk or cheese and animal exposure, especially cattle, hogs, and goats via contact with infected meat (slaughterhouse workers).

SiSx—Typically, the disease comes to attention during a work-up for an FUO, classically with an intermittent nightly fever (undulant fever). Otherwise, symptoms are nonspecific, including sweats, malaise, anorexia, arthralgias (especially sacroiliitis), weight loss, and depression. Many patients have lymphadenopathy, but hepatosplenomegaly is rare. Epididymitis may be seen in men. Meningoencephalitis may also occur.

Dx—Routine laboratory test results are nonspecific. Cultures and serologic tests are used to make the diagnosis. It is better to use a site that is involved (liver, bone marrow, CSF, lymph nodes) for culture if possible, but the culture can take a while to grow. Serum testing includes agglutination testing and/or and ELISA. Polymerase chain reaction is less commonly used. Diagnosis is made with an appropriate positive titer in the right clinical setting.

Tx—Doxycycline is given for 6 weeks, plus streptomycin or gentamicin. Other regimens include ofloxacin and rifampin. Neurobrucellosis may require additional agents such as trimethoprim-sulfamethoxazole.

Anthrax

D—A condition caused by the bacterium *Bacillus anthracis*, formally a disease associated with exposure to animal hides, now a concern with regard to bioterrorism.

RF—It is caused by exposure to animal hides, usually those of sheep, calves, horses, goats, and swine, as well as bioterrorism.

P—The bacterium is a gram-positive, spore-forming aerobic rod. Spores, not the bacteria, are the infectious form. Transmission occurs via inoculation of broken skin, mucous membranes, or inhalation of spores. Disease by spore ingestion is rare. Spores are carried to regional lymph nodes, where they multiply, causing a hemorrhagic lymphadenitis with sepsis that kills the host.

SiSx—There are three major manifestations:

Skin—This occurs within 2 weeks of spore exposure. Erythematous papules vesiculate and ulcerate with necrosis, forming a classic purple/black eschar. Typically, this form is not purulent and usually is self limited.

Pulmonary—This starts with nonspecific viral flu-like symptoms, anterior chest pain, and mediastinitis that can result in overwhelming sepsis within hours. It may lead to meningitis.

Gastrointestinal—Several days after ingestion of meat contaminated with spores, there is abdominal pain, rebound tenderness, vomiting, and diarrhea. Gastrointestinal lesions may ulcerate, leading to blood in the stool or even bowel perforation.

Dx—It is necessary to isolate the organism from fluid (pleural, CSF, urine, blood) or tissue; cultures are usually positive if no prior antibiotic therapy was given. Organisms are boxcar-shaped rods in chains that and are encapsulated. The chest X-ray classically shows mediastinal widening if there is pulmonary involvement with mediastinitis.

Tx—The prognosis is good for patients with localized disease. The mortality rate for those with systemic disease is high. First-line therapy is a quinolone such as ciprofloxacin. Second-line therapy is doxycycline.

Babesiosis

D—A tick-borne illness causes by protozoa that is similar to malaria in many respects.

Epi—Areas of transmission are coastal areas of Massachusetts including Cape Cod, Nantucket, and Martha's Vineyard, as well as Long Island (New York), Connecticut, and island areas of Rhode Island. Most cases occur between May and August.

P—More than 100 species of protozoa have been identified, all using animals as a reservoir. The disease is spread by the *Ixodes* tick, which is also the carrier of Lyme disease and human ehrlichiosis. Most cases in the United States are due to *Babesia microti*; *B divergens* is more common in Europe and is more virulent. Tick larvae feed off rodents, and adult ticks feed off white-tailed deer. Severe disease occurs in immunocompromised hosts. After a bite, protozoa invade RBCs and differentiate into trophozoites, which replicate asexually by budding into merozoites that invade other RBCs, eventually leading to hemolysis.

SiSx—Disease ranges widely, from asymptomatic to massive hemolytic anemia with fevers, chills, headaches, and myalgias. Hepatosplenomegaly and hemoglobinuria may also be seen. Eventually, the disease may result in death. The incubation period is 1–3 weeks. Unlike malaria, there is no periodicity of symptoms.

Dx—Initial evaluation is by thin and thick smears showing round or oval forms. There can be up to eight parasites per cell, and sometimes parasites are found outside of RBCs. The classic "Maltese cross" form helps distinguish this disease from malaria. Thick smears have a lower yield since the parasites are small and hard to see. False-negative rates can be high in cases of low parasitemia. Serum IgM antibody testing can be used to confirm the diagnosis. Antibodies are usually present 1–4 weeks after the onset of symptoms. Other, less often used techniques include PCR-based methods.

Tx—*Babesia divergens* may require more acute therapy, including antimicrobials and exchange transfusion. Treatment of asymptomatic patients is also recommended. Regimens include atovaquone plus azithromycin or quinine plus clindamycin as second-line therapy. Other agents include primaquine and pyrimethamine. Treatment of concomitant conditions (Lyme disease and ehrlichiosis) transmitted by the same tick with doxycycline may also be indicated. In mild cases, the disease is self-limited and most patients recover without sequelae.

Common Infections in Travelers

Malaria

D—A protozoal disease transmitted by the anopheles mosquito.

Epi—It affects >1 billion people worldwide and causes 1–3 millions deaths per year. It has been eliminated from North America, Europe, and Russia. It is common in the developing world, specifically in Central and South America, Africa, Asia, and the South Pacific.

P—Four species of *Plasmodium* cause all infections, as shown in Table 8-23.

The disease is transmitted by some but not all anopheles mosquitoes. The life cycle is as follows. After the mosquito inoculates the *sporozoites* during a blood meal, they invade

Table 8-23. Characteristics of Four Major Types of Malaria

Species	Location	Comments
P. falciparum	Africa New Guinea Haiti South America	By far the most common overall Parasitemia is high usually Multiple parasites per RBC may be seen on smear
P. vivax	Central America India South America	Second most common form Has a dormant liver form Parasitemia is low because only infects young RBCs
P. ovale	Africa only, mainly West Africa	Has a dormant liver form Parasitemia is low because only infects young RBCs
P. malariae	Sub-Saharan Africa	The so-called "benign malaria." Not as virulent as the other three types.

hepatocytes and reproduce by the thousands, bursting open hepatocytes and releasing daughter *merozoites*. These invade RBCs, multiply every 48–72 hours, and grow into *trophozoites*, which consume hemoglobin and cause the RBCs to burst, releasing even more daughter merozoites. Symptoms occur when the parasitic concentration is high enough. *Plasmodium vivax* and *P. ovale* are different in that they have intrahepatic forms (*hypnozoites*) and can be dormant for years, causing disease relapse. After several cycles other forms are produced, which undergo sexual reproduction and can be used to transmit malaria to other organisms after other mosquitoes bite the host.

Plasmodium changes the RBC in several ways, altering the cell membrane transport properties, exposing new surface antigens, and inserting its own proteins. Therefore, RBCs become more irregularly shaped and less pliable and become sequestered in important organs, such as in the kidneys, causing acute renal failure, and also in the brain, causing cerebral malaria.

RF—Travel to endemic areas is a risk factor. The disease can also be transmitted by blood transfusion, needle-stick injury, sharing of needles by infected drug addicts, or organ transplantation. The incubation period in these settings is often short because there is no preerythrocytic stage of development.

SiSx—Initially, there is a nonspecific virus-like prodrome with malaise, fever, and muscle aches. The classically described cyclical malarial paroxysms with fever spikes and rigors are actually rare with *P. falciparum*, and may suggest *P. vivax* or *P. ovale* infection instead. There are few physical findings initially except mild hepatosplenomegaly. Jaundice from hemolysis can also be seen but resolves in several weeks; it is usually common among adults. There are, however, a number of recognized complications:

Cerebral malaria—can present with obtundation/coma or delirium/change in behavior. Onset may be gradual or sudden following a convulsion. It is associated with a 20% mortality rate. A diffuse encephalopathy without focal neurologic signs is classic. The exact cause is unclear but may involve nitric oxide and induction of sticky knobs on the surface of parasitized cells that promote cytoadherence to endothelial cells. This is usually a clinical diagnosis.

Renal impairment—the cause is unclear. It may be related to RBC sequestration causing acute tubular necrosis. It may occur simultaneously with other vital organ dysfunction (in which case mortality is high) or it may progress as other disease manifestations resolve.

Hypoglycemia—more common in children and pregnant women due to failure of hepatic gluconeogenesis and an increase in the consumption of glucose by both the host and the organisms.

Lactic acidosis—commonly coexists with hypoglycemia and is an important contributor to death from severe malaria.

Anemia—results from accelerated RBC destruction. Slight coagulation abnormalities are common in falciparum malaria, and mild thrombocytopenia is usual. Only <5% of patients with severe malaria have significant bleeding with evidence of disseminated intravascular coagulation. Hematemesis from stress ulceration or acute gastric erosions may also occur.

Liver dysfunction—mild hemolytic jaundice is common in malaria. Severe jaundice is associated with *P. falciparum* infections and is more common among adults with hemolysis, hepatocyte injury, and cholestasis. Hepatic dysfunction contributes to hypoglycemia, lactic acidosis, and impaired drug metabolism. Occasional patients with falciparum malaria may develop deep jaundice (with hemolytic, hepatic, and cholestatic components) without evidence of other vital organ dysfunction.

Dx—The gold standard is thick and thin blood smears repeated three or four times if the diagnosis is suspected. Thick smears are more sensitive, allowing a scan of more blood for organisms; thin smears allow species determination. First smears are usually positive in most cases; if they are negative, they should be repeated every 6–12 hours to exclude the diagnosis. Other methods, including fluorescent microscopy, PCR-based testing, and antibody testing, have lower sensitivity or specificity and require more time, training, and/or equipment. *Plasmodium falciparum* has classic ring forms with chromosome dots and is more likely to be the diagnosis, producing higher parasitemia and multiple ring forms per cell

Tx—Many different drug classes exist. Chloroquine resistance is quite common. Common treatments include quinine and doxycycline or clindamycin, atovaquone-proguanil, and artemisin-based regimens where available. Other agents include mefloquine, primaquine, certain sulfonamides, doxycycline, and clindamycin, among others. In multiorgan involvement, supportive care is required with IV hydration, dialysis as needed, frequent monitoring of blood glucose, and exchange transfusion when there is high parasitemia. Smears should be checked daily until the parasitemia clears and weekly thereafter for a month to assess for recrudescence of infection.

Dengue Fever

D—An acute arbovirus infection that presents with fever, rash, and lymphadenopathy.

Epi—It is most common in the tropics and subtropics, especially Africa and Southeast Asia. It is a common diagnosis in the returning traveler.

P—Dengue is a member of the flavivirus family of single-stranded RNA viruses. Four serotypes exist. Transmission is by *Aedes* mosquitoes, which remain infected for life, as the virus replicates in their salivary glands. The second infection is typically much worse than the first, more likely to cause hemorrhagic fever. The incubation period is typically 5–10 days.

SiSx—There are three overlapping clinical forms:

Classic dengue—mild to moderate febrile illness, called *breakbone fever*, with headache, retroorbital pain, arthralgias, back pain, and rhinopharyngitis. After several days, a second peak of symptoms occurs with a maculopapular rash on the trunk that spreads to the arms and legs, sparing the palms and soles. Then tender lymphadenopathy erupts, followed by decreased WBCs and platelets. Fatigue may persist for weeks.

Dengue hemorrhagic fever—a more severe form including abdominal pain. Patients bruise and bleeding easily. Melena, hematemesis, epistaxis, and bleeding gums may be seen. It can progress to shock.

Dengue shock syndrome—increased vascular permeability and leakage leads to vascular compromise.

Dx—Viremia is detected within 3–5 days with all three types. IgM antibodies are nonspecific.

Tx—There is no mortality from the classic infection. Supportive care is the only treatment for more serious types.

Typhoid Fever (Enteric Fever)

D—Severe multisystemic illness caused by two types of *Salmonella*, *S. typhii* and *S. paratyphii,* which are found in developing countries.

Epi—There are 500 cases a year in the United States, generally from travel abroad, most commonly to India. Worldwide, there are 22 million cases and 200,000 deaths each year.

P—The cause is a motile gram-negative bacillus found only in humans. It is important to differentiate nontyphi salmonella from other types that cause acute, self-limited gastroenteritis. The infectious dose is at least 10,000 bacteria. They multiply within the lymph nodes, spleen, and elsewhere. The clinical phase begins in 1–3 weeks of incubation. The *S. typhii* and *S. paratyphii* strains are pathogenic only in humans.

RF—Risk factors include poor sanitation (fecal-oral transmission from contaminated food or water or contact with an acutely ill patient or asymptomatic carriers), antacid use (prevents bacterial killing in the stomach), and an immunocompromised status.

SiSx—During the incubation period (1–10 days), patients may have mild diarrhea. With bacteremia, patients develop high fevers, abdominal pain, and anorexia. Constipation may also be seen from hypertrophy of Peyer's patches. Pulmonary and oropharyngeal involvement may also occur, including a sore throat, a cough, and lobar pneumonia. Classically, there may be a pulse–temperature dissociation (relative bradycardia) as well as rash appearing during the second week, with papules on the trunk called *rose spots* (bacterial emboli to the skin) seen in about one-third of patients. If untreated, the illness lasts for 4 weeks. A response starts within a few days of beginning antibiotic therapy.

Dx—Stool culture with speciation usually makes the diagnosis. IgM and IgG antibodies are now more commonly used as well. Blood cultures are usually positive in the first week of illness.

Tx—An oral quinolone usually is needed, although resistance is reported, so that susceptibility testing may be needed to guide appropriate antibiotic selection. This is different from the treatment of nontyphoid strains of salmonella gastroenteritis, in which antibiotic treatment may not be needed.

Schistosomiasis

D—A condition caused mainly by three blood flukes—*Schistosoma mansoni, S. haematobium*, and *S. japonicum*—primarily due to a hypersensitivity reaction to the organism.

Epi—Over 200 million individuals are affected worldwide, 20 million annually, with 200,000 deaths. *Schistosoma mansoni* is found mainly in Africa and South America, *S. haematobium* mainly in the Middle East and Africa, and *S. japonicum* mainly in China and the Philippines.

P—Schistosomes infect susceptible freshwater snails in endemic areas. Snails release cercariae (small 1-mm larvae), which live in fresh water, and with exposure attach to human skin with their oral suckers. They migrate through veins into the lungs and worms eventually migrate through the pulmonary capillaries into the systemic circulation, affect other organs, mature, and produce eggs. The eggs are highly antigenic, induce an intense granulomatous response, and eventually are shed via feces or urine.

RF—Freshwater exposure in endemic areas is the risk factor.

SiSx—Many patients are asymptomatic, with few organisms. Symptoms are divided into acute and chronic phases:

Acute phase (Katayama fever)—an allergic response after 2–7 weeks of incubation. Fever, bloody diarrhea, myalgias, malaise, and dry cough can be seen, as well as hepatosplenomegaly, weight loss, and eosinophilia.

Chronic phase—occurs months to years after infection. Patients can have chronic abdominal pain, irregular bowel movements, persistent hepatosplenomegaly, and develop cirrhosis/portal hypertension. Immune complex–related GN can occur. *Schistosoma haematobium* favors urinary tract disease and can cause hematuria, and proteinuria. This chronic bladder infection predisposes to squamous cell bladder cancer.

Dx—Screening involves testing for eggs in stool. Definitive diagnosis is by mucosal or tissue biopsy. *Schistosoma haematobium* eggs may be found in the urine. Early in the infection, the stool examination may be negative. Enzyme-linked immunosorbent assay (ELISA) or serologic testing for antigens may be positive, however. Serum and urine antigen titers may correlate with the degree of infection.

Tx—Praziquantel can be used to treat all species. Metrifonate can be used for *S. haematobium* and oxamniquine for *S. mansoni* as alternatives. Steroids can be considered for life-threatening acute disease.

Spirochete-Related Infections

Lyme Disease

D—A systemic disease caused by the spirochete *Borrelia burgdorferi* transmitted to humans by the *Ixodes* tick.

Epi—It is the most common vector-borne disease in the United States. The incidence is unclear but is perhaps approximately 15,000 cases a year. Most cases occur in the northeastern, mid-Atlantic, and north central United States.

P—The *Ixodes* tick has three life cycle stages. As nymphs and larvae, they prefer the white-footed mouse as a host. As adults, they prefer the white-tailed deer. Most human infections occur in the spring and summer. Ticks must feed for 24 hours or longer to transmit the infection. If left alone, the tick will drop off at 2–4 days of feeding. Nymphs are much smaller and are often the vehicle of transmission.

RF—Working in endemic areas is the risk factor.

SiSx—There are three recognized stages of disease:

Stage 1—early localized: A prodrome with flu-like symptoms (fever, chills, and myalgias) and a characteristic rash (erythema migrans) are usually seen 1 week after a tick bite. The rash starts as a raised red lesion with eventual central clearing as it expands. Usually it is found in the groin, axilla, or thigh. Twenty percent may not have this classic finding. Some nonclassical rashes may also occur, which are vesicular or without central clearing. The constitutional symptoms resolve on their own without treatment, usually in a few weeks.

Stage 2—disseminated infection: The spirochete spreads in the blood and lymph several weeks after inoculation. Fatigue, malaise, and migratory arthralgias are common. Systemic symptoms affect the skin, heart, and CNS. One can see more erythema migrans lesions or reddish nodules or plaques. Conjunctivitis and keratitis are also seen. Cardiac manifestations include myopericarditis, arrhythmias, and heart block. Neurologic manifestations vary and can include aseptic meningitis. Bell's palsy, encephalitis, peripheral neuropathy, and transverse myelitis can be seen.

Stage 3—late persistent: This stage occurs months to years after infection. Joint and articular pain or frank arthritis and synovitis are common. Subacute encephalopathy and a host of neurologic manifestations similar to those in stage 2 can occur. More common in Europe is the skin finding of *acrodermatits chronicum atrophicans,* involving bluish-red skin discoloration with swelling.

Dx—This is a clinical diagnosis, especially early on, as serologic tests are not useful until after several weeks of infection. Immunofluorescence assay (IFA) or ELISA can detect antibodies in serum; the latter is more specific. Western blot looking for IgM and IgG antibodies is used as a confirmatory test. IgM is seen usually 2–4 weeks after erythema migrans occurs. IgG takes 6–8 weeks to appear. Serologic tests are also not highly reproducible. Physician-documented erythema migrans in endemic areas makes the diagnosis in early disease. Late disease requires a known clinical manifestation and serologic evidence. Patients with nonspecific symptoms should not be tested, as false positives are high. Empiric antibiotics are given to those with a high pretest probability of disease.

Tx—Tick bites needs no treatment, especially if it is less then hours old. Some suggest that a single dose of doxycycline within 72 hours of the bite can help prevent Lyme disease, however. For first-stage disease, doxycycline is the treatment of choice. Amoxicillin is a second-line agent used in pregnant women. Longer courses of therapy are used for second- or third-stage disease. Chronic Lyme disease is difficult to treat.

Leptospirosis

D—Severe infection caused by *Leptospira interrogans.*

Epi—It has a worldwide distribution. In the United States, it is seen in returning freshwater adventure travelers.

P—It is transmitted to humans by food contaminated with urine of the reservoir animal. It can also enter through mucosal lesions following swimming in contaminated water. The incubation period is up to 2 weeks.

SiSx—The anicteric type is more benign and has two phases. The first phase, the septicemic phase, begins with fever, chills, abdominal pain, headache, and myalgias (classically of calf muscles). Symptoms improve after 3 days. In the second phase, the immune phase, is characterized by meningitis, uveitis, rash, and adenopathy. All of these infections are usually self-limiting. Icteric leptospirosis (Weil syndrome) is the most severe form, with renal and liver dysfunction, changes in mental status, and a 10% mortality rate. Complications include myocarditis, aseptic meningitis, and pulmonary infiltrates with hemorrhage.

Dx—A WBC count as high as 50,000 may be seen. The CK level is also usually elevated. Darkfield microscopy exam of blood can show organisms early on. Cultures can take up to 6 weeks so diagnosis is made by serologic tests. The ELISA can be positive in 2 days.

Tx—The treatment of choice is penicillin. Prophylaxis is with doxycycline.

Relapsing Fever

D—An infection classically spread by rodents and tics caused by the spirochete *Borrelia recurrentis.*

P—Spread from human to human is via infected lice. Thus, crowded conditions, cold climate, and lice-infested populations propagate the disease.

SiSx—There is an abrupt onset of constitutional symptoms including nausea, vomiting, severe headache, hepatosplenomegaly, and rash. The attack stops after 3–10 days and, after 1 week, returns in a milder form. Up to 10 relapses can occur before recovery.

Dx—During the acute episodes, spirochetes can be seen in blood smears or cultured in special media. The nontreponemal test for syphilis may also be falsely positive. There also false positive result in those who have *Borrelia burgdorferi.* Serologic studies with antibodies are available to make the diagnosis.

Tx—A single dose of tetracycline or procaine penicillin usually is adequate treatment.

Rat Bite Fever

D—An acute infectious disease caused by the spirochete *Spirillum minus* transmitted by a rat bite.

RF—Rat-infected slums and laboratories are risky environments.

SiSx—One week after the original rat bite heals, the site become swollen and painful and may ulcerate. Lymphadenopathy and lymphadenitis with fever, malaise, and signs of systemic infection can occur. Splenomegaly and a rash on the trunk/extremities as well as arthritis can be seen. Symptoms subside but reappear after several days, and this process continues.

Dx—Nontreponemal tests of syphilis are falsely positive. Darkfield exam of the ulcer or lymph node material can show the organism. It cannot be cultured, but blood inoculation into a laboratory animal can help make the diagnosis.

Tx—Treatment consists of penicillin or tetracycline. The mortality rate is as high as 10%.

Ehrlichiosis

D—A disease that describes two conditions including human monocytic ehrlichiosis (HME) which is caused by *Ehrlichia chaffeensis* or human granulocytic anaplasmosis (HGA) which is caused by *Anaplasma phagocytophilum* (formerly called *human granulocytic ehrlichiosis*) and is seen in western Japan.

P—The disease is spread by small tick-borne, gram-negative obligate intracellular bacteria. Dogs are the main nonhuman hosts. The main vector in the United States is the Lone Star tick (*Amblyomma americanum*). Other ticks, including those of the genus *Ixodes,* are also vectors.

SiSx—After an incubation period of about 10 days there is a prodrome of fever and malaise. Rash, headache, stiff neck, and rigor can occur and lymphopenia and thrombocytopenia usually develop. Serious consequences include acute respiratory distress syndrome (ARDS), encephalopathy, and acute renal failure.

Dx—Indirect fluorescent antibody assay from the CDC makes the diagnosis, as does a rapid PCR assay. Culture is difficult. On the buffy coat examination, one may see the classic intracytoplasmic inclusions (morulae) within neutrophils.

Tx—Doxycycline is given for at least 1 week.

Q Fever

D—Disease spread by inhalation or ingestion of the rikettsial bacterium *Coxiella burnetii*, usually while dealing with cattle, sheep, and goats.

P—Transmission is via animal milk and feces. It is resistant to heat because of its ability to form endospores.

SiSx—The incubation period is up to 3 weeks. A febrile viral prodrome occurs with a nonproductive cough. Granulomatous hepatitis and pneumonitis can be seen. Endocarditis, most commonly of the aortic valve and characterized by large vegetations, is a rare but serious form of infection. Other rare findings include acute renal failure, mediastinal lymphadenopathy, and hemolytic anemia.

Dx—Abnormal LFTs and elevated WBCs can be seen in the acute phase. A serum ELISA can help make the diagnosis. IgG titers of >1:200 are seen in endocarditis. Chest X-ray may show patchy pulmonary infiltrates.

Tx—Treatment usually involves tetracycline or doxycycline. Endocarditis treatment is often necessary for years, with doxycycline, trimethoprim-sulfamethoxazole, quinolones, or rifampin. Heart valves usually need replacement.

Rocky Mountain Spotted Fever (RMSF)

D—A condition caused by *Rikettsia rickettsii* characterized by fever and rash.

Epi—It is most common in the southeastern and south central United States and the northern Rocky Mountains. Cape Cod (Massachusetts) and Long Island (New York) are hot spots.

Disease occurs mostly in spring and early summer.

P—*Rikettsia rickettsii* is a gram-negative obligate intracellular bacterium with a predilection for human endothelial cells. The vector is the American dog tick, *Dermacentor variabilis* or *D. andersonii.* Infection is via tick bite. Up to one-third of patients do not recall having had a recent tick bite or contact.

SiSx—Symptoms begin 2–14 days after a bite. At first, patients have fever, headache, and malaise. Children may have abdominal pain that can be misdiagnosed as other conditions. A rash develops in 3–5 days (not seen in up to 10% of patients), classically beginning on the ankles and wrists and spreading centrally to the palms and soles, usually as a macular and then as a petechial rash. It is not pruritic. Seizures and focal neurologic deficits can be seen in many cases along with bleeding and edema. Low platelet levels can become prevalent as the disease progresses; this is thought to be caused by increased destruction at areas of vascular injury. Disseminated intravascular coagulation is rare. Low sodium, elevated transaminases, bilirubin, and acute renal failure can be seen in advanced cases.

Dx—There is no completely reliable diagnostic test early on. Later, skin biopsy can be done with direct immunofluorescence or immunoenzyme methods; it has 70% sensitivity and 100% specificity. Other tests include the indirect fluorescent antibody test but this test not helpful during the first 5 days of symptoms. Blood cultures can be done for rickettsia as well.

Tx—Treatment usually involves doxycycline for all patients and continues for at least 3 days until after the patient has become afebrile. Most patients need antibiotics for 5–7 days. Early treatment is important.

Fungal Infections

Histoplasmosis

D—*Histoplasma capsulatum* is a dimorphic fungus. Despite its name, the fungus is unencapsulated.

Epi—It occurs in the Ohio and Mississippi river valleys (i.e. the southeastern, mid-Atlantic, and central states).

P—*Histoplasma capsulatum* prefers moist surface soil, particularly that enriched by droppings of certain birds and bats. The fungus persists in contaminated soil for years and becomes airborne when the soil is disturbed. In many endemic areas, ≥80% of residents have been exposed. Fungus is acquired by inhalation of spores. Microconidia, or small spores, reach the alveoli and transform there into budding forms. With time, an intense granulomatous reaction occurs. Transient dissemination may leave calcified granulomas in the spleen and other organs. In adults, a rounded mass of scar tissue, with or without central calcification, called a *histoplasmoma*, may remain in the lung. In a small proportion of patients, histoplasmosis becomes a progressive, potentially fatal infection. The disease occurs either as chronic fibrocavitary pneumonia or, less commonly, as disseminated infection. A history of tobacco use or the presence of emphysema is elicited from nearly all patients with chronic progressive pulmonary histoplasmosis. Acute, rapidly fatal, disseminated infections are encountered in children and immunosuppressed patients.

RF—Immunocompromised hosts are at risk.

SiSx—The primary infection is similar to influenza. Systemic signs include cough, fever, and weight loss. Other presentations include skin and mouth lesions, and adrenal lesions are common. The disease can sometimes cause adrenal insufficiency. Cavitary pulmonary lesions may also be seen. Cough, fever, malaise, and chest X-ray findings of hilar adenopathy, with or without one or more areas of pneumonitis, are typical features. Approximately one-third of patients stabilize or improve spontaneously early in the course of disease. The remainder progress insidiously. *Disseminated histoplasmosis* has many features in common with hematogenously disseminated tuberculosis. Presumed ocular histoplasmosis syndrome is a clinical syndrome characterized by discrete atrophic choroidal scars in the macula or mid-periphery, peripapillary atrophy, and choroidal neovascularization. These changes lead to a severe loss of central vision.

Dx—Blood cultures should be performed in all cases. Cultures of bone marrow, mucosal lesions, liver, and bronchoalveolar lavage fluid are diagnostically useful in disseminated histoplasmosis in the appropriate setting. Diagnosis is based on Giemsa-stained smears of blood/bronchoalveolar lavage fluid or tissue specimens. Anti-*Histoplasma* antibodies are positive in most cases. *Histoplasma* antigen can be detected in the urine of 90% and in the serum of 70% of disseminated cases; less frequently, it is found in other sterile body fluids.

Tx—Acute pulmonary histoplasmosis requires no specific therapy. Oral itraconazole may shorten the course of the illness. All patients with disseminated or chronic pulmonary histoplasmosis should receive antifungal therapy. Amphotericin B (conventional or lipid formulation) is the drug of choice for the initial treatment of patients with disseminated histoplasmosis. Patients with AIDS should receive long-term itraconazole following treatment to prevent relapse. Immunocompetent patients with disseminated or chronic pulmonary histoplasmosis are treated for 6–12 months.

Coccidiomycosis

D—An infection caused by the fungi *Coccidioides immitis* or *C. posadasii*.

P—Infection is via inhalation of the organism, which enlarges within the lung and produces endospores. Reinfection commonly occurs in already infected hosts.

RF—It is found in the southwestern United States, the San Joaquin Valley of California, and central Arizona, in addition to Mexico, Central America, and South America. Filipino and black males, pregnant females, and immunocompromised hosts are at risk for meningitis and more severe disease.

SiSx—Two-thirds of the infections are subclinical and do not come to medical attention. Dry cough and fever are similar to those

HITCHHIKER'S GUIDE TO INTERNAL MEDICINE

occurring with the flu and are self-limited. Chest pain may be seen. One can see pleural effusions, coin lesions, or cavities causing hemoptysis. Dissemination to the CNS, causing meningitis, is possible, as is spread to the skin, bones (including ribs and vertebrae) and joints. Erythema nodosum is not uncommon in women and indicates an active immune system. One may see eosinophilia in 25% of patients and ipsilateral hilar adenopathy on chest X-ray, though in many patients the chest X-ray will be normal.

Dx—Culture or biopsy with silver stain is performed, as this is virtually always a laboratory diagnosis. IgG and IgM antibody testing is also available.

Tx—In many cases, resolution of illness occurs without medical therapy. Fluconazole or itraconazole, or amphotericin B in immunocompromised or pregnant hosts, can also be used. Fluconazole is used for meningitis. Chronic suppressive therapy may be needed in certain individuals.

Blastomycosis

D—Fungal infection geographically limited to the south central and midwestern United States and Canada.

P—Disease occurs commonly in the lungs of immunocompetent individuals. Dissemination is more common in immunocompromised hosts.

SiSx—It may be asymptomatic, however symptoms of cough, fever, dyspnea, and chest pain can be seen. Patients may also have bloody/purulent sputum, pleurisy, and weight loss. Disseminated disease can involve the skin, bones, or urogenital system. Skin lesions are verrucous and may mimic those of skin cancer.

Dx—Chest X-ray or CT may show diffuse pulmonary infiltrates; rarely, enlarged lymph nodes are seen. Skin findings include raised verrucous cutaneous lesions with an abrupt downward-sloping border and a central atropic scar. As in coccidiomycosis, bones, including ribs and vertebrae, are commonly involved. The organism is found in sputum or tissue as a thick-walled cell with a single broad-based bud, which readily grows on culture. Serologic tests typically are not useful.

Tx—Itraconazole, used for several months, has a good response rate. Amphotericin B is used for CNS disease or in cases of treatment failure.

Paracoccidioidomycosis (South American Blastomycosis)

D—A dimorphic fungus that is limited in scope to South and Central America and Mexico.

P—Primary infection is via inhalation.

RF—Travel to endemic areas is risky.

SiSx—Most patients are asymptomatic for a long time. Ulceration of the nasopharynx and oropharynx is usually the first presenting symptom, which helps distinguish it from other infections. Ultimately, there can be destruction of other tissues, including the epiglottis, vocal cords, and uvula, with lesions on the face and lips as well. Other organ systems are also affected, causing hepatosplenomegaly and CNS disease. Pulmonary symptoms are usually nonspecific.

Dx—Laboratory tests are nonspecific. Serologic tests are diagnostic and positive in almost all cases. Sputum may show *P. brasiliensis* in sputum, pus, or tissue (spherical cells with many buds).

Tx—Itraconazole is given for at least several months, with monitoring for several years after therapy. Second-line therapy is amphotericin B or sulfonamides.

Mucormycosis/Zygomycosis

D—Opportunistic infection caused by the *Rhizopus, Muco, Absidia*, and *Cunninghamella* genera of fungi.

Epi—It is ubiquitous in nature and is found mostly on decaying vegetation and soil. The organisms grow quickly and release a large number of spores, which are airborne. In most cases, the infection is suppressed by a healthy immune system.

RF—Risk factors include DKA, renal insufficiency, iron chelation therapy, immunocompromised status, trauma, and burns.

P—The organisms have a key enzyme, ketone reductase, which allows them to thrive in high-acid and high-glucose environments.

SiSx—Invasive disease typically involves the sinuses, lungs, and orbits. Classic signs include a black necrotic lesion of the nose and sinuses with cranial nerve involvement, as CNS invasion can occur readily without treatment.

Tx—Treatment involves amphotericin B and control of the underlying condition, as well as holding of immunosuppressants. Surgical removal of necrotic, nonperfused tissues is necessary. Overall, the prognosis is poor, with up to 50% mortality in patients with localized disease.

Aspergillosis

D—An illness due to from allergic reaction to, colonization by, or tissue invasion by *Aspergillis*.

Epi—It is ubiquitous in the environment.

P—*Aspergillis* disease has a tropism for blood vessels. Most commonly, disease is caused by *A. fumigatus* and *A. flavus*, often introduced via the respiratory tract. Rarely, inoculation via skin can occur from trauma.

SiSx—There are several clinical manifestations. Pulmonary involvement is the most common presentation in immunocompromised hosts. Allergic bronchopulmonary aspergillosis (ABPA; see Chapter 3) is seen in asthmatics, accompanied by hard-to-control exacerbations, eosinophilia, and high IgE levels. Invasive infections can cause chronic sinusitis or colonization of a preexisting cavity. In immunocompromised hosts, especially those who are neutropenic, the disease can be life-threatening, causing a necrotizing pneumonia. Classically, patients present with pleuritic chest pain. There can be hematogenous spread to the CNS and other organs. Chronic invasive forms may include aspergillomas ("fungus ball") that are slowly progressive; they are usually seen with an intact immune system but with underlying lung or sinus disease. The disease can present similarly to mucor of the sinuses and can also cause a tracheobronchitis in lung transplant or AIDS patients. It is second only to *Candida* as a cause of fungal endocarditis.

Dx—Blood cultures have a low yield. Enzyme-linked immunosorbent assay can be used to detect galactomannan, which is a major constituent of cell walls. Isolation from pulmonary secretions does not imply invasive disease. The mainstay of diagnosis is through biopsy. Biopsy of the involved organ shows acute angle branching septate hyphae. Imaging studies sometime may be characteristic, eliminating the need for biopsy, especially in critically ill patients.

Tx—Treatment is with amphotericin B or caspofungin or voriconazole; the latter may be most effective.

Candidiasis

D—One of the most common fungal infections. It is due to an ubiquitous yeast.

P—It is part of the common normal flora but is also considered an opportunistic pathogen.

RF—Risk factors include neutropenia, immunocompromised status, indwelling catheters, and IVDU.

SiSx—Candida can affect many different parts of the body. Skin and mucosal involvement is most common. Esophageal involvement can present with substernal odynophagia, GERD, or nausea and dysphagia. Oral lesions (thrush) may or may not be present. Thrush is distinguished from other conditions causing white plaques on the tongue because usually it can be wiped off. Vulvovaginal candidiasis is a common candidal infection, usually presenting with pruritis, a burning vaginal discharge, and dyspareunia (painful intercourse). Candiduria is usually asymptomatic and resolves with the removal of indwelling catheters. Disseminated disease is a problem, although blood cultures are not always positive even with disseminated disease. An important finding is possible endophthalmitis in cases where fluffy white retinal infiltrates are seen that can extend into the vitreous. All patients with candidemia should be evaluated for retinitis, as it affects the duration of treatment and monitoring. Hepatosplenic disease can be seen in patients who are profoundly neutropenic. Endocarditis, which occurs increasingly with the use of prosthetic valves, can be hard to eradicate and portends a poor prognosis.

Tx—Non-*albicans* forms are typically resistant to fluconazole, which is otherwise the treatment of choice. Echinocandins, amphotericin B, and voriconazole can be used.

Sporothricosis

D—A chronic fungal infection caused by *Sporothrix schenckii*.

Epi—It is commonly found in soil, moss, and decaying wood.

P—Organisms are inoculated via skin, classically during gardening.

SiSx—It is characterized by a hard, nontender nodule, adherent to skin, that ulcerates. More ulcerating nodules then develop within the lymphatic drainage area. Disseminated disease can involved the lung, bone, joints, and CNS.

Dx—Cultures are needed for diagnosis, though antibody testing is helpful in disseminated disease, including that of the CNS.

Tx—Itraconazole is given for several months. An alternative is terbinafine. Amphotericin B IV is used for severe systemic infection.

Protozoal Infections

Protozoans are unicellular eukaryotes and are responsible for several important, clinically relevant diseases in humans. These are summarized in Table 8-24.

Helminthic Infections

Helminths are worm-like parasites that live inside their host, in contrast to external parasites such as lice. Common human conditions are presented in Table 8-25.

CHAPTER 8 APPENDIX

Organism Classification

This section focuses on proper classification of common bacteria (Table 8-26) and viruses (Table 8-27). Finally, Table 8-28 serves as a quick reference guide to common bacterial infectious organisms.

Table 8-24. Noteworthy Protozoal Infections

Organism	Epi/P/RF	SiSx	Dx	Tx
Amebiasis *Entamoeba histolytica* and *E. dispar*	Most prevalent in subtropical and tropical areas with poor sanitation. 500 million are infected worldwide; 100,000 die each year. Humans are the only host. Virulence varies from commensal to invasive; seen in up to 10%. Transmission is via ingestion of cysts.	Presents as colitis, dysentery, and diarrhea with abdominal cramping, with or without bloody stool. May form hepatic lesions or abscesses. Can also produce localized granulomatous lesions of the colon (amebomas). Rare metastatic infection of lungs, brain, and genitalia.	Stool specimens for antigen. ELISA useful. Serologic testing can be used as an adjunct only for *E. histolytica*. Microscopic examination of the stool is not useful. Eosinophilia is rare. Percutaneous aspiration of liver abscesses may be needed for diagnosis.	In most patients, infection clears in 1 year. Asymptomatic patients can be treated with diloxanide furoate or iodoquinol with a single course. Endemic, asymptomatic patients are not treated because of frequent reinfection. Tinidazole or metronidazole is used for mild intestinal disease or severe disease. The regimen may also include chloroquine and dehydroemetine.
Coccidosis, Cryptosporidiosis, Isosporiasis, Cyclosporiasis and Microsporidiosis	Intracellular infections of intestinal epithelial cells. Mostly occur in the tropics or in developing countries; a cause of diarrhea outbreaks. Spread is fecal-oral from person to person. Microsporidiosis is zoonotic, however. Pathogenesis unclear; not enterotoxin based.	Small bowel and colon are most common sites of infection. May present as voluminous secretory or malabsorptive diarrhea. Types of diarrhea caused by these organisms are indistinguishable. Diarrhea typically is not bloody.	Usually by stool specimen analysis. Cryptosporidiosis is highly infective and is seen by modified acid-fast staining.	Self-limited disease in immunocompetent people; supportive care only. Immunocompromised patients are treated with trimethoprim-sulfamethoxazole or sulfadiazine/pyrimethamine/leucovorin for isosporiasis or trimethoprim-sulfamethoxazole or ciprofloxacin for cyclosporiasis. Albendazole is used for microsporidiosis. There is no clearly successful treatment for cryptosporidiosis, though many agents are tried. The main concern is to treat the immunosuppression.
Giardiasis *Giardia lamblia*	Areas of poor sanitation. Up to 2.5 million infections/year in the United States. Exists as a heart-shaped flagellated trophozoite and cyst form that is infectious by the fecal-oral route.	Most cases are asymptomatic. Otherwise can present with acute/chronic bulky, greasy, non-bloody diarrhea with abdominal cramps and distention.	Standard microscopy of stool to visualize cysts/trophozoites or immunoassay.	Treat asymptomatic patients to prevent transmission. Some infections, however, clear spontaneously. Metronidazole or tinidazole (one-time dose) are effective.

continued

Table 8-24. *(continued)*

Organism	Epi/P/RF	SiSx	Dx	Tx
Leishmaniasis Visceral Form (kala azar) Mucocutaneous Form (espundia)	A zoonosis transmitted by female sand flies that feed on wild animals and domestic dogs and then bite humans. Human-to-human transmission is only with kala azar (transfusions, congenitally). More common in temperate/tropical zones. 1–2 million cases occur yearly, mostly cutaneous. India, Bangladesh, Nepal, and Sudan are the most common locations for visceral leishmaniasis. Most cutaneous disease occurs in Afghanistan, the Arab states, Brazil, and Peru.	Visceral leishmaniasis has mortality of 90% if untreated. Starts with nodule at bite site, with fevers, chills, sweats, weakness, weight loss, cough, diarrhea, and an enlarged, hard, nontender spleen. Hyperpigmentation and petechiae are seen. Cutaneous disease appears weeks to month after bite as single or multiple papules that evolve to ulcerations with central depressions and can persist as nodules or plaques.	Giemsa stain used to find the intracellular organism in biopsy specimens from skin, mucous membranes, liver, or lymph nodes. Classically, Leishman-Donovan bodies are seen within mononuclear cells. ELISA is not very sensitive or specific.	Sodium stibogluconate or meglumine antimoniate is the drug of choice, given for 1 month or longer. Amphotericin B or pentamidine are second-line agents.
American Trypanosomiasis (Chagas' disease)	Occurs mainly in rural areas. Accounts for up to 45,000 deaths per year from heart disease. Usually affects immigrants from Latin America.	Acutely, most patients are asymptomatic. Those with symptoms (usually children) may have fevers, malaise, hepatosplenomegaly, lymphadenopathy, acute myocarditis, meningoencephalitis, and skin and eye findings. Chronically, there can be heart failure, GI involvement (megacolon and megaesophagus) with dysphagia, constipation, and sigmoid volvulus.	Organism can be found in blood culture or via animal innoculation in the acute phase. Rarely found directly in the chronic phase using animal culture. IgG testing should be repeated three times since the false-negative rate is high. Clinically, the diagnosis may be made with right GI and cardiac findings. Characteristically, apical aneurysms are found.	Treatment is usually not completely helpful in chronic cases because of medication toxicity. Benznidazole and nifurtimox are the two main drugs of choice. Acute infection should be treated. Treatment of chronic infection is controversial given the risks vs. benefits of treatment. Amiodarone is the antiarrhythmic drug of choice in these patients.

Table 8-25.   Noteworthy Helminthic Infections

Organism	Epi/P/RF	SiSx	Dx	Tx
Strongylodiasis *Strongyloides stercoralis*	Endemic in tropical and subtropical areas. Occurs in Appalachia and the southeastern United States. Larvae from soil enter the skin, migrate to lungs via blood, ascend the respiratory tract, and are swallowed. Worms mature and live in the SI mucosa, laying eggs. Humans are needed to propagate the disease.	Waxing and waning symptoms that go on for years. Feet are the most common site of initiation infection. Skin reaction: *larva currens*. Abdominal pain, duodenitis. Enterocolitis and malabsorption. Dry cough, dyspnea, wheezing, hemoptysis. Loeffler's-like eosinophilia. Steroids or immunosuppression can precipitate a hyperinfection syndrome due to massive dissemination of larvae into lungs, liver, heart, and elsewhere, causing multiorgan disease and shock.	The diagnosis should be suspected in any patient from an endemic area with unexplained eosinophilia and skin or pulmonary manifestations as described. Diagnosis made by detecting larvae in stool or via serology. In disseminated disease, it can be found in other organ fluid. (peritoneal, pleural, bronchoalveolar lavage, and so forth). ELISA is available.	Ivermectin is the treatment of choice, with albendazole given as a second-line therapy. Hyperinfection syndrome or disseminated disease needs longer treatment.
Enterobiasis (Pinworms)	Temperate and tropical climates. More commonly found in children. This is the most common helminthic infection in the United States and Europe from 20 to 40 million cases in the United States. Closed, crowded conditions facilitate disease transmission. Humans are the only host. Adults live in GI tract and produce thousands of eggs. The female migrates out through rectum to lay eggs on perianal skin. Fecal-oral contamination ensues.	Most patients are asymptomatic. The most common symptom is perianal itching from inflammatory reaction to presence of eggs and worms. Scratching increases transmission. Large worm burdens can cause abdominal pain, nausea, and vomiting. Eosinophilic enterocolitis can also result. In women, disease can enter the genital tract, causing vulvovaginitis.	Stool exam is not useful since eggs are not passed in the stool. Scotch tape test over perianal skin can help detect eggs. Test is done at night or first thing in the morning. The eggs have a characteristic bean-shaped appearance.	Mebendazole or albendazole are first-line treatments for pinworm infection. A single dose can have a high cure rate. A second dose is given weeks later. Reinfection is common given the means of spread and prevalence among families.

continued

Table 8-25. (*continued*)

Organism	Epi/P/RF	SiSx	Dx	Tx
Cysticercosis	Pork tapeworm infection. Yearly, 20 million people infected. Larvae can live for months to years.	Most patients are asymptomatic. Neurocysticercosis has protean manifestations, including encephalitis, parenchymal cysts, or meningeal, ventricular, or spinal cord cysts, even affecting the eye. It can also affect subcutaneous tissue and striated muscle.	Head CT or MRI may show the classic hole with dot images in addition to positive immunologic tests such as the electro-immuno-transfer blot (EITB) test.	Medical treatment is most effective for parenchymal cysts. Sometimes cysts die and resolve on their own. Albendazole or praziquantel are used otherwise. One-half die if untreated.
Echinococcosis	Parasitism by the larva stage of four *Echinococcus* species. Risk factors include exposure to dogs/ livestock in endemic regions (Europe, Russia, Australia, India, the United Kingdom the lower Mississippi Valley, Alaska, Canada) that are part of the life cycle.	Cysts are asymptomatic for years until they are large enough. Liver cysts may present as RUQ masses, biliary obstruction with rupture causing potential allergy/anaphylaxis. Cysts can metastasize to many other tissues.	Immunoblot test is the best. ELISA/ Western blot can also be used. Dead cysts, however, can be seronegative. Eosinophilia is common. LFTs usually normal. CT or MRI can show classic hydatid cysts with daughter cysts.	Albendazole is used to treat asymptomatic patients with small cysts not in danger of rupture. Otherwise, partial hepatic resection or percutaneous aspiration is needed in addition to medical treatment.
Paragonimiasis	Lung flukes that use humans and many animals for hosts. Primarily found in the Far East, West Africa, Southeast Asia, Pacific Islands, Indonesia, and New Guinea.	Most pulmonary infections are asymptomatic. Symptomatic patients may have pleuritic chest pain with small- or large-volume hemoptysis. CNS disease is rarely acute, as in meningitis; more commonly, it presents as space-occupying lesions or chronic meningoencephalitis.	Eggs can be found in sputum, gastric aspirates, bronchial washings, or biopsy or pleural specimens. Eosinophilia is common. CT may show small, round cystic lesions filled with fluid or gas.	Praziquantel is the drug of choice. Bithionol is an alternative drug. Chronic CNS disease is hard to treat.

Table 8-26. Classification of Clinically Significant Bacteria

	Gram Positive	Gram Negative
Cocci	*Staphylococcus, Streptococcus, Enterococcus*	*Neisseria, Moraxella*
Rods	*Bacillis, Corynebacterium, Listeria, Clostridium, (Rhodococcus, Erysipelothrix)*	*Shigella, Salmonella, Haemophilus, Enterobacter, Pseudomonas, Vibrio, Campylobacter, Brucella, Gardnerella, Pasteurella, Helicobacter, Acinetobacter, Yersinia, Bordetella, Legionella,* and so forth
Spirochetes	—	*Treponema pallidum, Leptospira, Borrelia, Spirillum*
Other	*Nocardia, Actinomyces*	—
Acid Fast	*Mycobacterium tuberculosis, Mycobacterium avium-intracelulare* complex (MAC)	—
Distinguishing Features of the Cell Wall	Teichoic acid, a potent antigen capsule with peptidoglycan. Has no porins and a low lipid content. It is vulnerable to lysozyme.	Lipid A of lipopolysaccharide (LPS) induces an inflammatory response. It has porin channels and is resistant to lysozyme because of its outer membrane which also has a high lipid content

Note: Endospores are made only by *Bacillus* and *Clostridium* and are resistant to boiling. *Listeria, Salmonella, Yersinia, Francisella tularensis, Brucella, Legionella,* and *Mycobacterium* all have phagolysosome fusion inhibitors that allows them to live inside cells without being killed by the superoxide radical pathway.

Table 8-27. Categorization of Clinically Significant Viruses

		(Strand) Virus Family	Examples
RNA	Non-enveloped	(+) Reovirus	Rotavirus (made of dsRNA segments)
		(+) Calcivirus	Norwalk and HEV
		(+) Picornavirus	Poliovirus, echovirus, rhinovirus, coxsackievirus, HAV
	Enveloped	(+) Togavirus	Western equine encephalitis (WEE), eastern equine encephalitis (EEE), Venezuelan equine encephalitis (VEE), and rubella
		(+) Flavivirus	Yellow fever, West Nile, dengue, St. Louis encephalitis, HCV
		(–) Orthomyxovirus	Influenza A, B, C
		(–) Paramyxovirus	Parainfluenza, measles, mumps, RSV
		(–) Rhabdovirus	Rabies
		(–) Filovirus	Ebola, Marburg
		(+) Retrovirus	HIV1 and –2, HTLV–1 and –2
		(+) Coronavirus	Common cold, severe acute respiratory syndrome (SARS)
		(–) Arenavirus	Lymphocytic choriomeningitis virus (LCMV)
		(–) Bunyavirus	Hanta, California encephalitis, Rift Valley fever
DNA	Non-enveloped	Adenovirus	Adenovirus
		Parvovirus	B19, HHV (ssDNA)
		Papovavirus	JC virus, human papilloma virus, BK virus
		Poxvirus	Smallpox, molluscum contagiosum
	Enveloped	Hepadnavirus	HBV
		Herpesvirus	HSV–1, –2, VZV, EBV, CMV, HHV–6, –7, –8

Table 8-28 Quick Reference to Bacteria and Their Associated Conditions

Bacterium	Source	Diseases
Streptococcus pyogenes, group A beta-hemolytic	Normal flora of skin and oropharynx	Impetigo, cellulitis, necrotizing fasciitis, pharyngitis, scarlet fever, post streptococcal glomerulonephritis, acute rheumatic fever, toxic shock syndrome
Streptococcus agalactiae, group B beta-hemolytic	Normal flora of vagina, vertical transmission	Neonatal meningitis and pneumonia, postpartum endometriosis
Streptococcus pneumoniae	Upper respiratory tract flora that seeds elsewhere	Lobar pneumonia, meningitis, sinusitis, otitis media
Streptococcus viridans	Flora of oropharynx	Subacute bacterial endocarditis, dental cavities, abscess of organs
Enterococcus faecalis	Normal bowel flora	UTI, subacute bacterial endocarditis, biliary tract infections
Staphylococcus aureus	Skin, nose	Impetigo, infective arthritis, osteomyelitis, sepsis, acute endocarditis, scalded skin syndrome, toxic shock syndrome, food poisoning, parotitis
Staphylococcus saprophyticus	Normal flora or GU tract, skin	UTI in sexually active women
Staphylococcus epidermidis	Normal skin flora, trauma	Subacute bacterial endocarditis, especially with prosthetic devices, bacteremia
Bacillus cereus	Reheated rice	Food poisoning
Bacillus anthracis	Animal hide, wool, goat, cow hide	Skin (malignant pustule respiration), Woolsorter's disease
Clostridium tetani	Soil, entry through wound	Tetanus with severe spasms
Clostridium difficile	Normal colon flora	Pseudomembranous colitis with overgrowth
Clostridium perfringens	Soil, dust, air, wound entry, in feces of all people	Gas gangrene, toxic enteritis, cellulitis, wound infection, myonecrosis
Clostridium botulinum	Spores in food ingestion of preformed toxin	Botulism food poisoning, floppy baby syndrome in infants' in adults, cranial nerve palsies
Corynebacterium diphtheriae	Colonizes pharynx in human carriers,	Myocarditis, neurologic toxicity, classic posterior pharynx pseudomembrane
Listeria monocytogenes	Unpasteurized milk, vertical transmission, food. Tropism for neural tissue.	Neonatal, immunocompromised, elderly people with meningitis, spontaneous abortion
Neisseria meningitides	Respiratory droplets	Meningitis if young adults and kids. Petechiae classic. Waterhouse-Friderichsen syndrome with bilateral adrenal hemorrhage, DIC.
Neisseria gonorrhoeae	Human-to-human transmission via sex, birth	Septic arthritis, conjunctivitis in babies, urethritis, prostatitis, epididymitis, DGI, pelvic inflammatory disease, endometritis, salpingitis, oophoritis, and cervicitis.
Moraxella catarrhalis	Upper respiratory tract, vagina	Otitis media, respiratory problems in COPD patients
Enterotoxigenic *Escherichia Coli* (ETEC)	Fecal-oral	Traveler's diarrhea—watery. Non invasive secretory diarrhea.
Enterohemorrhagic *Escherichia coli*	Fecal-oral, GI tract, undercooked hamburgers	Hemorrhagic colitis, bloody diarrhea. HUS from O157:H7
Klebsiella pneumoniae	Normal GI flora	Number two cause of gram-negative sepsis. Lobar pneumonia common in alcoholics for pneumonia. Currently jelly colored sputum is classic. High mortality rate

Organism	Transmission	Disease/Notes
Proteus mirabilis	Normal GI flora	UTI
Shigella	Fecal-oral	Bacillary dysentery, bloody diarrhea, reactive arthritis
Salmonella	GI tract of animals, feca-oral contamination	Typhoid fever: fever, RLQ pain, splenomegaly, rose spots on abdominal, diarrhea. Osteomyelitis in sickle cell patients
Vibrio cholerae	GI tract reservoir, fecal-oral spread, contaminated water	Rice water painless diarrhea. Death by dehydration
Vibrio parahaemolyticus	Uncooked seafood, sushi	Number one cause of diarrhea in Japan
Yersinia enterocolitica	Fecal-oral	Acute gastroenteritis, mucosal ulceration
Yersinia pestis	Flea bite	Bubonic plague
Pseudomonas aeruginosa	Obligate aerobe, everywhere, skin, mucosa, and so forth.	Opportunistic infection. Pneumonia (especially in cystic fibrosis patients), burn or wound infection, UTI, endocarditis, osteomyelitis, malignant otitis externa, corneal infections for contact lens wearers
Helicobacter pylori	Unclear; person-to-person transmission	Duodenal ulcers, chronic gastritis, gastric ulcers (second most important after use of NSAIDs)
Campylobacter jejuni	Fecal-oral, zoonotic, unpasteurized milk	Third most important cause of diarrhea worldwide along with rotavirus and ETEC
Bacteroides	GI flora, vagina flora, surgical wounds	Abscess or systemic infection
Haemophilus influenzae	Person-to-person only via respiratory droplet	Pneumonia (COPD, young or old people), meningitis (now uncommon with vaccine), epiglottitis, sinusitis, otitis media, conjunctivitis
Haemophilus ducreyi	STD	Chancroid, painful unilateral swollen lymph nodes, rupture exuding pus
HACEK group of organisms *Haemophilus parainfluenzae, Actinobacillus, Cardiobacterium hominis, Eikenella corrodens, Kingella kingii*	Normal oropharyngeal flora	Subacute bacterial endocarditis
Gardnerella vaginalis	Normal vaginal flora	Bacterial vaginalis, clue cells are diagnostic
Bordetella pertussis	Direct contact with discharge from mucous membranes	Whooping cough
Legionella pneumophila	Inhalational spread via aerosolized droplets	Community acquired pneumonia, Legionnaire's disease, Pontiac fever

CHAPTER 9

Hematology

ANATOMY AND PHYSIOLOGY

Bone Marrow

- The bone marrow has an architecture designed for cell–cell and cell–matrix interactions that are required for cell maturation and the deliverance of mature cells into the circulation.
- There are three major pools of cells: stem cells; proliferating and developing cells; and terminally developing cells, which also serve as a reserve pool to replace circulating elements.

Spleen

- The functions of the spleen are blood filtration, immunomodulation, and, in some cases, hematopoiesis.
- The spleen stores about one-third of the body's platelets. Ten percent of the circulating blood volume is present in the spleen, and this percentage increases as the spleen enlarges.

Hematopoiesis

- It starts in the yolk sac of the embryo during the first month in utero.
- The liver and spleen become the sites of blood production in the third month.
- The bone marrow acquires this function in the fourth month, while the other organs gradually lose it.
- In the adult, most of the marrow production occurs in the long bones, pelvis, ribs, and vertebrae.
- When the marrow is unable to produce enough cells (e.g., with myelofibrosis),

extramedullary hematopoiesis can occur in other organs (liver, spleen) or in areas of the bone marrow not usually seen as active in adulthood (such as the skull).

The Pro- and Anticoagulation Pathways

Hemostasis pathways activate after blood vessel wall damage, specifically with damage to the endothelium. Platelets plug the area (*primary hemostasis*), after which clotting factors respond to form cross-linked fibrin strands to strengthen the platelet plug and form a clot (*secondary hemostasis*).

Platelet Activation (Primary Hemostasis)

Exposed proteins after vessel wall injury, such as collagen, bind to glycoprotein Ia/IIa receptors and von Willebrand factor (vWF), which causes adhesion and activation of platelets, releasing many more factors from stored granules such as adenosine diphosphate (ADP), serotonin, even more vWF, platelet factor 4, and thromboxane A2, among others. Eventually, glycoprotein IIb/IIIa, a membrane receptor, is activated on platelets to bind to fibrinogen and allows aggregation of platelets.

Coagulation Cascade (Secondary Hemostasis)

There are two major pathways that cause fibrin cross-linking. It is important to know the factors involved and which ones are affected by anticoagulant drugs and acquired and inherited deficiencies. Many of these factors

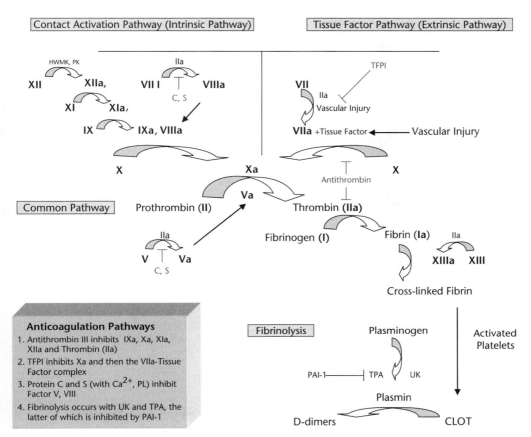

Figure 9-1. The Coagulation Cascade.
HMWK, high molecular weight kininogen; PAI-1, plasminogen activator inhibitor type 1, made in the liver; PK, prekallikrein; PL, platelet phospholipids; TFPI, tissue factor pathway inhibitor; TPA, tissue plasminogen activator, released by endothelial cells; UK, urokinase; α2-AP, α2-antiplasmin, cross-linked to α-chains of fibrin by factor VIIIa.

Note: Factor IV is calcium, and there is no factor VI for historical reasons; factors II, VII, IX, X, C, and S are vitamin K dependent.

(classified by roman numerals) are serine protease enzymes that are transformed into their active form (labeled with an *a*). See Figure 9-1.

DIAGNOSTIC AND THERAPEUTIC MODALITIES

The Peripheral Blood Smear

A peripheral smear is indicated for patients suspected of having hemolytic anemia (to examine RBC morphology), thrombocytopenia (to exclude signs of platelet consumption), and WBC disorders or malignancies. Smears are made directly from unclotted blood and can be "thin" or "thick" (for increased depth resolution). Rules of thumb: RBCs should be about same size as a lymphocyte; platelet counts are estimated as 10,000 for every platelet seen on a high-power field. Common RBC abnormalities are described in Table 9-1.

Table 9-1.   Common Peripheral Blood Smear Findings

Cell Type	Picture	Description	When Seen
Segmented Neutrophil		Multisegmented, usually not more than four or five lobes unless there is pathology. Much larger than an RBC.	As part of the normal blood smear.
Monocyte		Mast cell (in periphery) releases histamine.	As part of the normal blood smear.
Lymphocyte		A mature lymphoid cell with dense chromatin at the edge of the nucleus in a clock faced pattern. It is slightly larger than an RBC.	As part of the normal blood smear.
Basophil		A darker stippled cell with many granules, usually multilobed.	As part of the normal blood smear, usually rare.
Eosinophil		A bright red, heavily granulated cell.	Increased in IgE mediated responses (i.e. allergies).
Platelets		Short-lived (lives 7–10 days).	As part of the normal blood smear.
Normal RBC		Biconcave disk-shaped and compressible, with an area of central pallor.	Should be the predominant component of any peripheral blood smear. 2×10^{11}/L made per day.
Reticulocyte		Large, somewhat bluish RBC due to the RNA of polyribosomes. It is an RBC precursor that has already lost its nucleus.	Normal finding if <1% of total cells. Otherwise seen in states of bleeding, hemolysis, or B12/folate administration in someone with deficiency.
Nucleated RBC		More immature RBC form than the reticulocyte, with a small, condensed nucleus.	Indicates severe degree of hemolysis, profound stress, hypoxemia, or myelofibrosis.
Burr Cell or Echinocyte or RBC Crenation		Numerous regular, scalloped projections on the surface of the RBC.	Liver disease, severe renal disease, or artifact of preparation.
Schistocytes		Fragmented RBCs from physical damage in circulation.	TTP, DIC, severe vasculitis, or HUP, preeclampsia, eclampsia, mechanical heart valve.
Target Cell		Bulls-eye appearance of the cell with a central disk of hemoglobin.	Thalassemia or chronic liver disease, though in the latter, target cells are less uniform.

continued

Table 9-1. *(continued)*

Cell Type	Picture	Description	When Seen
Teardrop Cell or Dacryocyte		Pointed end on one side, round on the other.	Infiltration of bone marrow, infection, or TB.
Basophilic Stippling		Punctate dark spots on RBCs representing residual RNA. They are present when RBCs are prematurely released from the bone marrow.	Reticulocytosis, thalassemias, lead poisoning.
Acanthocyte		RBC with spiny projections.	Spur cell anemia, severe liver disease, or abetalipoproteinemia.
Stomatocyte		RBC with a slit-like central pale area, having lost the normal indentation on one side of the biconcave disk.	Alcohol abuse, inherited disease.
Spherocyte		Small RBC with little or no central pallor.	Hereditary or acquired membrane defect with clipping of membrane via spleen.
Heinz Body		Precipitate of denatured hemoglobin usually attached to the RBC surface. It forms secondary to an oxidative or chemical insult to the RBC and is suggestive of hemolytic anemia. Resembles a protuberance on the RBC under light but is detected easily with methylene blue staining.	G6PD or methemoglobinemia.
Howell-Jolly Body		Single circular black dot seen in the periphery of an RBC. These bodies are large DNA fragments, nuclear remnants that are normally removed by the spleen.	Seen after splenectomy or with hyposplenism. Also seen in some hemolytic anemias when the spleen becomes overwhelmed and cannot completely clear these forms.
Bite Cell or Degmacyte		"Bite" along the periphery.	Oxidative damage such as G6PD.
Pappenheimer Body		Dark blue iron-containing granules in RBCs that are hypochromic.	Seen in sideroblastic anemia, after splenectomy, and occasionally in severe hemolytic anemia.
Coin Stacked Cells or Rouleaux		Agglutination of multiple RBCs together in stacks.	Abnormal serum proteins such as in multiple myeloma.

APPROACH TO COMMON PROBLEMS

Approach to the Diagnosis of Anemia

Anemia is defined as a low hematocrit (Hct) in women (<36%) and in men (<41%) or low hemoglobin in women (<12 g/dL) or in men (<14 g/dL). It occurs from (1) increased RBC destruction, (2) decreased RBC production, or (3) blood loss. Findings on the history and exam are shown in Table 9-2.

1. Work-up: Obtain a reticulocyte count. If it is >2%, this is appropriate in an anemia of increased RBC destruction. If it is <2% with anemia, this is abnormal and indicates decreased production. Correction of the reticulocyte count for Hct should be done before interpretation, as reticulocytes circulate longer in the bloodstream when the Hct is lower (i.e., a very low Hct will have a higher percentage of reticulocytes if uncorrected).

$$\text{Corrected reticulocyte count} = \frac{\text{Measured Reticulocyte Count}}{\text{Maturation Factor}^*} \times \frac{\text{Patient's Hct}}{\text{Normal Hct}}$$

2. Evaluate the **mean corpuscular volume** (MCV) to determine the cause of anemia, as shown in Table 9–3.
3. Use additional tests to distinguish unclear cases:

Perform "iron studies" for most microcytic/normocytic anemias, which include ferritin, serum iron, total iron-binding capacity (TIBC), and transferrin (see Table 9-4).

- If hemolysis is suspected, check a blood smear to look for schistocytes and membrane defects. A Coombs test should also be done to evaluate for autoimmune hemolytic anemias. Increased LDH, increased indirect bilirubin, and decreased haptoglobin will also be seen if this test is performed. Intravascular bleeding is associated with hemoglobinuria and hemosiderinuria.
- Thalassemia is evaluated by hemoglobin electrophoresis.
- In macrocytic anemias, leukopenia and thrombocytopenia may also be seen, especially with vitamin B_{12} and folate deficiencies. Often the LDH is >500 IU/L and a blood smear shows hypersegmented neutrophils and oval macrocytes.

Table 9-2.   The History and Exam Findings of Anemia

Note the Following in the History:	Note the Following on Exam:
Blood loss—heavy menstrual periods, possibility of pregnancy, recent surgery, or a history of peptic ulcer disease.	Weakness or fatigue; pallor (best evaluated from the mucous membranes and skin).
Diet—vegan diet without vitamin supplements, heavy alcohol use.	Jaundice from indirect bilirubin or dark urine suggests hemolysis.
Infections—known history of HIV, chronic infections, chronic renal disease, any chronic inflammatory disease.	Tachycardia, decreased pulse pressure, orthostasis, and a systolic flow murmur may be seen if the anemia is acute.
Genetic causes—family history of anemia (e.g., sickle cell disease, G6PD, thalassemia).	Positive stool guiac test.
Malignancy—weight loss, fever, chills, night sweats. Ask about the most recent colonoscopy if the patient is >50 years old.	Patients with low Hct can be surprisingly asymptomatic if anemia has occurred over a long period of time (months).

---

* Maturation Factor = 1.5 for Hct of 35%, 2.0 for Hct of 25%, and 2.5 for Hct of 15%.

Table 9-3. Causes of Different Anemias by RBC Size

Type of Anemia	Microcytic (MCV <80 fL)	Normocytic (MCV 60–80 fL)	Macrocytic (MCV >100 fL)
Decreased Production	Chronic disease anemia Heavy metal (lead, and aluminum toxicity, copper deficiency) Iron deficiency anemia Thalassemias Sideroblastic anemia	Chronic disease anemia Renal disease Hypothyroidism Aplastic anemia Congenital red cell aplasia Acquired red cell aplasia Myelophthisic anemia	Megaloblastic anemia (MCV > 115 fL), as seen in vitamin B_{12} and folate deficiencies. Liver disease, alcoholism Hypothyroidism Drugs (AZT, methotrexate) Myelodysplastic syndrome
Increased Destruction/Loss	—	Hemorrhage Hemolysis 1. Hemoglobinopathy (sickle cell disease), unstable hemoglobin 2. Enzymatic defects (G6PD deficiency) 3. Membrane defect (spherocytosis) 4. Acquired membrane defect (PNH, liver disease) 5. Traumatic (DIC, TTP, stenotic valvular heart disease) 6. Infection (sepsis, clostridium, malaria) 7. Autoimmune	Autoimmune hemolytic anemia Reticulocytosis

DIC, disseminated intravascular coagulation; PNH, paroxysmal nocturnal hemoglobinuria; TTP, thrombotic thrombocytopenic purpura.

Table 9-4. Iron Study Results and Common Anemias

	Ferritin	Serum Iron	TIBC
Chronic Disease Anemia	Normal to ↑	↓	Normal to ↓
Iron Deficiency	If <10 ng/mL, very suggestive If >100 ng/mL, unlikely	↓	↑
Thalassemia	Normal to ↑	Normal to ↑	Normal
Sideroblastic	↑	↑	↓

Table 9-5. Causes of Thrombocytopenia and Thrombocytosis

Thrombocytopenia	Thrombocytosis
Decreased production (i.e., bone marrow suppression) 1. Drug related—chemotherapy, radiation therapy, long-term alcohol use, trimethoprim-sulfamethoxazole, valproic acid, among many others. 2. Infectious—post viral infection (parvovirus, rubella, varicella, hepatitis C, HIV, and others). 3. Nutritional—vitaminB_{12} deficiency, folic acid deficiency, late iron deficiency. 4. Congenital—Bernard-Soulier syndrome (lack of glycoprotein 1b), Alport's syndrome, Wiskott-Aldrich syndrome (X-linked). 5. Infiltrative—cancer, myelofibrosis, Gaucher's storage disease, granulomatous disease.	*Reactive*—infection, postsurgical, malignancy, postsplenectomy, acute blood loss. *Autonomous*—CML, polycythemia vera, myelodysplastic syndrome, essential thrombocythemia, agnogenic myeloid metaplasia. *Spurious*—mixed cryoglobulinemia, cytoplasmic fragments counted as platelets.

Increased destruction
1. Autoimmune—idiopathic thrombocytopenia purpura, thrombotic thrombocytopenic purpura, posttransplantation alloimmune destruction, antiphospholipid antibody syndrome, HELLP syndrome (near the time of pregnancy).
2. Mechanical—after cardiac bypass machine use, vascular malformations, prosthetic valve, severe valvular stenosis (all can destroy platelets).
3. Sequestration (from splenomegaly) —myeloproliferative disorders; lymphoma; portal hypertension, splenic or hepatic vein thrombosis or other causes; hemolytic anemia.

Iatrogenic
1. Distributional/dilutional—massive blood loss with packed RBC-only transfusions, diluting out platelets.
2. Pseudothrombocytopenia—platelet clumping in the tube from insufficient anticoagulation, EDTA-dependent agglutinins (in 0.1% of normal people) leading to platelet clumping.

Table 9-6. Differential Diagnosis of Common Cytopenias and Cytoses

Neutrophilia	Neutropenia
Infection	*Acquired*
Infarction (heart or lung)	Infection
Gout flare	Collagen vascular disease (lupus, Felty's syndrome)
Vasculitis	Drug induced
Drugs (steroids, epinephrine, lithium)	Autoimmune
Hypermetabolic (hyperthyroid)	Transfusion reaction
Myeloproliferative disorders	Bone marrow suppression (leukemia, aplastic anemia)
Diabetic ketoacidosis	
Intense exercise	*Congenital*
Stress	Chediak-Higashi syndrome
Burns	Cyclic neutropenia
Postsplenectomy (less sequestration)	Shwachman-Diamond-Oski syndrome
	Severe infantile agranulocytosis
Eosinophila	**Basophilia**
Drug reaction	Allergic disease
Parasitic infections, mostly helminths	Myeloproliferative disease, especially CML
Fungal infections	Occult carcinoma
Adrenal insufficiency	Chronic inflammatory conditions
Allergic/atopic-related disease	Tuberculosis (rare)

continued

Table 9-6. *(continued)*

Eosinophila *(continued)*	**Pancytopenia**
Rheumatic disease (e.g., Churg-Strauss syndrome)	Aplastic anemia
Malignant neoplasm	Drug induced
Hypereosinophilic syndromes	Radiation
Leukemia/lymphomas	Infection (bacterial sepsis, viral infection, fungal,
Mastocytosis	tuberculosis)
Transplant rejection	Leukemia/lymphoma with marrow involvement
	Myelofibrosis
Monocytosis	Vitamin B_{12} deficiency
Infections (subacute bacterial endocarditis, tuberculosis,	Systemic lupus erythematosus
brucellosis, malaria, and others)	Hypersplenism
Granulomatous disease	Sarcoidosis
Collagen vascular disease	AIDS
Leukemia, lymphoma	Congenital (Fanconi's anemia)
Myelodysplastic syndrome	
Malignant neoplasia	

Approach to Common Cytopenias and Cytoses

Aside from anemia, other cytopenias and cytoses are common laboratory findings, and it is important to have a differential diagnosis ready at hand for each. Platelet abnormalities tend to be the most common. There are numerous causes, as shown in Table 9-5. The differential diagnoses for all other cell line conditions are shown in Table 9-6.

HEMATOLOGIC DISEASES

The Anemias

Iron Deficiency Anemia

D—A condition marked by inadequate iron for the normal production of RBCs.

Epi—The most common cause is blood loss from menstruation (as many as 20% of young women are affected) or a GI bleed. The most common cause worldwide is parasitic infection.

P—The body has no mechanism to eliminate iron. Therefore, blood loss of some sort is usually the cause when the loss exceeds the dietary replacement rate. Iron stores in bone marrow are depleted first (ferritin decreases); subsequently, transferrin is upregulated. Later, there is a decrease in serum iron, then an increase in TIBC, and thus a decrease, in the percentage of transferrin saturation (ratio of serum iron to TIBC). At this point, RBCs become microcytic. In addition, RBC distribution width (RDW) increases since many smaller cells with widely varying sizes are produced.

RF—Any condition predisposing to bleeding or iron loss is a risk factor.

SiSx—In addition to those seen in generalized anemia, signs and symptoms more specific to iron deficiency include brittle nails, atrophic tongue, and pica (craving for metal, ice, and nonfood objects), which may lead to lead toxicity by enhancing lead absorption. Other symptoms, such as glossitis (inflammation of the tongue), spooning of the nails, or koilonychia, are consistent with but not specific for the condition.

Dx—In the appropriate setting, finding microcytic, hypochromic RBCs on a blood smear makes the diagnosis. The ferritin level is the single best test, with values <10 ng/mL for women and <30 ng/mL for men highly suggestive of iron deficiency. The plasma iron test has low specificity. Once the diagnosis has been made, the *underlying cause must also be found.* In patients >50 years old who are hemoccult positive, colonoscopy and esophagogastroduodenoscopy (EGD) are necessary to rule out tumors causing bleeding.

Tx—Treat the underling disease, if found. Administer oral iron as ferrous sulfate, though it can be constipating. Alternatives are ferrous gluconate or fumarate forms. These are best absorbed with an acid gastric pH; therefore, PPIs may hinder absorption. Addition of vitamin C may help, as well as taking other medications several hours apart. Intravenous formulations are given to patients on hemodialysis.

Anemia of Chronic Disease

D—Anemia that is associated with any chronic inflammatory condition, such as inflammatory arthritis, serious infections, and malignancy.

Epi—This is the second most common cause of anemia after iron deficiency in hospitalized patients.

P—Patients have adequate levels of body iron; however, its utilization by the bone marrow is decreased. A putative mechanism involves bone marrow insensitivity to erythropoietin due to the effect of inflammatory cytokines.

SiSx—Patients may be asymptomatic, as this is generally a slowly progressive anemia. They may have nonspecific findings of anemia such as pallor, weakness, and increased heart rate. They may or may not have an obvious inflammatory condition.

Dx—The patient must have a concomitant chronic inflammatory condition. Rarely is hemoglobin <7 g/dL. Red blood cells will be hypochromic and normocytic to microcytic on a blood smear. Serum ferritin is normal or high; serum iron and TIBC are low. Bone marrow biopsy, if done, shows adequate iron stores, though this is rarely necessary.

Tx—Correction or treatment of the underlying disease may reverse anemia within a month. Exogenous erythropoietin may also be appropriate, although high doses may need to be administered due to its decreased efficacy.

Sideroblastic Anemia

D—Anemia from aberrant synthesis of the heme moiety leading to diminished hemoglobin production and hypochromic, microcytic RBCs.

P—There is a defect in one of the multistep enzymatic reactions in the protoporphyrin ring synthesis pathway occurring in and around mitochondria. Unincorporated iron accumulates in and destroys these organelles. The ringed appearance of cells seen on an iron-stained marrow biopsy specimen arises from the perinuclear iron collection in nucleated RBCs. The condition may be inherited or acquired. In the former case, mutations may be found in either the nuclear (X-linked) or mitochondrial genomes. Etiologies of acquired forms include alcohol, lead, INH, and use of chloramphenicol. Idiopathic refractory sideroblastic anemia occasionally occurs after chemotherapy. This entity is clonal and thus is a subgroup of myelodysplastic syndrome (MDS).

SiSx—Aside from the usual symptoms of anemia, there may accompanying problems with the pancreas, liver, and kidney (Pearson's syndrome) if the disorder is of mitochondrial origin. The X-linked form does not manifest until early adulthood.

Dx—Blood smear reveals hypochromic, microcytic RBCs. Rarely, RBCs with Pappenheimer bodies may be seen. In patients with idiopathic refractory sideroblastic anemia, the RBC population may be dimorphous. Laboratory tests show a hemoglobin level of 8–10 g/dL, elevated ferritin levels, low TIBC, and high percent transferrin saturation. The diagnosis is confirmed by bone marrow biopsy showing ringed sideroblasts, which is the heme staining in and around mitochondria, as well as erythroid hyperplasia.

Tx—Treatment depends on the etiology. Inherited forms usually respond to high doses of pyridoxine. Certain acquired forms warrant discontinuation of the causative agent. There are no curative measures for the idiopathic refractory form, which may develop into leukemia. Patients are usually transfusion dependent. Exogenous erythropoietin is used in 20% of patients.

Megaloblastic Anemia

D—Condition due to either lack of the cofactors vitamin B_{12} or folate or the inability to use them in RBC production.

Table 9-7. Components of the Schilling Test

Part I	Saturate binding sites with 1 mg IM unlabeled vitamin B_{12}. Give tracer dose of radioactive cyanocobalamin (0.5–2 µg). Collect urine for 24 hours. Normally, >9% of the radioactive dose is excreted in the urine. In the context of vitamin B_{12} deficiency, such a finding points to dietary deficiency or malabsorption. Otherwise, go to part II.
Part II	Repeat part I with a dose of intrinsic factor. If urine levels are >9%, vitamin B_{12} deficiency is due to decreased intrinsic factor. Otherwise, go to part III.
Part III	Repeat part II after administering antibiotics. If urine levels are >9%, vitamin B_{12} deficiency is due to bacterial overgrowth, a sequela of blind loop syndrome.

Note: An extra step may be added between parts II and III to test for pancreatic sufficiency by administering exogenous enzymes.

P—Mammalian cells require vitamin B_{12} and folate for DNA synthesis, both of which must be acquired exogenously. In deficient states, cytoplasm development outstrips that of the nucleus, causing macrocytosis. Causes of vitamin B_{12} deficiency include pernicious anemia (most common), total gastrectomy, lye ingestion, ileal resections, Crohn's disease, drugs such as AZT, methotrexate, pancreatic insufficiency, blind loop syndrome, and tapeworms. Pernicious anemia results from the destruction of parietal cells by autoimmune antibodies, resulting in gastric atrophy, achlorhydria, and failure to secrete intrinsic factor. Folate deficiency is more nutritional and results from alcoholism, malabsorptive states, use of drugs such as anticonvulsants, methotrexate, and oral contraceptives, hemodialysis, pregnancy, cancer, and increased hematopoiesis.

SiSx—In addition to the general symptoms associated with other anemias, neurologic changes may also be seen in vitamin B_{12} deficiency: paresthesias in a stocking glove distribution, loss of vibratory sensation, ataxia, weakness, and reversible dementia. Folate deficiency does not present with neurologic symptoms.

Dx—Marked macrocytosis (>110 fL) makes megaloblastic anemia more likely. The complete blood count (CBC) also reveals thrombocytopenia and leukopenia. Blood smear shows RBC anisocytosis (variation in cell size), poikilocytosis (irregularly shaped RBCs), hypersegmented polymorphonuclear leukocytes (PMNs), and misshapen platelets. Serum vitamin B_{12} and folate levels should be measured. A vitamin B_{12} level <100 pg/mL indicates a vitamin B_{12} deficiency; a folate level <4 ng/mL indicates a folate deficiency. Homocysteine is increased in folic acid deficiency. Homocysteine and methyl malonic acid are increased in vitamin B_{12} deficiency. The pathogenesis of vitamin B_{12} deficiency is usually easy to identify. One can do the Schilling test, shown in Table 9-7. Although it is rarely performed today, it is a classic test that is worthwhile to know.

Tx—Besides addressing any underlying disorder, one must replace vitamin B_{12} and folate to eliminate deficiencies. require replacement. Keep in mind that folate administration may correct the symptoms of vitamin B_{12} deficiency except for the neurologic ones. Also, patients with pernicious anemia have an increased incidence of gastric polyps and gastric cancer. In vitamin B_{12} deficiency, neurologic recovery occurs with replacement.

The Thalassemias

The thalassemias are a group of congenital conditions due to point mutations in the α- or β-globin chains resulting in abnormal formation of hemoglobin tetramers. There is no substitute for α subunits, but β subunits can be substituted for by δ or γ types. In the normal individual, there are several forms:

HbA (α2β2)—predominant normal adult hemoglobin (>95%)

HbA2 (α2δ2) —comprises 2% of normal adult hemoglobin

HbF (α2γ2)—fetal isoform, which predominates in utero. One half of 1% of normal hemoglobin in adults is fetal.

β-Thalassemia Syndromes

D—A group of inherited hypochromic, microcytic anemia in which biosynthesis of β-globin is aberrant. There are several types, depending on how many of the two β-globin genes (one on each chromosome 11) are mutated.

β-*Thalassemia major*: The patient has two defective β-globin genes and has severe clinical manifestations. The baby is normal at birth, but after 1 year, transfusions are required. This anemia can cause growth failure, bony deformities, splenomegaly, and jaundice.

β-*Thalassemia intermedia*: The patient has two defective β-globin genes but has milder clinical manifestations. There is a chronic hemolytic anemia that usually does not require transfusions. It can cause splenomegaly.

β-*Thalassemia minor* (*or trait*): The patient has one defective β-globin gene (and is generally asymptomatic).

Epi—Ten percent of Italians and Greeks carry β-thalassemia alleles. To a lesser extent, these alleles are seen in Chinese, other Asians, and blacks.

P—The anemia is usually due to point mutations instead of deletions. Aberrant synthesis of one type of globin leads to diminished production of hemoglobin tetramers. α-Globin accumulates and interferes with most developing erythroblasts. Those that survive retain inclusion bodies and are detected by the spleen, which leads to hemolytic anemia. Compensatory erythroid hyperplasia in the marrow, liver, and spleen can lead to bone deformities, as can marrow expansion. Diversion of nutrients for ineffective erythropoiesis results in infection, endocrinopathies, and general wasting.

Conditions of variable clinical severity arises from phenotypic modifiers, including coinheritance of aberrant α-globin alleles (reduces unbalanced α-globin production) and increased γ-globin synthesis.

SiSx—Children present with "chipmunk" facies and deformities of long bones. Symptoms of hemolytic anemia—splenomegaly, jaundice, leg ulcers, gallstones, and CHF—may also be seen.

Dx—The diagnosis should be considered when there is microcytosis out of proportion to the degree of anemia, generally when the MCV <60, though severe iron deficiency can cause this condition. A positive family history is helpful as well. The diagnosis of β-thalassemia major is usually made in childhood from (1) evidence of anemia with hepatosplenomegaly, (2) a characteristic blood smear, and (3) elevated levels of HbF/HbA$_2$. Serum hemoglobin electrophoresis can help make the diagnosis. An individual with β-thalassemia minor will have no clinical features of anemia, but a blood smear will show marked microcytosis and hypochromia with target cells. In β-thalassemia minor, the Hct is usually 28–40. The MCV is usually 55–75; basophilic stippling may be present. Hemoglobin electrophoresis will show increased Hemoglobin A2 and F. In β-thalassemia major, anemia is so severe that without transfusion the Hct can fall to <10. Variable amounts of Hemoglobin A2 and Hemoglobin F are seen.

Tx—Patients with β-thalassemia major require chronic transfusions; splenectomy may be necessary. Vaccinate the patient with pneumococcal vaccine, administer folate, and watch for sequelae of hemolytic anemia and endocrinopathies. Allogeneic bone marrow transplants are the only cure. Patients with β-thalassemia intermedia may have the aforementioned symptoms but can usually survive without transfusions. Note that patients with both types may develop secondary hemochromatosis from chronic transfusions, which commonly causes death from cardiac failure. Deferoxamine is usually given as an iron chelating agent.

α-Thalassemia Syndromes

D—A group of inherited hypochromic, microcytic anemias in which biosynthesis of α-globin is aberrant. There are several types, depending on how many of the four α-globin genes (two on each chromosome 16) are mutated.

Hydrops fetalis: The stillborn fetus has four defective α-globin genes.

Hemoglobin H (HbH): The patient has three defective α-globin genes and anemia of variable severity. Pallor and splenomegaly are prominent.

α-Thalassemia-2 trait: The patient has two defective α-globin genes (is asymptomatic and has normal life expectancy).

α-Thalassemia silent carrier: The patient has one defective α-globin gene (is asymptomatic).

P—HbH disease arises from unbalanced production of β-globin, which forms β_4 tetramers (HbH). HbH inclusions can be found in circulating blood cells but do not precipitate.

RF—The condition is most common in Southeast Asia and China and less common in people of African descent.

SiSx—HbH disease has a clinical course similar to that of β-thalassemia intermedia, with symptoms consistent with hemolytic anemia but milder, ineffective erythropoiesis.

Dx—People with the α-thalassemia-2 trait usually have Hct of 28–40% with MCV of 60–75 fL. Electrophoresis shows no increase in the percentage of Hemoglobin A2 or F and no HbH. α-Globin gene analysis is the only way to diagnose the trait and the carrier. Usually, therefore, this is a diagnosis of exclusion. The reticulocyte count is normal. Iron studies are normal. A blood smear can be stained to detect HbH. Electrophoresis shows more rapidly migrating H. HbH disease has a Hct of 22–32% with MCV of 60–70 fL. The reticulocyte count is elevated.

Tx—Thalassemia-2 trait and silent carrier alpha thalassemia-1 do not require therapy. Treatment of HbH disease is similar to that for β-thalassemia in requiring chronic transfusions.

Sickle Cell Anemia

D—An autosomal recessive condition that involves a mutated β-globin gene in which glutamic acid is substituted for valine at the sixth amino acid of the protein product (denoted by 6E→V). Different forms exist.

Sickle cell trait: This is an asymptomatic individual who has a single $\beta^{6E \to V}$-globin gene and thus produces ~40% HbS ($\alpha_2\beta_2^{6E \to V}$).

Sickle cell disease: The patient has two copies of the defective gene and produces HbS exclusively.

S/β⁰ thalassemia: The patient is a compound heterozygote with a $\beta^{6E \to V}$-globin and a null β-globin gene resulting in no HbA production.

S/β⁺ thalassemia: The patient is a compound heterozygote with a $\beta^{6E \to V}$-globin and a mildly defective β-globin gene resulting in some HbA production.

HbSC: The patient is a compound heterozygote producing both HbS and HbC($\alpha_2\beta_2^{6E \to K}$, meaning a substitution of glutamic acid by lysine at the 6th position).

Epi—Eight percent of African Americans are carriers of HbS; 2–30% of some West Africans carry HbS or HbC.

P—Deoxygenation causes HbS polymerization and sickling RBCs that become stuck in capillaries, leading to microvascular vaso-occlusion, ischemia, and infarction. The spleen is responsible for hemolysis of the malformed cells but usually autoinfarcts by early childhood in most patients with pure sickle cell disease.

SiSx—Acute vaso-occlusive episodes cause sickle cell disease. Patients can present with acute pain episodes, acute chest syndrome (see below), and fever. So-called *pain crises* may be precipitated by infection, dehydration, or hypoxia. Patients may also present with stroke or priapism. Up to 50% of children <3 years old will develop painful swelling of the hands and feet (dactylitis). Splenomegaly, jaundice, and pallor are manifestations of splenic and hyperhemolytic crises. Patients with S/β⁺-thalassemia have milder symptoms. HbSC patients have fewer features consistent with hemolytic anemia but are more prone to develop aseptic bone necrosis, retinopathy, and complications of pregnancy.

Dx—Clinical features and blood smear lead to suspicion of the condition. Diagnosis is confirmed by hemoglobin electrophoresis. "Fish mouth vertebrae" may be seen on radiographs of the lumbar spine, due to compression of the vertebral endplates.

Tx—Administer hydration, oxygen, and analgesia during the acute crisis. For severe attacks or chest syndrome with respiratory distress, exchange transfusion or simple transfusion may be warranted. Chronic hydroxyurea may decrease the frequency of crises by increasing the amount of HbF. Vaccinate the patient with pneumococcal vaccine to prevent infection.

Complications include chronic hemolytic anemia, parvovirus B19 infection leading to aplastic crisis, high-output cardiac failure, and splenic sequestration of RBCs. Vaso-occlusive complications include pain crises, widespread organ damage [i.e., retinopathy, splenic infarction, GB disease (pigment gallstones), and chronic renal failure], priapism, stroke, avascular necrosis of the femoral head, and acute chest syndrome. Osteomyelitis is classically thought to be due to *Salmonella,* but *Staphylococcus aureus* is actually more common.

Acute Chest Syndrome of Sickle Cell Disease

D—A syndrome commonly seen in sickle cell patients characterized by
1. Presence of a new pulmonary infiltrate in at least one complete lung segment.
2. Chest pain.
3. Temperature >38.5°C.
4. Tachypnea, wheezing, or cough.

Epi—It may occur in up to 50% of sickle cell disease patients. Mortality is high.

RF—Underlying pulmonary infarction and pneumonia are risk factors.

P—The episode begins with sickling within the lung leading to lung dysfunction. The subsequent drop in arterial oxygen saturation may lead to widespread sickling.

SiSx—Symptoms include chest pain, temperature >38.5°C, tachypnea, wheezing, and cough.

Dx—The condition must be distinguished from PE, pneumonia, and MI. Chest X-ray shows the presence of a new pulmonary infiltrate involving at least one complete lung segment (not atelectasis).

Tx—Chronic transfusion lowers the percentage of HbS in patients with sickle cell disease by three mechanisms: (1) dilution;

(2) suppression of erythropoietin release by the rise in hematocrit, thereby reducing the production of new sickle erythrocytes; and (3) a longer circulating life span of normal compared to sickle erythrocytes. Exchange transfusion is necessary. Repeated episodes may lead to pulmonary hypertension and cor pulmonale.

Glucose-6-Phosphate Dehydrogenase (G6PD) Deficiency

D—An episodic hemolytic anemia caused by X-linked recessive deficiency of the G6PD enzyme.

Epi—There are several classes based on the level of enzyme activity, the most common of which are A, A-, and B. Whites have mostly G6PB-B. Most people of African descent have G6PD-A, but 15% have the G6PD-A- allele, where enzyme activity is about 15%. The G6PD Mediterranean allele is more severe.

P—Glucose-6-phosphate dehydrogenase is involved in the disposal of oxygen radicals in RBCs. Mutations cause G6PD to have a shorter half-life. Oxidative stress, from leukocyte products released during infection, drugs (e.g., sulfa drugs like trimethoprim-sulfamethoxazole, dapsone, sulfonamides, quinine, and quinidine), or ingestion of fava beans leads to oxidation of hemoglobin and formation of precipitates seen microscopically as Heinz bodies. Macrophages remove these bodies as RBCs pass through the spleen, which gives rise to bite cells.

SiSx—Patients are usually asymptomatic but can present with an acute, self-limited hemolytic anemia when under RBC oxidative stress, during which jaundice, pallor, tachycardia, and other signs of hemolysis may manifest.

Dx—Between episodes there are no specific findings. During hemolysis there is reticulocytosis, increased LDH, and indirect bilirubin. The blood smear shows RBCs with Heinz bodies and degmacytes (bite cells). A quantitative G6PD enzyme test is diagnostic. The assay should be repeated weeks after a hemolytic episode resolves.

Tx—The episodes are usually self-limited. The patient should avoid the aforementioned drugs. Severe anemia may warrant transfusion.

Methemoglobinemia

D—Condition in which the iron in heme becomes oxidized from Fe^{2+} to Fe^{3+}, forming what is called *methemoglobin* (metHb). In this state, oxygen does not bind to hemoglobin, causing a functional anemia.

P—It usually occurs usually in the setting of any oxidizing stress that overtaxes the NADH-dependent metHb reductase system that removes 99% of the MetHb which the body naturally produces. Abnormal forms of hemoglobin, such as *hemoglobin M* (HbM), cause a predisposition to MetHb.

RF—A number of drugs have been implicated, including local anesthetic agents (e.g., benzocaine, lidocaine, prilocaine), chloroquine, dapsone, nitrates (oxidizing agents), primaquine, quinones, and sulfonamides.

SiSx—Classically, patients are cyanotic out of proportion to their pulse oximetry readings. Skin changes can be seen with at little as 1.5 g of metHb (10%), whereas cyanosis from other causes usually requires 5 g/dL of deoxyhemoglobin. Other symptoms vary, including anxiety, tachycardia, DOE, fatigue, confusion, palpitations, coma, seizure, acidosis, and even death in severe cases.

Dx—In a cyanotic patient, at the bedside one can view a drop of blood on white filter paper. Deoxyhemoglobin will brighten after exposure to atmospheric oxygen, whereas metHb will stay dark. Pulse oximetry is misleading, as it uses absorbance from only two wavelengths of light to distinguish oxyhemoglobin from deoxyhemoglobin. Methemoglobin absorbs both of these wavelengths equally. Even a regular ABG will be misleading, as the pO2 is an extrapolation from the non-hemoglobin-bound oxygen. Therefore, co-oximetry on the ABG specimen is needed. It uses four different wavelengths of light to differentiate metHb, oxyhemoglobin, deoxyhemoglobin, and carboxyhemoglobin. Hemoglobin eletrophoresis should be done if hereditary causes of metHb are suspected.

Tx—Treatment depends on the severity of the deficiency. Any offending medications must clearly be stopped. Supportive care with supplemental oxygen is enough for many patients. Other treatment is needed in sicker patients or those with levels of MetHb >20%. The first-line antidote for methemoglobinemia is methylene blue, provided that there is no history of G6PD deficiency, in which case the response is minimal. Methylene blue facilitates the reduction of methemoglobin (Fe^{+3}) to hemoglobin (Fe^{+2}), provided that NADPH is present. Dextrose is needed for the formation of NADPH and for removal of metHb; it can also be administered along with *N*-acetylcysteine. Vitamin C can be used to reduce chronic metHb, but has no role acutely.

Hereditary Spherocytosis

D—An autosomal dominant disorder of the RBC membrane leading to chronic hemolytic anemia.

P—There is an abnormality of spectrin, which provides the scaffolding for RBC membranes. The surface-to-volume ratio is decreased, resulting in a spherical shape of the RBC as part of the membrane is clipped off while passing through the spleen. Hemolysis occurs because of trapping within the spleen.

SiSx—Hemolysis can cause jaundice; a palpable spleen may be felt. Anemia may or may not be present, as the bone marrow may be able to compensate for increased destruction.

Dx—Reticulocytosis is always present. A blood smear will show spherocytes, but they usually make up only a small percentage of the smear. The mean corpuscular hemoglobin concentration (MCHC) is usually greater than 36g/dL. The Coombs test will be negative. Spherocytes are abnormally vulnerable to swelling with hypotonic media; therefore, an osmotic fragility test can reflect the presence of spherocytes.

Tx—Folate supplementation should be given. Splenectomy is reserved for symptomatic patients, but it will not correct the membrane defect. It will, however, eliminate the site of hemolysis. In mild cases, splenectomy is not necessary.

Microangiopathic Hemolytic Anemia (MAHA)

This condition occurs when there is mechanical shearing of RBCs as they pass through the microvasculature. Blood smear shows schistocytes. This may occur from a variety of conditions and is seen in TTP/HUS, eclampsia, mechanical or prosthetic heart valves, and certain vasculitidies. Thrombotic thrombocytopenic purpura and HUS are discussed below.

Thrombotic Thrombocytopenic Purpura (TTP)

D—A microangiopathic hemolytic anemia characterized by formation of platelet aggregates in the microvasculature that leads to shearing of RBCs and organ dysfunction.

Epi—It is rare as a primary condition (4 in 1 million incidence) and is found more commonly as an acquired condition. The peak incidence is in the fourth decade.

P—Primary and acquired conditions have similar pathophysiology involving dysfunction of the vWF cleaving protease, which normally prevents large vWF aggregation. Dysfunction allows large multimers of vWF to form that the body cannot eliminate, causing overactivation of platelets and clumping in the microvasculature—a process independent of most coagulation factors. Clumping occurs primarily in the small vessels: arterioles and capillaries. Venules are spared. As the platelets partially occlude vessels, RBCs are sheared as they pass through. In the primary or familial form, the vWF cleaving protease activity is deficient; in the acquired form, there are antibodies that neutralize the protease. Other acquired causes are cancer related (usually adenocarcinoma), BMT-associated, drug induced, and HIV or pregnancy-associated.

SiSx—Classically, symptoms consist of the pentad of fever, thrombocytopenia, microangiopathic hemolytic anemia, transient neurologic deficits (change in mental status, headache, aphasia, vision changes seizures and hemiparesis from microinfarcts), and acute renal failure (hematuria/proteinuria). Stigmata of thrombocytopenia may include petechiae and purpura. Bleeding is quite rare, however, and the most worrisome outcomes are from platelet aggregate clotting. On autopsy, lesions are found to have spared no organ, as all of the microvasculature can be involved.

Dx—This is mainly a clinical diagnosis with presenting features and MAHA without any other known cause. Blood smear will show schistocytes (RBCs that have parts of their membrane sheared off), thrombocytopenia, and perhaps nucleated RBCs. Biopsy of the gingiva, skin, or bone marrow has a 30–50% diagnostic yield and may show vascular injury from platelet aggregation. Hemolysis will always be seen (increased indirect bilirubin and elevated LDH). The coombs test and coagulation studies are normal. The PT and aPTT are usually normal but can be elevated.

Tx—Before the advent of plasma exchange [in which the patient's plasma is removed and replaced with fresh frozen plasma (FFP)], survival was 10%; now it is upwards of 80%. Because this is a clinical diagnosis, one should err on the side of immediate plasma exchange. Plasma exchange is useful in primary and acquired conditions since it removes vWF aggregates as well as antibodies. Other therapies include steroids and immunosuppressives, which only have modest benefit and no clear data to support their use alone. When patients are subjected to immediate large-volume exchange, improvement occurs over a few days to 1 week. Splenectomy is considered if symptoms are recurrent or refractory to medical treatment.

Hemolytic-Uremic Syndrome (HUS)

D—A microangiopathic hemolytic anemia very similar to TTP in that it includes thrombocytopenia and more marked renal failure (early) but no neurologic symptoms, as seen with TTP. The pathophysiology is quite different from that of TTP.

Epi—It is more common in young children.

P—There are two types:

1. D+ is usually spread in epidemics, more common in children, and due to ingestion of undercooked hamburgers harboring

verotoxin-producing *Escherichia coli*. The toxin binds to Gb3 receptors on endothelial cells (especially those of the glomeruli), which leads to cell injury, cytokine production, endothelial swelling, endothelial detachment, and thrombosis.

2. D− is sporadic and can be seen in adults; the cause is unknown.

SiSx—The classic triad is fever, MAHA, and renal failure. Acute renal failure is seen in up to 90% and anuria in up to one-third of patients. One can find diarrhea or bleeding of the GI tract; rarely, acute abdominal perforation is seen. It can cause pancreatitis from microinfarction. Acute rhabdomyolysis is also seen. Cardiac symptoms include CHF and arrhythmias. Retinal, choroidal, or vitreous hemorrhage is also observed in patients with HUS or TTP, so all patients should have an eye exam.

Dx—Results of the blood smear and laboratory tests are similar to those of TTP. Renal biopsy or biopsy of GI or skin lesions can also be of use to look for vascular injury. Hemolytic-uremic syndrome is a clinical diagnosis of exclusion. A history of recent GI illness may help make the diagnosis.

Tx—As with TTP, the patient should receive plasma exchange. If the disease is untreated, the mortality rate is about 90%. Adults have a worse prognosis than children. The degree of renal failure and the presence of vascular lesions on biopsy are also poor predictors of survival.

Autoimmune Hemolytic Anemia

D—Condition in which antibodies are directed against RBC membrane polysaccharide antigens, resulting in hemolysis. Classically, there are two types, differentiated on the basis of the two type of antibody involved: cold agglutinins or warm agglutinins. These are distinguished in Table 9-8.

Table 9-8.   Distinguishing Features of Cold and Warm Agglutinin Hemolytic Anemias

	Cold Agglutinin Hemolytic Anemia	Warm Agglutinin Hemolytic Anemia
P	This condition is mostly due to IgM antibodies to polysaccharides on RBCs. The reaction occurs only below core body temperature. Destruction of RBCs is due mainly to direct lysis by complement, as IgM is efficient at activating complement. Therefore, it is more likely to cause intravascular hemolysis (hemoglobinemia, hemoglobinuria, and hemosiderinuria) in cases of widespread hemolysis. Very rarely, it is possible to have IgG or IgA cold agglutinins.	This condition is mostly due to IgG antibodies to proteins on RBCs. The reaction occurs at body temperature. The Rh complex and glycophorin antigen are the most common RBC antigens. Direct lysis by complement is less common but can occur. Lysis more typically occurs with immune-mediated destruction in the spleen. Rarely, IgA or IgM antibodies are seen.
RF	This condition is classically seen in *Mycoplasma* infection and in infectious mononucleosis, usually 2 weeks after disease onset. It is seen with *Listeria* infection and also viral illnesses, including CMV and VZV. Persistent cold agglutinins may be seen in lymphoid malignancies.	Most cases are idiopathic, however this condition can be seen after viral infection (mostly in children), SLE, malignancy-such as CLL, purine analogues, drugs (penicillin, methyldopa) where a haptene reaction occurs (the drug bound to a protein creates a new antigen).
Sx	Signs of hemolysis (jaundice) or severe anemia (i.e., orthostasis, DOE, pallor) or intravascular hemolysis (dark urine). May present with dark purple discoloration on distal parts with cold exposure that disappears with warming. In severe cases, there can be skin ulceration. Splenomegaly can be seen.	Symptoms depends on the degree of hemolysis and range from none to severe symptomatic anemia, jaundice, and splenic enlargement.

continued

Table 9-8. *(Continued)*

	Cold Agglutinin Hemolytic Anemia	Warm Agglutinin Hemolytic Anemia
Dx	Increased LDH, reduced haptoglobin, and elevated indirect bilirubin will be seen. The sample must be kept warm before testing to prevent RBC clumping. A specimen is taken at body temperature until a clot has formed and the serum is removed. In the direct Coombs test (also known as a *type and screen*), RBCs washed and prepared with anti-C3d will clump in the presence of the antibody. The test is negative with anti IgG. Macrocytosis may be seen spuriously on a CBC because of RBC clumping.	Increased LDH, reduced haptoglobin, and elevated indirect bilirubin will be seen. The direct Coombs test is reactive with IgG and C3d.
Tx	Avoid cold and take special precautions (avoid hypothermic surgical procedures, warm IV solutions and blood products, avoid products containing complement). Treatment is cyclophosphamide and other agents such as chlorambucil or the anti-CD-20 antibody, rituxan. Steroids typically are not efficacious unless a rare IgG antibody is present. Plasmapheresis can be used to remove IgM, is short-lived (5 days), and is used for severe disease such as hemolytic disease or in preparation for surgery. Splenectomy is not helpful, as the spleen is not an organ of RBC destruction here. Erythropoietin can be used to augment RBC production.	Usually, if due to a self-limited reaction after a viral infection in children, the condition resolves in several weeks. In adults the condition is more chronic. Treat the underlying disease, if found. Steroids are much more effective than cold IgM and are first-line therapy. Cyclophosphamide or azathioprine are second-line therapy, as are danazol and rituximab. Splenectomy is also effective, as the spleen is an organ of RBC destruction. IVIG is sometimes useful. Transfusion is made difficult until compatibility is achieved in the presence of the autoantibody.

Aplastic Anemia

D—A condition in which there is anemia in the setting of pancytopenia, that is, a decrease in all cell lineages (WBCs, RBCs, and platelets) from hypocellular bone marrow.

P—It is thought to occur from injury or loss of pluripotent hematopoietic stem cells. The bone marrow becomes hypocellular. Causes are idiopathic, drug related (chemotherapy most commonly, also sulfa drugs, phenylbutazone, gold salts, phenytoin, and chloramphenicol), and due to whole-body irradiation, infections (CMV, EBV, HAV and HAC), and Fanconi's anemia, which involves an inherited defect in DNA repair.

SiSx—Neutropenia tends to be of greater consequence than anemia. Patients can present with myriad infections. Thrombocytopenia can present with mucosal hemorrhage and increased menstrual flow in women. People with anemia can be asymptomatic or present with a spectrum of symptoms ranging from fatigue to cardiopulmonary collapse. No splenomegaly is found on exam.

Dx—A CBC will show pancytopenia. If the cause is not obvious and cessation of drug use does not help, then bone marrow biopsy should be done. It will show hypocellularity and aplasticity.

Tx—Discontinue using the offending agent if possible. Early treatment of infection with antibiotics or antifungals is critical in patients who are neutropenic. Supportive transfusions of platelets and RBCs can be done until counts return to normal. Resolution of the infection may reverse the pancytopenia in infectious causes. Antithymocyte globulin and cyclosporine is the treatment for idiopathic aplastic anemia.

Paroxysmal Nocturnal Hemoglobinuria

D—A rare acquired clonal stem cell disorder in which the RBC membrane is prone to lysis by complement.

P—The defect in the *PIG-A* gene causes the absence of two proteins involved in complement: CD59, also known as a protector against membrane attack (complex inhibitory factor), and CD55, known as a decay-accelerating factor. This makes RBCs sensitive to destruction by complement and causes hemolysis. Hemolysis is mediated by complement. There may also be delayed fibrinolysis, which results in a hypercoagulable state.

SiSx—Classically, the first morning urine voided may be reddish-brown, as there is enhanced complement activity at night. There may be progression to aplastic anemia, MDS, or acute myelogenous leukemia (AML). Symptoms of anemia may also be present. Renal failure can occur. Venous thrombosis can occur, with a special predilection for mesenteric and hepatic veins, sometimes resulting in cirrhosis, as thrombosis tends to recur at the same site in organs. Deep vein thrombosis and pulmonary hypertension can also be seen.

Dx—Flow cytometry makes the diagnosis by identifying deficiencies in the CD55 and CD59 proteins. These deficiencies are seen on RBCs, WBCs, and platelets. The blood smear is nondiagnostic but may show macroovalocytes. The LDH is usually elevated. Iron deficiency is usually present.

Tx—Iron replacement may improve the anemia but can also cause transient hemolysis. Allogeneic bone marrow transplantation may be necessary in cases of transformation to AML or MDS. A new anticomplement antibody that binds to C5 and inhibits terminal complement activation is the treatment of choice.

Hemophilia

D—An X-linked hereditary disease of factor deficiency characterized by serious bleeding. There are two types: hemophilia A-factor VIII deficiency and hemophilia B-factor IX deficiency (also known as *Christmas disease*).

Epi—Hemophilia A is more common (1/10,000 births) than hemophilia B (1/30,000 births). Thirty percent of cases arise from new mutations.

P—Both types are X-linked recessive disorders. Internal bleeding may lead to large collections of blood, which puts pressure on adjacent tissues and results in compartment syndromes, pseudophlebitis (venous congestion), and nerve damage (e.g., femoral neuropathy arises from retroperitoneal hematoma). Human immunodeficiency virus and viral hepatitis are common complications of contaminated blood transfusions.

SiSx—Symptoms range from excessive bleeding to minor trauma. Hemarthrosis (bleeding into joints) and intramuscular bleeding are classic findings. Gastrointestinal bleeding is also seen. Over time, a hemophilic arthopathy can occur.

Dx—Order a platelet count, bleeding time, PT, and an activated partial thromboplastin time (aPTT). In hemophiliacs, only the aPTT will be abnormal. In this case, specific assays for factors VIII and IX are required.

Tx—Administer factor VIII or IX concentrate as needed. Recombinant and monoclonally purified factor concentrates are available. In mild hemophilia A, DDAVP may be administered before minor surgical procedures to increase endogenous factor VIII production. Consider an HIV and hepatitis screening and vaccination for patients who received replacement factors in the 1970s and 1980s. Aspirin is contraindicated.

Von Willebrand's Disease (vWD)

D—The most common bleeding disorder, resulting from a deficiency of vWF. There are several different types:

Type I (most common)—autosomal dominant form in which vWD level is decreased.

Type II (rare)—autosomal dominant form in which the vWD level is normal but the protein is dysfunctional.

Type III (rare)—autosomal recessive form in which the vWD level is undectectable.

Type IIN—due to a defect at the factor VIII binding site.

Acquired—due to anti-vWF antibodies, destruction of vWF multimers, or vWF-absorbing tumors (e.g., Wilms' tumor).

Epi—The prevalence is 1/800–1000.

P—Von Willebrand factor is produced by megakaryocytes and endothelial cells. Deficiency or dysfunction prevents the factor from linking platelets after binding to the GP IB receptor to the vascular subendothelium and carrying factor VIII in blood plasma, leading to bruising and bleeding (mucosal) similar to that seen with thombocytopenia.

SiSx—There is easy bruising and mucosal bleeding, including bleeding of the GI tract. More severe symptoms are seen in patients taking aspirin. Type III patients have, in addition, features of mild hemophilia. Type IIN patients have features of mild hemophilia exclusively.

Dx—Patients will have a combination of the following test abnormalities, depending on the specific type of disease: increased bleeding time, decreased factor VIII activity, reduced vWF concentration, and decreased vWF activity as measured by the ristocetin cofactor assay. The assay places platelet-rich plasma mixed with varying concentration of ristocetin in different tubes. Those with certain vWD forms will aggregate at lower than normal concentrations of ristocetin.

Tx—Intervention is necessary during surgery, after major trauma, during prolonged bleeding episodes, and with severe menorrhagia. DDAVP, an analogue of ADH without the vassopressor activity, can increase vWF and factor VIII levels by promoting release from endothelial cell stores and is effective in patients with mild or moderate type I disease. Factor VIII concentrate, which harbors vWF, or Humate-P (human vWF complex), is given to patients with type I, II, or III disease. The dose depends on the degree of bleeding.

Idiopathic Thrombocytopenic Purpura (ITP)

D—An acquired condition of thrombocytopenia due to autoantibodies against platelets, targeting them for destruction in the spleen. There are two types: chronic (adult form) and acute (usually pediatric). The disease is also called immune thrombocytopenic purpura.

RF—Chronic ITP may be associated with non-Hodgkin's lymphoma, Hodgkin's disease, chronic lymphocytic leukemia (CLL), HIV, lupus, and rheumatoid arthritis. Viral illness may precede the acute form.

P—It involves formation of anti-IIb-IIIa receptor or Ib-IX receptor IgG, which leads to platelet destruction after splenic sequestration. It may be precipitated by viral infections in children and occurs acutely. In adults, the condition is chronic.

SiSx—The disease has a variable presentation but is usually due to complications of thrombocytopenia. Bleeding of mucous membranes, petechiae, ecchymoses, easy bruising, epistaxis, gingival bleeding, menorrhagia. Gastrointestinal bleeding, and hematuria are uncommon, as is intracerebral hemorrhage, though this can be seen in older patients. There is no splenomegaly.

Dx—There are two diagnostic criteria:

1. Isolated thrombocytopenia with normal blood counts.
2. No other causes found for thrombocytopenia (diagnosis of exclusion) or intercurrent illness.

No standard test is available, and the diagnosis is made by exclusion. Low platelet counts but no anemia may be seen on CBC. A blood smear shows megathrombocytes and no schistocytes. The antiplatelet antibody test is not informative.

Tx—Acute ITP in children resolves spontaneously within 6 months. If the thrombocytopenia is severe, corticosteroids may be administered and tapered over 6 weeks. Platelet transfusions may be necessary for ITP patients only when there is mucosal bleeding. Usually transfusion is considered when the platelet count is <30,000 or if there is significant bleeding. Note that transfusions do not increase the platelet count in most cases. Corticosteroid treatment will produce remission of the disease and is the mainstay of therapy, but two thirds of patients will relapse if maintenance therapy is discontinued. Intravenous immune globulin also increases the platelet count within several days to weeks. Anti-D immunoglobulin (WinRho) can be used in RH-positive patients, minimizing the removal of antibody-coated platelets. Consider splenectomy (as second-line therapy) if thrombocytopenia is refractory to steroids. Rituxamab, danazol, cyclosporine, and azathioprine are used in relapsed/refracted patients.

Diseases of Hypercoagulability

Antiphospholipid Antibody Syndrome (APS)

D—A condition of arterial and venous thrombosis in which antibodies are made to various plasma proteins that bind to phospholipids and affect the clotting cascade. It can be a primary or secondary condition when it occurs together with SLE, other rheumatic conditions, infection, or drug-related conditions. Patients with *Sneddon's syndrome*, a condition involving livedo reticularis and multiple ischemic strokes, also have a large number of such antibodies.

Epi—Half of the patients have primary APS. It is estimated that up to one-third of SLE patients have APS.

P—The exact mechanism by which these autoantibodies lead to a hypercoagulable state is unclear. Some suggest that antibodies may interfere with coagulation homeostasis or lead ultimately to a T-cell immune response to serum phospholipid-binding proteins. The antibodies may be against epitopes on proteins uncovered after they bind phospholipids interfering with their action. Other antibodies are directed against specific phospholipids. The most common antibodies seen are anticardiolipin (ACL), anti-$\beta2$ glycoprotein I, the lupus anticoagulant, and the antiprothrombin antibody.

SiSx—The disease usually presents with venous (more common) or arterial thrombosis and its sequelae: DVTs, PEs, CVAs, nonhealing ulcers, livedo reticularis, digit ulceration, thrombocytopenia, and, classically, multiple miscarriages in young women. Multi-infarct dementia, stroke, and retinal artery occlusion may be seen. Other sequelae include migraine headaches, valvular heart disease, adrenal insufficiency, pulmonary hypertension, avascular necrosis, and Raynaud's phenomenon. Multiorgan failure can be seen in severe cases with multiple vessel occlusions (catastrophic antiphospholipid syndrome). On occasion, patients may develop Libmann-Sacks endocarditis (aseptic valve vegetations). Thrombocytopenia may also be seen.

In patients who present with bleeding, there may be antibodies to prothrombin. Those with SLE and lupus anticoagulant activity are at increased risk of arterial thrombosis.

Dx—Any one of the following tests for autoantibodies or combinations thereof may be positive: anticardiolipin antibodies, the Venereal Disease Research Laboratory (VDRL) test, and the lupus anticoagulant. However, detection of these antibodies alone in the serum does not necessarily make the diagnosis, as up to 2% of normal people have detectable antibodies. Hence, use of the Sapporo criteria include both clinical and laboratory data. One needs both a clinical condition and laboratory test findings to make the diagnosis:

Clinical: One or more vascular thromboses in any tissue or organ confirmed by pathology findings.

One or more unexplained miscarriages.

Lab: Presence of ACL antibody, either IgG or IgM, on two or more occasions.

Presence of the lupus anticoagulant on two or more occasions.

Inability to correct a prolonged screening test by mixing with normal platelet-poor plasma.

The paradoxically prolonged aPTT seen in these patients is an artifact of coagulation assays. There are several ways to test for the lupus anticoagulant, which causes an otherwise unexplained prolongation of the aPTT that is not reversed when the patient's plasma is diluted 1:1 with normal platelet-free plasma. Tests using Russell viper venom time (RVVT) can be done in patients using warfarin, as Russell viper venom is a factor X activator that activates the clotting cascade using a heparin- and warfarin-independent mechanisms. Patients with a lupus anticoagulant will still have prolonged clotting times.

Tx—Administer aspirin, and anticoagulate with heparin and then warfarin. Lifelong anticoagulation is necessary. Steroids and cytotoxic drugs have no proven benefit, though hydroxychloroquine may provide some protection from thrombosis in secondary causes of APS. Avoidance of other procoagulant factors such as OCPs is important as well.

Disseminated Intravascular Coagulation (DIC)

D—A serious systemic disorder characterized by pathologic consumptive coagulation that leads to widespread thrombosis as well as bleeding and ultimately to multiorgan failure. It can be either acute or chronic.

P—It usually occurs as a complication of an underlying illness. Causes include sepsis, transfusion reaction, trauma (burns or head injury), neoplasia, and obstetric complications. Sequelae result from overproduction of thrombin and plasmin. The opposing effects of these two proteases result in both thrombosis and bleeding in different areas of the body. Without early intervention, the condition leads to systemic collapse, shock, ARDS, or death. Two types are described:

Acute DIC—from exposure to large amounts of tissue factor at once, such that generation of thrombin overwhelms control mechanisms to prevent coagulation. Fibrin deposition can occur everywhere, causing ischemic tissue injury and microangiopathic hemolytic anemia.

Chronic DIC—usually due to continuous or intermittent exposure to small amounts of tissue factor such that the liver and bone marrow are able to partially replenish depleted products. The most common cause is malignancy, especially solid tumors more so than liquid tumors.

RF—Risk factors include infection, trauma, and malignancy [patients with acute promyelocytic leukemia (APML), a type of AML, are especially prone to this condition].

SiSx—Acute DIC usually presents with bleeding, classically from venipuncture sites or incisional wounds. Acute renal failure is quite common (2–40%), as is liver failure, respiratory failure, shock, and thromboembolic events. Central nervous system bleeding, GI tract bleeding, and digital gangrene can also be seen. Jaundice may result from hemolysis and hepatocellular injury. Chronic DIC may be asymptomatic or present with bleeding or thromboembolism.

Dx—Diagnosis is based on clinical information and laboratory test results. In acute DIC there is usually an obvious precipitant, but the key is evidence of thrombin generation and fibrinolysis: decreased fibrinogen, elevated fibrinogen degradation products (FDPs), and elevated d-dimer levels are seen. With consumption of coagulation factors there is an elevation of PT and aPTT, usually with thrombocytopenia. The blood smear may show microangiopathic anemia. In chronic DIC, the aPTT and PT may be within normal limits because of compensation. In such cases, the blood smear will show evidence of microangiopathic anemia, and there will be increased FDP and d-dimer and decreased fibrinogen.

Tx—Treat the underlying disorder and complications [e.g., IV antibiotics and IV fluids for shock or infection, mechanical ventilation for ARDS, all-trans-retinoic acid (ATRA) for APML (see Chapter 10), and so forth]. Transfusion of platelets is necessary for marked thrombocytopenia or for patients with bleeding, though the response to transfusion may not be marked. Cryoprecipitate is given to replenish fibrinogen, usually to a level >100 mg/dL. Fresh frozen plasma is give if INR is elevated (usually if it is above 1.5) to replace coagulation factors. There is no role for heparin per se except in patients with chronic or low-grade DIC who have mainly thrombotic manifestations.

Inherited Prothrombotic Disorders

This group of disorders is characterized predominantly by venous thrombosis, arising from autosomal dominant genetic defects in the innate anticoagulation systems.

Factor V Leiden/Activated Protein C (APC) Resistance

D—Hypercoagulable state wherein factor V cannot be cleaved by protein C, resulting in venous thromboembolic.

RF—The condition is worse in patients who are taking OCPs or hormone replacement therapy or who are pregnant.

Epi—It is the most common cause of inherited thrombophilia, accounting for 40–50% of cases in patients with a secondary cause. The carrier frequency is up to 5% in whites, and the rate of homozygotes is 1%. Patients also carry an increased risk of developing another inherited thrombophilic disorder.

P—The most common mutation is an R504Q substitution that renders factor V impervious to activated protein C cleavage, thus inhibiting the common pathway. Patients can develop APC resistance by other mechanisms, but this is the most common.

SiSx—Patients present primarily with venous thromboses, usually in the lower extremities. There is an increased risk of cerebral vein thrombosis, and it may play a role in some cases of recurrent miscarriage from presumptive thrombosis of placental vessels.

Dx—The screening test is the aPTT, which will be prolonged with APC resistance. Patients should then be genotyped for the mutation.

Tx—Anticoagulation should be used as appropriate. This condition in itself does not merit lifelong anticoagulation unless patients fulfill the criteria based on other considerations. There is no evidence that heterozygosity for factor V Leiden increases mortality. During high-risk periods, anticoagulation may also be appropriate.

Prothrombin (Factor II) Mutation

D—An autosomal dominant condition leading to increased prothrombin levels and, in some cases, a hypercoagulable state.

Epi—It is the second most common cause of inherited thrombophilia. Two percent of whites are heterozygous for the mutation. The highest prevalence is seen in Spain, where up to 6% of the population are heterozygotes. It carries a two to three times increased risk of developing a DVT.

P—The most common mutation is G20210A, which is thought to cause slower mRNA degradation and increased circulating prothrombin levels.

SiSx—Venous thromboembolism is the most common presentation. The reason for the increased predilection for arterial thromboses (i.e., stroke and MI) is still unclear. Heterozygotes have an increased risk of DVT. There is also increased risk of cerebral vein

thrombosis and perhaps arterial thrombosis in younger patients.

Dx—Use PCR methods to detect the G20210A mutation. This is usually a standard part of a hypercoagulable state work-up.

Tx—There is no data regarding lifelong anticoagulation in these patients. Those with multiple thrombotic episodes should be considered for it; otherwise, patients are treated with anticoagulation for any thromboembolic episodes.

Protein C Deficiency

D—Condition in which the naturally occurring anticoagulant, protein C, is deficient, resulting in an increased risk of thromboses.

Epi—It is rare, with a gene frequency of 1/200–500. Not all patients are symptomatic.

P—Protein C is a vitamin K–dependent protein made in the liver that is activated from its zymogen into activated protein C by thrombin or thrombomodulin. It inactivates factor Va and factor VIIIa, which are needed for factor X activation. Its activity is enhanced by protein S. More than 160 genetic defects have been identified. Either enzyme activity is decreased (type I mutations) or there are normal levels with decreased function (type II mutations). Acquired causes include severe infection and septic shock, liver disease, DIC, and ARDS or medication-related conditions such as chemotherapy. Inheritance is autosomal dominant in primary disease.

SiSx—Patients present with venous thrombosis, usually at an early age. Pregnancy or OCP use may also precipitate a thromboembolic event. There are no clear data on the increased risk of arterial thromboses.

Three main presentations are seen:

1. Venous thromboembolism in heterozygous or homozygous individuals. Seventy percent of the time it is spontaneous, with no obvious risk factors.
2. Neonatal purpura fulminans in homozygous newborns, occurring on the first day of life.
3. Warfarin-induced skin necrosis in adults, can occur after several days in association with large loading doses of warfarin without

the initial use of heparin. It usually occurs in areas of where there is significant subcutaneous fat from localized hypercoagulability. The most accepted etiology is that warfarin initially also decreases the vitamin K dependent factor protein C (which is anti-coagulative) leading to a transient hypercoagulable state. Others postulate the mechanism is a direct toxic effect of warfarin or a drug hypersensitivity related event.

Dx—Given the aforementioned presentation and a strong family history, assays for ATIII, proteins C and S, and factor V Leiden should be conducted on patients with unexpected venous thrombosis. Functional, immunologic, and DNA-based tests for protein C are available.

Tx—All patients should receive standard heparin followed by a course of warfarin for several months, as with any thromboembolic event. If skin necrosis develops, one must immediately stop warfarin therapy and give vitamin K and heparin, even though lesions may continue to progress. Patients can be started on warfarin only after they have been safely anticoagulated first with heparin for several days. Protein C can be given to patients with suspected or documented primary protein C deficiency.

Protein S Deficiency

D—An inherited or acquired condition in which the vitamin K–dependent anticoagulation factor protein S is deficient.

P—Protein S, named after its discovery in the city of Seattle, serves as a cofactor for protein C. It is made in both hepatocytes and megakaryocytes. From 40% to 50% circulates as free protein (acting as a cofactor) and the rest is bound to C4b-BP, a complement-binding protein. As with other factors, mutations have been identified in which the protein is decreased either in amount (type I) or in activity (type II). Causes can be primary or acquired, such as pregnancy and OCP use, DIC, acute thromboembolism, HIV infection, nephrotic syndrome, liver disease, and chemotherapy with l-asparaginase.

SiSx—Like ATIII and protein C deficiency, protein S deficiency usually manifests as venous thrombosis. There are little data to support this condition as a separate risk factor for arterial thrombosis.

Dx—Assays are readily available to measure total and free protein S and protein S function. It is important to do these tests while the patient is off warfarin. Being on heparin does not affect the tests.

Tx—Anticoagulation is needed for specific venous thrombosis. Lifelong anticoagulation for protein S deficiency alone is not indicated unless the patient fulfills the usual criteria for it.

Antithrombin III (ATIII) Deficiency

D—Deficiency of the major inhibitor of thrombin, antithrombin (AT), leading to thrombosis.

Epi—It is less common than factor V Leiden or protein C mutations. The most common variant can be found in 1/2000 individuals. The condition is thought to account for 1% of all thrombotic events.

P—Antithrombin III is an important serine protease inhibitor made by the liver that acts as a physiologic inhibitor of coagulation. Antithrombin normally inactivates thrombin, and in the presence of heparin does so at a faster rate. As with the other factors, there are two types of deficiency: reduced synthesis of normal AT (type I) or normal AT levels but reduced functional activity (type II).

RF—Acquired conditions include ARDS, eclampsia, liver disease, nephrotic syndrome (ATIII is lost in urine), drug-induced conditions (use of heparin, OCPs), and hepatic veno-occlusive disease.

SiSx—Severe thrombotic diseases such as DVT and PEs may be seen. Involvement of other vessels, such as the IVC, renal veins, and brachial or axillary veins, is not uncommon. Cerebral sinus or arterial thrombosis may also be seen. Sixty percent of patients develop recurrent thrombotic episodes. Forty percent have evidence of PE.

Dx—As part of the hypercoagulable work-up, immunoassays are used to detect the amount of AT and functional assays are used to detect its activity. Specimen collection should be avoided when the patient is on heparin or during an acute illness.

Tx—When heparin does not achieve a therapeutic response, an AT concentrate may be needed, especially in the setting of a surgical procedure. Otherwise, lifelong anticoagulation in patients with even one episode of DVT is necessary, especially in those with thromboses at atypical sites, such as mesenteric vessels.

Heparin-Induced Thrombocytopenia (HIT)

D—Condition in which administration of heparin not only causes a decrease in platelet level (<150,000/μL or a 50% decrease in patients with preexisting thrombocytopenia) but also may lead to life-threatening thrombosis. Two types exist, type I and type II, with the latter being the more serious and of clinical consequence.

Epi—It occurs in up to 1–5% of all patients placed on heparin.

P—The two types are distinguished in Table 9-9.

RF—The risk factor is exposure to heparin, even in quite small quantities, as subcutaneous heparin or in IV flushes.

SiSx—Type I is asymptomatic. Presenting symptoms of type II HIT can be thrombotic events that are both venous and arterial: MI, DVT, PEs, limb ischemia, renal failure (from renal artery thrombosis), and mesenteric ischemia. Skin necrosis in fat-rich areas may be seen. Adrenal hemorrhage has been reported. Type II rarely produces symptoms after 2 weeks on heparin.

Dx—The key is to recognize the clinical syndrome in the appropriate context: a drop in platelet levels in a patient with recent or current exposure to heparin with an associated thrombosis or hypercoagulable state, excluding other causes of thrombocytopenia. Diagnosis is made by either of three tests:

1. Serotonin release assay (the gold standard): Normal platelets are labeled with 14C-serotonin and washed. The patient's serum is added with a different heparin concentration. 14C-Serotonin is released with a supratherapeutic concentration of heparin, but if this occurs with a therapeutic concentration, the test is positive. This test has high sensitivity.
2. An ELISA specific for the heparin-platelet factor 4 complex can detect and quantify the amount of antibodies made, which can be followed over time.
3. The platelet aggregation test: washed normal platelets are added to the patient's serum with varying concentrations of heparin and the degree platelet aggregation is measured compared to that of a control. This test is specific but not as sensitive as the serotonin release assay.

Tx

Type I—no treatment is needed. There is no risk of thrombosis. Heparin can be discontinued, and counts should return to normal within a few days.

Table 9-9. Distinguishing Feature of Type I and Type 2 HIT

Type	Type I	Type II
Mechanism	Due to heparin-mediated platelet activation	Due to formation of antibodies to the heparin-platelet factor 4 (PF4) complex.
Time Course	Occurs 1–2 days after administration	Occurs 3–10 days after first-time administration, but may even occur within 12 hours in patients with preformed antibodies from previous exposure.
Platelet Count	Platelet level usually >100,000.	Platelet level rarely <20,000; usually around 60,000.
Comments	There is usually no clinical significance.	Life-threatening thrombosis since the heparin-PF4 complex leads to platelet activation and subsequent further PF4 complex formations, causing platelets to aggregate and form thromboses through as yet unclear mechanisms. These platelet aggregates are removed from the circulation and therefore leads to thrombocytopenia.
		Variants include *delayed-onset HIT*, which can occur up to 2 weeks after heparin is discontinued, as it takes longer to form the antibodies in some patients.

Type II—Treatment involves immediate discontinuation of heparin in all suspicious cases, including any flushes of lines. Use of another anticoagulant is mandatory, as the risk of thrombosis is 40–50% in the next 30 days. Alternative anticoagulants until diagnostic study results are positive or negative are:

1. Hirudin, a direct thrombin inhibitor, or lepirudin, a form of recombinant hirudin.
2. Argatroban, another direct thrombin inhibitor, is smaller than hirudin and interacts only with the active site of thrombin. It has a short half-life (24 minutes) and reaches a steady state in 3 hours. The aPTT is used to monitor its effects.
3. Danaparoid (dermatan sulfate and low-sulfated heparin sulfate), which is not approved by the Food and Drug Administration and has 10% cross-reactivity with the antibody causing HIT. One must measure antifactor Xa levels to monitor its effect.

Warfarin should also be avoided until the platelet count is over 100,000, since it can induce skin necrosis or worsen thromboembolism that has occurred due to its initial hypercoagulable effects.

For prevention, use of low molecular weight heparin (LMWH) is associated with a much lower incidence of HIT than unfractionated heparin and should be preferred in patients needing anticoagulation when possible. Starting warfarin earlier will also decrease exposure to heparin.

Myeloproliferative Disorders (MPD)

These are conditions caused by the clonal proliferation of a myeloid stem cell with overproduction of mature myeloid cell lines. These diseases have the potential to transform into acute leukemia.

Polycythemia Vera

D—Characterized by a marked increase in the production of RBCs, platelets, and sometimes WBCs (in two-thirds of patients).
P—A clonal proliferation may be due to an aberrant signal transduction pathway in myeloid stem cells. Cells may proliferate without erythropoietin; in fact, serum erythropoietin is decreased because of negative feedback. The disease represents an absolute erythrocytosis or a true increase in RBC mass as opposed to a relative one from decreased plasma volume. JAK-2 mutations occur in 95% of patients.
RF—People >60 years old are at risk. Men are more commonly affected than women.
SiSx—Symptoms include pruritis, typically after a warm bath (classically), tinnitus, blurred vision, headache and epistaxis. Signs of vascular sludging include stroke, angina, and claudication. Plethora (hypervolemia), large retinal veins on fundoscopy, and splenomegaly are also seen.
Dx—New World Health Organization (WHO) criteria are as follows:

Major criteria

(1) Hemoglobin >18.5 g/dL in men and >16.5 g/dL in women
or
(2) Hemoglobin or hematocrit level > 99th percentile
or
(3) Hemoglobin > 17 g/dL in men or > 15 g/dL in women or an increase of ≥2 g/dL from baseline
or
(4) Elevated red cell mass greater > 25% above mean normal value
(5) Presence of JAK2 mutation

Minor criteria

(1) Bone marrow trilineage myeloproliferation
(2) Low erythropoietin levels
(3) Endogenous erythroid colony growth
One needs two major and one minor or the first major criterion plus any two minor criteria.
Tx—Patients should be subjected to serial phlebotomy. Myelosuppressive agents such as hydroxyurea may be helpful. Patients should also be put on daily aspirin. Five percent of patients progress to leukemia and 20% to myelofibrosis.

Essential Thrombocytosis (ET)

D—Characterized by a persistent thrombocytosis (platelets >600,000/μL) that is neither reactive to another disease entity nor part of another myeloproliferative disorder.

Epi—The incidence is 1.5/100,000. The median age of occurrence is 60 years. Female patients slightly outnumber males.

P—The cause is unclear, but somehow proliferation of megakaryocytes in the bone marrow occurs.

SiSx—The most common presentation is with thrombosis. Less commonly, asymptomatic thrombocytosis is found on routine laboratory tests. Vasomotor symptoms, such as headache, erythromelalgia (burning pain and erythema of hands), paresthesia of the digits, and visual defects, may be seen. Thrombosis can occur in strange sites such as the mesenteric, hepatic, or portal veins. Hemorrhagic events may also be frequent. Splenomegaly is found in one-third of patients on physical exam. Bleeding occurs, is usually mucosal, and is caused by a qualitative platelet defect.

Dx—The platelet count is elevated, usually to over 2 million per microliter. The WBC count is also elevated, but usually not >30,000 per microliter. The hematocrit is usually normal. The blood smear shows enlarged platelets. The bleeding time is prolonged in 20% of patients. One must rule out secondary causes of thrombocytosis such as iron deficiency, inflammatory disease, and malignancy. Tests for ferritin and CRP and a blood smear may be helpful to this end. Bone marrow biopsy and cytogenetic studies will help distinguish ET from CML. The RBC mass is normal, and there is no Ph chromosome. JAK-2 mutations are positive in 40–60% of patients.

Tx—Aspirin is usually sufficient to alleviate vasomotor symptoms. In patients who have had a thrombosis or are >60 years old, hydroxyurea may be required; the potential leukemogenicity of the drug has yet to be determined. Patients are expected to have a normal life span, with <5% progressing to either leukemia or myelofibrosis. Alpha interferon may also control the platelet count. If there is severe bleeding, the platelet count should be lowered emergently with platelet pheresis. Usually an indolent course allows for long-term survival. Thrombosis is the major source of morbidity. There is a 5% risk of transformation to acute leukemia over 20 years.

Agnogenic Myeloid Metaplasia and Myelofibrosis

D—A syndrome in which clonal proliferation of an unknown cell type leads to ineffective hematopoiesis, fibrosis of the bone marrow, and extramedullary hematopoiesis (liver, spleen, and lymph nodes) with marked splenomegaly.

Epi—The incidence is 0.5/100,000. The median age of occurrence is 60–70 years.

P—A multipotent hematopoietic cell gives rise to a clonal population of megakaryocytes, which secrete transforming growth factor-β (TGF-β). Fibroblasts respond by secreting collagen. Fibrosis may occur in response to cytokine secretion.

SiSx—Usually this is an insidious process. Patients may present with anemia; a feeling of fullness is due to splenomegaly or massive hepatomegaly in most cases. Splenomegaly can cause portal hypertension, a hypercatabolic state, and mechanical discomfort. Later, anemia can become severe, and further thrombocytopenia can lead to bleeding. Splenic infarction can also occur. Transverse myelitis, from myelopoiesis in the epidural space, can also occur.

Dx—The blood smear is dramatic and shows poikilocytosis and many teardrop forms. Nucleated RBCs are present. The triad of teardrop poikilocytosis, leukoerythoblastic blood, and giant abnormal platelets is highly suggestive of myelofibrosis. The bone marrow usually cannot be aspirated ("a dry tap"), and early in the course of the disease there is hypercellularity with an increased population of megakaryocytes. Marrow fibrosis is demonstrated with a silver stain. Nucleated RBCs, tear drop cells, and immature granulocytes may also be seen. The diagnosis is confirmed by bone marrow biopsy. Other myeloid, lymphoid, and nonhematologic disorders that cause myelofibrosis also need to be ruled out.

Cytogenetic analysis may be helpful. One-third of patients with agnogenic myeloid metaplasia have del(13q) and del(20q). The JAK-2 mutation is seen in 50% of patients.

Tx—Except for allogeneic bone marrow transplantation, treatment is palliative. Such treatment for anemia may include use of androgen and corticosteroids which have been shown to decrease transfusion requirements. Erythropoietin may also be used, and splenectomy may need to be performed in transfusion-dependent patients. Patients have 5 year median survival. In some patients, the disease may convert to (AML).

Transfusion Medicine

Blood Products

Blood products must be separated, as they need to be stored at different temperatures for optimal use and because, if left alone, products will interact with one another. Table 9-10 describes the uses of common blood products.

Adverse reactions to transfused blood components can be of several types, as shown in Table 9-11.

Transfusion-Related Acute Lung Injury (TRALI)

D—A complication of transfusion that results in an ARDS-type presentation. It is also called *pulmonary leukoagglutinin reaction.*

Epi—It is seen in 2–4 in 1000 units of blood given and is a leading cause of transfusion-associated fatalities in the United States.

P—It is thought to be caused by antigranulocyte antibodies either from the donor (90% of cases) or from the recipient. Most such donors are multiparous women who became sensitized to fetal antigens during pregnancy. Recipient antibodies usually result from prior transfusions or pregnancies. The severity of symptoms is unrelated to the source of the antibodies. There appear to be sequential insults that prime neutrophils and activate endothelial cells.

Table 9-10. Uses of Blood-Derived Products

Product	Storage	Indications for Using Transfusing	Comments
Packed RBCs	Stored at 4°C for up to 42 days.	Massive symptomatic blood loss. To increase oxygenation in certain conditions, such as in patients with active or imminent cardiac ischemia. In general keep >7 g/dL in most ICU patients although there are no hard and fast rules for many other patients in which case treat based on symptoms, especially those with chronically low hemoglobin (i.e., sickle cell patients).	One unit should increase the hemoglobin by 1 g/dL or the Hct by 3%. It may take a full 24 hours for the body to re-equilibrate fluid shifts. Note that each RBC also contains a small number of WBCs, trapped plasma proteins, and added preservative, usually citrate, which during a large transfusion can chelate calcium. Some centers leukocyte deplete the RBCs to further prevent allergic reactions.
Whole Blood	Not typically stored.	When a massive transfusion is needed with acute blood loss.	Rarely used today. Resuscitation is commonly done with normal saline or lactate Ringer's solution and then packed RBCs.

continued

Table 9-10. *(continued)*

Product	Storage	Indications for Using Transfusing	Comments
Platelets	Stored at –18°C. Useful up for up to 5 days	Given in the following conditions: Bleeding patients with platelet count <50,000/μL. Preoperatively if <50,000/μL or <100,000/μL in certain neurosurgical procedures. Platelets <10,000/μL in all patients to prevent intracerebral hemorrhage from spontaneous bleeding.	A 6-pack should increase the platelet level by 60,000/μL. Patients who do not respond may have preformed antibodies that can be tested for. Acutely thrombocytopenic patients can bleed spontaneously even if serum platelet levels are >50,000/μL, since platelets may be old, making them less functional. Those with ITP can do quite well with surprising low platelet levels. Those with uremic platelets can be given DDAVP or fresh frozen plasma prior to a procedure. Some centers leukocyte deplete the platelets to further prevent allergic reactions. Do not give in patients with HIT, HELLP, or TTP.
Fresh Frozen Plasma	Stored at –18°C. Useful for up to 1 year.	Given with massive transfusion as coagulation factors are diluted out. Given for elevated INRs preprocedurally to prevent bleeding or to reverse warfarin. Also may be given in factor deficiency, DIC, or TTP.	A transient correction of coagulopathy that lasts for only 2–4 hours.
WBCs	—	Used rarely in patients with neutropenia, usually from chemotherapy with overwhelming infections.	No good data on its utility. WBCs also have a very short half-life. Antibiotics, G-CSF, and GM-CSF are used in most of these situations instead.
Cryoprecipitate	Stored at –18°C. Useful for up to 1 year.	For bleeding in vWD, in factor XIII deficiency, and to replace fibrinogen in DIC (usually when <100 mg/dL).	Contains factor VIII, fibrinogen, vWF, and factor XIII. Made by letting FFP thaw at 4°C. These cold-insoluble proteins separate out from the rest first. Usually 10–15 cc for each unit.
Cryoprecipitate-poor Plasma	Stored at –18°C. Useful for up to 1 year.	For infusion or plasma exchange in TTP-HUS. Also used for bleeding due to warfarin or vitamin K deficiency.	Can be used to manufacture albumin or globulin.

Table 9-11.   Adverse Transfusion Reactions

Reaction Type	Cause	Sx	Dx	Tx
Acute Hemolytic	Due to ABO incompatibility and destruction of donor cells by preformed recipient antibodies.	Fever, nausea, vomiting, wheezing, dyspnea, flank and back pain, pink or red urine (from hemoglobinuria). Major sequelae include shock, DIC, and acute renal failure.	Confirm blood type match of donor and recipient. Obtain a sample of blood for direct antiglobulin Coombs test and plasma free hemoglobin. Check urine for hemoglobin.	Stop the transfusion immediately. Maintain intravascular volume with IV fluids. For renal protection, also give diuretics or mannitol to keep urinary output > 100 mL/hr. Adding sodium bicarbonate to IV fluids for alkalinization of urine may facilitate excretion of hemoglobin. Monitor electrolytes for hyperkalemia.
Febrile Nonhemolytic	From cytokines such as IL-1, IL-6, IL-8 and TNFα that have accumulated in the blood components and are released after an interaction between donor leukocytes and recipient antibodies.	Occurs 1–6 hours after transfusion of RBCc or platelets. Headache, chills, fevers, and mild dyspnea.	A clinical diagnosis. One must distinguish it from a hemolytic process by looking for hemoglobinemia and hemoglobinuria.	Usually quite benign. Treatment requires antipyretics and supportive measures only. Less than 15% of patients suffer recurrence in subsequent transfusions. Can be minimized, however, with leuko reduced RBCs or platelets.
Allergic	Host IgE recognizes donor plasma antigen.	Urticaria, pruritis. IgA-deficient patients may have anaphylactic reactions with wheezing, swelling, and SOB.	Usually a clinical diagnosis.	Treatment depends on the severity. Stop the transfusion. In severe cases, protect the airway, use IV epinephrine, give IV fluids and pressors if needed, and maintain the airway.
Bacterial Sepsis	Contamination of donor blood by a bacterial pathogen.	Chills, rigors, and vomiting.	Obtain Gram stain or culture of noninfused blood.	Halt transfusion at first suspicion of bacterial sepsis and administer broad-spectrum antibiotics.
Delayed Hemolytic Transfusion Reaction	From an anamnestic antibody response due to reexposure of an antigen encountered from a prior transfusion. It is usually due to an Rh or Kidd type antigen.	Occurs 2–10 days after transfusion; hemolysis is seen. Less severe than with an acute reaction. Slight fever.	Elevated bilirubin, evidence of hemolysis. Positive direct Coombs test and antibody screen in blood bank.	No treatment is needed unless hemolysis is severe. It is necessary to document this reaction in the event of future transfusions.

RF—Risk factors include the number of transfusions and the age of transfused blood products.

SiSx—Patients may experience a sudden onset of respiratory distress after the transfusion of blood products, as well as fever, tachycardia, and hypoxemia sometimes requiring mechanical ventilation. Resolution occurs rapidly, usually in 24 hours.

Dx—This is a clinical diagnosis. In the appropriate clinical setting, the finding of granulocyte leukoagglutinating or lymphocytotoxic antibody in the serum from a donor or recipient is strong evidence. A decrease in complement C3 or C5 levels 12–36 hours after onset with a rise in C3 or C5 thereafter is also evidence. The sensitivity and specificity of these tests are unclear.

Tx—Treatment is supportive. Clinical improvement should occur spontaneously as the lung injury resolves. Usually the patient needs mechanical ventilation for several days. Diuretics may be used in fluid overload. Intravenous steroids may be beneficial, but the evidence is still anecdotal. Subsequent transfusions should not be from the same donor.

Chapter 9 Appendix: Common Laboratory Tests

Tests Related to Anemia

Ferritin—the iron-binding protein for storage in cells. Although it never transports iron in the bloodstream, a small amount does exist in the serum in proportion to its cellular concentration. Hemosiderin is a denatured aggregate of ferritin molecules in crystal form, which hold even more iron. Ferritin is an acute phase reactant, so it can be falsely elevated in the setting of acute inflammation. Iron deficiency, however, is unlikely to be present with a ferritin level of >100 ng/mL even in the setting of inflammation.

Total iron binding capacity (TIBC)—estimate of serum transferrin, the iron transport protein in the blood (free iron is toxic).

Percent transferrin saturation—calculated by dividing the serum iron level by the TIBC and multiplying by 100. When the value is above 80%, iron accumulates in other tissues.

Tests Related to the Coagulation System

Prothrombin time (PT)—depends on the concentrations of factors of the extrinsic and common pathways (II, VII, IX, X, and I). Isolated PT prolongation suggests liver disease, warfarin anticoagulation, or vitamin K deficiency.

INR (international normalized ratio)—a way to normalize the sensitivity of the thromboplastin used in the test to eliminate causes of variation between different tests.

Activated partial thromboplastin time (aPTT or PTT)—depends on concentrations of factors of the intrinsic and common pathways (VIII, IX, XI, XII, I, II, V, X, PK, and HMWK). An isolated prolonged aPTT suggests vWD, hemophilia, or heparin anticoagulation.

Fibrinogen—decreased in DIC, severe liver disease, with thrombolytic agent therapies, and in congenital conditions.

Less Commonly Used Tests

Thrombin time—used to monitor fibrinolytic therapy, detect heparin resistance, and diagnose hereditary fibrinogen deficiencies.

Reptilase time—used to detect FDP even in the setting of anticoagulation because it is not greatly affected by anticoagulants.

FDPs—sometimes used to detect early DIC. High levels are seen in DIC, cancer, cirrhosis, PE, and DVT.

D-dimer—used to screen for DIC as well as in arterial and venous thromboses. It is also used in low-probability PE algorithms and has good negative predictive value.

CHAPTER 10

Oncology

APPROACH TO COMMON PROBLEMS

Approach to Screening for Cancer

Cancer has now become one of the most common causes of death in both men and women in the United States, equaling or surpassing deaths from atherosclerotic heart disease. At current rates, one in two men and one in three women will develop cancer in their lifetime. Over 500,000 cancer deaths occur each year, and one in four Americans will die from cancer. The most common causes of cancer deaths are shown in Table 10-1.

Different guidelines are provided by the American Cancer Society (ACS) and the United States Preventative Service Task Force (USPSTF) for cancer screening in asymptomatic individuals; they are shown in Table 10-2. The latter organization tends to be more conservative and less specific. Note that these guidelines are not intended for patients who have signs or symptoms suspicious for cancer or who have a familial syndrome or a strong family history of malignancy.

ONCOLOGIC DISEASES

Oncologic Emergencies

A variety of urgent or emergent clinical situations can occur in patients with oncologic tumors. A range of metabolic disturbances can be seen, such as hypercalcemia (as from bone destruction), hyponatremia (SIADH), hypoglycemia (pancreatic and neuroendocrine malignancies), and hyperuricemia (tumor lysis). Furthermore, space-occupying lesions can impinge upon the airway or the spinal cord, resulting in rapidly progressing neurologic symptoms. Intracranial metastases can cause edema or hemorrhage; pericardial tamponade, neutropenic fever, leukostasis, pulmonary embolism, and disseminated intravascular coagulation (DIC) can all be the result of tumors that can cause death or serious debility within 24 hours of clinical suspicion if not emergently treated. Some of these are conditions considered in other chapters. Following are four specific entities that any clinician should be able to recognize in the cancer patient, as they require urgent or emergent treatment.

Table 10-1. Seven Most Common Cancers: Incidence and Mortality* in 2008 (American Cancer Society)†

Men—Incidence (new cases/year)	Men—Mortality (deaths/year)	Women—Incidence (new cases/year)	Women—Mortality (deaths/year)
1. Prostate (186.3)	1. Lung (90.8)	1. Breast (182,4)	1. Lung (71)
2. Lung (114.7)	2. Prostate (28.7)	2. Lung (100.3)	2. Breast (40,5)
3. Colon/rectum (77.1)	3. Colon/rectum (24.3)	3. Colon/Rectum (81.5)	3. Colon/rectum (25.7)
4. Urinary bladder (51)	4. Pancreas (17.5)	4. Uterus (51.2)	4. Pancreas (16.8)
5. NHL (35.5)	5. Liver (12.6)	5. NHL (30.7)	5. Ovary (15.5)
6. Melanoma (35)	6. Leukemia (12.5)	6. Thyroid (28.4)	6. NHL (9.4)
7. Renal (33.1)	7. Esophageal (11.3)	7. Melanoma (27.5)	7. Leukemia (9.3)

* Numbers are in thousands per year
† Taken from www.cancer.org.
NHL, non-Hodgkin's lymphoma.

Table 10-2. Recommendations for Screening of Asymptomatic Individuals

	American Cancer Society*	United States Preventative Service Task Force†
Cancer-Related Check-Ups	For people aged >20 years, health counseling about tobacco, sun exposure, diet and nutrition, risk factors, and environmental/occupational exposure is recommended. Perform a complete physical exams every 3 years at ages 30–39, and annually at 40 and older for cancers of the thyroid, testicles, ovaries, lymph nodes, oral cavity, and skin.	Ask all adults about tobacco use and provide tobacco cessation interventions for those who use tobacco products. There is not enough evidence for or against whole-body skin examination by a primary care clinician or patient skin self-examination. Do not screen for ovarian, thyroid, or testicular cancer.
Breast Cancer	Women should perform a monthly breast self-examination beginning at age 20. Clinical breast examination (CBE) should be done every 3 years from ages 20–39, annually after age 40. A mammogram following CBE should be done every year after age 40.	No recommendation for or against breast self-examination. No recommendation for or against routine clinical breast examination. Screening mammography every 1–2 years for women aged 40 and older.
Colon/Rectum	At age 50 and over: Annual fecal occult blood test or fecal immunochemical test plus 1. Flexible sigmoidoscopy every 5 years or 2. Double-contrast barium enema every 5 years or 3. CT colonography (virtual colonoscopy) every 5 years. Alternatively, colonoscopy every 10 years beginning at age 50.	At age 50 and over: Annual fecal occult blood testing yearly is recommended plus 1. Flexible sigmoidoscopy or 2. Double-contrast barium enema (there is insufficient evidence to determine appropriate intervals). 3. There is insufficient evidence for use of colonography. Alternatively, one can use colonoscopy every 10 years starting at age 50. At ages 76–85, screen based on the individual patient. Over age 85, do not screen.
Prostate	Offer annual digital rectal examination (DRE) and the prostate-specific antigen (PSA) test annually to men over 50 years, to African American men over 45 years, and to men 40 years of age and over with several first-degree relatives who had prostate cancer at an early age. Patients should have at least a 10-year life expectancy.	There is insufficient evidence for screening in men <75 years. Do not screen in men ≥75 years.
Cervix	Screen yearly with a routine Pap test or every 2 years with liquid-based Pap test in sexually active women. At age 30, if there are three normal Pap tests, screening can be lengthened to every 2–3 years with the routine Pap test and every 3 years with the liquid-based Pap test, plus the human papillomavirus (HPV) DNA test. Women >70 years with three or more normal Pap tests in a row and no prior abnormal Pap test within 10 years can stop having cervical cancer screening. Women with risk factors (e.g., HIV infection, immunocompromised state) should be screened annually even >70 years of age. After total hysterectomy, continue to screen if removal was done for cervical cancer or if the cervix is still present. If hysterectomy without removal of the cervix was done for benign conditions, woman can choose not to have screening.	Screen yearly with Pap smears for those who are sexually active. There is insufficient evidence for or against routine use of HPV testing as a primary screening test for cervical cancer. Do not screening women >65 for cervical cancer who have had adequate recent screening with normal Pap smears and otherwise are at low risk for cervical cancer. Do not screen with Pap smear in women who have had a total hysterectomy for benign disease.

Sources: *CA Cancer J Clin. 2008;58 and †http://www.ahrq.gov/.

Spinal Cord Compression

D—Compression of the spinal cord secondary to direct tumor vertebral destruction by bony metastases.

Epi—About 25,000 cases occur every year. This may be the first presentation of cancer in many patients.

RF—Risk factors include cancers of the breast, lung, prostate, renal system, and GI tract, as well as lymphoma and myeloma. A history of known metastatic disease is also important.

P—A vertebral body is the most common site of metastases producing spinal cord injury. The most likely sites are the thoracic spine (70%) and then the lumbar spine (20%). In general, lung and breast cancers metastasize to the thoracic spine and GI and pelvic tumors to the lumbosacral spine. Weakening of the vertebral body's bony support by solid tumors causes compression fracture with extension of tumor posteriorly into the epidural space, compressing the cord from anterior to posterior. Lymphomas, by contrast, typically spread through an intervertebral neuroforamen. There may be edema and hemorrhage of the cord in the vicinity.

SiSx—Fifty percent of patients have back pain, 70% have motor deficits, and 30% have sensory deficits. Loss of bowel and bladder continence or the presence of sensorimotor deficits requires immediate attention. Back pain worsens, usually over weeks, before the onset of compression (invasion of vertebral soft tissues elicits pain). Classically, the pain is more severe when supine and also worsen with increased intra-abdominal pressure. Weakness is seen in up to 60–80% of patients at the time of diagnosis. Radiculopathy can be seen at the level of a vertebral body injury. Autonomic dysfunction (e.g., bladder and bowel dysfunction) is a late finding in these patients. Painless urinary retention may be seen.

Dx—Diagnosis requires a high level of suspicion. Any cancer patient who complains of new-onset back pain should be evaluated. Plain films can help make the diagnosis in >66% of cases, but they have poor negative predictive value. Patients suspected of having cord compression should have an emergent MRI with gadolinium (the gold standard, with >90% sensitivity and specificity). This is one of the few indications for an emergent MRI. In patients who absolutely cannot have MRI, a CT myelogram is another option, in which contrast is injected via a lumbar puncture (LP) into the epidural space.

Tx—Immediately administer dexamethasone (e.g., 4 mg IV every 6 hours) to reduce inflammation and edema at the time of the suspected diagnosis. Obtain radiation oncology and neurosurgery consultations as appropriate. Less commonly, chemotherapy may be given. Radiation can help stabilize the majority of neurologic deficits and reduce pain; commonly, there is residual autonomic dysfunction and paralysis.

Superior Vena Cava Syndrome

D—Obstruction of the superior vena cava (SVC) by extrinsic compression or internal blockage, usually due to malignant tumors (most commonly lung cancer and lymphoma). Nonneoplastic causes of SVC obstruction include tuberculosis and thrombosis (e.g., iatrogenic from a central line).

Epi—It is seen in 5–10% of patients with right-sided intrathoracic masses. Most tumors which cause this condition are of the right lung, much less commonly from esophageal or breast carcinoma or aggressive lymphomas.

SiSx—Early symptoms include facial plethora, distended neck veins, and hoarse voice. Later and more severe symptoms include facial swelling, cyanosis, increased intracranial pressure, and changes in mental status. Lying flat may aggravate the symptoms. If obstruction occurs gradually, followed later by acute thrombosis, there may be time for collaterals to form and reduce the pressure.

Dx—Chest CT/MRI can visualize lesions and distinguish an acute process from a chronic one (the latter is characterized by the presence of collateral vessels). Venography can also be used to localize obstruction in slower-onset cases. There may be an upper extremity venous pressure discrepancy. Tissue diagnosis should be made by the least invasive method possible.

Tx—Avoid anesthesia or heavy sedation and provide respiratory support. Acute treatment with intraluminal stenting of the SVC, usually with acute radiation therapy/chemotherapy, is indicated in patients with severe central nervous system (CNS) manifestations and is an effective solution. Anticoagulation after stenting should be provided in cases of SVC thrombosis.

Tumor Lysis Syndrome

D—Spontaneous or, more frequently, chemotherapy-induced tumor cell lysis with subsequent release of intracellular contents, especially uric acid, phosphate, and potassium, into the bloodstream.

RF—It is associated with a large tumor burden, high sensitivity to chemotherapy, and cancers with rapid doubling times, especially leukemia and highly aggressive lymphoma (e.g., Burkitt's non-Hodgkin's lymphoma).

SiSx—Many are asymptomatic. Oliguria and crystalluria may occur in severe lysis. Nausea, vomiting, and changes in mental status can result from renal failure. Muscle cramps are caused by hypocalcemia resulting from acute hyperphosphatemia.

Dx—Diagnosis is most commonly made by abnormal laboratory test results in asymptomatic patients or at the start of chemotherapy. Check baseline and serial WBC counts, serum LDH, uric acid, basic metabolic panel (BMP), phosphorus, and calcium levels. Repeat tests every 4–6 hours. In the appropriate clinical setting, one will see elevated LDH, uric acid, potassium, phosphorus, and creatinine levels. The calcium level will be low.

Tx—Delaying chemotherapy until electrolyte abnormalities are controlled is the mainstay of therapy. In some cases (e.g., Burkitt's lymphoma) this is not possible. Hydration with large volumes of IV fluid (>2.5–3.0 L/m^2/day) is needed to keep urine output >150 cc/hr (the body surface area for a 70-kg, 6-ft man is ~1.8 m^2). Furosemide may be used to help facilitate this if necessary, especially in patients with volume overload or heart failure. Prophylactic treatment with allopurinol (ideally started 2–3 days prior to chemotherapy) is used to prevent uric acid buildup. If uric acid rises rapidly to above >8 mg/dL despite prophylaxis, rasburicase (a recombinant urate oxidase enzyme) can be given. Aluminum hydroxide should be used to treat or prevent hyperphosphatemia. Hypocalcemia is not reversed unless the patient is symptomatic; however, watch for calcium and phosphorus deposition and acute obstructive uropathy during correction. Correct hyperkalemia with binding resins (i.e., sodium polystyrene sulfonate, otherwise known as Kayexalate). Hemodialysis may be necessary in refractory cases.

Neutropenic (NTP) Fever

D—Single temperature ≥38.3°C (101°F) or three temperatures ≥38.0°C (100.4°F) in 24 hours with an absolute neutrophil count (ANC) <500 [ANC = WBC × (% Bands + % PMNs)].

P—Malignancy or cancer treatment reduces the body's immune function and the ability to fight bacterial, viral, and fungal infections. Aerobic gram-positive cocci and aerobic gram-negative cocci are the most common pathogens. Patients treated with long-term antibiotics are susceptible to fungal infection or antimicrobial-resistant bacterial pathogens.

SiSx—Often there is a paucity of symptoms due to blunting of the inflammatory response. Infections and symptoms usually center on indwelling catheters, as well as the GI tract and the skin, particularly if these barriers are compromised.

Dx—Attempts should be made to identify the source of fever and the responsible pathogen. Initial evaluation includes chest X-ray, urinalysis, urine culture, and blood cultures. The time of the last chemotherapy session is important for recovery, as neutrophil counts usually reach their nadir at 7–10 days after therapy, but the timing of recovery varies, depending upon the regimen and the underlying tumor. Often an exact source of fever is not found.

Tx—Cultures should be obtained as soon as possible so that therapy can begin immediately (ideally, within 1 hour of temperature elevation). As in meningitis or other imminently life-threatening infections, the inability to draw cultures should not delay antibiotic treatment. All patients should receive broad-spectrum IV antibiotics. The antibiotic initially chosen must cover *Pseudomonas aeruginosa,* as this organism is common in these patients and rapidly produces sepsis with a high case fatality rate. Acceptable monotherapy includes cefepime, ceftazidime, piperacillin/tazobactam, meropenem, or imipenem-cilastatin. If the patient is allergic to penicillin, vancomycin plus aztreonam or levofloxacin plus gentamicin can be given. Vancomycin should be included if the patient is unstable or if the port or peripherally inserted central catheter (PICC) line looks infected. Patients with hemodynamic instability should receive aggressive fluid resuscitation and broader antibiotic coverage (including *Candida,* MRSA, and resistant gram-negative organisms), and urgent central venous catheter removal should be considered. The treatment duration for stable patients is not well established; therapy is usually maintained until resolution of neutropenia. Low-risk patients (those with solid tumors who are clinically well at the time of presentation, lack mucositis, and have no identifiable source) can usually be converted to oral antibiotic treatment if fever resolves within 3 days. Those with an identifiable source should receive a full course of IV antibiotics. Persistent fever after 3 days of initial therapy should prompt expansion of coverage with additional antibiotics (such as vancomycin). Antifungals should be considered after 3–7 days of persistent fever, particularly in patients with hematologic malignancies, chronic neutropenia prior to chemotherapy, or long-term immunosuppression (e.g., allogeneic stem cell recipients). Use of granulocyte colony-stimulating factor (G-CSF) in neutropenic patients has been shown to reduce the nadir period, but does not affect the course of disease or patient survival.

Cancers of the Head, Neck, and Thorax

Primary Central Nervous System Tumors

D—Primary CNS tumors may develop from brain parenchyma, meninges, cranial nerves and their associated myelin-producing cells, or glands, such as the pituitary or pineal. These tumors are classified by the cell type of origin.

Epi—The most common intracranial tumor is a meningioma. The most common parencyhmal tumor is an astrocytoma. Other primary CNS tumors include oligodendrogliomas, ependymomas, pituitary adenomas, neurofibromas, and schwannomas. Other rarer causes are not discussed in this section. Primary CNS tumors cause 13,000 deaths per year. Metastasis of CNS tumors outside the CNS is rare. Metastases to the brain are much more common than primary CNS tumors and usually arise from lung, breast, melanoma, renal, and colon cancer (in order of decreasing frequency).

SiSx—The presentation varies based on the tumor's location and aggressiveness. Personality changes, seizures, headaches that worsen when supine (due to elevated intracranial pressure), nausea, and malaise can be nonspecific symptoms. Frontal lobe tumors may present with intellectual decline and personality changes. Temporal lobe tumors may present with seizures. Occipital lobe tumors can present with visual field defects. Brainstem tumors can present with cranial nerve palsies, ataxia, or pyramidal and sensory deficits.

Dx—Neuroimaging demonstrates a mass lesion usually associated with edema. An MRI scan with gadolinium is the preferred neuroimaging modality for most tumors. The signal characteristics vary, depending on the type of tumor. Metastases are multiple and usually occur at the junction of the gray and white matter. Grade II astrocytomas appear hyperintense on T2 imaging and have minimal or no enhancement. Grade III or IV astrocytomas are often multifocal, may cross the corpus callosum (butterfly lesion), and have ring-shaped enhancement (the necrotic core does not enhance). Meningiomas are extra-axial with a dural tail, isointense on T1 imaging, and enhance homogeneously. Meningiomas are often calcified, allowing identification on head CT scans. Advanced forms of neuroimaging such as MR spectroscopy, perfusion imaging, or PET, may help differentiate tumors from other mass lesions. The gold standard diagnostic test is a brain biopsy in order to confirm a diagnosis and guide treatment or gross surgical resection.

Tx—Treatment depends on the tumor type and grade. High-grade astrocytomas are treated with partial surgical resction, chemotherapy, and whole brain radiation. Many meningiomas are resectable with a curative intent. Table 10-3 shows some common CNS tumors and their characteristics.

Head and Neck Cancer

D—These cancers encompass five basic areas:
Oral cavity (lips, buccal mucosa, gingiva, tongue, hard palate)
Pharynx (oropharynx, nasopharynx, and hypopharynx)
Larynx
Nasal cavity
Salivary glands

Epi—Head and neck cancers account for 3% of adult malignancies. There are 40,000–50,000 cases per year. Most patients are >50 years old.

P—Most of these cancers are squamous cell in origin and arise from mucosal surfaces.

RF—Alcohol and tobacco (smokeless products as well) are the most common risk factors,

Table 10-3. Classification and Features of Common Central Nervous System Tumors in Adults

Class	Type	Features	Comments
Astroctyic Tumors	Diffuse astrocytoma	Grade II: defined by the absence of mitotic figures, endothelial proliferation, and necrosis.	Progresses to a higher-grade astrocytoma. Median survival of 5–6 years with treatment.
	Anaplastic astrocytoma	Grade III: defined by the presence of mitotic figures without endothelial proliferation or necrosis.	Treated the same as glioblastoma.
	Glioblastoma (formerly called *glioblastoma multiforme*)	Grade IV: defined by the presence of either endothelial proliferation or necrosis.	Managed with steroids, partial surgical resection, whole brain radiation and chemotherapy, which prolongs survival by an average of 9 months. The course is rapidly progressive, with a poor prognosis. Median survival of 1 year.
Oligodendroglial Tumors	Includes oligodendroglioma and anaplastic oligodendroglioma	Have classic appearance of round cells with perinuclear halos on microscopy.	More benign course than astrocytomas and more responsive to chemotherapy. For grade III or anaplastic oligodendrogliomas, median survival is ~5 years.
Ependymal Tumors	Ependymoma	Arise from ependymal cells lining the ventricular system.	Low-grade tumors. On CT or MRI, appear as diffusely enhancing, well-demarcated masses. Prognosis is good, with >80% 5-year disease-free survival after resection.
Meningeal Tumors	Meningioma	Arise from the arachnoidal cap cell, a type of meningothelial cell in the arachnoid membrane.	Usually benign and attached to the dura. A smaller number may invade the brain and can be malignant or anaplastic. Total surgical resection of benign meningiomas is curative.

involving a 200 times increased risk. Others include orogenital sexual exposure to human papillomavirus (HPV, especially HPV 16), as well as marijuana, woodworking, and textile fiber exposures. Human papillomavirus is strongly associated with oropharyngeal location and basaloid histology. Epstein-Barr virus is associated with nasopharyngeal cancer, especially in the Mediterranean area and the Far East.

SiSx—Symptoms include the following:

Oral cavity: nonhealing ulcers, painful lesions, changes in speech (if the lesion is located at the tongue base).

Pharynx: symptoms are rare; they may cause sore throat and/or otalgia.

Nasopharynx: unilateral serous otitis media, unilateral or bilateral nasal obstruction, epistaxis, cranial nerve neuropathy.

Larynx: hoarseness.

In some cases, the cancer may present as cervical lymphadenopathy without a symptomatic primary tumor.

Dx—Biopsy is performed. Staging may involve a CT scan of the head and neck. Lymphadenopathy should prompt chest imaging and a bone scan. Definitive staging is performed under anesthesia and may include laryngoscopy, esophagoscopy, and bronchoscopy with additional biopsy.

Tx—Treatment is multidisciplinary, involving ear, nose, and throat (ENT) specialists, radiation oncologists, medical oncologists, and sometimes plastic/reconstructive surgeons. Surgery (preferred in oral cancer to avoid xerostomia) or radiation therapy (preferred in laryngeal cancer to preserve the voice) with or without chemotherapy is performed for localized disease. Surgery, radiation therapy, and chemotherapy are required for locally or regionally advanced disease. A feeding tube may be necessary to provide nutrition. The thyroid may be damaged during surgery, so its function should be monitored.

Thymoma

D—Tumor that originates from the thymic epithelial cell (if the lymphoid cells of the thymus become neoplastic, the result is a lymphoma). Most thymomas are benign growths that, by definition, lack cellular atypia and generally do not invade outside of the tumor's capsule. Invasive thymic epithelial neoplasms are rare, show cytologic atypia, and are generally not associated with autoimmune paraneoplastic disorders.

Epi—This is a rare condition classically associated with paraneoplastic phenomena, including myasthenia gravis and cytopenias (classically pure RBC aplasia). It is the most common cause of anterior mediastinal masses.

P—Thymomas develop from epithelial cells of the thymus. Seventy percent of patients have other systemic diseases: 30% have associated myasthenia gravis; 5–8%, RBC aplasia; and ~5%, Good syndrome (combined immunodeficiency and hypogammaglobulinemia). Rarely, the condition is associated with polymyositis, lupus, thyroiditis, Sjögren's syndrome, ulcerative colitis, pernicious anemia, Addison's disease, scleroderma, and panhypopituitarism.

SiSx—Most tumors are asymptomatic and are found incidentally on chest X-ray. One-third of symptoms are due to esophageal, bronchial, or SVC compression by a mass causing dysphagia, cough, or plethora.

Dx—Generally, the tumor is inaccessible by bronchoscopic biopsy and requires mediastinoscopy or limited thoracotomy. Fine needle aspiration usually cannot distinguish thymoma from lymphoma. A CT scan is used for staging. Other causes of an anterior mediastinal mass include lymphomas, germ cell tumors and substernal thyroid tumors, which are important to distinguish from this entity.

Tx—Complete surgical resection is performed in most cases, followed by radiation therapy if complete resection is not possible or if the tumor is stage II or III. Anesthetic/postoperative ICU monitoring for thymectomy can be challenging for patients with myasthenia. Neoadjuvant chemotherapy is used (to shrink the tumor). Adjuvant chemotherapy with or without radiation therapy is used in patients with unresectable or metastatic tumors. The immunologic consequences of thymectomy in an adult are generally inconsequential, and resection can improve or resolve the accompanying autoimmune disorders (e.g., myasthenia gravis or RBC aplasia).

Thyroid Cancer (see Chapter 7)

Lung Cancer

D—There are four major histologic subtypes: squamous cell carcinoma (20–30%), adenocarcinoma (30–40%), large cell carcinoma (10%), and small cell carcinoma (20%). See Table 10-4 for a comparison of these types. For purposes of staging, treatment, and prognosis, lung cancer is divided into small cell lung cancer (SCLC) and non–small cell lung cancer (NSCLC). Bronchoalveolar cell carcinoma, also called *broncholoalveolar cell carcinoma*, is a subtype of adenocarcinoma. Oat cell carcinoma is the most common subtype of small cell carcinoma. Adenocarcinomas are particularly likely to harbor activating epidermal growth factor receptor (EGFR) mutations, especially among nonsmokers and Asian patients. Such mutations have

Table 10-4. Comparison of Common Types of Lung Cancer

Type of Lung Cancer	Adenocarcinoma	Large Cell	Squamous Cell	Small Cell
Prevalence	40–50%	10–15%	30–40%	20–30%
Location of common lesion	Peripheral	Peripheral	Central	Central main stem/lobar
Aggressive features	Worse prognosis than squamous cell cancer. Bronchoalveolar cell carcinoma is more indolent.	Rapid growth and early metastasis.	Slow-growing over 3–4 years. Most likely to cavitate.	Worst prognosis. Rapid growth & early metastasis. Most cases associated with smoking and paraneoplastic syndromes (ACTH, SIADH, Eaton-Lambert syndrome).
Histology	Four subtypes: bronchoalveolar, acinar, papillary, solid with mucin production.	Mostly poorly differentiated. Two variants: giant cell and clear cell.	Wide range of differentiation. Make keratin pearls.	Three subtypes: oat cell, combined (a mixed type), and intermediate.
Subtypes	Bronchoalveolar carcinoma can present as a single nodule, multifocal disease, or diffuse (like pneumonia) on radiograph, with preservation of the alveolar architecture.	No relevant difference among subtypes.	Pancoast tumor: tumor at the apex of the lung or superior sulcus that involves the brachial plexus and sympathetic ganglion vertebral bodies; causes Horner's syndrome (miosis, ptosis, anhydrosis).	No relevant difference among subtypes.

prognostic importance, as they predict the response to kinase inhibitors of EGFR.

Epi—Lung cancer is the second most common cancer in the United States in incidence and is the leading cause of U.S. cancer deaths in men and women. In the United States, the incidence and mortality are declining in men but rising in women; 89,000 men and 74,000 women develop lung cancer every year. Mortality is 60% at 1 year and 86% at 5 years. The majority of lung cancer (in 90% of men and 80% of women) develops in smokers. Smoking cessation decreases the risk. The incidence in nonsmokers is about 1/10,000 overall. At diagnosis, 15% of patients have local disease, 25% have disease that has spread to lymph nodes, and >55% have metastases.

P—Lung cancer originates in the cells lining the bronchi. It is not uncommon to have separate primary tumors. Small cell cancer metastasizes early to the brain, bone, lung, liver, adrenal, and skin.

RF—Smoking is the most important risk factor (up to a 30% risk in heavy smokers, <1% in nonsmokers). There is a 10 times increased risk with smoking one pack per day and a 20 times increased risk with smoking more than two packs per day. Asbestos exposure causes a 6 times increased risk, and the risk is synergistic in smokers (53 times increase). Tuberculosis may predispose to the disease, as cancer is found at the site of old tuberculosis scars (adenocarcinoma most commonly). Also implicated are ionizing radiation, air pollution with arsenic, nickel, chromium, and vinyl chloride.

SiSx—The great majority of lung cancers are symptomatic at presentation. Ten percent are found incidentally. The most common symptoms are cough, dyspnea, hemoptysis, pneumonia (central, postobstructive), chest, shoulder, or arm pain (due to invasion of the chest wall), weight loss (a poor prognostic factor usually signifying the spread of disease), bone pain (distant metastases), hoarseness (due to left recurrent laryngeal nerve paralysis), headaches or seizures (CNS metastases), and swelling of the face or neck (via SVC syndrome). One may also see pleural effusion (dissemination of tumor into pleura or a postobstructive process), a single lobar collapse (LUL collapse is a classic symptom, as little else can do this), a paralyzed diaphragm (the phrenic nerve is affected), and clubbing. Paraneoplastic neuroendocrine syndromes include SIADH or Cushing's syndrome from ectopic ADH or ACTH secretion (SCLC), Eaton-Lambert syndrome (SCLC), and hypercalcemia from parathyroid hormone–related protein (PTHrP) in squamous cell cancer. Gynecomastia can be seen in large cells from β-human chorionic gonadotropin (β-hCG) secretion. Clubbing is most common in adenocarcinoma. The constellation of pain along C7 to T1, an apical tumor, and Horner's syndrome (ipsilateral ptosis, anhydrosis, and miosis from C8 to T1 involvement) make up Pancoast's syndrome.

Dx—Chest X-ray is often the first-line screening procedure, but large-scale screening is not recommended. Thereafter, a CT scan can be used to better define the lesion. Once the lesion is identified, the method of diagnosis depends on how accessible it is.

1. Sputum cytology, which is useful in patients who have a lung mass visible on chest X-ray. It is 70–80% sensitive. It is never used to rule out cancer.

2. Thoracentesis for pleural fluid cytology (when an effusion is seen on chest X-ray).

3. Bronchoscopy for washings, brushing, and direct biopsy of central lymph nodes or masses.

4. Mediastinoscopy, CT-guided transthoracic needle aspiration, or video-assisted thorascopic surgery (VATS) to perform biopsy and visualize the lesion to evaluate for resectability in NSCLC.

5. Percutaneous needle biopsy when surgery and thoracotomy are not possible. It may also be less invasive than bronchoscopy to access lymph nodes.

Work-up for all patients should include CBC, LFTs panel 7, CT or PET-CT of the chest, abdomen, and pelvis (where adrenal metastases commonly occur), and pathologic confirmation of malignancy. A CT or MRI scan of the brain is done only if there are CNS symptoms. Consider performing a head CT scan even if there are no symptoms in SCLC. Pulmonary function tests are needed if lung resection is planned.

Patients who have unresectable tumors with airway compromise can be given palliative care with local brachytherapy, airway stents, or cryotherapy.

Tx—Treatment depends on tumor histology and stage (see Tables 10-5a and 10-5b).

Limited SCLC is treated with combined radiation therapy and chemotherapy. Extensive SCLC is treated with chemotherapy alone. Half of all patients with NSCLC are inoperable at the time of diagnosis. Generally, surgery in NSCLC is of benefit up to stage IIIA, though neoadjuvant therapy in stage IIIB may allow otherwise unresectable patients to undergo surgery. Spirometry determines whether patients can tolerate major pulmonary resection (preoperative FEV_1 of >800 mL).

Table 10-5A. Staging of Small Cell Lung Cancer

Stage	Features	Treatment	5-Year Survival
Limited Disease (30%)	Confined to ipsilateral hemithorax, including contralateral mediastinal lymph nodes.	Radiation therapy and chemotherapy (cisplatin and etoposide). Prophylactic whole brain radiation therapy. Surgical resection if there is a solitary nodule.	20%
Extensive Disease (70%)	Extends beyond thorax, malignant effusion.	Palliative chemotherapy.	<1%

Table 10-5B. Staging of NSCL*

Stage	Features	Treatment	5-Year Survival
0	Carcinoma in situ.	Surgical resection.	
I	Isolated lesion. No invasion, no nodes involved.	Surgical resection, with or without adjuvant chemotherapy if stage IB, or radiation therapy if patient is not a surgical candidate.	50%
II	Spread to ipsilateral hilar or peribronchial lymph nodes.	Surgical resection with or without adjuvant chemotherapy or radiation therapy.	25%
IIIA	Spread to mediastinum, chest wall, pleura, or pericardium but is resectable.	Surgical resection plus chemotherapy with or without radiation therapy.	12%
IIIB	Includes presence of any of the following: contralateral or supraclavicular lymph nodes, a *malignant pleural effusion*, involvement of cardiac great vessels, trachea, or esophagus.	No surgery; unresectable; chemotherapy with or without radiation therapy; palliative therapy.	5%
IV	Metastatic disease, including several lesions in the opposite lung.	Palliative therapy; palliative chemotherapy.	2%

*Uses the AJCC/TNM staging system.

Table 10-6. Classification of Breast Cancer Types

Common Types*	Comment
Ductal Carcinoma in Situ (DCIS)	Noninvasive cancer. Treatment varies very widely, including breast conserving therapy (wide excision alone, or lumpectomy plus radiation therapy) and mastectomy. Adjuvant tamoxifen may lower the relapse rate or the incidence of contralateral breast cancer.
Lobular Carcinoma in Situ (LCIS)	Considered a marker for increased risk of invasive disease. Thirty percent of patients have invasive disease at 20 years. Treatment options include prophylactic bilateral mastectomy in high-risk patients vs. watching and waiting or tamoxifen use.
Invasive Ductal Carcinoma (80%)	The most common malignant cancer. Either tubular, colloid, medullary, or true papillary cancer. Can appear as a firm, irregular mass on exam.
Invasive Lobular Carcinoma (5–10%)	The second most common type. A mass lesion usually is not evident, just small cells infiltrating mammary stroma on microscopy. No microcalculi; usually bilateral and multifocal. Has a slightly better prognosis then ductal cancer. May accompany LCIS and DCIS.
Inflammatory Breast cancer (1–4%)	Most rapid and lethal; poorly differentiated. The majority lack estrogen receptor or progesterone receptor (PR) expression and show HER-2 overexpression. Presents with diffuse induration, erythema, warmth, edema, and peau de orange skin with or without a mass. Metastasis is common. Higher mortality; only 25% of patients are alive at 5 years.
Paget's Disease of the Nipple (1–3%)	The dermis is infiltrated by cells of ductal origin. Virtually always associated with DCIS or invasive cancer.

*Other types include tubular carcinoma, mucinous carcinoma, and medullary carcinoma, among others.

Breast Cancer

D—Cancer that affects either the ducts (ductal cancer) or lobules (lobular cancer). Classification of the different types of breast cancer is shown in Table 10-6.

Epi—Breast cancer is the third most common cancer in world and the most common cancer in women. Lifetime incidence in women is 13% and somewhat. This cancer is the leading cause of death in women 40–55 years of age. Seventy-five percent of patients have no known risk factors. Five-year survival is 85%; it is 97% if the cancer is diagnosed while it is still localized.

RF—Risk factors include age >40 years, a personal history of breast cancer (including ductal carcinoma in situ), a personal history of atypical hyperplasia or lobular carcinoma in situ, a family history (primarily first-degree relatives; inactivating mutations of *BRCA* genes), early menarche, late menopause, late first pregnancy, exogenous estrogen use, thoracic irradiation, and alcohol use.

SiSx—Often a painless breast mass is detected, most commonly in the upper outer quadrant. There is a change in the shape of the breast. New-onset nipple retraction or a discharge is seen. Skin changes are apparent. Axillary adenopathy develops. Otherwise, the mass is asymptomatic and is picked up on routine mammography.

Dx—For masses detected on physical exam, if the patient is premenopausal, recheck in 2–4 weeks, ideally 5–7 days into the follicular phase. If the mass persists or the patient is menopausal, further work-up is necessary. Consider mammography and fine needle aspiration with microscopic examination of fluid. Persistence or recurrence of a lesion after aspiration or recovery of bloody fluid all prompt further study. The decision to perform core or excisional biopsy depends on the risk of cancer. Core biopsy provides information about cellular architecture. Excisional biopsy involves fully defining tumor margins, and allows definitive diagnosis at the time of the procedure and molecular analysis of the tumor.

Tx—Treatment options are listed in Table 10-7. Adjuvant therapy may be included, depending on the risk of recurrence. This may include chemotherapy, endocrine therapy (with tamoxifen with or without an aromatase inhibitor) for estrogen receptor– or progesterone receptor–positive tumors, and/or trastuzumab (a HER2 antibody) for HER-2/neu-positive tumors.

Prognostic Factors

- Lymph node involvement is most important; the prognosis is worse with increased lymph node positivity.
- Increased cellular differentiation improves the prognosis.
- An increased number of cells in S-phase is associated with a poorer prognosis.

Table 10-7.   Staging of Breast Cancer

Stage	Criteria	Treatment	5-Year Survival
—	Lobular carcinoma in situ	Observation or Tamoxifen or Bilateral prophylactic total mastectomy	>99%
0	Ductal carcinoma in situ	Breast conserving surgery and radiation with or without tamoxifen or Total mastectomy with or without tamoxifen or Breast conserving surgery without radiation	>99%
I	Tumor < 2 cm	Breast conserving therapy (lumpectomy, radiation and surgical staging of the axilla) or Modified radical mastectomy (entire breast removal and axillary node dissection) Adjuvant radiation may be used post mastectomy in node positive tumor Chemotherapy in intermediate and higher risk individuals with or without tamoxifen. Monoclonal antibody therapy as appropriate*	>99%
II	A: smaller less local lymph node involvement B: larger, more local lymph node involvement		85%
IIIA	A: any tumor size, significant local lymph nodes involvement		57% (for all stage III types)
IIIB or IIIC	B: peau de orange, breast skin ulcer, chest wall invasion, satellite lesions with metastases to none, moveable, or fixed/matted axillary lymph nodes C: spread to ipsilateral infraclavicular, supraclavicular or internal mammary and axillary lymph nodes	Multimodality therapy with curative intent	
IV	Distant metastases often to lung, liver, bone, and brain	Palliative surgery (for metastases or recurrent effusions), palliative radiation therapy, hormone therapy, and cytotoxic chemotherapy. Depends on extent of tumor; treatment usually has palliative intent.	20%

*Examples of monoclonal antibodies include trastuzumab, a humanized monoclonal antibody that binds to the HER-2/neu receptor, and lapatinib, an orally administered tyrosine kinase inhibitor of both HER2/neu and the epidermal growth factor receptor. Testing for tumor production of these receptors prior to use is important.

Table 10-8. Common Nonmalignant Breast Conditions

	D/SiSx	Epi/RF	Dx	Tx
Fibroadenoma	Freely movable adenoma in the breast; 50% are <3 cm.	Very common young women; hormone dependent	FNA for cytology, but most tumors resolve spontaneously. Usually well circumscribed.	Resect if large or observe.
Fibrocystic Change of the Breast	Lumpy, with discrete masses and usually associated with changes in the menstrual cycle. Significant pain; a green-brown discharge may be seen on aspiration. Usually worse a few days after menses.	Seen in women 30–40 years old; associated with caffeine, tobacco, NSAIDs	A clinical diagnosis.	Can give danazol, tamoxifen or observe. Tell patient to stop using aggravating agents such as tobacco or coffee.
Breast Cyst	Seen commonly with changes in the menstrual cycle.	Seen in women 40–50 years old	FNA	Needle drainage to remove it if needed.

- Estrogen and progesterone receptor positivity confers a better prognosis due to the patient's response to hormone-targeted therapy.
- Overexpression of some molecular markers, including HER-2/neu, is associated with a poor prognosis but predicts the response to HER-2-directed therapies.

Benign Breast Masses
There are a number of benign conditions that present as breast lumps or masses. It is important to be able to distinguish them from malignant conditions. These benign conditions are presented in Table 10-8.

Gastrointestinal Cancers

Esophageal Cancer

D—Malignant esophageal tumors include adenocarcinoma and squamous cell cancer.
Benign tumors are rare. Of these, leiomyomas are the most common. They are intramural and usually asymptomatic.
Epi—The incidence is 4/100,000. Seventy-five percent of esophageal cancers are node positive at presentation.

RF—Risk factors include tobacco and alcohol use, vitamin A deficiency, nitrates, fungal toxins in pickled vegetables, lye ingestion, achalasia, Barrett's esophagus (10% of patients develop adenocarcinoma), Plummer-Vinson or Paterson-Kelly syndrome (esophageal web with glossitis and iron deficiency), and tylosis (hyperkeratosis of the palms and soles). Adenocarcinoma is more common among Caucasians and squamous cell carcinoma is more common in African Americans.
SiSx—There is constant pain in the midback. Progressive dysphagia for solid food develops, with persistent dysphagia when the lumen of the esophagus becomes <12 mm. Dysphagia for liquids may then ensue in advanced cases, accompanied by pain, hoarseness, and weight loss. Adenocarcinoma tends to occur at the bottom third of the esophagus from GERD and subsequent Barrett's metaplasia; squamous cell cancer develops at the top third of the esophagus from squamous cell metaplasia (e.g., with smoking). Tracheoesophageal fistulas may develop in severe disease.
Dx—Barium swallow is done when obstruction is likely. Esophagogastroduodenoscopy with

Table 10-9. Staging of Esophageal Cancer

Stage	Degree of Invasion	5-Year Survival
I	Lamina propria and submucosa	80%
II	Muscularis propria or adventitia	33%
III	Adventitia and nodes or direct invasion	15%
IV	Distant metastases	0–5%

biopsy identifies smaller lesions. Chest CT scans with or without PET scans are performed for staging, which is shown in Table 10-9.

Tx—Patients amenable to surgery are usually those with disease within the lower esophagus, though long-term survival is low. Radiation therapy is done for more proximal lesions in combination with chemotherapy. Esophageal bougienage or stent therapy can be undertaken in selected patients to maintain esophageal patency for palliation. Metastatic disease is common at the time of diagnosis, with associated poor survival. Overall, fewer than 5% of patients diagnosed with esophageal cancer survive for 5 years.

Gastric Cancer

D—Eighty-five percent of gastric cancers are adenocarcinomas. Other types include gastrointestinal stromal tumors (GISTs), GI lymphomas, and leiomyosarcomas. Benign tumors are less common, including a hyperplastic polyp, leiomyoma, gastric adenoma, and hypertrophic pancreatic tissue. There are two types of adenocarcinoma:

1. Diffuse type: Cancerous cells infiltrate the stomach and thicken the gastric wall, leading to a "leather bottle" quality of the stomach, the so-called *linitis plastica*.
2. Intestinal type: Cancerous cells form gland-like tubular structures, which are often ulcerative.

Epi—Gastric cancer is the second most common cancer worldwide and the eighth leading cause of cancer in the United States. It was the most common cancer until the 1940s. Male patients outnumber females by 2:1. The most common age of occurrence is 50–75 years.

RF—Risk factors include a family history (20%), hereditary nonpolyposis colorectal cancer (HNPCC, also called *Lynch syndrome*), low socioeconomic status, blood type A, tobacco use, vitamin C deficiency, eating salted or smoked foods, nitrosamines, pernicious anemia, atrophic gastritis, postgastrectomy status, gastric polyps, common variable immunodeficiency (CVID), and *Helicobacter pylori* infection. There is a higher incidence in China, Japan, and Finland.

SiSx—When superficial and surgically curable, most of these cancers are asymptomatic. As cancer spreads, patients may feel vague upper abdominal discomfort that increases to become more severe and persistent. Weight loss and anorexia may develop. Patients with linitus plastica experience early satiety. Metastases may spread to intra-abdominal lymph nodes, left supraclavicular lymph nodes (Virchow's node), the ovaries (Krukenberg's tumor), the periumbilical region (Sister Mary Joseph node), or the peritoneal cul-de-sac (Blumer's shelf, palpable on a digital rectal or vaginal exam). Other associations include iron deficiency anemia and occult blood in the stool.

Dx—An upper GI series will show most tumors. Any ulcers found on radiography should be followed with EGD and biopsy. A CT scan is 70% accurate for regional lymph node spread. The carcinoembryonic antigen (CEA) level may be elevated. Staging follows the TNM classification, with T1 disease invading the lamina propria or submucosa, T2 invading the muscularis propria, T3 invading the serosa (visceral peritoneum) but not adjacent structures, and T4 invading any adjacent structure.

Tx—Surgery provides the only chance of cure for carcinomas or sarcomas. but only one-third of patients are appropriate for this treatment. Radiation therapy and chemotherapy may be administered before and after surgery or for palliative treatment of unresectable or metastatic disease. Even with widely metastatic and bulky disease, GISTs typically have a dramatic clinical response to imatinib (a tyrosine kinase inhibitor) and other drugs targeting c-KIT and/or platelet-derived growth factor (PDGF) tyrosine kinases. These oncogenes are mutated in essentially all cases of GIST. Treatment of *H. pylori* may cause regression of localized gastric mucosa-associated lymphoid tissue (MALT) lymphomas.

Colorectal Cancer

D—A common malignancy of the large bowel.

Epi—It affects up to 5% of the population. It is the third most common cancer in the United States and the second leading cause of cancer death. There are 150,000 cases a year.

P—Most cancers develop from adenomatous polyps by accumulating genomic mutations. The probability that a polyp will develop into a cancer depends on its gross appearance, histology, and size. Grossly, polyps may be sessile or pedunculated, the former type being more closely associated with malignancy.

Histologically, polyps may be, from best to worst in terms of prognosis, tubular, tubulovillous, or villous. Cancer is found in <1% of tumors <1 cm and in 45% of those >2 cm.

RF—Risk factors include adenomatous polyps, carcinogen exposure, older age, a low-fiber, high-fat diet, personal history, inflammatory bowel disease, and genital tract cancer. It occurs with equal frequency in males and females until after age 50, when it becomes more common in males. A family history is also quite important, especially since there are well-described familial syndromes associated with colon cancer, as shown in Table 10-10.

SiSx—The cancer may be asymptomatic and picked up by screening colonoscopy or the fecal occult blood test. Symptoms include GI bleeding, change in bowel habits, anemia, anorexia, malaise, and weight loss. Right-sided colon cancer presents more often with fatigue, weakness, occult blood loss, and late obstruction because of increased compliance of the right colon. Left-sided cancer present

Table 10-10. Autosomal Dominant Familial Syndromes Associated with Colon Cancer

Condition	Defect	Comment
Familial Adenomatous Polyposis (FAP)	[APC or MUTYH gene]	Autosomal dominant. Colon has hundreds of polyps, which invariably leads to cancer. Treatment is colectomy.
Gardner's Syndrome	[APC gene]	Risk of developing cancer in small or large intestine approaches 100%. Also associated with soft tissue and bone tumors. Considered a variant of FAP.
Turcot's Syndrome	[Unclear: APC gene or mismatch repair gene?]	Risk of developing cancer in large intestine approaches 100%. Also associated with brain tumors.
Hereditary Nonpolyposis Syndrome Colorectal Cancer (HNPCC or Lynch syndrome)	[DNA repair defect]	80% lifetime risk of developing colorectal cancer. Women have increased risk of developing endometrial and ovarian tumors as well.
Peutz-Jeghers Syndrome (hereditary intestinal polyposis)	[STK11 gene]	Hamartomas of small and large intestines and stomach with small malignant potential. Associated with melanin pigmentation of oral mucosa, lips, hands, and genitals. Also, tumors in ovary, breast, pancreas. and endometrium.
Juvenile Polyposis	[Unclear. May be SMAD4 or PTEN gene]	Hamartomas of small and large intestines and stomach with small malignant potential.

Table 10-11.   Staging of Colorectal Cancer

Stage	Features	TNM Staging*	5-Year Survival
I	Cancer penetrating through submucosa (T1) and muscularis (T2)	T1–2, N0, M0	T1: >95% T2: >90%
II	Tumors penetrating through muscularis	T3, N0, M0	70–85%
III	Tumors involving regional lymph nodes	Tx, N1–2, M0	N1 (one to three lymph nodes): 50–70% N2 (more than three lymph nodes): 25–60%
IV	Metastatic disease	Tx,Nx,M1	<5%

*x represents any number.

with "apple-core" lesions that encircle the bowel and cause more bleeding and early obstruction.

Dx—Colonoscopy with biopsy is used to diagnose a suspected lesion or polyp. Screening should be performed in all average-risk patients and may include one of several options, given current guidelines: annual fecal occult blood testing (FOBT), flexible sigmoidoscopy every 5 years, double-contrast barium enema every 5 years, or colonoscopy every 10 years. If cancer is confirmed, LFTs should be checked for liver metastases. The CEA level should be obtained to follow the cancer. Staging includes chest X-ray, CT scan of the abdomen and pelvis, and colonoscopy to view the whole colon if the cancer is found by other method. If rectal cancer is found, use endoscopic ultrasound to evaluate the tumor stage and perirectal lymph node involvement. The different stages of colorectal cancer are shown in Table 10-11.

Tx—Resection is the treatment for many patients, with regional lymph node dissection for staging. Resection of solitary liver or even lung lesions may cure a minority. Regarding chemotherapy, no adjuvant chemotherapy is given for stage I cancer. Adjuvant therapy is controversial in stage II. Chemotherapy improves survival in stage III and IV patients. 5-Fluorouracil (5-FU, a pyrimidine analog) with leucovorin (folinic acid) is commonly administered after surgical resection. Chemotherapy usually is based on 5-FU. Monoclonal antibodies directed against vascular endothelial growth factor (VEGF) (bevacizumab) and EGFR (cetuximab) have also been shown to improve survival in combination with chemotherapy in patients with metastatic disease. Neoadjuvant chemotherapy with or without radiation therapy is often used in rectal disease to decrease the need for abdominoperineal resection of the rectum.

Carcinoid Tumors and Carcinoid Syndrome

D—Tumors primarily of the GI tract that secrete a number of vasoactive humoral substances and can cause a specific syndrome when these compounds are not metabolized.

Epi—Most tumors are found incidentally during radiographic procedures. Most commonly, carcinoids occur in the appendix (35%), ileum (28%), rectum (13%), and bronchi (13%). The mean age of occurrence is 50–70 years.

P—Carcinoid tumors, found most commonly in the GI and respiratory tracts, secrete a large number of compounds, mostly commonly serotonin, histamine, kallikrein, and prostaglandins (PGs). The presence of symptoms depends on whether these compounds are metabolized before they can act. The liver and lung are primary mediators of metabolism; hence, most tumors of GI origin do not cause symptoms unless they metastasize to the liver. Histamine (mainly from gastric tumors) causes flushing and pruritis.

Kallikrein causes vasodilation and flushing in some patients. The role of PGs is not clear. Serotonin is the most prominent compound secreted and is the cause of diarrhea. It is not made in foregut carcinoids, which lack an amino acid decarboxylase. On the other hand, hindgut tumors cannot convert tryptophan to serotonin, so they typically do not cause the syndrome either. After spreading to the liver, carcinoids can metastasize to the lungs, bone, skin, or almost any organ.

SiSx—Classic symptoms of the syndrome are unexplained cutaneous flushing, severe watery diarrhea, and occasionally bronchospasm. Flushing lasts less than a minute and usually affects the face and upper chest, with or without a burning sensation. It can be provoked by various foods, alcohol, strongly emotional events, or pressure on the tumor. Anesthesia-induced episodes can be prolonged and have concomitant hypotension. Telangiectasias may appear after repeated episodes of prolonged vasodilation. Secretory diarrhea occurs in up to 80% of patients, with as many as 30 bowel movements per day, the timing of which is usually unrelated to the flushing. From 20% to 30% of patients have bronchospasm. Rarer findings are right-sided fibrous cardiac valvular lesions (less commonly found are left-sided valvular lesions due to pulmonary metabolism). Some tumors may causes signs of tryptophan deficiency (dry skin, glossitis, angular stomatitis) as much more tryptophan is converted into serotonin. The most severe symptoms may be present in carcinoid crisis, where there is bronchospasm and arrhythmia with delta MS. This can occur spontaneously after palpation of tumor masses.

Dx—The initial diagnostic test is a 24-hour urine 5-hydroxyindoleacetic acid (5-HIAA) excretion (the end product of serotonin). Most symptomatic patients have levels >100 mg/day (normal, 2–8 mg/day). The test is 75% sensitive and nearly 100% specific, but it can be affected by other syndromes such as celiac disease, malabsorption, and a high tryptophan diet (precursor of serotonin). Lower levels will be seen in patients with metastatic carcinoid tumors but without the carcinoid syndrome. In suspected foregut carcinoid (bronchial and gastric) there may be no amino acid decarboxylase, and therefore serum serotonin needs to be measured. If the 5-HIAA test result is equivocal, plasma chromogranin A or a mean fasting serum serotonin test can be used. Provocation tests with epinephrine and pentagastrin are used in those cases where flushing is prominent, but they have equivocal results otherwise. Confirm these test results by finding increased 5-HIAA product in urine. Once the biochemical diagnosis is made, localization is carried out using CT and indium-111 octreotide, a somatostatin analogue (can be used since these tumors almost always contain somatostatin receptors). The CT scan is useful for detecting liver metastases most easily.

Tx—The treatment of choice for localized disease is surgery. Appendix tumors <2 cm are unlikely to have metastases, but patients with metastatic disease have 5-year survival of 50%. Metastases of small bowel tumors require lymph node dissection since they metastasize regardless of size. Small gastric tumors are treated with local excision and follow-up. Symptomatic care involves avoiding foods that cause flushing or pressure trauma to the tumor. Bronchodilators are given for wheezing. Octreotide can be used in patients with severe disease, especially those with carcinoid crisis, and helps to relieve flushing and diarrhea. Cyproheptadine, a serotonin antagonist, is also used. Chemotherapy has been used but has shown minimal effect to date.

Liver and Biliary Tree Cancers

Hepatoma or Hepatocellular Carcinoma (HCC)

D—Primary malignant neoplasm arising from parenchymal liver cells.

Epi—It is more endemic to China and sub-Saharan Africa, where there are high hepatitis B carrier rates, and aflatoxin produced by *Aspergillus* in food stored without refrigeration. In the United States, HCC is a common sequela of cirrhosis.

RF—Usually there is an underlying cirrhotic disease of any cause: HCV (10% of patients develop cirrhosis and of those, 5% develop cancer), chronic alcohol consumption, and HBV. Hemochromatosis and α_1-antitrypsin deficiency are other risk factors.

SiSx—Jaundice, encephalopathy, ascites, and any signs of cirrhosis may give a clue to the disease, as may deterioration in an otherwise stable cirrhotic patient. Exam may show an enlarged, palpable liver. Vascular invasion is common, leading to satellitosis or multifocal tumors.

Dx—Diagnosis is made by ultrasound, CT, and MRI. The α-fetoprotein (AFP) level is increased in 60–80% of cases. In the context of a cirrhotic liver, a liver mass and an AFP level >500 ng/mL (normal, 0–30 ng/mL) is diagnostic of HCC.

Imagining is important. One can perform either MRI or triple-phase CT (initially non-contrast, then venous and arterial contrast phases), which helps determine tumor vascularity and size. Ultrasound is not very sensitive. Liver biopsy is done; however, seeding is a potential risk, so it may not be done if other studies are diagnostic. It is important to distinguish HCC, which is staged as shown in Table 10-12a, from benign hepatic tumors, described in Table 10-12b.

Tx—Resection with negative margins of solitary tumors may be possible. Transplantation may be done in patients with cirrhosis if the tumor is small (<5 cm). Chemotherapy alone does not prolong life. Chemoembolization is palliative, using ethanol, radiofrequency ablation (RFA) or cryotherapy. There is a 50% recurrence rate in such cases, and the procedure is much harder to do in patients with cirrhosis, as regeneration is limited.

Table 10-12a. Staging of Hepatocellular Tumors

T0	No primary tumor
T1	Solitary tumor, no vascular invasion
T2	Vascular invasion or multiple tumors <5 cm
T3	Tumor >5 cm or one involving a major branch of the portal or hepatic vein
T4	Direct invasion of other organs

Table 10-12b. Benign Hepatic Tumors

Cavernous Hemangioma	Found in 5–10% of adults. Can be >4 cm. Ultrasound scan showing hyperechoic areas is diagnostic. No treatment is necessary, as rupture is rare. Resect if painful.
Hepatic Adenoma	Seen most commonly in females 30–50 years old. Estrogen exposure (OCP use) is a common risk factor. Tumor is usually solitary and unencapsulated. Treatment is resection because of malignant potential.
Focal Nodular Hyperplasia	Central scar with fibrous septa, nodular hyperplasia. No premalignant potential. Hard to diagnosis with CT or ultrasound. Can remove it or watch.

Cholangiocarcinoma

D—Tumor of the bile ducts. Adenocarcinoma is the most common type.

Epi—It accounts for 3% of all cancer deaths and is more common in people >50 years old. Two-third of these cancers arise from the perihilar extrahepatic ducts (called *Klatskin's tumor* if it is located at the bifurcation of the common duct) and the rest from the intrahepatic or distal bile duct.

RF—Risk factors include chronic hepatobiliary parasitic infections, ectatic ducts, primary sclerosing cholangitis, and chronic ulcerative colitis.

SiSx—Painless jaundice is the most common presenting sign. With obstruction of the extrahepatic biliary system, RUQ pain is a late finding. Anorexia and weight loss may be seen. Hemobilia can occur if there is erosion into a blood vessel or with fistula formation.

Dx—Conjugated hyperbilirubinema is seen in many cases with elevated alkaline phosphatase. Cancer 19-9 may be positive. Ultrasound or CT can show a mass. Magnetic resonance cholangiopancreatography (MRCP) or endoscopic retrograde cholangiopancreatography (ERCP) may be needed to show vascular invasion.

Tx—Curative surgery may be possible only in limited stage disease. Usually liver resection is needed, especially the caudate lobe, with multiple margins. In general, there is a limited response to chemotherapy. Few patients survive for more than 1 year.

Pancreatic Cancer

D—Tumor of the pancreas, mostly ductal adenocarcinomas; overall, the prognosis is poor.

Epi—It is the fourth most common cause of cancer-related mortality. Male patients outnumber females. Disease usually occurs >50 years.

RF—Risk factors include tobacco use, a family history, obesity, and chronic pancreatitis.

P—Usually adenocarcinoma or islet cell tumors are found. Most are in the head of the pancreas rather than in the body or tail.

SiSx—Painless jaundice, usually from biliary obstruction, is the classic presentation. Weight loss and back or abdominal pain that improves with bending forward may be seen. Severe pain may suggest retroperitoneal involvement. Other findings include clay-like stools, pruritis, and glucose intolerance, perhaps as a direct consequence of the tumor. Other rare presentations or findings are venous thrombosis and migratory thrombophlebitis (Trousseau's syndrome), splenomegaly, and GI hemorrhage from varices when there is portal venous system compression by the tumor.

Dx—Most tumors are metastatic or locally aggressive at the time of diagnosis. Carcinoembryonic antigen and cancer 19–9 markers may be elevated. Ultrasound is done to visualize the gallbladder and pancreas. A CT scan can detect a malignant pancreatic lesion in >80% of cases. An MRI scan can sometimes help distinguish benign from malignant neoplasms; otherwise, it is not better than CT. Ultimately, surgical laparotomy and/or endoscopy ultrasound with biopsy is needed to make the diagnosis.

Tx—Complete surgical resection (Whipple procedure or pancreaticoduodenectomy, done if the lesion is in the pancreatic head) is the only effective treatment for this disease. Cure is possible in only 10–15% of patients with pancreatic head tumors. Median survival for patients with unresectable tumors is 6 months. External beam radiation does not prolong survival, but it may reduce pain in patients with unresectable or metastatic disease. Chemotherapy regimens include 5-FU with or without radiation therapy or gemcitabine (a pyrimidine antimetabolite). These regimens have a modest impact upon survival but a more important role in symptom control or improvement of the patient's quality of life.

Gynecologic and Genitourinary Cancers

Bladder Cancer

D—Common urologic cancer that is mostly epithelial in developed countries and primarily squamous cell cancer (SCC) in developing countries.

Epi—It is the second most common urologic cancer, as well as the fourth most common cancer in men and the tenth most common cancer in women. Fifteen percent of patients present with metastases; 40% will have metastases within 2 years after the start of treatment. African Americans have a worse prognosis than Caucasians. Eighty percent of bladder cancers are associated with environmental exposure (i.e., tobacco use).

RF—Risk factors include tobacco use, industrial dye exposure, chronic Foley catheter use, bladder stones, Schistosoma haematobium infection, and radiation to the pelvis.

SiSx—Patients usually present with gross or microscopic hematuria of any sort. There may be increased urinary frequency or urgency. Signs of metastases include hepatomegaly or lymphadenopathy.

Dx—Urinalysis may show hematuria and pyuria. Anemia may be seen. Urine cytology should be done, but has low yield in diagnosing superficial lesions. Computed tomography urography, MRI, or ultrasound may be useful to visualize a mass, Intravenous pyelography (IVP) can image the upper urinary tract but not the renal parenchyma. Cystoscopy with biopsy is needed to make a diagnosis. Grading is based on histology, and staging follows the typical TNM cancer staging system

Tx—Treatment options include complete resection of the bladder, intravesical or systemic chemotherapy, intravesical BCG immunotherapy, and/or external beam irradiation.

Renal Cancer

D—Cancer arising from the kidneys, 95% of which is renal cell carcinoma that arises from the proximal renal tubule.

Epi—It accounts for 3% of all cancers. There are 52,000 cases per year and 13,000 deaths per year. It is more common in Caucasians.

RF—Risk factors include Von Hippel–Lindau disease, hereditary renal cell syndromes, tobacco use, obesity, cystic kidney disease, and tuberous sclerosis.

SiSx—The classic triad of flank pain, hematuria, and flank mass is actually uncommon (10%)—except on board exams. Many tumors are asymptomatic and are found incidentally on imaging. Constitutional symptoms such as weight loss, fever, and sweats may be seen. Paraneoplastic hypercalcemia, erythrocytosis, neuropathy, and hypertension may also be found. Rarely, a left-sided varicocele can be seen in men due to obstruction of the left testicular vein. Thirty percent of patients have metastases at diagnosis, mostly to the lung, liver, bone, and soft tissue.

Dx—Imaging via contrast CT scan is the most useful test, although ultrasound, MRI, or PET can suggest a diagnosis. Computed tomography–guided biopsy can be done in patients with cystic lesions. Staging follows the TNM staging system.

Tx—Over 50% of patients with early-stage disease are cured with surgical resection. Tumor confined to the renal parenchyma portends a 60–70% 5-year survival. For advanced disease, options include VEGF-inhibiting antibodies (bevacizumab) or kinase inhibitors (Sunitinib or Sorafenib), and mammalian target of rapamycin (mTOR) inhibitors (temsirolimus and everolimus). Other options include radiation therapy, chemotherapy, and hormonal or immunotherapy, but these have less impact on the disease course.

Prostate Cancer

D—Usually an adenocarcinoma, which is the most common cancer in men and the second leading cause of death from cancer.

Epi—It is the most common cancer in men after skin cancer, accounting for 29% of new cancer cases and 11% of cancer deaths in men. The incidence of this cancer increased dramatically in the 1980s and 1990s, likely secondary to prostate-specific antigen (PSA) screening. It is a very common finding at autopsy, discovered in >70% of men over 80. There are 230,000 cases per year and 30,000 deaths per year.

RF—Risk factors include a family history and a Western diet. African Americans are more at risk than Caucasians.

SiSx—Many tumors may be asymptomatic. A mass may be felt on digital rectal exam. In more advanced disease symptoms of obstruction, impotence, and hesitancy in voiding may be found. Bone pain at sites of metastatic disease is also common. Cord compression is also possible as a result of epidural metastases.

Dx—Digital rectal exam may find tumors in the posterior aspects of the prostate gland; overall, this exam has low positive predictive value. Most cancers are diagnosed after routine screening with PSA. In patients with PSA values >4 ng/mL, the tumor is generally followed by transrectal biopsy. However, the PSA can be mildly elevated by other conditions, such as BPH. The PSA velocity test is also useful; a fast rate of rise (usually >2 ng/mL per year) is considered a high-risk feature. Cystoscopy is not routinely done, but transrectal ultrasound is used for staging, and MRI can help demonstrate if lymph nodes are involved. Bone scan can help assess for metastatic disease. Computed tomography plays little role in evaluation. Grading is via the Gleason score, which is based on histology.

Tx—Screening has not been shown to improve survival in most trials. Treatment is based on the patient's age and other factors, as prostate cancer in general is more indolent than other solid tumors. For localized disease, radical prostatectomy can be done, either open or laparoscopically. Radiation therapy can also be done with curative intent, using either external beam therapy or radiation seeds. Most tumors are initially hormone dependent and respond to androgen deprivation. Prostate-specific antigen surveillance is done after treatment. For metastatic disease, docetaxel-based regimens improve survival. Radiation can be an important adjuvant to treat bone pain from metastases. Since prostate cancer is an indolent disease, many patients opt for watchful waiting and treatment of symptoms, especially if they have other significant comorbid conditions.

Ovarian Cancer

D—Common female cancer with varying cell types that carries a poor prognosis.

Epi—It is the fifth most common female cancer and the fifth most common cause of death from cancer. There are 23,000 cases per year and 14,000 deaths.

P—Serous (50%), mucinous (20%), endometrioid, clear cell, transitional cell, and undifferentiated adenocarcinoma are common histologic types. Tumor spread can be intraperitoneal via lymphatics or hematogenous.

RF—Risk factors include Turner's syndrome, breast and ovarian cancer syndromes, HNPCC, endometriosis, unopposed estrogen therapy, and a family history.

SiSx—Symptoms are usually nonspecific, with most women having advanced disease at the time of diagnosis. Ovarian torsion is rare. Abdominal distention, ascites, anorexia, or dyspnea with pleural effusions may be seen. Paraneoplastic conditions such as hypercalcemia, Trousseau's syndrome (migratory thrombophlebitis), or multiple seborrheic keratoses (sign of Leser-Trelat) are rare but can be seen. Pelvic exam may reveal an adnexal mass.

Dx—Ultrasound is the first useful test in diagnosing an adnexal mass. A CT or MRI scan can show metastases. Note that metastases to the ovary can occur from colon, gastric, breast, and other GI tumors, so these must be looked for as well if appropriate. Endometrial cancer is found in 10% of patients with concomitant ovarian cancer. Ultimately, surgery is needed for diagnosis and staging. Serum cancer antigen 125 (CA-125) will be elevated in 80% of women.

Tx—Bilateral salpingo-oophorectomy at the time of hysterectomy for benign uterine disease in women over age 40—and after childbearing has been completed in younger women with strong family histories—is advocated by many to prevent the development of ovarian cancer. Cytoreduction surgery (removing all visible tumor) is a cornerstone of metastatic disease therapy, which also includes debulking of peritoneal metastases. Postoperative chemotherapy usually includes platinum-based compounds such as cis-platin or carboplatin. Although it is more toxic, intraperitoneal chemotherapy is preferred over IV chemotherapy in optimally debulked patients with advanced ovarian cancer due to its survival benefit.

Endometrial Cancer

D—The most common pelvic malignancy in women; most tumors are adenocarcinomas.

Epi—There are 40,000 new cases per year and 7000 deaths. This is mainly a disease of postmenopausal women 50–70 years of age.

RF—Risk factors include obesity, altered menstruation, late menopause, anovulation, postmenopausal bleeding, and use of *tamoxifen*.

SiSx—Symptoms include an abnormal vaginal discharge (90%); abnormal bleeding (80%), which is usually postmenopausal; and leukorrhea (10%).

Dx—The Pap smear is usually negative. Vaginal ultrasound may show a thickened endometrium. Endometrial biopsy or aspiration curettage is used but is not always positive. Staging requires surgery to assess the degree of myometrial invasion.

Tx—Uncomplicated carcinoma is treated with total abdominal hysterectomy and bilateral salpingo-oophorectomy. Pre- or postoperative radiation therapy may be used, but survival is not significantly altered. Patients with stage IV disease (outside the abdomen or invading the bladder or rectum) are treated palliatively with radiation, surgery, and/or progestational agents.

Cervical Cancer

D—Cancer of the cervix that is unique in that it is generally an STD.

Epi—There are 10,000 invasive cases per year with 3900 deaths; 50,000 cases of carcinoma in situ occur yearly.

P—Venereal transmission of HPV has a major etiologic role.

RF—Risk factors include early sexual activity, multiple partners, smoking, and low socioeconomic status.

Over 66 types of HPV have been isolated, many associated with genital warts. Those associated with cervical carcinoma are mainly types 16 and 18 as well as types 31, 45, and 51 to 53. The protein product of HPV-16, the E7 protein, binds and inactivates the tumor-suppressor gene Rb. The E6 protein of HPV-18 has sequence homology to the SV40 large T antigen, and has the capacity to bind and inactivate the tumor-suppressor gene p53. Proteins E6 and E7 are both sufficient to cause cell transformation in vitro. Eighty percent of invasive cervical cancers are squamous cell tumors, and 10–15% are adenocarcinomas,

SiSx—Symptoms generally consist of metrorrhagia (spotting unrelated to menstruation), postcoital spotting, and cervical ulceration. A bloody or purulent, odorous, nonpruritic discharge may appear after invasion. Bladder and rectal dysfunction or fistulas and pain are late symptoms. Many tumors are asymptomatic and are picked up on screening.

Dx—The Pap smear is 90–95% accurate in detecting early lesions such as cervical intraepithelial neoplasia (CIN) but is less sensitive in detecting cancer when frankly invasive cancer or fungating masses are present. Inflammation, necrosis, and hemorrhage can produce false-positive smears, and colposcopic-directed biopsy is required when any lesion is visible on the cervix, regardless of Pap smear findings.

Tx—For in situ disease, cone biopsy or cryotherapy can be done versus total abdominal hysterectomy, if women have completed childbearing. Stage I disease (microinvasive) is treated with either radical hysterectomy or radiation therapy. Stages II to IV involve radical resection and radiation therapy or other combined-modality therapies. Platinum-based chemotherapy with radiation therapy improves survival. Overall five-year survival is 50–70% on average for all of those diagnosed with the disease. Quadrivalent HPV 6/11/16/18 vaccine (Gardasil) can be given to prevent the most common HPV serotypes, but it does not eliminate all carcinogenic HPV serotypes or the need for Pap smear screening.

Testicular Cancer

D—Ninety-five percent of primary testicular cancers are germ cell tumors (GCTs). Half of them are seminomatous and half are nonseminomatous. Nonseminomas include mixed GCTs (40%), teratomas (30%), and embryonal cell tumors (20%) and choriocarcinoma (1%), which has the worst prognosis. The 5% of non-GCT tumors include Leydig cell and Sertoli cell tumors.

Epi—Testicular cancer is the most common solid tumor in males aged 18–35 years. There is an incidence of 7,000 cases and 400 deaths per year, representing 1% of all male cancers. This cancer is more common in Caucasians. Nonseminomatous and seminomatous types are equal in incidence. A family history may be important. A testicular mass at age >50 is considered lymphoma until proven otherwise.

P—Excess copies of chromosome 12p is a marker seen in almost all GCTs. Tumor spread is via the para-aortic and renal hilar lymph nodes (not the inguinal lymph nodes).

RF—A history of undescended testes confers a 14 times increased risk. Orchiopexy (removal of undescended testes) decreases the risk of GCT. However, a risk is still present even if the condition is surgically corrected. If there is tumor on one side, there is a 25% chance of developing cancer in the contralateral testis in a patient with bilateral undescended testes. Klinefelter's (47 XXY syndrome) and complete androgen insensitivity syndrome (androgen receptor defect) are also important risk factors.

SiSx—An asymptomatic or painless testicular mass is the classic finding. Pain may signify tumor hemorrhage. Symptoms of metastases to the lung (hemoptysis, DOE), brain (CNS symptoms), and abdomen (back pain) are common. Gynecomastia may occur if the tumor secretes β-hCG.

Dx—Palpation and transillumination are done first, followed by ultrasound to rule out other causes of a testicular mass (hydrocele, spermatocele). Relief of pain with elevation is more indicative of epidydimitis. Ultrasound is used for equivocal cases. Work-up then includes a CT scan of the abdomen and pelvis, as well as serum tests for AFP and βHCG. Look for involved lymph nodes, most commonly the para-aortic lymph nodes. Never biopsy the testes directly, as this will cause seeding to the inguinal lymph nodes. If there are no lymph nodes to biopsy by CT guidance, then careful removal of the testes and examination of tissue will make the diagnosis. The inguinal approach is used to prevent additional pathways of spread to the abdomen. There are no strong recommendations regarding screening with self-exams. Staging is shown in Table 10-13. Note that there is no stage IV, unlike many other cancers.

Tx—Orchiectomy with vascular control of the spermatic cord in most cases is done for diagnosis in addition to treatment. Treatment options are shown in Table 10-14. Importantly, seminomatous tumors are quite radiation sensitive.

Table 10-13. Staging of Testicular Cancer

Stage 0—In situ disease

Stage I—Tumor limited to testes or spermatic cord

Stage II—Metastasis to any regional lymph node

Stage III—Any metastasis to another organ

Cancer of Unknown Primary

D—Condition in which a metastatic tumor site is found with a clearly identifiable primary tumor origin after an appropriate work-up. Management is based on the specific cancer subgroup type.

Epi—This accounts for 2% of all cancers.

P—Usually the cancer is placed into one of several histologic categories (see Table 10-15) that determine their work-up for identification of a primary site and their treatment.

SiSx—Symptoms vary widely, depending on the location of the metastatic lesion. Many patients are asymptomatic and notice a swollen lymph node or the disease is picked up on routine diagnostic testing for another condition.

Dx—Much of the diagnosis focuses on the work-up of identifying the primary site and depends on the type of histology obtained from the metastatic tissue, as this will strongly influence treatment (see Table 10-15).

Tx—Median survival is 6–10 months. Systemic chemotherapy is given in many cases based on the resemblance to the type of primary tumor of origin. There are several favorable groups for treatment:

1. Women with isolated axillary adenopathy are treated as though they have stage II or III breast cancer after evaluation by breast mammography, ultrasound, and/or MRI.

2. Women with peritoneal carcinomatosis are treated as though they have ovarian cancer even though no primary is identified. They have cytoreductive surgery followed by platinum-based chemotherapy.

Table 10-14. Treatment Differences Between Nonseminomatous and Seminomatous Testicular Cancers

Nonseminomatous	Seminomatous
In early-stage disease, 75% are cured by orchiectomy. Confined tumors without invasion may be watched.	Early-stage disease is treated by orchiectomy and radiation therapy. Later-stage disease is treated with chemotherapy; many patients will have a complete response and cure.
Large nodes or metastases require chemotherapy and resection of any residual lymph nodes.	These tumors are typically exquisitely sensitive to radiation.
Lung and liver metastases can be treated in many cases.	

Table 10-15.   Different Types of Cancer of Unknown Primary

Type	Features and Diagnostic Work-up
Adenocarcinoma (70%)	Typically involves the liver, lungs, bones, and lymph nodes. In only 20% is the primary site ever found. Evaluate for lung, prostate, breast, and ovarian cancer, among others. Use of tumor markers (CEA for colon cancer, CA-19–9 for pancreatic cancer and cholangiocarcinoma, CA-15–3 for breast cancer, and CA-125 for ovarian cancer) usually is not helpful diagnostically but can be used to follow the tumor during treatment.
Poorly Differentiated Carcinoma (15–20%)	Usually involves the mediastinum and retroperitoneum. Chest, abdominal, and pelvic imaging is important, as is immunohistochemistry.
Poorly Differentiated Neoplasia (5%)	Unable to differentiate by light microscopy between carcinoma, sarcoma. and lymphoma. Necessary to use additional measures such as immunohistochemistry, chromosomal analysis, or electron microscopy to try to further categorize the tumor.
Squamous Cell Carcinoma (rare)	Usually associated with a head and neck cancer or a neck mass. Immunohistochemical studies and electron microscopy are of little value in identifying the primary site in patients with squamous cell carcinoma of unknown primary site. With inguinal adenopathy genital or anorectal area cancers are suspected, so a careful exam of the vulva, vagina, cervix, or penis should be performed. Digital rectal examination and anoscopy should done in all patients. Upper and midcervical adenopathy most likely suggests a head or neck cancer. Evaluate with head and neck CT, ENT evaluation with direct laryngoscopy, and nasopharyngoscopy. A PET scan can be done if these scans are unrevealing. Lower cervical or supraclavicular adenopathy, or other metastases, suggest lung cancer. Consider chest CT and/or bronchoscopy.
Neuroendocrine Carcinoma (rare)	There are three types: 1. Low-grade neuroendocrine carcinomas such as carcinoid or islet cell tumors can have metastases to the liver or other organs. 2. Small cell carcinoma types suggest a bronchogenic malignancy. CT scan of the chest or bronchoscopy can help identify the primary. Other possible organs can be the origin of non-lung-related small cell cancer and include the bladder, ovary, cervix, esophagus, and salivary glands. 3. Poorly differentiated neuroendocrine carcinoma suggests a high-grade or aggressive malignancy, usually with many sites. A specific primary site is rarely ever found.

3. Poorly differentiated carcinoma with midline adenopathy suggests extragonadal germ cell malignancy, which is usually quite responsive to platinum-based chemotherapy (>50% response).

4. Patients with SCC with cervical adenopathy are treated as though they have head and neck cancer with node dissection and radiation therapy.

5. Patients with low-grade neuroendocrine carcinoma usually can be treated with somatostatin analogues. Some with high-grade disease are treated as though they have SCLC, with one-fourth showing a complete response.

Leukemias and Lymphomas

Although they have common histologic and immunophenotypic characteristics, by convention leukemic malignancies are diseases that primarily involve the marrow and blood, whereas lymphomas primarily infiltrate lymph nodes and/or the spleen. In several cases, the same condition can have both leukemic and lymphoma components.

Hodgkin's Disease

D—A type of lymphoma characterized by Reed-Sternberg (RS) cells in the appropriate clinical setting. There are four major types based on the histology:

Nodular sclerosing—the most common form; there are areas of necrosis, and RS cells are rare.

Lymphocyte predominant—mainly lymphocytes, with rare or no eosinophils; it has the best prognosis.

Lymphocyte depleted—hypocellular because of fibrosis; large numbers of RS cells are seen; this is more common in HIV.

Mixed cellularity—a combination of lymphocytes, histiocytes, eosinophils, and plasma cells.

Epi—There are bimodal peaks at two age ranges: in the 20s and >50s. There is an annual incidence of 8000 cases.

P—The tumors are of B-cell origin. Classically, lymphadenopathy initially involves a single lymphoid area followed by orderly spread to contiguous lymph nodes. Widespread dissemination suggests that the disease is aggressive/late in its course.

SiSx—Commonly present is a painless mass, usually in the neck, or an asymptomatic mediastinal mass found on chest X-ray. The patient may have constitutional ("B") symptoms as well (fevers weight loss, sweats, pruritis). Other findings are rare.

Dx—Diagnosis is usually made by biopsy of available tissue or lymph node excision, demonstrating the classic owl-eye RS cells (see Figure 10-1), which are giant multinucleated cells seen under LM. They can also be seen in

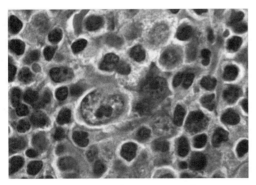

Figure 10-1. The Reed Sternberg Cell.

Note: the giant multinucleated cell seen under light microscopy toward the middle of the figure. Courtesy of Dale Frank, M.D., Hospital of the University of Pennsylvania.

Table 10-16. Stages of Hodgkin's Disease

Stage		10-Year Survival
I	One lymph node area	80%
II	Two lymph node areas, same side of diaphragm	80%
III	Two lymph node areas, both sides of diaphragm	50–60%
IV	Bone marrow or other extranodal involvement, disseminated	50–60%

other conditions, however, such as infectious mononucleosis; hence, other clinical features are needed. Fine needle aspiration of a lymph node is not usually adequate for diagnosis. Staging is primarily clinical, using the Ann Arbor classification scheme shown in Table 10-16. Letters added to the stage are "A" if there are no constitutional symptoms and "B" if constitutional symptoms exist, specifically fevers, night sweats, and unintentional weight loss >10% within 6 months.

Tx—Radiation therapy or a short course of chemotherapy plus radiation therapy is given for early-stage, low-risk disease. Later stages are commonly treated with full-course chemotherapy such as ABVD (adriamycin, bleomycin, vincristine, dacarbazine), among others. Autologous bone marrow transplant can cure patients who fail to respond to initial therapy or relapse. The prognosis is worst in those who are older or who have mixed-cellularity or lymphocyte-depleted types of tumors. The lymphocyte-predominant type has the best prognosis (>70% cure rate) even with disseminated disease.

Non-Hodgkin's Lymphoma (NHL)

D—A large group of cancers that involve both B lymphocytes (90% of cases) and T lymphocytes (10% of cases) with varying presentations and prognoses. Some forms have overload with specific leukemias. The most common types of NHL are classified roughly as shown in Table 10-17.

Epi—Overall, there are 50,000 cases per year. There is an increasing incidence of diffuse large cell lymphoma.

Table 10-17.   Classification of Non-Hodgkin's Lymphoma

Common B-Cell Lymphomas (% of total)	Comments
Small Lymphocytic Lymphoma (SLL) (6%) (*indolent*)	This is the lymphoma form of CLL; they are considered to be the same disease but at different stages.
Marginal Zone Lymphomas (5%) (*indolent*)	• Includes three types: (1) nodal marginal zone lymphoma, (2) extranodal MALT, and (3) splenic marginal zone lymphomas. • Most common extranodal MALT lymphoma is that of the stomach. Some are associated with inflammatory (*Helicobacter pylori*)/autoimmune conditions (Sjögren's syndrome, Hashimoto's thyroiditis).
Mantle Cell Lymphoma (6%) (*indolent*)	• Median age of occurrence is 60–65 years; usually widespread at time of diagnosis; 50% of patients are alive at 3 years. • 70% have a characteristic chromosomal translocation: t(11;14), cyclin D1, and immunoglobulin heavy-chain genes. • High relapse rate with subsequently more aggressive behavior
Diffuse Large B-Cell Lymphoma (30%) (*aggressive*)	• Most common type in the United States and worldwide. Caucasian patients outnumber African Americans. • Neck and abdomen are common sites. Potentially curable with chemotherapy, with 40% long-term disease-free survival in all those presenting with the disease. • In cases of posttransplant lymphoproliferative disorder EBV is strong associated with this entity.
Follicular Lymphoma (25%) (*aggressive*)	• Neoplasia of follicular center B cells. Female patients outnumber males. • Abdominal disease common; CNS disease rare. There is 40% 5- year disease-free survival with treatment. • In about 85%, the t(14,18) translocation causes bcl-2 overexpression and protection from apoptosis.
Precursor B-Cell Lymphoblastic Lymphoma (rare) (*highly aggressive*)	This is the lymphoma form of precursor B-cell ALL and is considered the same disease with a different presentation.

Burkitt's Lymphoma (3%) (*highly aggressive*)	• Three forms are recognized:
	  1. Endemic (African), presenting with jaw/facial bone tumors, strongly associated with EBV infection.
	  2. Sporadic (more common in the United States; presents mainly with abdominal masses, ascites).
	  3. Immunodeficiency associated.
	• Limited disease forms have a 90% cure rate in adults with chemotherapy alone.
	• c-myc protooncogene translocation occurs [most commonly t(8;14)], causing overexpression and malignant transformation.

Common T cell lymphomas	Comments
Cutaneous T-Cell Lymphoma (CTCL) (*Mycosis fungoides* and Sézary syndrome) (*indolent*)	• Heterogeneous group of lymphomas involving the skin primarily. African Americans > Caucasians > Asians. *M. fungoides* is most common variant (50%), and Sezary syndrome is an end-stage variant. Cutaneous lymphocyte antigen (CLA) expression helps infiltrate the skin. • Can present with dermatitis unresponsive to therapy. • More skin involved = more likely to have extracutaneous disease. • Cure is rare and is possible only in the early course. Most patients die of infection.
Anaplastic Large Cell Lymphoma (*aggressive*)	• More common in children and adolescents. Presents with advanced disease. • The t(2,5) translocation of nucleophosmin and a tyrosine kinase gene make the new fusion protein p80 in 50% of cases.
Peripheral T-Cell Lymphoma (*aggressive*)	• Considered a wastebasket term for otherwise undesignated T-cell lymphoma. Occurs mostly in lymph nodes. Accounts for 50% of cases of T-cell lymphoma.
Adult T-Cell Leukemia/ Lymphoma (*highly aggressive*)	• Highest incidence in Japan, the Caribbean, tropical Africa, and South America. • Associated with HTLV-1 infection that is transmitted by sexual and blood-borne routes.
Precursor T-Lymphoblastic NHL (*highly aggressive*)	• Lymphomatous presentation of pre-T-ALL. • Typically seen in teenage boys and young adult men; often presents with aggressive and bulky anterior mediastinal masses.

RF—People with HIV, transplant patients, and other immunosuppressed individuals have a much higher risk. Epstein-Barr virus has been linked to Burkitt's lymphoma, a disease found in Africa. Human T-cell lymphoma/leukemia virus-1 (HTLV-1) is associated with T-cell lymphoma in Japan and the Caribbean. In the United States, Caucasians outnumber African Americans for most lymphomas. An increased incidence is seen in farmers, gardeners, and certain industrial exposures such as organophosphates.

SiSx—Most patients are asymptomatic and have painless lymphadenopathy. Twenty percent have B-type symptoms of fever, night sweats, and/or weight loss. Indolent lymphomas can have waxing and waning lymphadenopathy, but persistent nodal enlargement is more common. Depending on the sites of involvement, some patients may present with abdominal pain or fullness (common with Burkitt's lymphoma, which tends to involve the abdomen).

Dx—The blood smear is normal unless the lymphoma has a leukemia phase or involves extensive marrow replacement. A CT scan of the abdomen or pelvis with contrast can identify suspicious lesions. Bone marrow biopsy, excisional lymph node biopsy, or biopsy of the tissue is needed for diagnosis. Fine needle aspirates of lymph nodes should be avoided due to their poor specificity, similar to that in Hodgkin's disease. Additional tests include flow cytometry, cytogenetic studies, and specific studies looking for classic gene rearrangements, as mentioned in Table 10-17. All patients with neurologic symptoms should have a MRI scan of the brain and CSF analysis.

Tx—Treatment varies widely, based on the type and distribution of disease, and involves either single or combination chemotherapy with radiation therapy as well as bone marrow transplant in certain cases. Intrathecal chemotherapy may be needed for CNS prophylaxis with aggressive lymphomas. There are many common regimens of chemotherapy, including R-CHOP [rituxan, cyclophosphamide, hydroxydaunomycin (doxorubicin),

Oncovin (vincristine), and prednisone], used commonly for diffuse large B-cell lymphoma. Radiation therapy can be curative in selected localized disease. Lymphoblastic lymphoma, Burkitt's lymphoma, and other highly aggressive NHLs require even more aggressive chemotherapy regimens. For the prognosis, the Ann Arbor staging system for Hodgkin's lymphoma can be used, although is not ideal. Survival is highly variable and largely dependent upon tumor histology and clinical aggressiveness.

Chronic Myelogenous Leukemia (CML)

D—Condition of proliferation of mature myeloid cells, predominantly neutrophils. It has a triphasic course that marks increasing disease severity, as shown in Table 10-18.

Epi—It accounts for 15–20% of adult leukemia. The incidence is 1/100,000. The median age of occurrence is 50 years.

P—The pathophysiology is linked directly to the initial causative mutation in a myeloid stem cell: formation of the so-called *Philadelphia chromosome (PhCr)*, which is a fusion protein formed from the translocation (t9;22) that forms the fusion protein BCR-ABL. BCR-ABL has novel oncogenic tyrosine kinase properties that can transform normal cells into proliferative states and perhaps also delay apoptosis. Acquisition of additional mutations causes the accelerated and blast crisis phases. Commonly seen are trisomy 8, trisomy 19, and duplication of the PhCr in these phases.

RF—No risk factors are known except perhaps radiation exposure.

SiSx—One-half of these lesions are asymptomatic and are discovered on routine blood tests. Otherwise, patients may have B-type symptoms, abdominal fullness (up to 75% have splenomegaly), and bleeding from thrombocytopenia, which is more common in the accelerated and blast crisis phases.

Dx—In addition to the clinical findings described above, and bone marrow biopsy and smear (Figure 10-2) showing proliferation of mature myeloid cells, demonstration of t(9;22) (Philadelphia chromosome) by

Table 10-18.   Triphasic Course of Chronic Myelogenous Leukemia

Chronic Stable	Accounts for 85% at diagnosis; the most indolent form; >95% responsive to BCR-ABL inhibitors (e.g., imatinib, Gleevec).
Accelerated	Neutrophil differentiation is further impaired. Escalating WBC levels are harder to control with chemotherapy.
Blast Crisis	Resembles either ALL or AML in nature. Prior to the use of BCR-ABL kinase inhibitors, blast crisis was expected to occur 3–5 years after diagnosis of the chronic stable phase and up to 18 months after onset of the accelerated phase. It will occur in almost all untreated patients. Transformation to blast crisis is very rare in the setting of chronic phase disease, provided that a complete cytogenetic response to BCR-ABL kinase inhibitors is achieved and maintained with ongoing therapy.

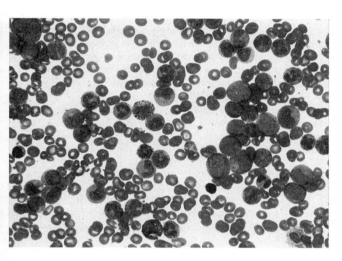

Figure 10-2. Peripheral Smear of Chronic Myelogenous Leukemia. Note the large number of mature myeloid cells, which are much larger than the RBCs on this slide. Courtesy of Dale Frank, M.D., Hospital of the University of Pennsylvania.

classical cytogenetics or fluorescent *in situ* hybridization (FISH) or reverse transcriptase-PCR (RT-PCR) detection of the BCR-ABL fusion gene's transcript confirms the diagnosis. There may also be low leukocyte alkaline phosphatase (LAP) activity in the circulating neutrophils in the chronic phase. The blastic phase is defined by (1) >20% of blasts in the peripheral blood smear or bone marrow biopsy, (2) large foci of blasts in the bone marrow biopsy, (3) extramedullary blastic infiltrates, and (4) clonal evolution [development of additional cytogenetic abnormalities in addition to t(9;22)].

Tx—Regardless of the treatment modality, extended survival is not expected in the absence of a complete cytogenetic response. Among those who receive an allogeneic transplant, complete molecular clearance

(e.g., undetectable BCR-ABL by RT-PCR) is a predictor of cure. A poor prognosis is classically associated with increased age, a higher percentage of blasts, a platelet count >700,000/μL, an enlarged spleen, and extreme eosinophilia and basophilia. In the current therapeutic era, the best predictor of survival is the initial response to imatinib. Patients who fail to achieve a complete cytogenetic response to imatinib within 12–18 months have a substantially higher risk of blastic transformation than those who achieve a complete cytogenetic response. Treatment options vary based on the patient's age and comorbid conditions, and on the mortality associated with each type of treatment. The different options are presented in Table 10-19.

Table 10-19. Treatment Options for Chronic Myelogenous Leukemia

Oral tyrosine kinase inhibitors including first-generation (imatinib) and second-generation (nilotinib and dasatinib) agents	• These drugs are the treatment of choice in the majority of patients with newly diagnosed CML in the chronic phase. Most patients respond to them initially. However, they do not cure the disease. Disease status needs to be frequently monitored to detect (1) lack of a significant initial response (primary resistance) or (2) failure of therapy after the initial response. This involves frequent laboratory tests and quantitative RT-PCR or FISH on the peripheral blood. Bone marrow cytogenetic studies are done in patients when peripheral blood FISH is 0–5% positive or every 18–24 months in those with a complete cytogenetic response. In those with a response, the drug is continued indefinitely. • These drugs are also used in patients with blast crisis. In lymphoid blast crisis, they are used in conjunction with combination chemotherapy. In myeloid blast crisis, they are preferred over stem cell transplantation as the initial therapy to attempt to return the patient to an earlier phase; thereafter, stem cell transplantation can be attempted.
Hematopoietic stem cell transplant	The only option that offers the chance of a cure; however, it carries the risk of significant morbidity and mortality. Can be considered in young individuals with CML who have a suitably matched sibling donor. Many patients and clinicians still opt to use an oral tyrosine kinase inhibitor first and stem cell transplant later if there is no response or if the accelerated or blast crisis phase has been reached. The mortality rate in young patients with fully matched HLA donors is 10–20%. Five-year overall survival is 60–80% compared to 90% in those treated with imatinib.
Chemotherapy as bridge to stem cell transplant	Used in accelerated or blast phases along with tyrosine kinase inhibitors with the goal of doing a stem cell transplant at some point.
Oral agents: hydroxyurea	Used rarely as a palliative adjunct in older patients with many comorbid conditions.

Chronic Lymphocytic Leukemia (CLL)

D—An indolent disease involving progressive accumulation of mature and monoclonal but functionally incompetent lymphocytes identical to the mature peripheral small lymphocytic lymphoma (SLL), an indolent type of NHL. The two conditions are just at different stages, one leukemia and the other tissue infiltration of the same cells.

Epi—It is the most common leukemia in Western countries. Thirty-one percent of all leukemias in the United States are CLL. This disease accounts for 1% of all cancers. The male:female patient ratio is 1.7:1. There is a higher incidence among Caucasians. In the United States, the incidence is 7,000 cases per year. It is a disease of the elderly; the median age of diagnosis is 70. The incidence is lower in Asian countries.

P—Ninety-five percent of cases are B-cell CLL; 5% are T-cell CLL with a different clinical course.

RF—No risk factors have been identified.

SiSx—Eighty percent of patients commonly present with lymphadenopathy, which can be large or small. Cervical, supraclavicular or axillary lymphadenopathy is most commonly seen. Splenomegaly, usually painless, is seen in 25–50% of patients. Hepatomegaly is seen less often, with small or moderate enlargement. The WBC count >100,000 in 30% of patients. Anemia and thrombocytopenia may also be seen. Twenty-five percent of patients have no symptoms and are found to have an abnormal WBC count on routine laboratory tests. Twenty percent present with B-type symptoms (weight loss, fevers, night sweats, extreme fatigue). Some may present with immunodeficiency complications such as infection. The skin is the most common nonlymphoid organ involved, but this involvement is seen in less than 5% of cases. Meningeal involvement is rare. High viscosity resulting from elevated WBC counts is not an issue compared to AML. ZAP-70 overexpression is associated with lack of somatic hypermutation in malignant cells and suggests clinically more aggressive disease.

Dx—There are three categorical requirements:

1. An absolute lymphocyte count >10,000 with mostly mature small lymphocytes sustained over at least 4–6 weeks.
2. Normocelluar to hypocellular bone marrow, with lymphocytes accounting for >30% of cells.
3. Lymphocyte phenotyping showing monoclonality of B-type lymphocytes.

Otherwise, the smear may show classic smudged WBCs because of their fragility (Figure 10-3). The bone marrow biopsy shows three types of bone marrow infiltration: nodular, interstitial, and diffuse. A diffuse pattern indicates a worse prognosis and more advanced disease. Biopsy of a lymph node shows a diffusely effaced node with naked germinal centers. The infiltrate consists of many mature small lymphocytes with prolymphocytes and paraimmunoblasts. Two staging systems are used, Rai and Binet, as shown in Table 10-20A and B. Many patients live for 5–10 years with a benign initial course; the terminal phase is due to complications of morbidity and therapy. Malignant transformation into another lymphoproliferative disease can occur, as shown in Table 10-21.

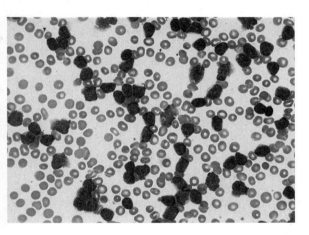

Figure 10-3. Peripheral Smear of Chronic Lymphocytic Leukemia.
Note the large number of mature lymphocytes that have very little clear cytoplasm. They are slightly larger than the RBCs on this slide. Courtesy of Dale Frank, M.D., Hospital of the University of Pennsylvania.

Table 10-20A. Binet Staging System for Chronic Lymphocytic Leukemia

A	Fewer than three involved lymphoid sites
B	Three or more involved lymphoid sites
C	Anemia and thrombocytopenia

Table 10-20B. Rai Staging System for Chronic Lymphocytic Leukemia

Stage	Feature	% at Diagnosis	Survival
0	Lymphocytosis only	25%	150 months
1–2	Lymphadenopathy, organomegaly	50%	71–101 months
3–4	Anemia, thrombocytopenia	25%	9 months

Table 10-21. Secondary Lymphoproliferative Disorders Complicating Chronic Lymphocytic Leukemia

Prolymphocytic Leukemia	Cells change to large ones with distinct nucleoli and less dense chromatin. Associated with refractoriness to chemotherapy. Seen in up to 10%.
Richter's Transformation	NHL, especially the diffuse large B-cell type, usually with sudden clinical deterioration and increased worsening of symptoms. There may be an elevated LDH, progressive lymphadenopathy, and monoclonal gammopathy. This is seen in 3% of cases. More rarely, there can be transformation to Hodgkin's disease.
Acute Myelogenous Leukemia	More likely due to chemotherapy rather than clonal progression of the disease itself.

Tx—Some patients with early-stage CLL need no treatment until symptoms begin, either (1) B-like symptoms, (2) the presence of anemia and thrombocytopenia, (3) rapidly progressing disease with increasing lymphocytosis and a doubling time <6 months, or (4) rapidly enlarging nodes, spleen, and liver. There is no evidence that CLL can be cured with any therapy except hematopoietic stem cell transplantation. The mainstay, therefore, is chemotherapy for symptomatic patients or those with rapidly progressing disease. Fludarabine-containing regimens (an purine analogue), often with rituximab (antibody to CD20 found on B cells), are most commonly employed in younger patients and alkylator-based regimens are typically used in less fit or older patients.

Acute Myelogenous Leukemia (AML)

D—A disease of myeloid lineage characterized by a clonal proliferation of myeloid precursors that cannot differentiate into more mature forms. Accumulation of leukemia cells in the bone marrow can lead to reduction in other cell lines; they can also cause pathology by accumulating in other tissue.

RF—A history of myeloproliferative neoplasm or myelodysplastic syndrome is a risk factor. Others include exposure to chemic solvents, insecticides, or petroleum products, previous cytotoxic therapy and radiation therapy for another disorder (secondary AML), Down syndrome, Fanconi anemia, and similar inherited defective DNA repair disorders.

P—The exact cause is unknown, but there are multiple genetic mutations associated with various forms. In general, the disease can be seen 5–7 years after treatment with alkylating agents or radiation therapy. Myelodysplasia is seen first, followed by marrow failure and pancytopenia. Half of such patients with therapy-related myelodysplastic syndrome (MDS) evolve to AML in 6 months; median survival is 8 months. Those treated with topoisomerase inhibitors have another type of AML that rarely features antecedent MDS and occurs with a much shorter latency period.

Common translocations include:

t(8:21)—the most frequent abnormality in children with AML, which causes the *AML1/ETO* gene fusion. Bone marrow eosinophilia, auer rods, and indented nuclei are commonly seen. It has a favorable prognosis.

Inv(16)—causes the CBFb/MYH11 gene fusion and is associated with extramedullary blast collections (often in gingiva or lymph nodes), dysplastic marrow, eosinophilia, and myelomonocytic blast morphology (M4Eo). It has a favorable prognosis.

t(15:17)—is highly specific for acute promyelocytic leukemia (APL) and is not found in any other type of leukemia or solid tumor. It forms a fusion of the PML and RARα (retinoic acid receptor gene) genes that causes reduced sensitivity to retinoic acid leading to persistent transcriptional repression. Pharmacologic doses of all-trans retinoic acid, used in treatment, can overcome this repression. Disease presents with profound bleeding tendencies due to DIC. It has the highest cure rate of any adult leukemia (approximately 80%).

SiSx—In patients who are symptomatic, the following may be seen:

Heme (usually due to cytopenias).

Anemia—fatigue, weakness, orthostasis, tachycardia.

Thrombocytopenia—ecchymoses, epistaxis, menorrhagia, gingival bleeding, poor wound healing.

Neutropenia—despite leukocytosis from circulating leukemic blasts, patients are frequently profoundly neutropenic and present with systemic infections related to lack of phagocytes.

Hyperleukocytosis/leukostasis (WBC counts >100,000 from excess blasts are seen)—in patients with many blasts cells, vascular sludging can occur as well as a hyperviscosity syndrome. Certain forms of AML (more common in M4/M5) can present with granulocytic sarcoma, which occurs when there is extramedullary leukemia, that usually deposits in the skin or gingival, where infiltration of leukemia cells occurs. Infiltration of many solid tissues causes organ dysfunction.

Palpable adenopathy is uncommon, as is an enlarged liver or spleen. If either condition is seen, consider ALL or evolution of AML from a prior disorder such as CML in blast crisis.

Pulmonary—WBC infiltration can lead to hypoxia.

CNS—Much less common than with ALL, but can cause increased ICP presenting with headache, lethargy, and occasionally cranial nerve deficits (more common in M4 or M5 patients). It is associated with higher mortality.

Renal—renal failure, especially in the setting of rapid cell turnover with elevated WBC levels.

Eye—hemorrhages or exudates in many patients.

Bone pain may occur, most commonly in the long bones.

Dx—Generally, diagnosis is made by the bone marrow biopsy specimen sent for pathologic studies, flow cytometry, and cytogenetic analysis. Technically, all three of the following are needed to make the diagnosis:

1. Infiltration of the bone marrow with blasts making up >20% of the cells visualized on bone marrow biopsy.
2. Blasts must be of the myeloid line, usually seen via cytochemical and immunophenotyping studies. The peripheral blood smear can be helpful if it shows classic Auer rods (see Figure 10-4), which are seen only in malignant myeloblasts.
3. The disease fits into one of the classification schemes shown in Table 10-22 for reference. The important things to note are that M2 and M4 forms of AML are the

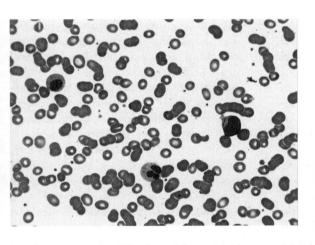

Figure 10-4. Peripheral Smear of Acute Myelogenous Leukemia.
Note the Auer rods in the myeloid cell in the right middle portion of the figure. Courtesy of Dale Frank, M.D., Hospital of the University of Pennsylvania.

Table 10-22. Classification of Acute Myelogenous Leukemia

FAB Classification	Associated Cytogenetics	Frequency (%)	Characteristics
M0		3	AML, minimally differentiated
M1		19	AML without maturation
M2	t(8:21)	30	AML with maturation
M3	t(15:17): (PML/ RAR-α)	7	Acute promyelocytic leukemia (APL) Treatable with all-trans retinoic acid Associated with hypercoagulability
M4	Inv(16) or t (6:16)	23	Acute myelomonocytic leukemia (AMML); variant is AMML with abnormal eosinophils
M5		12	Acute monoblastic leukemia subtypes: 1. Poorly differentiated (M5a) 2. Differentiated (M5b)
M6		3	Acute erythroleukemia
M7		3	Acute megakaryoblastic leukemia

most common and M3 AML has a specific treatment based which is based on the associated cytogenetic abnormality.

Without CNS symptoms, doing an LP is not necessary, though the CNS can be a site of occult disease (especially in M4/M5 AML).

Tx

Acute treatment: Any acute symptoms must be treated immediately. Symptoms resulting from leukocytosis require rapid cytoreduction with either chemotherapy (e.g., hydroxyurea) or leukapheresis. Tumor lysis syndrome and DIC are always concerns during initial therapy, especially with a bulky tumor burden. Disseminated intravascular coagulation can occur in all subtypes but is more likely to be clinically significant in APL. The decision to treat the stable patient is based on the patient's age and the ability of the patient with other comorbid conditions to tolerate treatment.

Chronic treatment: This occurs in several phases. In *induction,* the first phase, chemotherapy is designed to reduce the number of leukemic cells from $>10^{12}$ to below the cytologically detectable level of 10^9. The most common remission induction regimen is continuous infusion of cytarabine (an antimetabolite that inhibits DNA synthesis) for 7 days plus daunorubicin (an anthracycline) for the first 3 days (the so-called 7 + 3 regimen). If it works, this is called *complete remission,* defined by normal bone marrow biopsy that shows no blasts cell clusters, trilineage hematopoiesis, and normalization of peripheral neutrophil and platelet counts. From 60% to 80% of patients may achieve a complete remission, especially if they have favorable prognostic factors. After induction therapy, either *consolidation* therapy with further rounds of chemotherapy is given or patients are treated with hematopoietic stem cell transplantation. Different chemotherapy regimens are used for consolidation or for those who relapse or fail induction. Acute promyelocytic leukemia is different in that it can be cured with less intensive chemotherapy plus all-trans retinoic acid, which causes differentiation of promyelocytes.

Acute Lymphoblastic Leukemia (ALL)

D—A malignant monoclonal proliferation of lymphoid precursors that replaces normal bone marrow. It is also known as Acute Lymphocytic Leukemia.

Epi—It is the most common leukemia in children and is rarer in adults. It is the most common malignancy in children under age 15 years. There are 4,000 cases a year.

P—Arrest in early development of lymphoblasts occurs, causing accumulation in marrow and rapid marrow failure from lack of normal, maturing hematopoietic elements. The disease has many subtypes and can be classified by immunologic, cytogenetic, and molecular genetic methods. These methods can identify biologic subtypes requiring treatment approaches that differ in their use of specific drugs or drug combinations, dosages of drug, or duration of treatment required to achieve optimal results. Nearly 80% of children and 40% of adults can expect long-term, leukemia-free survival—and probable cure—with contemporary treatment. Presence of the Philadelphia chromosome (BCR-ABL) indicates high-risk disease, but this can be treated successfully with regimens including imatinib and similar kinase inhibitors.

RF—Risk factors include radiation therapy, chemotherapy, pesticides, insecticides, Fanconi's anemia and similar inherited syndromes of defective DNA repair, and Down syndrome. Some patients may have had a preexisting myeloproliferative disorder.

SiSx—Symptoms are due to decreased production of normal bone marrow elements: anemia (weakness, fatigue, dizziness), neutropenia (infections, DIC, sepsis), thrombocytopenia (bleeding), bone marrow infiltration (bone pain); LUQ pain (splenomegaly) is common in ALL (and, by contrast, rare in AML). Shortness of breath, hoarseness, or chest or back pain from mediastinal masses (usually T cell-ALL) may occur. Leukostasis with a very high WBC count may cause respiratory

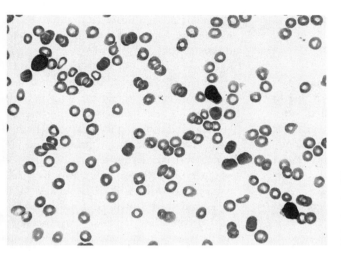

Figure 10-5. Peripheral Smear of Acute Lymphoblastic Leukemia. This is an example of T-cell ALL, which is indistinguishable from B-cell ALL by LM. Courtesy of Dale Frank, M.D., Hospital of the University of Pennsylvania.

problems and changes in mental status, though leukostasis is much less common compared to AML.

Dx—The CBC may show lowered counts or high numbers of atypical cells such as blasts that can be viewed on the smear (Figure 10-5). LDH levels may be high, along with elevated uric acid levels. The peripheral blood smear may show atypical blasts. Bone marrow biopsy is used to confirm the diagnosis. Classically, a negative myeloperoxidase stain is the hallmark. TdT is usually positive. Specific B- and T-cell markers can then be used to confirm the diagnosis.

Tx—Chemotherapy has an extremely high response rate, but relapse is common. Chemotherapy is prolonged (usually delivered over 2–3 years) but cures only 20–40% of adult patients. Induction is usually with multidrug regimens. Consolidation and bone marrow transplantation are performed in appropriate patients. Intrathecal therapy, regardless of CSF involvement, is typically done to reduce the risk of relapse as there is high risk of spread to the meninges.

Plasma Cell Dyscrasias

Monoclonal Gammopathy of Uncertain Significance (MGUS)

D—Condition involving the presence of a monoclonal protein but criteria are not met for other related conditions such as smoldering myeloma or multiple myeloma (presence of end organ damage).

Epi—It affects 1–2% of all adults; the percentage is higher in people over age 70. African American patients outnumber Caucasians.

P—The cause is unknown. Whether the condition is immune mediated or chronic inflammatory conditions predispose to its development is unclear. It is considered to be a precursor state to other conditions with monoclonal gammopathies such as primary amyloidosis, light chain deposition disease, plasma cell leukemia and multiple myeloma.

SiSx—By definition, MGUS is asymptomatic. It is picked up on routine laboratory tests.

Dx—For diagnosis, three criteria must be met:

1. Presence of a serum monoclonal protein (called an *M protein*, which is either IgA, IgM, or IgG) at a level of <3 g/dL.
2. Less than 10% cells in the bone marrow biopsy are plasma cells.
3. No evidence of related end organ damage (i.e., no lytic bone lesions, anemia, renal failure, or hypercalcemia due to the plasma cell dyscrasias).

In addition, there must be no evidence of another neoplastic plasma cell or lymphoproliferative disorder.

Tx—Watchful waiting and frequent reassessment with blood work and skeletal surveys with X-rays for progression to another disease is done. The risk of developing multiple myeloma is about 1% per year.

Waldenström's Macroglobulinemia

D—A lymphoplasmacytic lymphoma characterized by hyper-IgM production due to malignancy of lymphoplasmacytoid cells. Although IgM overproduction and marrow infiltration are similar to those in myeloma, some features more closely resemble indolent NHL (i.e., lymphadenopathy is more common than extensive bone/marrow disease).

Epi—It is a rare condition with an incidence of 0.3/100,000. The median age of occurrence is 64 years. The disease is one-seventh as common as multiple myeloma. Sixty percent of patients are male.

P—The cause is unclear; both somatic mutations and chromosomal abnormalities have been found.

SiSx—Weakness, fatigue, weight loss, and chronic oozing of blood from the nose and gums are the most common presenting features. Fever and night sweats may be present but not bone pain, as in multiple myeloma. In some patients, there is a demyelinating peripheral symmetric neuropathy that affects the lower and then the upper extremities. Cryoglubulinemia also occurs in some patients. Some show signs of the hyperviscosity syndrome with marked CNS disturbances. Fundoscopic exam may show a "sausage-link" appearance to the retinal veins in the presence of hyperviscosity. Anemia and hepatosplenomegaly may be seen. The quantity of light chains in the kidney is much less than in multiple myeloma, and cast nephropathy does not occur. Nephrotic syndrome is rare. Bleeding diathesis is secondary to hyperviscosity or coagulopathy from M-protein interactions that impair the activation of clotting factors or platelets.

Dx—Serum protein electrophoresis (SPEP) and urinary protein electrophoresis (UPEP) may demonstrate a monoclonal spike (of any size) and lymphocytic-plasmacytic infiltration of the bone marrow. Patients with IgM M protein and marrow lymphoplasmacytic infiltrates but no disease-related symptoms or significant laboratory abnormalities may have smoldering macroglobulinemia (akin to smoldering multiple myeloma) and should not be treated until symptoms develop. Although untreated, they may remain stable for long periods of time. Staging schemes use the level of $\beta 2$-microglobulin (higher stage with higher level), the amount of IgM protein, and the hemoglobin concentration.

Tx—Hyperviscosity can be treated by plasmapheresis, which will easily remove IgM. Long-term treatment to decrease IgM production includes systemic chemotherapy. Splenectomy is performed in select patients with massive splenomegaly to remove a large reservoir of immunoglobulin. Overall, however, median survival is only 5 years from the time of diagnosis.

Multiple Myeloma

D—Malignant disease of plasma cell proliferation of a single clone producing monoclonal immunoglobulins that have evidence of end organ damage (to be distinguished from other conditions involving monoclonal M proteins, such as MGUS and Waldenström's macroglobulinemia). Variants include:

1. Solitary bone plasmacytoma—a single lytic bone lesion without marrow plasmacytosis.
2. Extramedullary plasmacytomas—involve the submucosal lymphoid tissue of the nasopharynx or paranasal sinuses without marrow plasmacytosis.

Plasmacytomas are highly responsive to local radiation therapy.

Epi—It accounts for 1% of all malignant diseases and 10% of hematologic malignancies. The incidence is 4/100,000 per year in the United States. The disease is more common in men and African Americans (occurring twice as often as in Caucasians). The median age of occurrence is 65.

P—The monoclonal immunoglobulin is the M protein, usually IgG (53%) or IgA (23%); 20% of patients will only have light chains in serum or urine. The cause of the disease is unclear; it is associated with nonspecific genetic mutations. Hypogammaglobulinemia results from downregulation of immunoglobulins because of the excess M protein and the increased destruction of normal immunoglobulins through acceleration or upregulation of catabolic and clearance mechanisms. Bone lesions are caused by osteoclast activation, responding to factors made by myeloma cells, osteoclast activating factors that are mediated by several cytokines. Much calcium is liberated from bone as well as alkaline phosphatase, though little change is seen in the alkaline phosphatase level diagnostically. Excess urinary light chains (called *Bence Jones proteins*) cannot be reabsorbed and catabolized in the renal tubules and are excreted, causing proteinuria.

RF—Risk factors include exposure to toxic chemicals, radiation therapy, genetic abnormalities and a history of chronic inflammatory diseases.

SiSx—Bone pain is the most common symptom (presenting in two-thirds of patients at diagnosis), along with osteopenia and/or pathologic fractures. The pain is not like that of metastatic carcinoma, which is worse at night. This pain is worse with movement. One may also see normochromic normocytic anemia (80%), hyperuricemia, hypercalcemia, and renal insufficiency in 25% of patients caused by hypercalcemia and cast nephropathy. Recurrent bacterial infections in the form of pneumonias and pyelonephritis occur with immunosuppression. Extramedullary plasmacytomas can develop. Thoracolumbar radiculopathy is the most common neuropathologic complaint, either from compression of a nerve or degeneration of vertebrae. Peripheral neuropathy is uncommon prior to therapy. When it is disease related, it may be due to amyloidosis. Symptoms of hyperviscosity occur at paraprotein concentrations of >4 g/dL for IgM, >5 g/dL for IgG, and >7 g/dL for IgA, (see below).

Dx—The minimal criteria for the diagnosis of multiple myeloma include the following:

1. An M protein in the serum (>3 g/dL) or in the urine.

2. Bone marrow plasmacytosis with >10% of the cells being plasma cells.

3. Evidence of end organ damage from the plasma cell dyscrasia such as lytic bone lesions (as seen on X-rays), hypercalcemia, anemia, or renal failure.

If there is no end organ damage, the disease is considered to be smoldering multiple myeloma.

Basic laboratory tests may show an increased protein gap (total protein level more than twice the albumin level). Urine dipsticks that mainly measure albumin are not reliable for measuring urine light chains, but a low protein level on dipstick with a high urine protein level on SSA protein precipitation is very suggestive for light chain proteinuria. Serum protein electrophoresis shows a localized band or peak in 80%. About two-thirds of patients with serum M proteins have free urinary light chains. Those with IgM paraproteins are more likely to have hyperviscosity (50%). Among the 20% with no localized band on SPEP, hypogammaglobulinemia is seen in about one-half (due in part to suppression of normal gamma globulin production) and no apparent abnormality in the remainder. Bone marrow involvement may be focal or diffuse, so it is necessary to study multiple areas. Increased β2-microglobulin and low albumin are associated with more aggressive disease.

Conventional X-rays reveal punched-out lytic lesions, diffuse osteopenia, or fractures in nearly 80% of patients with multiple myeloma at diagnosis. The vertebral bodies, skull, thoracic cage, pelvis, and proximal humeri and femora are the most frequent sites of involvement. Bone scans are not diagnostically useful (unlike other cancers metastatic to bone).

Tx—The mainstay of treatment is chemotherapy. Active regimens include thalidomide (DNA intercalator) or its analogue, lenalidomide, in combination with dexamethasone with or without bortezomib (Velcade, a proteasome inhibitor) or doxorubicin (anthracycline).

Autologous bone marrow transplantation is done, usually in middle-aged or younger patients. Older, less fit patients are often treated with low-dose melphalan (an alkylating agent) plus prednisone. A 50% decrease in the serum or urine M protein plus clinical improvement suggests a response to chemotherapy. This is seen in 50–60% of patients, resulting in median survival of over 4 years. Treatment of the hypercalcemia with bisphosphonates is important, together with hydration and control of myeloma. Treatment of hyperuricemia with allopurinol is important as well. Plasmapheresis is the main treatment for hyperviscosity syndrome. Radiation therapy can be done for palliation of neurologic dysfunction, as well as for painful bony lesions and plasmacytomas. The prognosis

is as follows: overall, 15% of patients die in 3 months and 15% per year thereafter. There is a chronic course in some patients for 2–5 years before the development of an acute terminal phase marked by the development of pancytopenia, cellular marrow that is refractory to treatment.

CHAPTER 10 APPENDIX

Paraneoplastic Syndromes

These are condition mediated by tumor cells primarily by production of humoral factors (cytokines, hormones) or by an immune response generated against the tumor (usually via certain antibodies). Common syndromes are shown in Table 10-23.

Table 10-23. Commonly Recognized Paraneoplastic Syndromes

Organ System Affected	Condition	Classic Related Cancers	Mechanism
Endocrine	Cushing's syndrome	Small cell lung cancer (SCLC)	Ectopic ACTH secretion
	SIADH	SCLC	Ectopic ADH secretion
	Hypercalcemia	Squamous cell lung cancer Breast cancer Renal cell Ovarian cancer	Parathyroid hormone–related protein
	Hypoglycemia	Hepatocellular fibrosarcoma	Insulin secretion or insulin-like secretion
	Carcinoid syndrome	Bronchial carcinoid Metastatic carcinoid	Serotonin Bradykinin secretion
Hematologic	Polycythemia	Renal cell cancer Hepatocellular cancer	Erythopoetin secretion
Neurologic	Lambert-Eaton myasthenic syndrome	SCLC NHL	Antibodies to calcium channels
	Paraneoplastic cerebellar degeneration	Lung cancer Breast cancer Ovarian cancer	Anti-Yo and anti-Tr antibodies
	Limbic encephalitis	SCLC	Anti-Hu antibodies and anti-Ma proteins
Skin	Acathosis nigricans	Gastric cancer Lung cancer	EGF secretion
	Dermatomyositis	Lung cancer Breast cancer	Immune mediated
	Sign of Leser-Trélat (multiple seborrheic keratoses)	Gastric cancer Liver cancer Colorectal cancer Pancreatic cancer	Cytokine mediated

CHAPTER 11

Neurology

ANATOMY AND PHYSIOLOGY

The central nervous system (CNS) is divided into the brain and spinal cord. The brain is divided into the cortex, basal ganglia, thalamus, cerebellum, and brainstem. The peripheral nervous system consists of the spinal nerves, plexi, peripheral nerves, neuromuscular junction, and muscles.

Cortex

Functions of the cortex generally vary by location. Figure 11-1 and Table 11-1 show the location and functions of the major lobes.

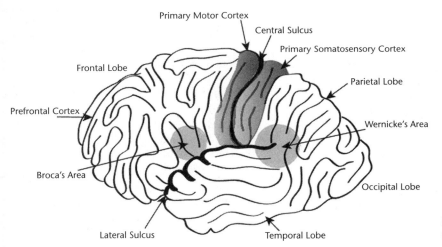

Figure 11-1.
Cerebral Lobes.

Table 11-1. Functions Associated with Cerebral Lobes

Cerebral Lobe	Key Structures	Function
Frontal Lobe	Motor area for speech (Broca's area)	Speech production (L)
	Primary motor cortex	Motor execution
	Frontal eye fields	Eye movements
	Orbitofrontal cortex	Executive function
Parietal Lobe	Primary sensory cortex	Somatosensory perception
		Attention (R)
		Integration of visual and somatospatial information
Temporal Lobe	Associative auditory cortex (Wernicke's area)	Language comprehension (L)
	Primary auditory cortex (Heschl's gyrus)	Auditory perception
		Long-term memory
	Hippocampus	Emotion
Occipital Lobe	Primary visual cortex	Vision perception and processing

R, right side; L, left side

Thalamus and Basal Ganglia

- These are two major subcortical structures that have specific roles.
- The thalamus is an egg-shaped mass of gray matter separated into two halves by the third ventricle and plays a major role in integration of motor and sensory systems by serving as a relay station to the cortex.
- Virtually all sensory systems (except for olfaction) project to the thalamus on their way to the cerebral cortex.
- The basal ganglia is a network of nuclei that modulate motor (speed and magnitude of movement) and cognitive functions of the cerebral cortex.
- The caudate and putamen receive excitatory input from the ipsilateral cortex and inhibit the globus pallidus.

Cerebellum

- The cerebellum controls the accuracy and rhythm of movements.
- The cerebellum is divided into two cerebellar hemispheres separated by the midline vermis.
- Each hemisphere receives information about ipsilateral limb movements via sensory neurons from the ipsilateral spinal cord and via motor neurons from the contralateral frontal lobe.
- Each hemisphere projects back to the contralateral frontal lobe to modulate ipsilateral limb movements.
- The vermis modulates axial movements.

Brainstem

- The brainstem is a collection of cranial nerve nuclei and axons traveling between the cortex, cerebellum, and spinal cord. It is divided into the midbrain, pons, and medulla.
- The cell bodies of cranial nerves 3–12 reside in the brainstem. Cranial nerves 3 and 4 are located in the midbrain. Cranial nerves 5–8 are located primarily in the pons. Cranial nerves 9–12 are located in the medulla. With the exception of cranial nerve 4, all of these cranial nerve nuclei innervate ipsilateral muscles or sensory receptors.

- Axons from primary motor cortex descend ipsilaterally in the ventral brainstem and cross in the medullary pyramids to innervate the contralateral body.
- Sensory axons from the body ascend contralaterally in the brainstem to the primary sensory cortex (via a synapse in the thalamus), carrying information from the contralateral body.
- Therefore, a brainstem lesion should be suspected when there is cranial nerve dysfunction and contralateral weakness or numbness. Further localization within the brainstem can be guided by the cranial nerves that are affected.

Spinal Cord

- The white matter of the spinal cord is a collection of axons descending from the motor cortex and axons ascending from the body to the primary sensory cortex (via a synapse in the thalamus).
- The cell bodies of the peripheral sensory neurons are not contained within the spinal cord but instead in the dorsal root ganglia in the neural foramina.
- Table 11-2 describes the tracts of axons based on their neurologic function, which are also shown in Figure 11-2.
- The spinal cord level is based on which spinal nerve root is projecting to and receiving axons from the gray matter. There are 30 clinically relevant spinal cord levels and spinal nerves; their names are based on where the nerve exits the spinal canal.
- There are eight cervical spinal nerves. The first seven exit *above* the vertebrae for which they are named (e.g., the C6 spinal nerve exits in the C5/C6 foramina above C6). The C8 spinal nerve exits above the T1 vertebra (there is no C8 vertebra).
- The 12 thoracic, 5 lumbar, and 5 sacral spinal nerves exit below the vertebrae for which they are named (e.g., the L4 spinal nerve exits the L4/L5 formina below L4). See Table 11-3.
- A coccygeal spinal nerve exists, but it does not have a clinical function.
- The spinal cord ends as the conus medullaris at the L1/L2 intervertebral space. Below level L1/L2, the lumbar and sacral spinal nerves

Table 11-2. Clinically Relevant Tracts of the Spinal Cord

Anterolateral System or Spinothalamic Tract	Axons convey sensory information regarding pain, temperature, and itch. These small-fiber peripheral sensory nerves synapse on neurons with cell bodies in the dorsal horn of the spinal gray matter. Axons from the dorsal horn cross anterior to the ventral horn (in the anterior commissure) and ascend in the anterolateral white matter on the contralateral side of the sensory input. See Figure 11-2A.
Posterior Column–Medial Lemniscus Pathway or Dorsal Column–Medial Lemniscus Pathway	Axons convey sensory information regarding position and vibration. These large-fiber peripheral sensory nerves do not synapse in the spinal cord but instead ascend in the dorsal columns ipsilateral to the side of sensory input to synapse at nuclei in the dorsal medulla. Axons from the nuclei in the medulla cross and ascend as the medial lemniscus contralateral to the side of sensory input. See Figure 11-2B.
Lateral Corticospinal Tract	Axons originating in the primary motor cortex (upper motor neurons) cross in the pyramids of the medulla and then descend in the spinal cord to synapse on the anterior horn of the spinal gray matter. Motor axons from the anterior horn (lower motor neurons) innervate ipsilateral muscles. See Figure 11-2C.

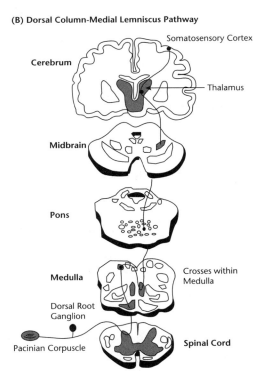

(A) Spinothalamic Tract

(B) Dorsal Column-Medial Lemniscus Pathway

Figure 11-2 (A–C). Tracts of the Spinal Cord.

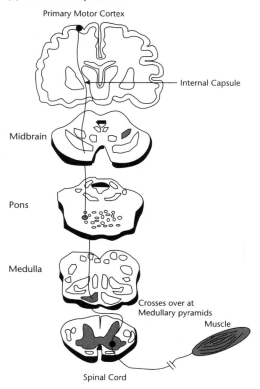

(C) Lateral Corticospinal Tract

Primary Motor Cortex

Internal Capsule

Midbrain

Pons

Medulla

Crosses over at
Medullary pyramids

Muscle

Spinal Cord

Figure 11-2 (A–C). (*Continued*)

Table 11-3. Clinically Relevant Spinal Cord Levels and Spinal Nerve Distributions

	Motor Innervation (myotomes)	Sensory Innervation (dermatomes)
Cervical Cord	C3-C5: respiration (diaphragm) C5-C6: shoulder movement, arm flexion C7-C8: arm extension, wrist extension and flexion, finger extension C8-T1: finger abduction, finger flexion, thumb abduction	C5: lateral upper arm C6: thumb and index finger C7: middle finger C8: fourth and fifth fingers
Thoracic Cord	T2-T12: trunk flexion and extension	T1: medial upper arm T4: nipples T10: umbilicus
Lumbosacral Cord	L2-L4: hip flexion and adduction, knee extension L4-L5: hip abduction, ankle dorsiflexion, inversion, and eversion L5-S1: knee flexion S1-S2: ankle plantar flexion	L2-L3: anterior thigh L4: medial lower leg and medial first toe L5: lateral lower leg, lateral first toe, and second to fourth toes S1: lateral posterior thigh and leg S2: medial posterior thigh and leg

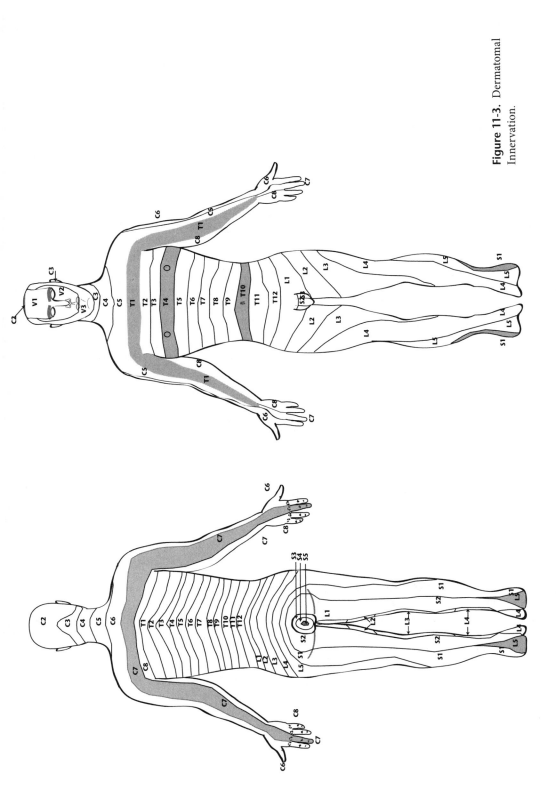

Figure 11-3. Dermatomal Innervation.

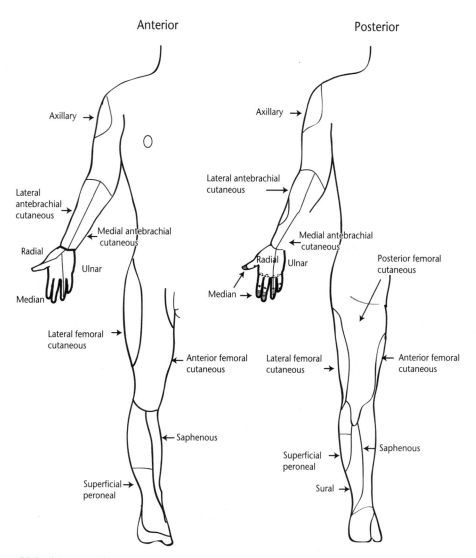

Figure 11-3. (*Continued*)

descend as the cauda equina to exit the spinal canal at their appropriate intervertebral level.
- There is a discrepancy among the spinal cord and vertebrae levels. The cervical spinal cord actually ends at the C6 level, the thoracic cord ends at the T10 level, the lumbar spinal cord ends at the T12 level, and the sacral spinal cord ends at the L1/2 intervertebral space.
- The spinal cord receives its blood supply from (1) the anterior spinal artery, which supplies the anterior horn cells, anterior lateral system, and lateral corticospinal tracts, and (2) paired posterior spinal arteries, which supply the posterior columns. These spinal arteries receive blood from the vertebral arteries in the cervical spine and from radiculomedullary branches of spinal arteries in the thoracic and lumbar spine. The thoracic spinal cord has a poor collateral blood supply, making it particularly susceptible to ischemia.
- Skin dermatome patterns are shown in Figure 11-3.

Cerebrospinal Fluid (CSF)

- The brain and spinal cord are surrounded by CSF that is produced by the choroid plexus in the lateral ventricles.
- The course of ventricular drainage is shown in Figure 11-4.
- Cerebrospinal fluid courses from the lateral ventricles to the *foramen of Monroe*, then to the third ventricle, then to the *cerebral aqueduct*, then to the fourth ventricle, then to the *foramina of Luschka* (lateral*)* and *foramen of Magendie* (midline), and then to the subarachnoid space surrounding the brain and spinal cord. Finally, it is absorbed into the venous sinuses through the arachnoid granulations.
- Obstruction of CSF drainage can cause hydrocephalus, defined as increased CSF volume.
- Two types of hydrocephalus exist. In *communicating hydrocephalus* there is improper absorption at the arachnoid granulations (e.g., due to previous meningitis or subarachnoid hemorrhage). Neuroimaging shows dilation of the entire ventricular system. In *obstructive hydrocephalus*, there is compression of either the foramen of Monroe or the cerebral aqueduct. Here, neuroimaging shows dilation of the ventricular system proximal to the compression.

Cerebral Blood Supply

- The blood supply to the brain is provided by the internal carotid arteries (anterior circulation) and the vertebral arteries (posterior circulation), which communicate with each other via the *circle of Willis*, as shown in Figure 11-5A.
- The internal carotid artery bifurcates into the middle cerebral artery (MCA), which supplies the lateral frontal, parietal, temporal lobes, and the basal ganglia, and the anterior cerebral artery (ACA), which supplies the medial frontal and parietal lobes, as shown in Figure 11-5B. The anterior cerebral arteries are connected by an anterior communicating artery.
- Prior to its termination, the internal carotid artery gives off the posterior communicating artery, which connects to the posterior cerebral artery, joining the anterior and posterior circulations.
- The vertebral arteries supply the medulla and give off the posterior inferior cerebellar arteries (PICA), which supply most of the cerebellum. The vertebral arteries join to form the basilar artery, which supplies the pons.
- The basilar artery terminates in the posterior cerebral arteries (PCA), which supply the midbrain, thalamus, and occipital lobes. The posterior arteries connect to the posterior communicating artery.

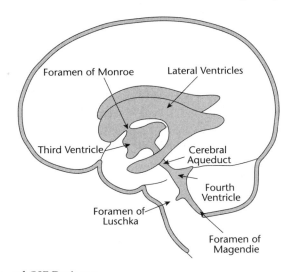

Figure 11-4. Ventricles and CSF Drainage.

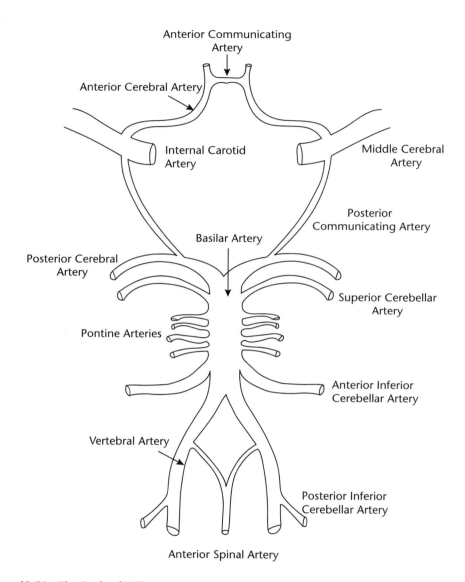

Figure 11-5A. The Circle of Willis.

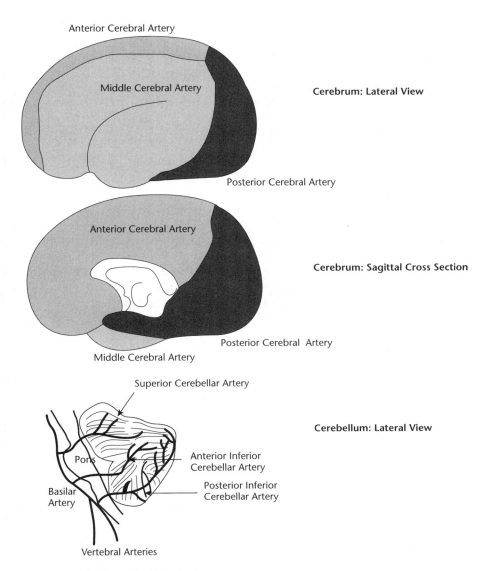

Anterior Cerebral Artery

Middle Cerebral Artery

Cerebrum: Lateral View

Posterior Cerebral Artery

Anterior Cerebral Artery

Cerebrum: Sagittal Cross Section

Posterior Cerebral Artery

Middle Cerebral Artery

Superior Cerebellar Artery

Cerebellum: Lateral View

Pons

Anterior Inferior
Cerebellar Artery

Posterior Inferior
Cerebellar Artery

Basilar
Artery

Vertebral Arteries

Figure 11-5 (B). Blood Supply of the Brain.

THE NEUROLOGIC EXAM

The neurologic exam can be divided into seven parts: mental status, cranial nerves, motor, sensation, motor coordination, reflexes, and gait. The examination is used to localize the site of neurologic dysfunction, which guides both the differential diagnosis and testing. Below, methods are described for basic neurological testing.

1. Mental Status Exam (MSE)

A well-performed MSE can provide valuable clues to localize cortical dysfunction. The basic clinical assessment focuses on the following:

a. **Level of Consciousness**—Impairments suggest either diffuse cortical dysfunction (as from an infection, toxin, or medication) or brainstem dysfunction. Test and divide into awake, arousable (to voice, touch, or a noxious stimulus such as sternal rub), or comatose based on your interaction with the patient.

b. **Attention**—Impairments are seen in delirium, dementias, depression, and frontal lobe lesions. Classically, attention is tested by asking the patient to perform serial 7 subtractions from 100 or to spell the word *world* backward.

c. **Orientation**—Disorientation usually indicates an inability to maintain consciousness or attention (delirium). In dementia, disorientation develops late in the course of disease. Test orientation to person, place, and time (date/day of the week).

d. **Language Function** (speech and writing)—This is categorized by either abnormal fluency or abnormal comprehension, which are easily tested while taking a history. Dysfunction of either category localizes to a different area of cortex (see Table 11-4 for classic aphasias). In most right- and left-handed people, language function localizes to the left hemisphere.

e. **Memory**—Present three words and ask for immediate repetition (tests attention). After a 5-minute delay, ask again for recall (assesses long-term memory, mediated by the hippocampus).

f. **Executive Function** (the frontal lobe)—This involves execution of higher-level tasks. Test by asking the patient to continue the pattern A1, B2, C3 (called the *oral trails* test). You can also give the patient 1 minute to list words that begin with the letter *F*. A number greater than or equal to 15 words is normal.

g. **Visual-Spatial Function** (the parietal lobe)—Ask the patient to draw a clock or bisect a line. Also ask the patient to identify where he or she is being touched: the right side, the left side, or both.

Neglect, a deficit of visual-spatial function, develops transiently after a right parietal stroke and can also be tested. Patients can correctly identify sensory (tactile or visual) stimuli on the left side when presented alone, but they ignore the same sensory stimuli when presented simultaneously with right sensory stimuli.

2. Cranial Nerve Examination

- The *cranial nerves* are so named because they emerge directly from either the brain or the brainstem (unlike spinal nerves, which come off of the spinal cord). All cranial nerves are named using roman numerals. A complete list of their names, functions, and testing is shown in Table 11-5 as well as in Table 11-6, which focuses specifically on the causes of visual field cuts seen with the course of the second cranial nerve.

3. Motor Examination

- Observe for atrophy (muscle wasting) and fasciculations (worm-like twitches at rest), both of which suggest lower motor neuron disease.
- Test for tone (resistance of relaxed muscle to passive movement). Spasticity is abnormal tone that increases with increased velocity of movement. For example, with the patient supine, lift the leg at the knee at different rates and observe the heel of the foot; normally, the knee bends freely, causing the heel to slide along the bed. When tone is increased, the heel will lift off the bed.
- Test the strength of individual muscle groups. These are graded as shown in Table 11-7.
  - Subtle arm weakness can be revealed by asking the patient to rotate the arms

Table 11-4. Types of Aphasia

Type of Aphasia	Characteristics	Associated Symptoms	Location
Broca's (nonfluent aphasia)	Poor fluency and normal comprehension. Paucity of speech, poor grammar, inability to write and name objects. Trouble with repetition. Able to follow commands.	Hemiparesis, hemisensory loss	Frontal lobe
Wernicke's (receptive aphasia)	Normal fluency but poor comprehension. May use incorrect words or make up words (neologisms). Trouble with repetition. This aphasia may be mistaken for delirium.	Hemianopsia	Posterior temporal lobe

Table 11-5. Summary of Cranial Nerve Function and Tests

Cranial Nerve	Function	How to Test/Comment
Olfactory (I)	Sensory—smell.	Hold out a substance for the patient to smell. Anosmia, the inability to smell, may be seen after brain injury, in Parkinson's or Alzheimer's disease, and with the Kallman syndrome of hypothalamic hypogonadism.
Optic (II)	Sensory—sight.	Test visual acuity and visual fields by four-quadrant confrontation of one eye at a time (see Table 11-6), and then test pupillary constriction. Assess for an afferent pupillary defect (APD): if one pupil constricts less or paradoxically dilates when quickly swinging light from eye to eye, that eye has an optic neuropathy. Perform fundoscopy to look for disc abnormalities, papilledema, hemorrhages, and so forth.
Oculomotor (III)	Motor—four extraocular muscles. Superior rectus (to look up), inferior rectus (to look down), medial rectus (to adduct the eye), and inferior oblique (to extort and look up). Innervates the levator palpebrae superioris, which helps the eyelid move up, and the pupillary constrictor.	Test extraocular movements (have the patient follow your finger up, down, left, and right) and ocular alignment (shine light from afar and see where the reflection of the light source is in each eye). Also test pupil constriction and check for ptosis.
Trochlear (IV)	Motor—innervates the superior oblique muscle (to intort and look down).	Test extraocular movements and ocular alignment as previously mentioned.
Trigeminal (V): Divided into three parts (V1, V2, V3)	Sensory of the face—forehead (V1), cheek (V2), jaw (V3). Motor—innervates muscles of mastication (masseter, temporalis, and medial and lateral pterygoid muscles).	Touch the forehead, cheek, and jaw. Ask the patient if he or she can feel this. In the unconscious patient, facial sensation can still be assessed by the corneal reflex. Saline or gauze that touches the edge of the cornea should cause eyelid closure. Jaw strength can be assessed by providing resistance to the chin. Jaw strength is decreased in bilateral V3 lesions or myopathy. If the jaw deviates to one side, then there is an ipsilateral V3 lesion.
Abducens (VI)	Motor—innervates the lateral rectus (abducts the eye).	Test extraocular movements and ocular alignment as previously mentioned.
Facial (VII)	Motor—innervates numerous muscles of facial expression and the stapedius muscle in the inner ear. Sensory—taste from the anterior two-thirds of the tongue. Secretomotor innervation of all salivary glands except the parotid gland; innervation of the lacrimal gland.	Ask the patient to smile and shut the eyes tightly to resist opening. All of these movements will be weak with peripheral and upper motor neuron facial nerve palsies. Forehead movement will be normal with a unilateral upper motor neuron lesion due to bilateral upper motor neuron innervation of the facial nucleus that supplies the forehead. In the unconscious patient, facial weakness can be assessed with the corneal reflex. Saline or gauze that touches the edge of the cornea should cause eyelid closure. Stapedius dysfunction causes hyperacusis (abnormally acute hearing).

(continued)

Table 11-5. (*continued*)

Cranial Nerve	Function	How to Test/Comment
Vestibulocochlear (VIII)	Sensory—sound, rotation, and balance.	Place a vibrating high-frequency (512-Hz) tuning fork in the middle of the forehead and ask the patient where he or she hears the vibration (Weber test). If the patient does not hear the vibration in the ear with hearing loss, there is a vestibulocochlear neuropathy (sensorineural hearing loss). If the patient hears the vibration louder in the ear with hearing loss, then there is an otologic disease (conductive hearing loss).
Glossopharyngeal (IX)	Sensory—taste from the posterior one-third of the tongue. Parotid gland secretory and motor innervation. Stylopharyngeus muscle (elevates the larynx and pharynx, helps swallowing).	Test the gag reflex. Even in the unconscious patient, oropharyngeal sensation can be assessed by the gag reflex.
Vagus (X)	Sensory—parasympathetic fibers to all thoracic and abdominal viscera (to the level of the splenic flexure). Motor—many laryngeal and pharyngeal muscles.	Palate and uvula elevation can be evaluated by asking the patient to say "aahh." The palate and uvula should elevate symmetrically. If the uvula deviates to one side, there is weakness of the contralateral palate. Vocal cord paralysis causing hoarseness or stridor (if bilateral) suggests laryngeal nerve injury.
Accessory (XI)	Motor—innervates the sternocleidomastoid (SCM) and trapezius muscles.	Ask the patient to shrug his/her shoulders. Weakness is associated with ipsilateral nerve disease. Ask the patient to turn his/her head against resistance. Weakness is associated with contralateral nerve disease, as the right SCM turns the head left.
Hypoglossal (XII)	Motor—innervates the tongue.	Look for fasciculations and bulk. Deviation of the tongue to one side suggests an ipsilateral XII nerve palsy.

Table 11-6. Causes of Specific Visual Field Cuts

Visual Field Loss	Localization
Entire visual field loss in one eye (monocular loss)	Optic nerve or retinal disease
Bitemporal hemianopsia (loss of the outer half of vision in each eye)	Optic chiasm disease
Homonymous field cut in any one quadrant (loss of the same section of vision in each eye)	Posterior to the optic chiasm from the contralateral optic tract to the occipital lobe

Table 11-7. Motor Strength Grading System

5/5—movement against gravity and full resistance

4/5—movement against gravity and partial resistance

3/5—movement against gravity only

2/5—movement but not against gravity

1/5—visible/palpable muscle contraction but no movement

0/5—no contraction

around each other. The weak arm will be relatively stationary, while the strong arm rotates around it like a satellite.

▫ Functional tests such as standing on heels/toes, rising from a chair, or deep knee bends can help assess leg muscle strength.

4.   Sensory Examination

- The sensory exam is highly subjective and may be unreliable in certain patients.
- Different sensory modalities need to be tested separately, as shown in Table 11-8.

Common patterns of sensory loss are shown in Table 11-9. This assessment often helps to localize the disease process.

5.   Motor Coordination Examination

The cerebellum controls the smoothness and accuracy of motion, with the vermis affecting truncal stability and the cerebellar hemispheres affecting limb movements. Tests include:

- Finger-to-nose: have the patient touch the nose and then an object such as your finger held out in front of the patient. Assess for tremor as the patient's hand approaches the target (intention tremor) and for an inability to touch the target (dysmetria).
- Heel-to-shin test: ask the patient to move the heel up and down the shin.
- Rapid alternating movements test (e.g., finger or toe tapping): assess for poor rhythm of these alternating movements (dysdiadochokinesia). Decreased speed and amplitude of

Table 11-8.   The Sensory Exam

	Example of How to Test	Possible Location of Defect
Proprioception	1. Romberg's test.* 2. Move a finger or toe up or down with the patient's eyes closed and ask the patient to state the direction of movement.	Large fibers Posterior column
Vibration	Apply a low-pitched (128-Hz) tuning fork to bony prominences; assess if and when the patient feels it vibrate.	Large fibers Posterior column
Light Touch	Touch skin with finger or cotton wisp.	Small or large fibers
Temperature/Pain	Touch skin with a hot/cold surface. Touch skin with a pin.	Small fibers Spinothalamic tract
Sensory Interpretation	1. Ask the patient to identify a letter written on the palm (graphesthesia). 2. Ask the patient to identify an object by feel only (stereognosis)	Both sensory nerve tracts and higher-level function

* In Romberg's test, the patient stands with the feet together and the eyes closed. The test is positive if the patient sways or falls. A positive Romberg's sign indicates poor proprioceptive sensation of the feet, which may be caused by polyneuropathy or dorsal column dysfunction. Romberg's test does not assess cerebellar function, as is often mistakenly believed. Patients with cerebellar disease will sway or fall with their feet together and their eyes open.

Table 11-9.   Patterns of Sensory Loss

Lesion	Pattern of Sensory Deficits
Spinal cord lesion	Ipsilateral vibration/proprioception loss (the posterior columns do not cross until the medulla) and contralateral pain and temperature loss (the spinothalamic tract crosses in the spinal cord).
Polyneuropathy	Sensory loss begins distally and ascends in a predictable fashion. By the time sensory loss reaches the knee, the fingertips have become affected (stocking and glove distribution).
Mononeuropathy—focal lesion of a peripheral nerve	Well-demarcated area of sensory loss in the sensory distribution of a peripheral nerve (not length-dependent, as in polyneuropathy).
Radiculopathy—spinal nerve root lesions	Poorly defined sensory loss because of overlap of adjacent spinal dermatomes.

these movements could also suggest disease of the basal ganglia/substantia nigra (extra-pyramidal system).

6.   Examination of Reflexes

• Reflexes test the afferent (sensory) and efferent (motor) fibers of the peripheral nerves and the central inhibition of these pathways. Commonly tested reflexes are shown in Table 11-10.

• Hyperreflexia is due to upper motor neuron disease and loss of normal inhibition.
   ◘ Movement of muscle groups that are not part of the reflex arc is known as *spreading of the reflex*. Example: striking the medial thigh of one leg causes adduction of both legs.
   ◘ Clonus, an extreme form of hyperreflexia, is a repetitive, rhythmic, and involuntary movement of the muscles tested by the reflex.

• Hyporeflexia is due to peripheral nervous system disease. Even mild dysfunction of the sensory nerve fibers may reduce the reflex, as is commonly seen in polyneuropathy. In contrast, there must be severe motor neuron or muscle disease to cause hyporeflexia.

• Reflexes are graded as follows:

   0   Absent
   1+ Hypoactive
   2+ Normal
   3+ Hyperactive with spreading to the other side, no clonus
   4+ Hyperactive with clonus

Primitive reflexes are usually suppressed in adults unless there is CNS pathology that releases this inhibition. Examples include:

   ◘ Babinski sign—Provide a noxious stimulus to the lateral sole of the foot and assess the initial movement of the large toe. Extension of the toe (up-going) signifies corticospinal tract (upper motor neuron) disease.
   ◘ Hoffman's sign—Flick the nail of the middle finger and assess for movement of the thumb. Flexion of the distal phalanx of the thumb signifies corticospinal tract disease.

7.   Stance and Gait Examination

• Have the patient walk normally and assess the distance between the feet (base), the length of the stride, the movement of the feet and legs, arm swing, and turning.

• Have the patient walk with one foot in front of the other (tandem gait).

• Common findings are shown in Table 11-11.

Table 11-10. Commonly Tested Reflexes

Basic Reflex	How to Test	Nerve Level
Jaw jerk	With the mouth partially open, tap the chin.	Trigeminal nerve
Biceps	With the arm supinated and partially flexed, tap the biceps tendon.	C5-C6
Brachioradialis	With the arm partially pronated, tap the distal radius.	C5-C6
Triceps	With the arm flexed, tap the distal triceps muscle.	C7-C8
Quadriceps (patellar, knee jerk)	With the knee flexed, tap the patellar tendon below the knee.	L2-L3-L4
Achilles (ankle jerk)	With the foot dorsiflexed and everted, tap the Achilles tendon.	S1

Table 11-11. Abnormalities in Gait

Characteristic Gaits	Description
Parkinsonian	Slow initiation/starting, narrow-based, short, shuffling steps with a tendency to accelerate (festinate), as if chasing the center of gravity, stooped posture, turns en bloc, with feet moving only in tiny steps.
Cerebellar	Wide-based, irregular, staggering, reeling (as if intoxicated).
Sensory-ataxic	Wide-based, uneven gait, with high steps and hard striking of the heel on the ground (due to proprioceptive sensory loss).
Antalgic	Favoring certain motions to avoid acute pain.

DIAGNOSTIC TESTS IN NEUROLOGY

Lumbar Puncture

Cerebrospinal fluid is obtained from the lumbar cistern (an enlarged subarachnoid space), usually entered at the L4-L5 interspace, using both right and left anterior superior iliac crests as an anatomic landmark. At this level, the cauda equina is traversing the subarachnoid space. The spinal cord terminates at the level of the L1-L2 interspace. Contraindications include an infection at the site of intended puncture and a space-occupying lesion in the brain that is causing mass effect. Interpretations of results are shown in Table 11-12 and 11-13.

Technique: The patient may sit with the legs flexed or lie in the lateral decubitus position with the legs flexed. An opening pressure can be measured only if the patient is lying down. After sterilization of the skin and injection of a local anesthetic, the needle is inserted toward the umbilicus. The needle will pass through the following layers: (1) skin and superficial fascia, (2) ligaments: supraspinous, interspinous, ligamentum flavum, (3) the epidural

Table 11-12. Interpretation of CSF Test Results

Finding	Interpretation
RBC with xanthochromia*	Subarachnoid hemorrhage, hemorrhagic encephalitis
RBC without xanthochromia	Traumatic tap
WBC: polymorphonuclear cells	Bacterial vs. early viral infection
WBC: lymphocytes	Infection (viral, fungal, mycobacterial); demyelination [multiple sclerosis (MS), acute disseminated encephalomyelitis (ADEM)]; CNS lymphoma
Elevated protein	Infection, demyelination, tumor, Guillain-Barré syndrome, advanced age
Low glucose†	Infection (bacterial, mycobacterial, fungal) or carcinoma
Oligoclonal bands	Demyelination (MS); CNS infections (e.g., Lyme disease); noninfectious inflammatory process (e.g., systemic lupus erythematosus)
Positive EBV PCR	Highly suggestive of CNS lymphoma in patients with AIDS or immunosuppression

*Xanthochromia: breakdown of RBCs with extravasation of iron content, tinting the CSF a yellow/straw color.

†The CSF glucose is decreased due to impairment of transport from the serum into the CSF (not because the organisms are consuming the glucose).

MS, multiple sclerosis; ADEM, acute disseminated encephalomyelitis

Table 11-13. CSF Findings in Common Neurologic Diseases

Disease	Pleocytosis	Protein	Glucose	Other
Guillain-Barré syndrome/CIDP*	Absent	High	Normal	
Viral meningitis/ encephalitis	Lymphocytes	High	Normal	Viral PCR +
Herpes simplex virus	Lymphocytes	High	Low/normal	Red blood cells, HSV PCR +
Bacterial meningitis	Polymorphonuclear cells	High	Low	
Multiple sclerosis	Few lymphocytes	High (IgG)	Normal	Oligoclonal bands
Acute disseminated encephalomyelitis (ADEM)	Lymphocytes or polymorphonuclear cells	Usually high	Normal	
Subarachnoid hemorrhage	In proportion to number of RBCs (1:750)	May be high	Normal	Xanthochromia

*CIDP: chronic inflammatory demyelinating polyneuropathy.

space, (4) the dural membrane, (5) the sub-dural space, and (6) the arachnoid membrane into the CSF-containing subarachnoid space. (Note: If there is blood seen while entering the subarachnoid space, be sure to collect at least 10 mL between tubes 1 and 4 to help differentiate a traumatic lumbar puncture from a subarachnoid hemorrhage.)

Indications for neuroimaging (CT of the head) prior to lumbar puncture include the following:

1. Focal neurologic deficit (including altered mental status)
2. Seizure
3. Immunocompromised patients
4. Patients >65 years old

Electroencephalography (EEG)

- Electroencephalography records the summation of electrical activity from cortical neuron postsynaptic potentials at standardized locations on the skull.
- The normal pattern is symmetric and varies, depending on the state of the patient (e.g. awake and alert, awake with eyes closed, asleep).
- Indications include:
  - Evaluation for epileptic activity (the most common reason). The sensitivity of EEG in epilepsy patients is only 50%, however, and only 30% for simple partial seizures. Sleep deprivation and continuous recording for several days may increase sensitivity to 60–80%.
  - Evaluation and management of suspected nonconvulsive status epilepticus; consider this in patients with prolonged postitcal states.
  - Titration of antiepileptic medications in status epilepticus.
  - Diagnosis of some syndromes based on classical features. For example:
    - Absence epilepsy EEG showing generalized spike and wave epileptiform discharges at a frequency of 3 Hz.
    - Creutzfeld-Jakob disease (CJD) with periodic slow wave complexes every second.
    - Subacute sclerosing panencephalitis (SSPE), a rare postmeasles infection syndrome, is marked by high-amplitude

bilateral, synchronous, periodic slow wave complexes every 4–15 seconds.
  - Monitoring for focal ischemia/vasospasm following aneurysmal subarachnoid hemorrhage.
  - Confirming the diagnosis of toxic/metabolic encephalopathies (e.g., hyperammonemia or uremia), which have triphasic waves.

Nerve Conduction Studies (NCS) and Electromyography (EMG)

- These are electrophysiologic tests of the peripheral nervous system that serve as an extension of the neurologic examination. They allow for a quantifiable assessment of peripheral nervous system (sensory neurons, motor neurons, nerve root, nerve, neuromuscular junction, and muscle) function. The findings of NCS/EMG studies must be interpreted in the context of the patient's history and examination.
- In NCS of motor nerves, an electrical stimulus is applied to the skin over a peripheral nerve and the subsequent electrical activity of a distal associated muscle is measured. In NCS of sensory nerves, an electrical stimulus is applied to the skin over a peripheral nerve and the subsequent electrical activity of a distal or proximal nerve is measured. The amplitude of the response and the speed of transmission are determined and compared to normative values.
- In EMG, a needle electrode is inserted into a muscle to assess the electrical activity of that muscle at rest and during active contraction. The amplitude, duration, and morphology of the response are determined and compared to normative values.
- Testing with NCS/EMG is useful in distinguishing the different disease processes that affect the peripheral nervous system, such as motor neuron disease, radiculopathy, mononeuropathy (e.g., carpal tunnel syndrome), polyneuropathy, diseases of the neuromuscular junction (e.g., myasthenia gravis), and myopathy.
- Clinical indications for NCS/EMG include weakness with atrophy, fasciculations, hyporeflexia, and numbness in a focal or

Table 11-14.   Situations in Which Nerve Conduction Studies and EMG Can Be Useful

Symptoms	Differential Diagnosis	Utility of NCS/EMG
Bilateral foot and/or hand numbness and weakness (stocking-glove distribution)	Axonal neuropathy Demyelinating neuropathy (e.g., CIDP)	The pathophysiology of polyneuropathies can be classified by NCS as either demyelinating or axonal. In addition, NCS/EMG can localize the type of neurons (motor, sensory, or both) affected. Both of these factors narrow the differential diagnosis.
Weakness of ankle dorsiflexion (footdrop)	Peroneal neuropathy Lumbar radiculopathy (L5) Sciatic neuropathy (uncommon)	NCS/EMG will localize the lesion, guiding management decisions.
Pain and paresthesias over thumb and index fingers	Carpal tunnel syndrome C6 radiculopathy Brachial plexopathy (uncommon)	NCS/EMG will localize the lesion, guiding the management decisions.
Proximal weakness without sensory symptoms	Myopathy NMJ* disorder	NCS/EMG will distinguish NMJ disorders and myopathy.
Bulbar weakness	Myopathy Amyotrophic lateral sclerosis NMJ disorder	NCS/EMG will distinguish LMN disease, NMJ disorders, and myopathy.

*NMJ, neuromuscular junction.

Table 11–15.   Comparison of Brain MRI and Head CT

	Advantages	Disadvantages
CT	Quick and relatively inexpensive. Certain pathologies are well evaluated and may appear hyperdense (white) or hypodense (dark). Hyperdense/white: acute blood, calcification, and thrombus. Hypodense/dark: most other pathology, including subacute infarction, demyelination, and masses with associated edema. Identification of skull fractures and herniation syndromes.	Radiation exposure Markedly worse resolution than MRI. Many pathologies without edema, including acute ischemic stroke, most demyelinating lesions, and small masses, are not well seen. Contrast: nephrotoxicity, allergic reactions.
MRI	Excellent resolution: acute ischemic strokes are easily demonstrated 15 minutes after symptom onset; previous asymptomatic hemorrhages are easily seen. Demyelinating lesions are easily identified. Brainstem is well visualized.	Time-consuming, expensive. Cannot be performed in patients with pacemakers or magnetic metal (e.g., plates, bullets). Claustrophobic patients have difficulty tolerating the study because the scanners are narrow cylinders. Contrast may rarely cause dermatologic disease in patients with renal failure.

length-dependent pattern. Such situations are shown in Table 11-14. The results of NCS/EMG testing will be normal in the evaluation of CNS disease.

- Complications are rare but may include bleeding, infection, nerve trauma, and local injury. Testing may be uncomfortable. Follow-up diagnostic studies may include nerve or muscle biopsy, genetic studies, blood studies, or neuroimaging.

Neuroimaging

Primary imaging modalities in neurology include CT and MRI. The advantages and disadvantages of each are summarized in Table 11-15. Figure 11-6 shows how to distinguish between types of MRI sequences. Other imaging modalities are shown in Table 11-16.

Table 11–16. Additional Imaging Modalities for the Nervous System

Procedure	Description	Advantages	Disadvantages
Computed Tomography Angiography (CTA)/ Venography	A spiral CT scanner rapidly captures multiple thin, overlapping sections. After IV contrast injection, images track the passage of the contrast through the vasculature.	Useful in examining carotid, vertebral, or intracranial disease such as stenosis, aneurysms, vascular malformations, and venous sinus occlusion.	Limited sensitivity in detecting small aneurysms. Radiation exposure. Patients may also need high-resolution imaging of the brain, making MRI/MRA more practical. IV contrast toxicity/allergic reaction.
Magnetic Resonance Angiography (MRA)/ Venography	The MR scanner visualizes blood vessels by detecting properties of blood (rate at which blood enters imaged area, velocity and relaxation time, absence of turbulent flow) to generate images. These images can be obtained with or without gadolinium. The sensitivity and specificity for carotid stenosis are higher with gadolinium.	Useful in examining carotid, vertebral, and intracranial disease such as stenosis, aneurysms, vascular malformations, and venous sinus occlusion. Often performed in conjunction with an MRI scan of the brain, which provides complementary information about the location of recent and remote strokes.	Limited sensitivity in detecting small aneurysms (<5 mm in diameter). Often overestimates the degree of stenosis of a vessel. Same disadvantages as standard MRI.
Angiography	A catheter is inserted into the femoral or brachial artery and passed into one of the major cervical vessels. Contrast material is then injected through the catheter, permitting visualization of the vessels.	Despite advances in CT and MRA, conventional angiography remains the gold standard for studying the cerebrovascular system. Indications include intracranial aneurysms, arteriovenous malformations, or fistulas; subarachnoid hemorrhages (SAH); TIAs to evaluate lesions for surgical intervention and/or risk stratification; vasculitis; and venous sinus thrombosis. In addition to diagnostic studies, angiography allows for interventions, such as intra-arterial TPA, intravenous sinus TPA, angioplasty or stenting of stenotic blood vessels, and coiling of aneurysms.	Complications include contrast anaphylaxis, stroke (1%), bleeding, and/or occlusion of the artery where the catheter was inserted.
Transcranial Doppler (TCDs)/ Carotid Ultrasound	Sonography uses a probe with one or more acoustic transducers to measure the difference between emitted and received ultrasound frequencies. Doppler assesses the movement of blood toward or away from the transducer and the velocity of flow.	These procedures are inexpensive and noninvasive and have a role in the work-up of both stroke and SAH. Carotid ultrasound is particularly useful for screening for stenosis of the carotid bifurcation. TCDs can screen the anterior circulation for vasospasm after aneurysmal subarachnoid hemorrhage and may help identify intracranial stenosis or occlusion.	Carotid ultrasound has low sensitivity for carotid dissection or atherosclerosis at atypical locations. TCDs are not effective for screening the posterior circulation. Both procedures are highly operator dependent.

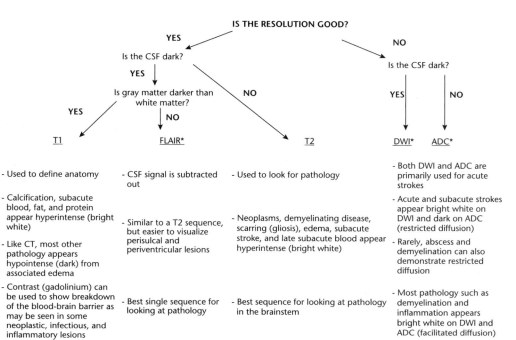

IS THE RESOLUTION GOOD?

YES — Is the CSF dark?

YES — Is gray matter darker than white matter?

YES → **T1** NO → **FLAIR***

NO → **T2**

NO — Is the CSF dark?

YES → **DWI*** NO → **ADC***

T1
- Used to define anatomy
- Calcification, subacute blood, fat, and protein appear hyperintense (bright white)
- Like CT, most other pathology appears hypointense (dark) from associated edema
- Contrast (gadolinium) can be used to show breakdown of the blood-brain barrier as may be seen in some neoplastic, infectious, and inflammatory lesions

FLAIR*
- CSF signal is subtracted out
- Similar to a T2 sequence, but easier to visualize perisulcal and periventricular lesions
- Best single sequence for looking at pathology

T2
- Used to look for pathology
- Neoplasms, demyelinating disease, scarring (gliosis), edema, subacute stroke, and late subacute blood appear hyperintense (bright white)
- Best sequence for looking at pathology in the brainstem

DWI* **ADC***
- Both DWI and ADC are primarily used for acute strokes
- Acute and subacute strokes appear bright white on DWI and dark on ADC (restricted diffusion)
- Rarely, abscess and demyelination can also demonstrate restricted diffusion
- Most pathology such as demyelination and inflammation appears bright white on DWI and ADC (facilitated diffusion)

* FLAIR: Fluid Attenuation Inversion Recovery; DWI: Diffusion Weighted Image; ADC: Apparent Diffusion Coefficient

Figure 11-6. Guide to Distinguishing Types of MRI sequences.

APPROACH TO COMMON PROBLEMS

Approach to the Patient with Acute Stroke

- Stroke is defined as the sudden onset of focal neurologic deficits caused by cerebrovascular disease and may be caused by either ischemia (80%) or hemorrhage (20%).
- The clinical presentation depends on the area of the brain involved. Common focal neurologic symptoms include aphasia, neglect, homonymous visual field deficits, hemiparesis, and hemisensory loss. Common presenting stroke symptoms and their localization are addressed in the Neurologic Diseases section under Ischemic Stroke.
- Acute stroke is a neurologic emergency carrying a mortality rate of 20%. Another 15–30% of patients have permanent neurologic disability. The outcome of ischemic stroke is primarily determined by the duration of ischemia. The outcome of hemorrhagic stroke is primarily determined by the volume of hemorrhage.
- Intravenous recombinant tissue plasminogen activator (TPA) given to patients with an ischemic stroke within 3 hours of symptom onset has been shown to double the likelihood of a complete neurologic recovery and decrease the number of patients with severe neurologic disability by 50%. There is a 6% risk of symptomatic intracerebral hemorrhage. Intravenous recombinant TPA given to patients with an ischemic stroke 3–4.5 hours[1] after symptom onset has been shown to increase the likelihood of a complete neurologic recovery by 7% with only a 2% risk of symptomatic intracranial hemorrhage. The earliest possible treatment is recommended.
- Table 11-17 suggests an algorithmic approach to the treatment of acute ischemic stroke, and hemorrhagic stroke.

[1] *N Engl J Med.* 2008;359(13):1317–1329.

Table 11-17.   Treatment Algorithm for Acute Stroke

Time	Action	Comment
0–30 minutes	Consider the possibility of stroke.	Ask about risk factors for vascular disease, such as hypertension, diabetes, hyperlipidemia, coronary artery disease, prior stroke or TIA, use of anticoagulant medications, tobacco use, drug use, and recent trauma.
	Determine the onset of symptoms.	This is key for use of TPA. If the time of symptom onset is unknown, use the last time the patient was seen to be normal.
	Airway—**B**reathing—Circulation.	As per the Advanced Cardiac Life Support (ACLS) protocol, maintain patient on telemetry and pulse oximetry monitoring.
	Perform a brief exam.	Level of consciousness? Aphasia? Neglect? Gaze preference? Visual fields? Facial weakness? Dysarthria? Arm or leg weakness/numbness? Ataxia?
	Obtain IV access × 2 and start normal saline at rate of 100 cc/hr.	Temper use of fluids if patient has congestive heart failure. Do not routinely add dextrose since hyperglycemia is associated with a worse outcome in stroke.
	Check blood glucose, basic metabolic panel, CBC, coagulation studies, and toxicity screen.	Hypoglycemia can cause focal neurologic deficits. Hyperglycemia needs to be treated. Look for thrombocytopenia or coagulopathies that can predispose to hemorrhage or increase the risk of hemorrhage after use of lytics. In a hemorrhagic stroke patient, thrombocytopenia or coagulopathies should be corrected emergently with appropriate blood products.
	Perform a head CT scan.	Rule out acute hemorrhage (hyperdensity on CT scan). If hemorrhage is not present, evaluate for early ischemic changes such as loss of differentiation of the tissue at the gray and white matter junction, sulcal effacement from edema, or focal hyperdensity in the middle cerebral artery (MCA) in the Sylvian fissure (hyperdense MCA sign). Note that an initial normal head CT scan can still be consistent with an acute ischemic stroke.
30 minutes–4.5 hours	Treat patients without hemorrhage on head CT with TPA if patient was last seen neurologically normal <**4.5 hours** ago and meets eligibility criteria.	If patient has had an ischemic stroke and is not eligible for TPA, give aspirin 325 mg. Most patients with ischemic stroke should not be treated with anticoagulants acutely.
After 30 minutes	Position the head of the bed flat for patient with ischemic stroke or elevated to 30 degrees for patient with hemorrhagic stroke.	Head positioning optimizes cerebral perfusion pressure.

(continued)

Table 11-17. (*continued*)

Time	Action	Comment
	Manage BP: For ischemic stroke, goal mean arterial pressure is <140 mmHg. For hemorrhagic stroke, goal systolic pressure is <160 mmHg. If BP is above these levels, begin titratable IV antihypertensive medication (e.g., nicardipine or labetalol) and decrease BP by <25%.	Increased BP may be a compensatory mechanism for elevated intracranial pressure. Goal BPs attempt to balance cerebral perfusion and risk of further injury. Do not augment low BP with pressors unless the patient's exam deteriorates with decreased BP.
	Maintain normoglycemia (blood glucose <150 mg/dL) with sliding scale insulin or IV insulin drip. Maintain normothermia with acetaminophen or ice. Perform infectious evaluation for fever.	Both hyperthermia and hyperglycemia have been associated with worse outcomes after stroke.
	Keep patient NPO until evaluation for dysphagia is done.	This can be performed by a trained physician, nurse, or speech therapist.
	Admit patient to ICU or floor with telemetry, depending on the severity of disease.	Telemetry will evaluate for atrial fibrillation, a common cause of ischemic stroke.
	Initiate appropriate DVT prophylaxis or GI prophylaxis.	Subcutaneous heparin or enoxaparin can be given to patients with ischemic stroke who do not receive TPA. In patients who receive TPA, subcutaneous heparin can be initiated 24 hours later. In patients with hemorrhagic stroke, subcutaneous heparin can be initiated 48 hours later. For these patients, appropriate initial prophylaxis includes pneumatic compression devices.

Important points to remember about TPA are the following:

◻ It should not be given to patients with recent major surgery (within 2 weeks), known intracerebral hemorrhage, or a recent history/high risk of bleeding from another source. Do not given TPA if the stroke symptoms are already improving significantly.

◻ Monitoring in the ICU and frequent neurologic checks are needed after the stroke, along with strict BP goals (<180/105 mmHg).

◻ Aspirin and subcutaneous heparin are held for 24 hours, at which time a repeat head CT scan is done to evaluate for hemorrhage.

Approach to the Patient with Status Epilepticus

• Status epilepticus (SE) is classically defined as 30 minutes of persistent seizure activity or multiple seizures without regaining normal consciousness. Most seizures last <5 minutes without treatment, and consciousness increases 20 minutes after seizure activity ceases.

• The presentation of SE differs, depending on the cortical location involved. Altered mental status (absence SE or complex partial SE) and convulsive activity (primary

Time	Action	Comment
0–5 min	Consider the possibility of convulsive status epilepticus in a patient who appears to be seizing.	Obtain a brief history (from family/friends if possible): duration of seizure activity, history of epilepsy, use of medications for epilepsy, alcohol use, drug use, recent trauma or stroke.
	Airway – Breathing – Circulation	As per ACLS protocol. Monitor with telemetry and pulse oximetry monitoring.
	Position on his/her side to prevent aspiration.	Perform a brief exam: Consciousness? Seizure? Focal neurologic deficits?
	Obtain IV access x 2 for fluids and therapy.	Start a normal saline drip.
	Check glucose and blood work: basic metabolic panel, CBC, drug levels, ABG, tox screen.	Hypoglycemia and hyponatremia can cause seizures. Also look for acidosis and hypoxia.
	Empirically may give 100 mg Thiamine IV then 50ml of 50% Dextrose IV.	Try to determine why patient seized: non-compliant with seizure meds? Stressor such as infection in the setting of epilepsy? If patient stops seizing, consider brain imaging in a first time seizure to look for mass/tumor/bleed. Consider an LP after brain imaging to rule out meningitis or encephalitis when the patient is stable.

⇨

Administer Benzodiazepine

Time	Action	Comment
If seizure continues		
6–9 min	Lorazepam 0.05 mg/kg IV (rate 2 mg/min IV) Repeat if convulsions persist after 5 min.	If the patient does not have IV access, give diazepam 20 mg rectally. Monitor respiratory status and vital signs to assess need for ventilatory support.

⇨

Administer Phenytoin or Fosphenytoin

Time	Action	Comment
If seizure continues		
10–30 min	Phenytoin OR fosphenytoin 20 mg/kg IV drip (rate of 50mg/min for phenytoin and 150mg/min for fosphenytoin).	Phenytoin should be given in an alkaline solution through its own line. Monitor BP during infusion, infuse slowly. If hypotension, arrhythmia, or bradycardia develop (more likely with phenytoin), decrease rate.
	Use an additional 10mg/kg of phenytoin or fosphenytoin if convulsions persist.	The goal is a free dilantin level of 2–2.5 micrograms/mL.

⇨

If seizure continues:

30 min

Order continuous EEG monitoring.

Intubate and Admit to the ICU

⇨

If seizure continues:

30–60 min

Midazolam 0.2 mg/kg IV every 5 minutes until convulsions stop (max 2.9 mg/kg), followed by 0.1 mg/kg/hr.

Propofol 1 mg/kg IV every 5 minutes until convulsions stop (max 10 mg/kg) then 1 mg/kg/hr.

Phenobarbitone 20 mg/kg IV (rate of 50-100 mg/min).

Administer Midazolam, Propofol, or Phenobarbitone

Note: this drug has a delayed clearance with renal failure.

Monitor for organ failure, infusion syndrome (acidosis, rhabdomyolysis, shock).

Delayed clearance with liver failure. Goal phenobarbitone level of 40 microgram/mL.

⇨

If seizure continues

>60 min

Pentobarbital 5 mg/kg IV (rate of 25 mg/min). May repeat if convulsions persist, then 1 mg/kg/hr.

Administer Pentobarbital

Patients may develop severe hypotension requiring pressors, ileus, immune suppression, and myocardial depression.

Figure 11-7. Treatment Algorithm for Status Epilepticus.

Table 11–18. Common Causes of Acute Mental Status Changes

Category	Examples	Clues on History or Exam	Basic Work-up	Comment
Infections	Aspiration pneumonia, urinary tract infection, decubitus ulcers, meningitis, and so forth.	Fevers, cough, increased urinary frequency, elevated WBC count. However, many patients may be asymptomatic and afebrile, especially if immunocompromised or on steroids.	Chest X-ray. Blood cultures. Urine studies. Consider LP if exam points to meningitis (meningismus, photophobia) or if work-up is unrevealing.	Treat the underlying infection. Much more common in the elderly, especially in nursing home residents. Can exacerbate mental status changes in combination with almost every other cause on this list.
Organ Failure Related	Renal failure	Changes in taste, anorexia, decreased urine output or change in urine sediment, asterixis.	Panel 7 for BUN/Cr, electrolyte abnormalities.	Correct the underlying cause of renal failure or initiate dialysis if indicated.
	Liver failure	Asterixis, features of cirrhosis and portal hypertension on exam (spider angiomata, ascites, edema), jaundice. Acute fulminant hepatic failure may not have signs of chronic liver disease.	LFTs, including transaminases, alkaline phosphatase, coagulation and protein studies. Ammonia level.	Consider a peritoneal fluid tap in anyone with ascites to assess for SBP. Treatment of hepatic encephalopathy with lactulose and antibiotics may help in those with chronic liver failure.
	Respiratory failure, hypoxia and hypercarbia	Basic vital signs will help show hypoxia. Hypercarbia should be suspected in any patient with a reason to have hypoventilation.	Urgent ABG and pulse oximetry. Chest X-ray or other imaging (PE protocol, chest CT) to help determine etiology.	Proceed cautiously in those with chronic lung disease such as COPD who live at lower PaO2. When given excessive oxygen, their drive to breathe decreases. Undiagnosed sleep apnea may also present this way.
Endocrine	Thyroid crises (both hyper- and hypothyroidism)	Thyromegaly, orbitopathy, thyroid acropathy, hyper- or hypotension. Hyper-reflexia or markedly delayed relaxation of reflexes.	Check TFTs.	Unrecognized thyroid storm can cause profound mental status changes and should be diagnosed and treated quickly. Similarly, severe hypothyroidism with myxedema coma can cause significant mental status changes. Treat the underlying condition.
	Adrenal insufficiency	Hypotension not responsive to fluids; low sodium and high potassium levels may be seen.	Consider cortisol stimulation.	Consider in the immunocompromised and those on chronic steroids. Usually precipitated by an acute illness in a patient who cannot mount an appropriate cortisol stress response.

Category	Cause/Condition	History/Assessment	Diagnostic Test	Treatment
Metabolic Derangements	Hypercalcemia	History of cancer? Metabolic bone disorder? Family history? Patient can also present with abdominal and bone pain.	Check serum calcium.	IV fluids, furosemide once the patient is euvolemic. Bisphosphonate therapy if indicated.
	Hyper- or hypoglycemia	Prior history of diabetic ketoacidosis (DKA) or Hyperosmolar Hyperglycemic State (HHS); history of insulin use.	Fingerstick glucose check.	Treat as appropriate.
	Hyper- or hyponatremia	Diuretic use, NPO with extensive free water losses. Reason to have syndrome of inappropriate antidiuretic hormone (SIADH).	Panel 7.	Treat as appropriate.
Medications	Prescription or illicit drug use (benzodiazepines, narcotics, steroids, anticholinergic medications, alcohol)	Thorough history of medications taken in the last 24 hours. Eye exam (pupils pinpoint or dilated), tremors, marks suggestive of IV drug use.	Toxicology screen. If unclear, one can assess the response to reversal agents such as naloxone.	Treat as appropriate.
CNS Related	Cerebrovascular diseases such as stroke (e.g., thalamic) Nonconvulsive SE Subdural hematoma Hypertensive encephalopathy Seizures with post-ictal states	Assess for focal neurologic deficits.	Consider brain imaging and EEG. Both tests are useful in those who remain undiagnosed. Ultimately, a brain MRI scan may be necessary.	Treat underlying conditions.
Other	Sundowning	A change in behavior at night without obvious medical illness. Thought to be due to impaired circadian regulation and changes in the environment; especially common in ICU patients.	Clinical diagnosis.	Most commonly seen in demented or elderly patients. Severely agitated patients may need physical restraints or medication.

or secondary generalized SE) are common possibilities.

- Although convulsive SE patients may cease to convulse, they may continue to have electrographic seizures as seen on EEG, manifesting clinically as persistent altered mental status.
- Convulsive SE is a neurologic emergency with a mortality of up to 25%. Another 10–20% of patients with convulsive SE develop persistent neurologic deficits. The outcome is primarily determined by the duration of seizure activity.
- Any seizure lasting >5 minutes should be treated as SE. An EEG should be done in any patient with persistently altered mental status 1 hour after cessation of the seizure to assess for ongoing seizure activity.

Figure 11-7 suggests an algorithmic approach to the treatment of status epilepticus

Approach to the Patient with Altered Mental Status (AMS)

- Most patients cannot tell you what is wrong; hence a thorough review of their history, especially medications, and a complete exam are necessary.
- Symptoms range from subtle memory changes to obtundation, and can be acute/subacute (as with delirium) or chronic (as with dementia). Major features may include impaired awareness, confusion, altered perception (e.g., hallucinations), memory difficulties, agitation, language difficulties, or any change from baseline.
- Elderly patients with mental status changes may manifest delirium as an initial sign of systemic illness.
- Chronic conditions (e.g., heart failure, anemia, cancer) make the patient more susceptible to stressors that cause delirium.
- If nonpharmacologic measures and treatment of the underlying condition do not control the delirium, typical or atypical antipsychotics may be used transiently. Consider whether constant supervision by a medical assistant is needed for patient safety.

- Common causes of mental status changes with a basic work-up are shown in Table 11-18.

NEUROLOGIC DISEASES

Vascular Disorders

Ischemic Stroke

D—Stroke is defined as the sudden onset of focal neurologic deficits caused by cerebrovascular disease. It can be ischemic (80%) or hemorrhagic (20%). If the ischemic symptoms resolve within 24 hours of onset, it is clinically called a *transient ischemic attack* (TIA). Hemorrhagic stroke can be either a subarachnoid hemorrhage or an intracerebral hemorrhage.

Epi—Stroke is the leading cause of disability and the third leading cause of death in the United States. There are 800,000 strokes per year in the United States, which account for >50% of all hospitalizations for neurologic disease. Lacunar infarcts account for 20–30% of ischemic strokes, atherosclerosis for 15–20%, and emboli from a cardiac source for 20–30%.

P—Ischemic strokes are caused by insufficient blood flow to focal areas of the brain, resulting in inadequate supplies of metabolic substrates necessary to maintain normal cellular function. This results in intracellular edema, production of toxic free radicals, and inappropriate activation of catalytic enzymes. Common causes of decreased cerebral blood flow include (1) artery-to-artery embolism of atherosclerotic plaques from either large vessels or, less commonly, small vessels; (2) thromboembolism from the heart or from venous clots that traverse to the arterial side via shunting; (3) deposition of fibrin and collagen in the vessel walls (lipohyalinosis), as seen in chronic hypertension that leads to thrombosis of small terminal arteries; this classically causes small (<1.5 cm) strokes in the internal capsule, corona radiata, thalamus, or pons (called *lacunar infarctions*); (4) direct thrombosis of large arteries (internal carotid, vertebral, and intracerebral) due to atherosclerosis at sites of arterial branching; (5) arterial dissection resulting in thrombosis of a large artery; and (6) hypoperfusion due to a combination of hypotension and chronic large vessel narrowing from atherothrombosis, causing a *watershed infarction*. Chronic thrombosis of a large artery even to the point of complete occlusion can be compensated for if there is enough time to form a collateral blood supply. Cardiac conditions that frequently cause ischemic stroke include atrial fibrillation, atrial flutter, endocarditis, ventricular akinesis after myocardial infarction, dilated cardiomyopathy, and intracardiac tumors (myxoma). Rare causes of ischemic stroke include vasculitis and venous sinus thrombo-

sis (VST). The etiology of 20–30% of ischemic strokes remains unclear (cryptogenic).

RF—The incidence of stroke doubles every 10 years over age 55. Males are affected more often than females. African Americans and Hispanics are affected twice as often as whites. Other risk factors include a family history, hypertension, hyperlipidemia, diabetes mellitus, atrial fibrillation, coronary artery disease, smoking, a sedentary lifestyle, and obesity. Patients who have had a TIA are at increased risk (10%) for ischemic stroke within 90 days of TIA onset.

SiSx—The clinical presentation of a TIA or ischemic stroke is dependent on the brain location involved. Common stroke presentations are described in Table 11-19.

Table 11-19. Common Stroke Presentations

Area of Brain Involved	Blood Vessel Involved	Clinical Presentation
Medial frontal and parietal lobes	Anterior cerebral artery (ACA)	Contralateral leg weakness and numbness Ipsilateral gaze preference
Left lateral frontal, parietal, and temporal lobes	Left middle cerebral artery (MCA)	Severe right face and arm weakness and numbness Mild right leg weakness and numbness Left gaze preference Global aphasia Right homonymous hemianopsia
Left lateral frontal and parietal lobes	Left superior division of MCA	Right face and arm weakness and numbness Left gaze preference Nonfluent (Broca's) aphasia Right inferior homonymous hemianopsia
Left lateral temporal lobe	Left inferior division of MCA	Receptive (Wernicke's) aphasia Right superior homonymous hemianopsia
Right lateral frontal, parietal, and temporal lobes	Right MCA	Severe left face and arm weakness and numbness Mild left leg weakness and numbness Right gaze preference Left-sided neglect Left homonymous hemianopsia
Occipital lobe	Posterior cerebral artery (PCA)	Contralateral homonymous hemianopsia, which may or may not spare central vision (macular sparing)
Internal capsule	Lenticulostriate branches of MCA	Contralateral face, arm, and leg weakness
Thalamus	Penetrating arteries from PCA	Contralateral face, arm, and leg numbness
Lateral medulla (Wallenberg's syndrome)	Posterior inferior cerebellar artery (PICA)	Ipsilateral loss of pain/temperature sensation on the face; contralateral loss of pain/temp sensation on the body Dysarthria/dysphasia, vertigo Ipsilateral Horner's syndrome Ipsilateral ataxia
Eye (amaurosis fugax)	Ophthalmic artery	Ipsilateral monocular vision loss

Dx—(Acute evaluation is addressed in the Approach to Common Problems section.) Differential diagnosis includes migraine headaches with focal neurologic symptoms and focal neurologic symptoms after partial-onset seizures. A brain MRI scan for an acute ischemic stroke will show hyperintensity on diffusion-weighted imaging (DWI) and hypointensity on apparent diffusion coefficient (ADC) imaging. Brainstem strokes may not be well seen on DWI but will be hyperintense on T2 imaging. Some TIAs have MRI evidence of an acute ischemic stroke, making this clinical distinction arbitrary from a pathologic perspective.

Patients with a TIA can be stratified according to the risk of an ischemic stroke within 2 days of TIA onset, as described in Table 11-20. However, a treatable etiology is identified in approximately 20% of low-risk TIA patients (ABCD$_2$ scores of 0–3); therefore, all TIA patients should undergo a complete stroke evaluation.

After the diagnosis of ischemic stroke is established, an etiology should be sought. Work-up includes the following:

1. Blood studies: lipid panel, rapid plasma reagin (RPR) for neurosyphillis, erythrocyte sedimentation rate (ESR) for systemic vasculitis.
2. Vascular imaging of the neck for large artery disease. A carotid ultrasound is a cost-effective screening test. A CT or MR angiogram of the neck can evaluate the entire carotid artery (important when a dissection is suspected) and evaluates the vertebral arteries for posterior circulation infarcts.
3. Vascular imaging of the head with a CT or MR angiogram may demonstrate intracranial large artery disease. However, this rarely changes the management and thus should be performed only when the etiology remains unclear or there is a concern about vasculitis.
4. Telemetry and an ECG are done to assess for atrial fibrillation. Consider outpatient cardiac monitoring for occult atrial fibrillation in patients without an obvious cause.
5. A transthoracic echocardiogram will assess for large valvular vegetations, left ventricle thrombus, and dilated cardiomyopathy. A saline bubble study can help assess for patent foramen ovale. If there is high suspicion for a cardioembolic source or the etiology remains unclear, a transesophageal echocardiogram should be performed to assess for left atrial masses, subtle valvular vegetations, and aortic atherosclerosis.
6. Young patients (<50 years old) without a clear etiology should have a hypercoagulable work-up.
7. If a patient presents with both hemorrhage and ischemic stroke, or in the appropriate clinical setting, consider a MR venogram for venous sinus thrombosis.

Tx—The acute treatment of ischemic stroke is addressed in the Approach to Common Problems section and Table 11-17. For large MCA infarcts, cerebral edema may be life-threatening. Hemicraniectomy has been shown to markedly reduce morbidity and mortality in these patients. Subacute and chronic therapy is aimed at preventing further strokes and includes the following:

1. Chronic antiplatelet therapy is recommended for cryptogenic strokes, for small vessel strokes, and while the patient is awaiting definitive treatment of large vessel disease. Antiplatelet therapy includes clopidogrel, a combination of dipyridamole and aspirin, or aspirin alone if cost is an issue. Clopidogrel and dipyridamole/aspirin are equivalent for secondary stroke prevention; both are slightly superior to aspirin.

Table 11-20.   The ABCD^2 Score for TIAs

Age >60 (1 point)	6–7 points: high
BP ≥140/90 mmHg (1 point)	2-day risk of 8.1%
Clinical: unilateral	4–5 points:
weakness (2 points),	moderate risk of
speech impairment	4.1%
without weakness	0–3 points, low risk
(1 point)	of 1.0%
Duration ≥60 minutes	
(2 points) or 10–59	
minutes (1 point)	
Diabetes (1 point)	

Source: Lancet 2007;369: 282–292.

Clopidogrel is better tolerated than dipyridamole/aspirin, as it is given daily and does not carry a 15% risk of headache. The combination of clopidogrel and aspirin does not provide greater benefit than clopidogrel alone, and it increases the risk of gastrointestinal hemorrhage.

2. Anticoagulation with IV heparin and warfarin is indicated in ischemic stroke caused by extracranial arterial dissection (i.e., cervical arteries or vertebral arteries), venous sinus thrombosis, basilar artery thrombosis, and recurrent stereotyped transient neurologic symptoms from large artery thromboembolism (stuttering TIA). Other indications include atrial fibrillation, cardiac thrombus, dilated cardiomyopathy with an ejection fraction <25%, hypercoagulable states, and aortic arch atherosclerosis >4 mm, especially if there is a mobile component. There is no benefit of anticoagulation over antiplatelet therapy for intracranial stenosis. Anticoagulation is typically started 7 days after the infarction, although this varies depending on the size of the infarction, the etiology, and the presence of hemorrhagic conversion.

3. Risk factor modification: a high-dose statin has been shown to decrease the risk of secondary stroke independent of the low-density lipoprotein (LDL) level. The goal LDL level for patients with an ischemic stroke is <70 mg/dL. Hypertension can be treated with hydrochlorothiazide and an ACE inhibitor or angiotensin receptor blocker, usually initiated 1 week after ischemic stroke. Other antihypertensive agents are added as clinically indicated with a blood pressure goal of <130/70 mmHg. Diabetes mellitus is aggressively managed from the time of hospital admission; patients should chronically be treated for a goal HgbA1c <7.0%. Cessation of smoking, and diet and exercise are important factors in secondary prevention.

4. Treat the underlying causes: symptomatic carotid stenosis (>70% carotid stenosis ipsilateral to an ischemic stroke in the anterior circulation) should be treated with carotid endarterectomy (CEA) or carotid stenting. Carotid stenting has not been shown to be equivalent to CEA by randomized clinical trials. Stenting of the vertebral or intracranial arteries may be performed in medically refractory patients, but these techniques have not been proven efficacious by randomized clinical trials.

Closure of the patent foramen ovale has not been proven efficacious by randomized clinical trials.

Bacterial endocarditis with septic emboli to the brain is treated with aggressive administration of antibiotics.

Epidural Hematoma (EDH)

D—Accumulation of blood in the potential space between the dura and the periosteum of the skull.

Epi—This condition complicates 1–4% of traumatic head injury cases. Skull fractures are present in 75–95% of patients.

P—Epidural hematoma is usually caused by an arterial injury. The most commonly affected artery is the middle meningeal artery as it courses through the foramen spinosum.

RF—The major risk factor is head trauma.

SiSx—Patients present with trauma and loss of consciousness. Classically, they regain consciousness for a few hours (*lucid interval*) followed by neurologic deterioration (headache, vomiting, drowsiness, seizures, hemiparesis) due to continued arterial bleeding and hematoma expansion. The lucid interval occurs in only 20% of patients with EDH.

Dx—The condition is diagnosed by head CT and appears as a biconvex (lens-shaped) hyperdensity that does not cross the suture lines of the skull (see Figure 11-8a). Lumbar puncture is contraindicated in the setting of an EDH.

Tx—Acute EDH is a neurologic emergency that requires neurosurgical intervention (craniotomy and hematoma evacuation; identification and ligation of the bleeding vessel when indicated) to prevent further brain injury and death secondary to hematoma expansion, elevated intracranial pressure, and brain herniation. Mortality is 10% in adults. Poor prognostic factors include severe neurologic deficits, the presence of pupillary

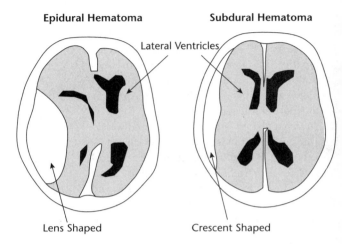

Figure 11-8. Subdural and Epidural Hematomas.

abnormalities, a large hematoma volume, a large degree of midline brain shift, and the presence of associated trauma.

Subdural Hematoma (SDH)

D—Accumulation of blood in the space between the dura and the arachnoid membranes.

Epi—Head trauma is the most common cause of SDH.

P—Subdural hematoma is usually caused by rupture of the veins draining the surface of the brain into the venous sinuses (*bridging veins*). In patients with marked cerebral atrophy, the bridging veins are stretched, making them more susceptible to rupture even from minor injury. Traumatic rupture of small arterioles on the surface of the brain accounts for 20–30% of SDH. Anticoagulation increases the risk of hematoma accumulation.

RF—Head trauma, especially in patients with brain atrophy (the elderly, alcoholics, patients with previous traumatic brain injury or dementia), is a risk factor.

SiSx—Subdural hematoma may present acutely (1–2 days after onset) or chronically (15 or more days after onset), depending on the rate of hematoma accumulation. Patients typically present acutely with focal neurologic deficits and progressive alteration of consciousness. As in EDH, 12–38% of SDH patients have a lucid interval. Patients with chronic SDH usually present with headaches, cognitive impairment, and somnolence mimicking delirium.

Dx—Subdural hematoma is diagnosed by head CT scan and appears as a crescent-shaped hyperdensity (see Figure 11-8). An MRI scan of the brain is more sensitive for smaller SDHs and acute or chronic SDH.

Tx—Acute symptomatic SDH is a neurologic emergency that often requires surgical intervention (hematoma evacuation) to prevent irreversible damage caused by elevated intracranial pressure, hematoma expansion, and brain herniation. The estimated mortality of patients with acute SDH requiring surgical intervention is 40–60%, which is likely determined by coexistent traumatic brain injury. Age and neurologic status are important prognostic factors in patients with SDH.

Subarachnoid Hemorrhage (SAH)

D—Accumulation of blood in the space between the arachnoid and pia membranes.

Epi—It accounts for 5% of all strokes. It is more common in women and African Americans.

P—Spontaneous SAH is usually caused by bleeding from a ruptured aneurysm. Less commonly, spontaneous SAH may be caused by bleeding from a vascular malformation. In addition, SAH may be caused by head trauma.

RF—Risk factors for spontaneous SAH include a family history of aneurysm/SAH, hypertension, smoking, cocaine and alcohol abuse, and connective tissue diseases (Marfan's syndrome, polycystic kidney disease, Ehlers-Danlos syndrome). Head trauma is the major risk factor for traumatic SAH.

SiSx—Most unruptured aneurysms are asymptomatic. A large aneurysm may exert a mass effect with focal neurologic symptoms, depending on its location (e.g., a pupil involving third nerve palsy from a posterior communicating artery aneurysm. Some patients develop an acute, severe, transient headache (*sentinel headache*) days to weeks before spontaneous SAH occurs. Spontaneous SAH typically presents with a sudden, severe headache ("like a thunderclap," "the worst headache of my life") as blood enters the wall of the aneurysm. As blood enters the subarachnoid space, patients develop nausea, vomiting, and nuchal rigidity. They may lose consciousness as intracranial pressure rises abruptly. Focal neurologic signs are typically absent.

Dx—In 95% of cases, SAH will be identified by head CT, demonstrating hyperdensities in the sulci and cisterns. If the head CT scan is unremarkable but there is a high clinical suspicion of SAH, then a lumbar puncture (LP) should be performed to assess for the presence of RBCs and xanthochromia. Once the diagnosis of spontaneous SAH is confirmed and the patient is hemodynamically stable, a four-vessel cerebral angiogram should be performed to locate the aneurysm and possibly intervene to prevent further bleeding (there is a 5% risk within the first 24 hours).

Tx—Initial management should follow the guidelines outlined in the section: Approach to the Patient with Acute Stroke. In aneurysmal SAH, surgical clipping or endovascular coiling of the aneurysm should be performed as soon as possible to prevent rebleeding. Following aneurysmal SAH only, patients are at risk for delayed (2 days to 3 weeks) ischemia secondary to blood vessel constriction (vasospasm). Patients with aneurysmal SAH are treated with nimodipine for 21 days to reduce the risk of vasospasm. Screening for preclinical vasospasm is performed with daily transcranial doppler (TCD) studies and continuous EEG monitoring. The definitive treatment for vasospasm is direct vasodilation of the arteries by catheter angiogram. Hydrocephalus commonly occurs after SAH and is treated with ventricular drainage. Hyponatremia (*cerebral salt wasting*) may occur after SAH and can be treated with free water restriction. The mortality in SAH is 50%, with 10–15% of patients dying prior to arrival at the hospital. Survivors usually have significant neurologic disabilities.

Spontaneous Intracerebral Hemorrhage (ICH)

D—Accumulation of blood within the brain parenchyma causing destruction of normal brain tissue and a mass effect on adjacent tissue.

Epi—It accounts for 10% of strokes.

P—The most common cause of ICH is chronic, poorly controlled hypertension, which causes fibrin and collagen deposition in the walls of arterioles, decreasing their elasticity (lipohyalinosis). In the elderly, ICH is frequently caused by amyloid deposition in the walls of small arteries (amyloid angiopathy). Other causes of ICH include vascular malformations and anticoagulation.

RF—The incidence of ICH increases with age. It occurs more commonly in African Americans. It is associated with hypertension and anticoagulation treatment.

SiSx—Like ischemic stroke, ICH presents acutely with focal neurologic deficits that depend on the location of the hemorrhage. Hypertensive hemorrhages most commonly occur in the putamen and present with contralateral hemiparesis from involvement of the adjacent internal capsule. Other common locations of hypertensive ICH include the thalamus (causing contralateral sensory loss), cerebellum (ipsilateral ataxia) and pons (contralateral hemiparesis, ipsilateral sixth and seventh nerve palsies). Anticoagulation and amyloid angiopathy usually cause lobar hemorrhages, which present with cortical symptoms such as aphasia, neglect, visual field deficits, and contralateral hemiparesis. The focal neurologic deficits worsen progressively as the hematoma expands. In addition to focal neurologic deficits, patients with ICH may have headache, decreased level of consciousness, or seizures. Since the presentation of ICH and ischemic stroke may be identical, these entities cannot be distinguished clinically.

Dx—Intracranial hemorrhage is diagnosed by head CT scan and appears as an intraparenchymal hyperdensity. Patients with ICH should be immediately evaluated for coagulopathy, with a CBC and coagulation studies. An MRI scan of the brain may be performed when the patient is stable to evaluate for previous subclinical hemorrhages in suspected amyloid angiopathy or an underlying vascular malformation.

Tx—Initial management should follow the guidelines outlined in the Approach to the Patient with Acute Stroke section. The initial goal of treatment is to minimize further hematoma expansion. Any patient with an underlying coagulopathy should be treated emergently with appropriate blood products such as fresh frozen plasma, cryoprecipitate, or platelets. Patients on warfarin should receive vitamin K. All patients should be treated with IV antihypertensive medications (labetalol or nicardipine) to reduce their systolic blood pressure (SBP) below 160 or by 15% of the baseline SBP. Surgical evacuation of the hematoma is clearly indicated in cerebellar ICH with a high risk of brainstem compression (diameter of the hemorrhage >2 cm) and should be considered for superficial cortical hemorrhages (within 1 cm of the cortex). Edema associated with the ICH peaks at 3–5 days and may cause life-threatening elevation of intracranial pressure (ICP). Intracranial hemorrhage into the ventricles may cause associated hydrocephalus, further increasing ICP. Intracranial pressure can be monitored and partially treated with ventriculostomy. Intracranial pressure may be transiently lowered by osmotic agents (mannitol or hypertonic saline) or definitively treated with hemicraniectomy. The mortality in ICH is 30–40%, with survivors usually having significant neurologic disabilities.

Venous Sinus Thrombosis (VST)

D—Occlusion of an intracranial vein by thrombus.

Epi—The condition is rare, with an incidence of <1/100,000.

P—A thrombus in the intracranial venous system may develop in the setting of vascular injury, venous stasis, and hypercoaguability (Virchow's triad).

RF—Risk factors include the postpartum period (the first 3 weeks after delivery), pregnancy (late second and third trimesters), OCP use, malignancy, local infection (e.g., mastoiditis), hypercoagulable states, and dehydration.

SiSx—The clinical presentation varies based on which venous structure is affected. Isolated involvement of either the superior sagittal or transverse sinus usually presents with a diffuse headache, which is generally worse when lying down or with straining. There may be associated nausea and vomiting. Papilledema is present in only 50% of patients. Involvement of cortical or deep cerebral veins causes venous infarction and hemorrhages, which present with focal neurologic deficits, seizures, or altered level of consciousness. Involvement of the cavernous sinus presents with conjunctival injection, proptosis, and ophthalmoplegia.

Dx—Diagnosis is made by an MRI scan of the brain, which demonstrates venous infarctions or hemorrhages, and by an MR venogram, which demonstrates an absence of venous drainage in the occluded dural sinus or vein. If an etiology is not apparent, the patient should be evaluated for hypercoagulable states.

Tx—Treatment is with hydration and acute anticoagulation with IV heparin or subcutaneous low-molecular-weight-heparin followed by warfarin for at least 3 months (permanently if the patient has an underlying hypercoagulable state). Even patients with venous hemorrhages should be treated with anticoagulation. After 3 months, follow-up MR venography assessing for recanalization will determine if anticoagulation should be continued. Antiepileptic drug therapy is recommended for at least 6 months in patients who developed clinical seizures from VST. Mortality in adults with VST is approximately 5–10%. Only 15–25% of patients have persistent neurologic deficits.

Seizure Disorders

Seizures/Epilepsy

D—Seizures are transient episodes of neurologic dysfunction caused by inappropriate synchronous depolarization of cortical neurons. They are classified into seizures that arise from a focal group of cortical neurons (partial/location related) or those that arise diffusely from the entire cortex (generalized). They are also categorized by etiology. Provoked seizures occur as a direct result of an acute illness and manifest clinically as generalized tonic-clonic seizures. Unprovoked seizures have no clear precipitating illness. Epilepsy is a heterogeneous group of diseases characterized by at least one unprovoked seizure and a persistent predisposition to future seizures (previously, epilepsy was defined as at least two unprovoked seizures). Epilepsy can be categorized into different epilepsy syndromes, which are characterized by similar age of onset, seizure types, EEG findings, neuroimaging findings, and etiology.

Epi—Epilepsy is the third most common neurologic disorder. The prevalence is about 2 million in the United States. The incidence is 44/100,000 people per year, with peaks in childhood and in the elderly. Most patients have focal seizures (partial/location related), and 12% of patients have generalized seizures.

P—Seizures are manifestations of inappropriate increased synchronous electrical activity in cortical neurons. The underlying pathophysiology is dependent on the etiology. Provoked seizures can be caused by infections (meningitis, encephalitis), metabolic derangements (hypoglycemia, hyponatremia, uremia, hypercalcemia, hepatic encephalopathy, and so forth), head trauma, and substance withdrawal (e.g. alcohol, benzodiazepines). In genetically inherited epilepsy syndromes, mutations in neuronal ion channels, such as sodium channel mutations producing prolonged depolarization or potassium channel mutations producing decreased hyperpolarization, cause hyperexcitability of neurons. In structural epilepsy syndromes, seizures are believed to be caused by inappropriate neuronal connections resulting in self-excitatory circuits.

RF—Age is a strong risk factor. Children are more likely to have an inherited epilepsy syndrome and thus a family history. Elderly patients are more likely to have a structural abnormality (e.g., previous stroke or neoplasm). Other risk factors for epilepsy include febrile seizures as a child, developmental abnormalities (CNS malformation, cerebral palsy, genetic/metabolic syndromes), head trauma with loss of consciousness, or previous CNS infection.

SiSx—Symptoms vary based on the cortical location involved and whether the seizure propagates to other areas of cortex. As a general rule, routine seizures are brief (30 seconds to 5 minutes) and stereotyped. Focal seizures are subdivided into those that affect cognition (complex) and those that do not (simple). Abnormal cognition is not synonymous with loss of consciousness; instead, it may manifest as an inability to interact during the seizure (e.g., answer a question) or amnesia for the seizure. Focal seizures may present with normal cognition (simple) or abnormal cognition (complex) or may evolve from a simple focal seizure to a complex focal seizure as the epileptic activity spreads. If the epileptic activity spreads diffusely throughout the brain, patients with focal seizures will develop generalized tonic-clonic activity (secondary generalization). Seizures that originate from diffuse areas of cortex (generalized) are categorized by their clinical manifestations. The most common generalized seizures are generalized tonic-clonic and absence seizures. Uncommon generalized seizures include tonic, atonic, clonic, and myoclonic seizures. Both partial and generalized seizures are described in Table 11-21.

Dx—The diagnosis of a seizure is usually based on the description of the event. The differential diagnosis depends on the type of seizure but most commonly includes syncope and conversion disorder (psychogenic nonepileptic spells). If the history is consistent with seizure in a patient without known epilepsy, the patient should be evaluated for an acute etiology. This evaluation often includes:

1. A CT scan of the head to exclude hemorrhage or acute stroke.
2. Routine laboratory studies, including a urine toxicology screen, glucose level, and electrolytes.
3. Lumbar puncture to exclude meningitis if the patient is febrile.

Table 11–21. Classification of Seizures

Focal (Location-Related) Seizures	Signs and Symptoms
Simple Sensory/ Psychic	Since patients have normal cognition during these seizures, they can recall and describe the purely subjective sensory/psychic manifestations that they experience. If these seizures arise from the temporal lobe, patients commonly report unpleasant odors, unpleasant tastes, nausea, vomiting, a rising epigastric sensation, fear/feelings of impending doom, and familiarity with unfamiliar places (déjà vu). If seizures arise from the occipital lobe, patients usually describe flashing colors or lights and geometric patterns in the contralateral visual field. If seizures arise from the parietal lobe, patients describe electric shock or abnormal temperature sensations in the contralateral limbs, most prominently in the hand or face due to their large representation on the sensory homunculus. These seizures are usually brief, lasting for 30 seconds, and patients do not experience postevent fatigue. These simple sensory/psychic seizures are also called *auras*. Only patients with focal epilepsy have auras.
Simple Motor	Since patients have normal cognition during these seizures, they can also recall and describe them. However, these seizures have objective manifestations apparent to an observer. They typically arise from primary motor cortex in the frontal lobes and present as slow (3-Hz), rhythmic jerking of the contralateral limb, most prominently in the hand or face due to their large representation on the motor homunculus. If the seizure spreads along the motor homunculus, the rhythmic jerking will spread to adjacent muscles (Jacksonian march). These seizures are usually brief, lasting for 30 seconds, and patients often experience postevent weakness in the involved limbs (Todd's paralysis) lasting for minutes to hours. Only patients with focal epilepsy have postevent focal weakness.
Complex	Patients have impaired cognition, usually without recollection of the seizure. Thus, the clinical description is dependent on a witnessed account. If seizures arise from the temporal lobe, patients stop any activity (behavioral arrest), stare blankly, and have purposeless movements of the mouth/tongue. Next, patients develop purposeless activities of the ipsilateral arm such as picking at their clothes. The contralateral limb assumes a fixed, stiff posture. Routine complex temporal lobe seizures last for 1–3 minutes, and patients are confused for minutes to hours afterward. Patients may also have postevent weakness or aphasia. If seizures arise from the frontal lobe, patients may have simple or complex movements of contralateral or bilateral limbs. These seizures often appear bizarre and are not followed by postevent confusion, making it quite difficult to distinguish them from psychogenic spells.
Secondary Generalized Tonic-Clonic (GTC)	As in complex partial seizures and most primary generalized seizures, patients have impaired cognition. It is often difficult to distinguish a primary GTC seizure clinically from a secondary GTC seizure. In secondary GTC seizures, the initial finding is often forced head and eye movements away from the side of the seizure followed by an involuntary scream (ictal cry) as the diaphragm contracts against a closed larynx. Tonic stiffening of the contralateral limb often begins before that of the ipsilateral limb, and the clonic jerking is usually asymmetric. Routine secondary GTC seizures last for 2–5 minutes, and patients are usually obtunded and incontinent following the seizure. Patients often experience postevent weakness in the contralateral limbs (Todd's paralysis) lasting for minutes to 48 hours. Only patients with focal epilepsy have postevent focal weakness.

Diffuse (Generalized) Seizures	Signs and Symptoms
Tonic-Clonic (GTC)	Patients have impaired cognition. The clinical description is dependent on a witnessed account. The seizure begins with 10–15 seconds of tonic stiffening of the axial and limb muscles and an involuntary scream (ictal cry) as the diaphragm contracts against a closed larynx. There is no turning of the head. The eyes deviate upward. This tonic activity is followed by rhythmic, symmetric flexion of the arms and extension of the legs. GTC seizures last for 2–5 minutes, and patients are usually obtunded and incontinent following the seizure. Patients do not experience postevent weakness.

continued

Table 11–21. (*continued*)

Diffuse (Generalized) Seizures	Signs and Symptoms
Absence	Patients have impaired cognition and do not recall these seizures. Patients stop any activity (behavioral arrest), stare blankly, and blink repetitively. Absence seizures last for 15–30 seconds, and patients are not confused after a seizure. Absence seizures are much more common in children than in adults. It may be difficult to distinguish an absence seizure clinically from a complex focal seizure.
Myoclonic	Patients have normal cognition during myoclonic seizures and thus can describe the symptoms. A myoclonic seizure presents with sudden, symmetric contraction of the arms (most commonly), legs, or face. These seizures recur at irregular intervals. Most commonly, they occur in the early morning. Clinically, myoclonic seizures cannot be distinguished from myoclonic jerks secondary to encephalopathy, brainstem disease, or spinal cord disease.
Atonic	Patients have impaired cognition and do not recall these seizures. Patients collapse suddenly due to diffuse loss of postural tone, which lasts for only 1–5 seconds. As a result, patients frequently have traumatic injuries. There is no postevent confusion.

If the patient has a history of epilepsy, this evaluation is often unnecessary unless there is clinical suspicion of a new acute illness. Instead, the evaluation of a patient with epilepsy and a breakthrough seizure only includes antiepileptic drug levels. The diagnosis of epilepsy also includes EEG. The classic findings on EEG in epilepsy are background (interictal) epileptiform discharges that may be focal or generalized, depending on whether the patient has location-related or generalized epilepsy, respectively. However, interictal EEG has many limitations in the diagnosis of epilepsy. When the diagnosis of epilepsy remains uncertain after routine EEG, patients may be further evaluated with inpatient continuous EEG and video recordings (done in epilepsy monitoring units). Patients with location-related epilepsy should have an MRI scan of the brain, often with thin slices through the suspected epileptic focus, to identify an underlying structural etiology. An epilepsy syndrome (e.g., childhood absence epilepsy) may be diagnosed based on the age of onset, seizure types, and EEG and neuroimaging findings. Diagnosis of epilepsy syndrome guides treatment decisions and provides prognostic information.

Tx—Many patients who have a single seizure do not require treatment with antiepileptic drugs (AEDs). Provoked seizures from alcohol withdrawal or drug abuse do not require antiepileptic therapy. Provoked seizures from transient CNS insults, such as meningitis, may be treated with a short course (2–3 months) of AEDs while the patient is acutely ill and recovering. In patients with an unprovoked single seizure, initiation of AED therapy is based on the patient's risk of a subsequent seizure and the potential impact of a second seizure. Patients with a structural lesion on MRI or epileptic findings on EEG have a higher risk (70–80%) of subsequent seizure, and AEDs are usually recommended. If a patient initially presents with status epilepticus, an AED is usually recommended. In patients with a low risk of recurrent unprovoked seizures (normal EEG and MRI), initiation of an AED is based on the patient's preference. There are numerous AEDs with similar efficacy. An AED is chosen based on the type of epilepsy (focal or generalized)/epilepsy syndrome, side effect profile, and potential interaction with other medications. Generally, AEDs can be divided into broad-spectrum (those that treat both focal and generalized seizures and narrow-spectrum (those that treat either focal or specific generalized seizures) types. The indications, metabolism, and side effect profile of commonly used AEDs are listed in Table 11-22.

Table 11-22. AED Metabolism and Side Effects

Narrow-Spectrum AEDs	Use	Metabolism	Side Effects
Phenytoin (Dilantin)	Partial and GTC seizures	Hepatic metabolism, reduces concentration of OCPs.	Acute toxicity includes lethargy, altered mental status, nystagmus, ataxia, and dysarthria. Chronic toxicity includes gingival hypertrophy, hirsutism, acne, polyneuropathy, and reduced bone density.
Carbamazepine (Tegretol)	Partial and GTC seizures	Hepatic metabolism reduces concentration of OCPs and carbamazepine itself (auto-induction).	Acute toxicity includes ataxia, vertigo, diplopia, drowsiness, blurred vision, nausea, diarrhea, constipation, Stevens-Johnson syndrome, and hyponatremia. Chronic toxicity includes reduced bone density.
Oxcarbazepine (Trileptal)	Partial seizures	Hepatic metabolism reduces concentration of OCPs.	Acute toxicity includes somnolence, headache, ataxia, vertigo, diplopia, blurred vision, nausea, tremor, and hyponatremia.
Phenobarbital	Partial and GTC seizures	75% hepatic/25% renal metabolism; reduces concentration of OCPs.	Acute toxicity includes sedation, memory loss, irritability, and depression. Chronic side effects include connective tissue disorders, such as a flexed finger that cannot be straightened (Dupuytren contracture).
Ethosuximide	Absence seizures	80% hepatic/20% renal metabolism.	Acute toxicity includes nausea, headache, anorexia, and drowsiness.

Broad-Spectrum AEDs	Metabolism	Side Effects
Valproic Acid (Depakote)	Hepatic metabolism.	Acute toxicity includes somnolence, nausea, tremor, weight gain, alopecia, pancreatitis, and hepatic failure. Has the highest known teratogenic toxicity, including neural tube defects.
Lamotrigine (Lamictal)	90% hepatic metabolism. Other drugs, including OCPs, and the state of pregnancy increase the metabolism of lamotrigine.	Acute toxicity includes tremor, headache, insomnia, Stevens-Johnson syndrome (decreased with slow upward titration).
Topiramate (Topamax)	60% renal clearance. At doses >200 mg, topirimate reduces the efficacy of OCPs.	Acute toxicity includes somnolence, cognitive dysfunction, tingling paresthesias of the fingers, weight loss, dizziness, nephrolithiasis, and open-angle glaucoma.
Levetiracetam (Keppra)	Renal clearance without significant drug–drug interactions. Levetiracetam is not FDA-approved for monotherapy, but studies have shown efficacy similar to that of carbamazepine. As a result, it is frequently used off-label as monotherapy.	Acute toxicity includes irritability, somnolence, headache, and psychosis.

Movement Disorders

Parkinson Disease (PD)

D—A progressive neurodegenerative disorder characterized by the following four cardinal features: (1) resting tremor, (2) cogwheel rigidity, (3) bradykinesia, and (4) postural instability.

Epi—The prevalence is 200–300/100,000. It is uncommon before the age of 40. The average age of diagnosis is 70.5 years.

P—The exact pathogenesis of PD is unknown; it may be caused by dysfunction in protein degradation leading to accumulation of protein aggregates. The final common pathway is loss of dopaminergic neurons primarily in the substantia nigra, resulting in loss of dopaminergic input to the caudate and putamen of the basal ganglia. On histologic exam, cytoplasmic inclusions of protein aggregations known as *Lewy bodies* are seen; they contain multiple different proteins, most importantly α-synuclein.

RF—Risk factors include a family history, increasing age, and the use of pesticides that inhibit dopamine production.

SiSx—Symptoms develop insidiously and progress gradually. Prominent motor symptoms include resting tremor (70%), stiffness, gait dysfunction, and decreased speed of movement. The tremor usually begins asymmetrically in the hands and occurs at rest, often described as "pill rolling" at a frequency of four to six times per second. Tremor may then develop in the other hand, the legs, and the chin. The classic rigidity of PD is an alternating pattern of resistance and relaxation as the patient's limb is passively moved (cogwheel rigidity). Like tremor, rigidity begins asymmetrically and worsens with disease progression. Patients with PD have a generalized slowness of movements (bradykinesia). Although patients often describe this slowness as "weakness," their strength is normal on neurologic examination. Decreased dexterity and difficulty with simple motor tasks may be seen. Bradykinesia can affect the face, causing decreased blinking and a blank facial expression. On exam there is also decreased amplitude and speed of rapidly alternating movements. With disease progression, patients may fail to initiate movements (freezing). The gait is narrow-based with decreased stride length, often described as "shuffling." Patients also have difficulty turning, requiring many small steps (en-bloc). Postural instability develops later in the disease course and can cause significant morbidity from frequent falls. It can be assessed by gently pulling the patient backward while he or she is standing; a normal patient should be able to maintain balance, whereas a patient with PD takes multiple steps backward or falls into the physician's arms. Other motor features of PD include hypophonia and micrographia.

Nonmotor symptoms include cognitive dysfunction, mood disorders (depression, anxiety, abulia/apathy), sleep disorders (insomnia, restless legs syndrome, REM-behavioral disorder), fatigue, mild autonomic dysfunction, and olfactory dysfunction. Many of these symptoms may present prior to the onset of motor symptoms and can significantly impact the quality of life.

Dx—Diagnosis is based on the clinical history and exam. The diagnostic criteria include the asymmetric presence of at least two of the four cardinal manifestations listed above and an excellent response to dopaminergic therapy. The presence of early falls, early autonomic dysfunction, early cognitive dysfunction, eye movement abnormalities, cerebellar signs, symmetric involvement, and a poor response to dopaminergic therapy would suggest an atypical parkinsonian disorder (*Parkinson-plus*), such as dementia with Lewy bodies, corticobasal degeneration, progressive supranuclear palsy, or multiple-system atrophy (see Table 11-23). Patients, who have drug-induced parkinsonism, and were treated with a medication that antagonizes the dopamine receptor (e.g., typical and atypical antipsychotics, metoclopramide) may be difficult to distinguish clinically from those with PD (drug-induced parkinsonism).

Table 11-23. Parkinson-Plus Syndromes

Syndrome	Clinical Features	Treatment
Progressive Supranuclear Palsy	• Rare (1.5 cases per 100,000) • Prominent features are postural instability, frequent falls within 1 year of symptom onset • Minimal to no response to levodopa • Other prominent parkinsonian symptoms include bradykinesia (especially affecting the face, producing a characteristic stare) and axial rigidity • Classically, there is an inability to voluntarily move the eyes vertically (down > up); the eyes will move vertically with an oculocephalic reflex, localizing this gaze abnormality to the supranuclear pathways • Severe frontal cognitive deficits (apathy, perseveration, disinhibition, difficulty shifting attention) • Severe dysarthria and dysphagia causing malnourishment • Late in the disease, the patient may develop involuntary neck extension (dystonic retrocollis)	No effective therapy Mean survival of 6 years after diagnosis
Multisystem Atrophy (formerly known as *Shy-Drager Syndrome*)	• May be seen in as many of 10% of individuals initially diagnosed with PD • Prominent autonomic dysfunction within the first year of symptom onset with profound orthostatic hypotension (the most frequent reason for seeking medical attention) • Other symptoms include erectile dysfunction, constipation, urinary symptoms, and decreased sweating • Most patients (80%) have asymmetric bradykinesia and rigidity; 30% of these patients may have a partial response to levodopa, which is not sustained • 20% of patients have signs and symptoms of cerebellar dysfunction (ataxia, dysarthria, and nystagmus) • Patients may also have upper motor neuron signs (hyperreflexia or a Babinski sign)	Symptomatic treatment for orthostasis includes a high-salt diet, midodrine (α agonist), or fludrocortisone (synthetic mineralocorticoid) Mean survival of 9 years after diagnosis
Corticobasal Degeneration	• Rare (5–7 cases per 100,000) • Presents with strikingly asymmetric limb dysfunction, usually of an arm • Abnormal posturing of the limb (dystonia) and involuntary movements ("alien limb" phenomenon); myoclonus may also be present • Significant focal cognitive deficits, especially difficulty performing learned movements (e.g., using a tool), known as *apraxia* • Other cognitive deficits include neglect for both visual and tactile stimuli and aphasia • There is bradykinesia and rigidity of the limb that does not respond to levodopa • There are upper motor neuron signs (hyperreflexia or a Babinski sign)	No effective therapy Mean survival of 7–8 years after diagnosis

continued

Table 11-23. (*continued*)

Syndrome	Clinical Features	Treatment
Dementia with Lewy Bodies	• Overlaps clinically with both Alzheimer's and Parkinson's disease • May account for up to 10–20% of dementia based on autopsy studies • Presents with cognitive dysfunction within the first year of symptom onset, characterized by a fluctuating level of consciousness with visual hallucinations and delusions • Prominent parkinsonian symptoms include bradykinesia and rigidity more than tremor • Symptoms tend to be symmetric and respond partially to levodopa	Cholinesterase inhibitors (e.g., donepezil) are used to slow cognitive decline but may worsen parkinsonism. Dopaminergic medications may improve parkinsonism but may worsen hallucinations. Patients are very sensitive to neuroleptics and antiemetics that antagonize the dopaminergic system; these medications should be avoided.

distinguishing features of drug-induced parkinsonism include symmetric involvement and subacute onset. A diagnosis of PD should not be made unless symptoms persist for more than 3 months after the offending drug is discontinued. An MRI scan should be performed to exclude other organic causes if symptoms began suddenly or focal neurologic deficits are present on exam.

Tx—There is no known cure. Treatment is aimed at improving symptoms and the quality of life, for which numerous medications are available: levodopa/carbidopa, dopamine agonists, monoamine oxidase-B (MAO-B) inhibitors, catechol-O-methyltransferase (COMT) inhibitors, anticholinergic agents, and amantadine. Each type of agent is described in Table 11-24. In general, mild symptoms can be watched closely; however, with disease progression, both levodopa/carbidopa and a dopamine agonist may be needed for symptomatic treatment of motor symptoms. Patients with PD without cognitive dysfunction who initially responded to levodopa but develop worsening motor symptoms and dyskinesias may benefit from deep brain stimulation. Since nonmotor symptoms of PD cause significant morbidity in PD, it is crucial that these symptoms also be treated symptomatically. If there is high clinical suspicion of PD but the patient does not respond to levodopa, an atypical parkinsonian disorder is more likely.

Huntington Disease (HD)

D—A relentlessly progressive inherited neurodegenerative disease that is currently incurable and universally fatal. It affects predominantly the basal ganglia, and its main features are chorea, cognitive impairment, and psychiatric symptoms.

Epi—The estimated prevalence is 5/100,000 in Europe and North America, with lower prevalence in non-European ethnic groups. The estimated incidence is 2–4.7/1 million per year. Typically, HD presents between 30 and 40 years of age, although it may present at any age.

P—It is an autosomal dominant disorder caused by a trinucleotide (CAG) expansion in the first exon of the huntingtin gene, located on chromosome 4p. The huntingtin gene encodes the protein huntingtin. Fragments of the abnormal huntingtin protein accumulate in the nucleus and cytoplasm of neurons, interfering with transcription of other genes and axonal transport. Huntington disease is completely penetrant if the patient lives long enough. There is a direct correlation between the number of trinucleotide repeats and the

Table 11-24. Medications Used to Treat Parkinson's Disease

Medication	Mechanism	Comment
Levodopa/Carbidopa	Levodopa, a precursor of dopamine, can cross the blood–brain barrier and be metabolized to dopamine (dopamine itself cannot cross). Levodopa is combined with carbidopa, a peripheral decarboxylase inhibitor that prevents systemic conversion (in the liver) of levodopa to dopamine before it crosses the blood–brain barrier.	The most effective therapy for motor symptoms. Started once quality of life is compromised. Adverse effects include nausea, somnolence, headache, and involuntary movements (dyskinesias). More serious reactions include agitation, hallucinations, and psychosis due to excess CNS dopamine.
Dopamine Agonists (ropinirole, pramipexole, bromocriptine)	Direct agonists that do not need conversion and do not depend on neuronal uptake or release, like carbidopa/levodopa.	An alternative to levodopa/carbidopa early in the course of the disease. May provide less symptomatic relief but also has a lower risk of dyskinesias. Side effects of dopamine agonists include nausea, confusion, hallucinations and problems with impulse control (e.g., hypersexuality, excessive gambling).
Catechol-O-methyl-transferase (COMT) Inhibitors (tolcapone, entacapone)	Prolongs the half-life of levodopa by preventing peripheral degradation.	Used for those who have a "wearing-off" period of their medications between doses. Can help reduce the dose of daily levodopa. Adverse effects include nausea, confusion, and hallucination. Orthostatic hypotension can result from increased dopaminergic stimulation. Diarrhea and orange discoloration of urine can also be seen.
MAO-B Inhibitors (rasagiline, selegiline)	Inhibit dopamine degradation; may be neuroprotective by blocking free radical formation from the oxidative metabolism of dopamine.	Can provide mild symptomatic relief early in the course of the disease. Adverse effects include confusion and interactions with other medications such as SSRIs.
Amantadine	An antiviral that has mild antiparkinsonian activity by increasing dopamine release, inhibiting dopamine reuptake, and stimulating dopamine receptors.	Best used as short-term monotherapy in those with mild disease. Side effects included edema, confusion, and hallucinations.
Anticholinergic Drugs (trihexyphenidyl benztropine)	Centrally acting anticholinergic drugs help maintain the balance of dopamine and ACh. In PD, depletion of dopamine allows for excessive cholinergic sensitivity, which can worsen symptoms.	Useful as monotherapy in nonelderly patients with disturbing tremors but without akinesia or gait disturbance. Used an adjunct to levodopa. Side effects limit use, especially in elderly patients, and include confusion, dry mouth, blurred vision, constipation, urinary retention, impaired sweating, and tachycardia.

age of onset of the disease. The trinucleotide expansion is unstable and expands from generation to generation, resulting in an earlier presentation in the subsequent generation. This phenomenon is called *anticipation*. In HD, individuals who inherit the disease from their father tend to have more pronounced anticipation.

RF—A positive family history is the risk factor.

SiSx—Patients initially present with the insidious development of movement disorders (60%), behavioral disease (15%), or both (25%) and are often unaware of their symptoms.

Movement disorders: The classic movement disorder of HD is chorea, which is defined as rapid, random, purposeless, jerky movements. Early in the disease, patients may only appear fidgety or restless. Other movement disorders in HD include bradykinesia, dystonia, abnormal eye movements, gait dysfunction, and motor impersistence, which can be demonstrated as an inability to maintain protrusion of the tongue or contraction of the fingers (*milkmaid grip*). The gait combines the chorea and motor impersistence, creating a complex appearance with bobbing and lurching. With disease progression the pharynx and larynx may be involved, resulting in dysarthria, dysphagia, and involuntary vocalizations.

Cognitive impairment: Executive function is the primary deficit. Patients have difficulty with attention, decision making, and multitasking. On exam, they are disinhibited, perseverate, and have difficulty shifting attention from one task to another.

Psychiatric symptoms: Virtually all patients have psychiatric manifestations. The earliest symptoms include irritability, moodiness, apathy, and denial. Disorders of mood are common, especially depression (about one-third of cases). Almost 10% of patients with HD are reported to die from suicide.

Dx—Diagnosis is based on clinical features and a family history. Neuroimaging is usually nondiagnostic, showing generalized atrophy. Occasionally, selective atrophy of the caudate may be seen. All suspected cases can be confirmed with genetic testing; repeat numbers of CAG expansion of 36 or greater are diagnostic for HD, with the normal number being fewer than 30 repeats.

Tx—There is no cure for HD; the disease is typically fatal within 10–20 years after onset of symptoms. Symptomatic treatment of chorea may respond to drugs that affect the dopaminergic system, especially atypical antipsychotics. Selective serotonin reuptake inhibitors (SSRIs) may help to reduce aggression and agitation.

Restless Legs Syndrome (RLS)

D—A condition characterized by an urge to move the legs caused by an unpleasant sensation in the legs. Symptoms occur at night or after prolonged inactivity and are relieved by movement.

Epi—The estimated prevalence of RLS is 10–15% and increases with age. However, only 2.5% of patients with RLS have symptoms that affect their quality of life. The condition is more common in women.

P—Primary RLS may be idiopathic or inherited. Familial RLS is an autosomal dominant disorder with four different chromosomes linked to RLS. The associated genes have not yet been identified. Idiopathic RLS appears to be related to iron deficiency in the substantia nigra and decreased activity of the dopaminergic neurotransmitter system.

RF—The only risk factor for primary RLS is a positive family history. Secondary forms of RLS are associated with various medical conditions, including iron deficiency, renal failure, multiple sclerosis, PD, pregnancy, rheumatoid arthritis, radiculopathy, and polyneuropathy.

SiSx—Patients may describe a sensation in their legs as creeping, crawling, itching, stretching, aching, or tingling that makes them want to move their legs. These sensations are relieved by movement. Symptoms worsen in the evening and are maximal at night; they typically appear within 15–30 minutes of resting. Most patients suffer from insomnia, and 80% have periodic limb movements during sleep. The neurologic exam is normal.

Dx—Diagnosis is made by the history. The International Restless Legs Study Syndrome Group proposed the following diagnostic criteria: (1) an urge to move the legs, usually accompanied by an uncomfortable or unpleasant sensations in the legs; (2) occurrence of this urge during periods of rest or inactivity; (3) partial relief obtained by continuous movement, and (4) worsening of the urge in the evening/night than during the day. Restless legs syndrome can be distinguished from akathisia due to antipsychotic medications by its nocturnal exacerbation and its predilection for the legs. Patients should be evaluated for associated medical conditions, especially iron deficiency (check the ferritin level).

Tx—The first-line treatment for RLS is a dopamine agonist (pramipexole, ropinirole). Alternative treatment options include levodopa, gabapentin, benzodiazepines (in particular, clonazepam), and opioids. Iron supplementation should only be offered to patients who have low ferritin levels and should be given in conjunction with one of the above medications.

Peripheral Nerve Disorders

Mononeuropathy

D—A focal lesion of a single peripheral nerve.

Epi—Median neuropathy at the wrist [carpal tunnel syndrome (CTS)] is the most common mononeuropathy, with a prevalence of up to 3.4%. Females are more frequently affected than males. Ulnar neuropathy at the elbow is the second most common mononeuropathy. The most common lower extremity mononeuropathy is peroneal neuropathy at the fibular head.

P—Mononeuropathies are usually caused by mechanical distortion of a nerve by surrounding connective tissue (entrapment). This mechanical distortion causes focal demyelination of the nerve. Other, less common causes of mononeuropathy include trauma, infarction, or focal compression by a mass lesion.

RF—Focal mononeuropathies, especially CTS, may be associated with general metabolic conditions, such as diabetes mellitus, acromegaly, and amyloidosis, among others.

SiSx—Mononeuropathy caused by trauma or infarction presents acutely, whereas mononeuropathy caused by entrapment or focal compression develops gradually. Weakness in the muscles innervated by the affected nerve is seen, along with well-demarcated sensory loss in the sensory distribution of the affected nerve. Paresthesias and pain occur frequently but are not restricted to the affected dermatome. See Table 11-25 for specific symptoms of common mononeuropathies.

Dx—Exclude alternative etiologies, such as plexopathy, radiculopathy, or a CNS lesion. Musculoskeletal injuries may cause pain that limits muscle strength, mimicking a mononeuropathy. A thorough exam can help the clinician localize the lesion to a single peripheral nerve. Nerve conduction studies/electromyography (NCS/EMG) relies on the same principles to localize the lesion but also provides quantitative data on the severity of nerve injury. In entrapment mononeuropathies, nerve conduction studies show decreased speed of conduction because of focal demyelination. Typically, EMG shows large, polyphasic motor unit action potentials with reduced recruitment in the muscles innervated by the affected peripheral nerve entrapment neuropathy.

Tx—Individualized therapy for each type of mononeuropathy differs and is shown in Table 11-25.

Radiculopathy

D—A focal lesion of a spinal nerve root.

Epi—Structural compression is more common in the lower cervical roots than in the upper cervical roots. C7 radiculopathy accounts for 70% of cervical radiculopathies, C6 radiculopathy for 20%. The mean age of diagnosis is 48 years, with men more frequently affected than women. L5 radiculopathy is the most common lumbosacral radiculopathy.

P—Most radiculopathies are caused by structural compression (herniated discs,

Table 11-25. Characteristics and Treatments of Common Mononeuropathies

Mononeuropathies	Clinical Manifestations	Treatment
Median neuropathy at the wrist from compression within the carpal tunnel (carpal tunnel syndrome).	Symptoms include pain in the wrist, forearm, or arm and numbness/tingling of the thumb, index, and middle fingers. It is worse with driving and typing. Pain may awaken the patient. Thenar atrophy, thumb abduction weakness, and decreased sensation on the thumb, index, and middle fingers is seen. Sensation over the thenar eminence is normal. There may be pain with tapping of the carpal tunnel (Tinel's sign at the wrist).	Wrist splinting, especially at night for mild to moderate disease; avoidance of activities that exacerbate symptoms. Steroid injection into the wrist or surgical release of the flexor retinaculum for moderate to severe disease.
Ulnar neuropathy from compression/trauma at the medial elbow.	Hand weakness, pain in the medial hand, forearm, or elbow and numbness/tingling of the fourth and fifth fingers are common symptoms. Hypothenar atrophy, weakness of finger abduction, and decreased sensation on the fourth and fifth fingers and hypothenar eminence is seen. Pain may be elicited with tapping of the medial elbow (Tinel's sign at the elbow). Normal thumb abduction distinguishes this from a C8 radiculopathy.	Conservative treatment is with an elbow pad and nocturnal splinting. Surgical repositioning of the ulnar nerve can be done for more severe disease.
Radial neuropathy from radial nerve compression, as seen in prolonged resting of the arm over the back of a chair (Saturday night palsy).	Presentation can be with wrist and finger drop and numbness/tingling over the dorsum of the hand. Weakness of wrist extension, finger extensors, and elbow flexion with the arm partially pronated (brachioradialis) and numbness over the dorsum of the hand is seen on exam. The brachioradialis reflex is reduced or absent. Normal triceps strength and reflex distinguishes a radial neuropathy at the spiral groove from a C7 radiculopathy.	This condition usually resolves spontaneously. Persistent weakness may require surgical exploration, but results are often poor.
Peroneal neuropathy at the fibular head due to external pressure on the peroneal nerve from prolonged lying (surgery, hospitalization), crossing the legs, protracted squatting, or leg casts.	Presents with footdrop and numbness/tingling over the lateral shin and dorsum of the foot. Patients report frequent tripping over the foot unless the patient compensates by flexing the hip when walking (steppage gait). On exam, there is weakness of foot and toe dorsiflexion and foot eversion and numbness over the lateral shin and dorsum of the foot. Foot inversion is normal, as it is innervated by the tibial nerve.	Conservative treatment to relieve pressure on the nerve (extra cushioning, avoidance of leg crossing). An ankle-foot orthotic splint should be used until the footdrop has disappeared. Surgical decompression should be considered for patients who do not recover.

degenerative arthritis or spondylosis, mass lesions) of the spinal nerve root. Other causes include infiltration (carcinoma, lymphoid, sarcoidosis), infection (Lyme disease, varicella-zoster virus, cytomegalovirus, herpes simplex virus), infarction (vasculitis), or demyelination (early Gullain-Barré syndrome) of the nerve root.

RF—Trauma/injury are implicated, as well as risk factors for associated conditions listed above.

SiSx—Radiculopathy caused by a herniated disc, infection, infarction, or demyelination presents acutely, whereas radiculopathy caused by spondylosis or infiltration develops gradually. Patients complain of neck/back pain

Table 11-26.   Common Radiculopathies

Radiculopathy Location	Clinical Manifestation
C7	Pain: neck, shoulder, middle finger Weakness: elbow, wrist, finger extension, forearm pronation Sensory loss: third finger Reflexes: decreased or absent triceps reflex Normal brachioradialis strength and reflex distinguish a C7 radiculopathy from a radial neuropathy
C8	Pain: neck, shoulder, medial forearm, fourth and fifth digits Sensory loss: medial hand, fourth and fifth digits Weakness: finger extension, finger abduction, thumb abduction Reflexes: normal Weakness of thumb abduction and finger extension distinguish a C8 radiculopathy from an ulnar neuropathy
L5 (sciatica)	Pain: back pain radiating down the lateral aspect of the leg into the foot Sensory loss: lateral shin and dorsum of foot Weakness: foot dorsiflexion, foot inversion, foot eversion, toe extension Reflexes: normal Weakness of foot inversion distinguishes a L5 radiculopathy from a peroneal neuropathy
S1	Pain: back pain radiating down the posterior aspect of the leg into the foot from the back Sensory loss: posterior aspect of the leg and lateral foot Weakness: leg extension, plantar flexion, toe flexion Reflexes: loss of ankle jerk

with radiating pain and paresthesias into a limb, with occasional limb weakness and numbness. Exam may show mild to moderate weakness of muscles innervated by the affected nerve root. Complete paralysis does not occur because most muscles are innervated by multiple nerve roots. Associated pain may limit the exam and mimic weakness. Classically, sensory loss has a dermatomal distribution; however, many patients present with more diffuse limb numbness secondary to the overlap of adjacent dermatomes. See Table 11-26 for detailed clinical manifestations of specific radiculopathies.

Dx—First, exclude alternative etiologies that may cause similar patterns of weakness and numbness, such as plexopathy, mononeuropathy or a CNS lesion. The diagnosis can be largely clinical, but neuroimaging or NCS/EMG often provides complementary data. Neuroimaging has high sensitivity for detecting structural lesions, but specificity that the lesion is causing a radiculopathy is low. By contrast, NCS/EMG has high specificity but low sensitivity for detecting radiculopathies.

The neuroimaging modality of choice for detecting radiculopathy is an MRI scan without gadolinium. An MRI scan will show significant foraminal narrowing, often from a herniated disc. Sensory NCSs are always normal in radiculopathies, whereas they are usually abnormal in mononeuropathy or plexopathy. The typical EMG findings of a radiculopathy are large, polyphasic motor unit action potentials with reduced recruitment in the muscles innervated by the affected spinal nerve root.

Tx—Treatment depends on the severity of the radiculopathy. Patients with pain and/or sensory loss and without weakness are managed conservatively with physical therapy and oral analgesics (e.g., NSAIDs, muscle relaxants, narcotics). Bed rest is not recommended for acute back pain. A short course of oral prednisone may also provide pain relief. For patients who do not improve with conservative therapy, epidural steroid injections are recommended. If the pain persists despite these interventions, surgery may be considered, although the results are often unsatisfactory. For patients with weakness, surgery should be offered to prevent further axonal injury. However, many patients with weakness who decline surgery gradually regain strength with conservative therapy.

Polyneuropathies

Polyneuropathies may progress rapidly (days to weeks), but more commonly they progress insidiously. The most common rapidly progressive polyneuropathy is Guillain-Barré syndrome, which is usually demyelinating. A common rapidly progressing axonal polyneuropathy is critical illness polyneuropathy, seen in a number of ICU patients to varying degrees. Axonal polyneuropathies of many varieties are quite common and are discussed as well in this section below.

Guillain-Barré Syndrome (GBS)

D—A clinical syndrome characterized by the subacute (days to weeks) onset of symmetric weakness with minimal sensory symptoms and areflexia. It is not a single disease but instead is caused by a heterogeneous group of autoimmune diseases described below.

Epi—The worldwide incidence of GBS is 2/100,000 per year. People of all ages are affected, with a peak incidence in young adults and the elderly. Acute inflammatory demyelinating polyneuropathy (AIDP) accounts for 85–90% of GBS in the United States.

P—An infection within 1–4 weeks of symptom onset occurs in 70% of patients with GBS. The immune response caused by this infection cross-reacts against peripheral nerve components (molecular mimicry). The immune system can either target epitopes on Schwann cells, causing AIDP, or on peripheral nerve axons, resulting in acute motor axonal neuropathy (AMAN) or acute motor and sensory axonal neuropathy (AMSAN). The latter two conditions are quite rare. Although axons are not the primary target in AIDP, severe inflammation will cause axonal injury. The inflammation is primarily mediated by immunoglobulins, complement, and macrophages.

RF—Common infections that precede GBS include *Campylobacter jejuni* (20–45% of cases), *Cytomegalovirus* (10–20%), EBV (10%), *Mycoplasma* (5%), and HIV. Less commonly, GBS is associated with immunization, surgery, trauma, Hodgkin's lymphoma, and bone marrow transplantation.

SiSx—The initial symptoms of GBS are typically tingling paresthesias in the hands and feet and severe back pain. After a variable time interval (hours to days), patients develop progressive symmetric weakness. The severity of weakness varies from mild to complete paralysis. In classic GBS, this weakness begins in the feet and ascends to involve the legs, arms, diaphragm, and face. Severe respiratory muscle weakness requiring mechanical ventilation occurs in 30% of patients. In 10% of patients with GBS, weakness begins in the arms. The Miller-Fischer variant of GBS is characterized by a descending weakness beginning in the extraocular and facial muscles. On exam, patients with GBS are found to have symmetric weakness and absent reflexes (90% of patients). The sensory exam may be normal or reveal mildly reduced vibratory and proprioceptive sensation. Dysautonomia occurs in 70% of patients with GBS, manifesting most commonly as tachycardia, but other arrhythmias, labile blood pressure, orthostatic hypotension, urinary retention, and ileus can also occur. Classically, GBS symptoms usually progress over a period of 2–4 weeks before reaching their nadir.

Dx—The diagnosis of GBS is clinical and is supported by classic abnormalities on ancillary tests such as LP and NCS/EMG. Such tests, however, may be normal early in the course of the disease. Elevated CSF protein is seen in 80–90% without a prominent pleocytosis (defined as <10 WBCs); this finding is termed *albuminocytologic dissociation*. In the common form of GBS (AIDP), 85% of patients have classic features of demyelination on NCS/EMG testing after 3 weeks of symptoms. Be sure to exclude other conditions such as (1) critical illness polyneuropathy (CIP), a condition of absent reflexes in sick ICU patients who also may fail to be weaned from the ventilator, (2) cervical myelopathy, which can present acutely with ascending weakness and decreased reflexes, and (3) chronic inflammatory demyelinating polyneuropathy (CIDP), which is the diagnosis if symptoms last for more than 8 weeks.

Tx—Urgent treatment is needed at diagnosis. Either plasma exchange or IVIG may be used; both have been shown to improve the rate of recovery. Some patients may relapse after 2 weeks of clinical improvement and are retreated. Otherwise, supportive care is the mainstay. Respiratory function is monitored frequently; as 30% of patients will eventually need mechanical ventilation. Spirometry is used to help assess for impending respiratory failure, and elective intubation can be considered. It is better than simple pulse oximetry and ABG alone. Other supportive care treats neuropathic pain, assesses for autonomic dysfunction that affects blood pressure and focuses on DVT and decubitus ulcer prophylaxis. Even with IVIG or plasma exchange, there is 5% mortality and an additional 5–10% of patients have a prolonged course with delayed or incomplete recovery. Poor recovery is more typical with the axonal variants of GBS (AMAN and AMSAN).

Chronic Inflammatory Demyelinating Polyneuropathy (CIDP)

D—A chronic, progressive, acquired, inflammatory, demyelinating disorder of peripheral nerves.

Epi—The estimated prevalence of CIDP is 0.8–3.6/100,000. Although it can affect patients at any age, the prevalence increases with age. There is a slight male predominance.

P—The etiology is unknown. This disorder is believed to be caused by an autoimmune inflammatory reaction against a still unidentified antigen on Schwann cells. The inflammation is primarily mediated by immunoglobulins, complement, and macrophages. Although axons are not the primary target in CIDP, chronic inflammation will cause axonal injury.

RF—Chronic inflammatory demyelinating polyneuropathy has been associated with many diseases, including HIV, diabetes, chronic hepatitis, and other autoimmune diseases. Unlike GBS, CIDP is not usually preceded by an infection.

SiSx—Typically, CIDP presents with insidious, progressive (>8 weeks) weakness and numbness. Patients report numbness and tingling in their hands and feet, difficulty climbing stairs or rising from a chair, hand clumsiness, and gait difficulties. On exam, the weakness is usually symmetric and affects proximal and distal muscles, differentiating CIDP from an axonal neuropathy, which begins distally. Muscle atrophy is initially absent due to the primary demyelinating disease pathology. From 10% to 20% of patients with CIDP will have facial weakness or ophthalmoparesis. Respiratory involvement is rare. On sensory examination, vibration and joint position sensation are decreased in a length-dependent pattern. Reflexes are diminished or absent. There are multiple clinical variants of CIDP, including a pure sensory syndrome, a pure motor syndrome, and a relapsing-remitting syndrome, which is more common in younger patients.

Dx—The diagnosis of CIDP is based on the clinical presentation and abnormal findings on ancillary tests such as NCS/EMG, CSF analysis, and nerve biopsy. The CSF analysis is similar to that of GBS, with increased protein (>60 mg/dL) and <10 WBCs (albuminocytologic dissociation). A CSF WBC count >50 raises concern about coexistent HIV. On NCS, sensory responses are usually absent. Motor responses demonstrate classic findings of acquired demyelination with nonuniform, prolonged distal latencies, markedly decreased conduction velocities, and conduction block. The presence of conduction block distinguishes CIDP from an inherited demyelinating polyneuropathy, such as Charcot-Marie-Tooth type 1 (CMT1). The presence of acute and chronic denervation on EMG indicates secondary axonal injury. Nerve biopsy is performed when the diagnosis remains unclear. In CIDP, there is segmental demyelination and remyelination (onion bulb formation) of the nerve. Nerve biopsy also excludes other conditions in the differential diagnosis such as vasculitis. A demyelinating polyneuropathy may also be seen in paraprotein disorders such as Waldenström's macroglobulinemia, monoclonal gammopathy of unclear significance (MGUS), and POEMS, the syndrome of polyneuropathy, organomegaly, endocrinopathy, monoclonal gammopathy, and skin changes. These entities should be further evaluated with serum protein electrophoresis with immunofixation.

Tx—For typical CIDP, initial therapy is high-dose oral prednisone (1 mg/kg/day) for several months followed by a slow taper of prednisone over months to a year. Ninety percent of patients with CIDP respond to this regimen, but patients develop the typical side effects of chronic steroid use. Most patients relapse off steroids and require low-dose maintenance therapy. In these patients, numerous immunosuppressant medications, most commonly azathioprine and cyclophosphamide, have been used to taper the steroid dose further. The chronic use of both IVIG and plasma exchange has been shown to have similar efficacy to prednisone in CIDP, and they are used in patients with severe CIDP or after failure of prednisone alone. The long-term prognosis is favorable for most patients, but 15% remain severely disabled despite treatment.

Axonal Polyneuropathy

D—A heterogeneous group of disorders that similarly affect the peripheral nerve axons. It may be caused by metabolic diseases (especially diabetes mellitus), genetic mutations, inflammatory diseases, infection, critical illness, or toxic exposures (including numerous medications).

Epi—The epidemiology is dependent on the etiology. Diabetic polyneuropathy is the most common chronic axonal neuropathy. After 10 years of diabetes mellitus, 42% of patients have polyneuropathy compared to 6% of nondiabetic age-matched controls. Thirty percent of patients with HIV/AIDS have polyneuropathy, usually in the later stages of disease.

P—The pathophysiology depends upon the underlying etiology. Diabetic polyneuropathy is believed to be caused by chronic microvascular ischemia of the peripheral nerves. Some medications, such as vincristine, interfere with microtubule aggregation in the axon, disrupting axonal transport.

RF—Diabetes mellitus is the most common risk factor for axonal polyneuropathy. Many other diseases are associated with axonal polyneuropathy, including alcoholism/malnutrition, HIV, uremia, vitamin B_{12} deficiency, critical illness, amyloidosis, and hypothyroidism. Numerous medications are associated with axonal polyneuropathy, including isoniazid, metronidazole, nitrofurantoin, cisplatin, vincristine, paclitaxel, amiodarone, and hydralazine. There may be a family history of axonal neuropathy in patients with Charcot-Marie-Tooth type 2 (CMT2).

SiSx—In polyneuropathy, longer axons are affected earlier in the course of disease; thus, symptoms begin symmetrically in the toes/feet and progress proximally. By the time symptoms have progressed to the knees, patients will develop symptoms in the fingertips (stocking and glove distribution). Depending on the underlying etiology, polyneuropathy may predominantly affect sensory axons, motor axons, or both. If only sensory axons are affected, the polyneuropathy may predominantly affect small-diameter axons (conveying pain and temperature sensation), large-diameter axons (conveying vibration and proprioception sensation), or both. Symptoms of large-diameter axonal injury include numbness and balance difficulties, especially in dark places or with the eyes closed. Symptoms of small-diameter axonal injury include painful dysesthesias such as burning or "pins and needles" sensations. Since autonomic axons are also small in diameter, patients with small-diameter sensory symptoms may also report autonomic dysfunction such as orthostasis, impotence, urinary retention, constipation, and decreased sweating. Motor symptoms include cramps and weakness, initially affecting toe movement followed by ankle dorsiflexion. Generally, sensory symptoms predominate over motor symptoms in polyneuropathy. Surviving motor axons have the ability to sprout collaterally and reinnervate deinnervated muscle, whereas surviving sensory axons cannot reinnervate sensory organs. On exam, patients may have distal hand and foot weakness and atrophy, decreased vibration, temperature, and pinprick sensation in a length-dependent pattern on the arms and legs, decreased or absent reflexes (only the ankle jerks are absent in mild-moderate polyneuropathy), and a positive Romberg sign.

Dx—A good initial step is NCS/EMG to assess if the underlying pathology is axonal or demyelinating. The NCS findings in axonal polyneuropathy include reduced/absent sensory responses and normal/reduced motor responses with normal or mildly slowed conduction velocity (>70% of normal conduction velocity). The classic EMG finding in axonal neuropathy is large, long, polyphasic motor units in distal arm and leg muscles. The NCS/EMG testing and the clinical presentation also distinguish polyneuropathy from mononeuritis multiplex, which presents subacutely, with asymmetric, non-length-dependent involvement of multiple peripheral nerves caused by vasculitis. For axonal polyneuropathy, routine studies for common etiologies include a 2-hour glucose tolerance test, vitamin B_{12} level, and SPEP with immunofixation. Additional tests may be indicated, depending on the results of the initial tests. Genetic testing for some causes of CMT2 is available. Sural nerve biopsy may be performed when the underlying pathology remains unclear despite electrophysiologic testing and there is a high clinical suspicion of vasculitis or CIDP. Sural biopsy is complicated by transient dysesthesias and permanent numbness over the lateral foot.

Tx—The primary treatment for axonal polyneuropathy is treatment of the underlying disease. In diabetes, tight blood glucose control prevents progression of symptoms and may result in mild improvement that develops over years. In toxic neuropathies, the offending agent should be withdrawn. Medications that cause polyneuropathy should be avoided in patients with preexisting polyneuropathy. For symptomatic relief, gabapentin, pregabalin, and tricyclic antidepressants (TCAs) reduce painful dysesthesias. There is no treatment for numbness. Patients with distal weakness should be treated with stretching to prevent contractures and may benefit from orthotic braces.

Motor Neuron Diseases

Amyotrophic Lateral Sclerosis (ALS)

D—A progressive neurodegenerative syndrome primarily affecting both upper and lower motor neurons that is currently incurable and universally fatal. Also known as *Lou Gehrig's disease*, it causes progressive painless weakness and disability, with median survival of 3–5 years. It can be sporadic (90%) or familial (10%).

Epi—Incidence rates in North America and Europe are 1.5–3/100,000 per year. Incidence peaks at 74 years of age. Both incidence and mortality have been increasing, perhaps as a result of longer life expectancy. The male:female ratio is 2:1.

P—The pathogenesis of ALS is unknown. Hypotheses include glutamate excitotoxicity, mitochondrial dysfunction, autoimmune-mediated inflammation, increased apoptosis, and toxic protein aggregation. In 2006, the major constituent of the protein aggregates found in all cases of sporadic ALS and some familial cases was identified as TAR DNA-binding protein (TDP-43). This protein aggregate was also identified in a substantial proportion of cases of frontotemporal dementia, another neurodegenerative disorder. Pathologically, upper motor neurons die, leading to axonal loss and gliosis in the corticospinal tract. The ventral roots of the spinal nerves, which are formed from the axons of lower motor neurons, thin. With the loss of both the axons of the lateral corticospinal tract and lower motor neuron cell bodies in the ventral horn, the spinal cord becomes atrophic. Muscles that are innervated by affected lower motor neurons atrophy and show evidence of acute and chronic denervation.

RF—Age, a family history, and participation in the Gulf War (a 2 fold increase due to some as yet unclear exposure) remain the only established risk factors for ALS.

SiSx—Asymmetric, painless, focal limb weakness is the most common presenting complaint in patients with ALS. Limb weakness typically begins in a single spinal myotome and spreads to adjacent myotomes. Upper extremity weakness typically presents with asymmetric hand weakness and difficulty performing fine motor tasks (manipulating buttons/zippers or turning keys). Lower extremity weakness typically presents with footdrop; proximal pelvis girdle weakness is less common. Bulbar-onset ALS occurs in 20% of patients and usually presents with dysarthria or dysphagia for thin liquids. As the disease progresses, patients have difficulty with thick liquids, secretions, and even solids. Muscles of respiration are usually affected late in the disease course; rarely, patients present with respiratory muscle weakness (1–3%). Older men with ALS may present with muscle wasting and weight loss without focal weakness. In addition to weakness, patients may describe muscle twitching (fasciculations) or cramps in weak muscles.

Both are nonspecific signs of lower motor neuron disease that may also be seen in radiculopathy, mononeuropathy, or polyneuropathy. Patients should not have prominent sensory symptoms. They may demonstrate inappropriate laughter or crying, known as *pseudobulbar affect*. Approximately one-third of patients have mild cognitive impairment and 1 in 20 have frontotemporal dementia. On neurologic exam there is some combination of upper and lower motor neuron signs, as described in Table 11-27.

Dx—There is no definitive diagnostic test for ALS. Instead, the diagnosis is based on clinical criteria that include the simultaneous presence of both upper and lower motor neuron signs in three of four body segments (bulbar, cervical, thoracic, lumbar) and relentless progression of disease. An EMG can demonstrate acute and chronic lower motor neuron disease in any body segment, but it does not evaluate upper motor neuron disease. An MRI scan of the brain, cervical spine, and lumbar spine should be performed to exclude a coexistent brainstem lesion or cervical myelopathy with cervical/lumbar radiculopathies. Early in the disease, patients may manifest upper or lower motor neuron signs only, which expands the differential diagnosis and evaluation to include ALS variants, inherited diseases, infection, and autoimmune diseases. Diffuse

Table 11-27. Differentiation of Upper and Lower Motor Neuron Defects

	Upper Motor Neuron	Lower Motor Neuron
Definition	Neurons that originate in the motor region of the cerebral cortex or brainstem and carry information downward but do not innervate the target muscle	Motor neurons that connect the brainstem and spinal cord directly to the muscle fibers.
Tone	Increased, with spasticity	Decreased flaccid muscles
Reflexes	Hyperreflexia	Hyporeflexic/areflexic
Babinski Sign	Present (toes upgoing)	Absent Babinski sign
Muscle Fasciculations	Absent	Present
Muscle Atrophy	Little or no atrophy	Atrophy seen with muscle wasting
Areas of Disease Process	Spinal cord, brainstem	Anterior horn cell, nerve
Examples of Specific Conditions	Primary lateral sclerosis Hereditary spastic paraparesis Multiple sclerosis	Progressive muscular atrophy Adult spinal muscular atrophy

fasciculations/cramps without weakness are seen in benign fasciculation cramp syndrome. The nonfocal distribution of fasciculations and the absence of weakness distinguish this syndrome from ALS.

Tx—The progression of ALS is quite variable. Currently, there is only one disease-modifying drug, riluzole. Riluzole is thought to reduce glutamate-induced excitotoxicity, but its exact mechanism of action in ALS is not known. It has been shown to prolong survival and/or time to tracheostomy by approximately 3 months. Beyond drug therapy, there are other medical interventions that prolong survival. Bivalve positive airway pressure (BiPAP) has been shown to improve quality of life and median survival and should be considered in those with reduced vital capacity below 50% of the predicted level. Percutaneous endoscopic gastrojejunostomy (PEG) may prolong survival by several months.

Disorders of the Neuromuscular Junction

Myasthenia Gravis (MG)

D—An autoimmune disorder of the neuromuscular junction (NMJ) resulting in fluctuating weakness of ocular, bulbar, limb, and respiratory muscles.

Epi—It is the most common disease of neuromuscular transmission. The most common ages of presentation are: (1) neonates (due to transfer of maternal antibodies), (2) 20–40 years of age, and (3) >50 years of age. Women are affected more commonly than men. The prevalence in the United States is 0.5–20/100,000.

P—Myasthenia gravis is due to autoantibodies directed against the acetylcholine (ACh) nicotinic receptors and, less commonly, receptor-associated proteins, such as muscle-specific receptor tyrosine kinase (MuSK), which are located in the postsynaptic membrane of the NMJ. Antibody-mediated inflammation reduces the number of ACh receptors. Despite this, enough ACh is usually released from a motor nerve to generate a single muscle action potential. In normal individuals, the amount of ACh released with repetitive motor nerve action potentials decreases but enough ACh remains to generate repetitive muscle action potentials. The reduced quantity of ACh released and the smaller number of ACh receptors result in failure to generate repetitive muscle action potentials. Skeletal muscle is affected, causing fluctuating weakness that worsens with sustained muscle contraction; smooth and cardiac muscles are spared due to different antigenicity. More than 50% of patients have thymic hyperplasia, and 10–15% have a thymoma, a low-grade malignant tumor. The reason for this association in unclear but is mostly likely related to the role of the thymus in the immune system.

RF—Risk factors include a family history, certain HLA types, and a personal history of autoimmune disease.

SiSx—There is fluctuating skeletal muscle weakness with muscle fatigue. Common symptoms include ptosis, diplopia, difficulty chewing/swallowing, nasal speech, head drop, shortness of breath (SOB), and proximal limb weakness. Symptoms can fluctuate, generally worsening as the day progresses. There are two types of MG: isolated ocular (15% of MG) and generalized MG, which also affects bulbar, limb, and respiratory muscles. More than 50% of patients present with ocular symptoms, making it difficult to distinguish ocular from generalized MG. Ocular findings include ptosis and extraocular muscle weakness. Ptosis is worsened by sustained upgaze for 60 seconds and may be partially relieved by eye closure for 30 seconds. With asymmetric ptosis, manual lifting of the affected eyelid may worsen ptosis of the other eyelid (curtaining). Pupil size and constriction are always normal in MG, differentiating it from a Horner's syndrome or a third nerve palsy. Bulbar findings may include weakness of eye and jaw closure, tongue and palatal movements, transverse smile, and nasal speech. Axial and appendicular findings may include weakness of neck flexion, shoulder abduction, and hip flexion. Rarely, neck extension is more affected than neck flexion. Findings of diaphragmatic weakness may include tachypnea, weak cough and sniff, use of accessory muscles of respiration, and multiple breaths to complete a sentence. It is not uncommon for patients to develop severe respiratory distress (*myasthenic crisis*) requiring intubation. Myasthenic crisis may be precipitated by infection, recent surgery, or medication changes and remains the most life-threatening complication of MG.

Dx—The diagnosis is primarily made by the history, the exam, and corroborative testing. Confirmatory tests include serum antibody measurement, use of agents that should improve NMJ conduction, and EMG/NCS testing. Acetylcholine receptor–binding antibodies are highly specific for MG and are present in 80–85% of patients with generalized MG, but in only 50% of those with isolated ocular MG. Muscle-specific receptor tyrosine kinase antibodies may be found in up to 40% of patients who are acetylcholine receptor antibody negative. Such patients have more severe facial, bulbar, and neck weakness and more frequent episodes of myasthenic crisis. However, MuSK antibodies are exceedingly rare in patients with isolated ocular MG.

Classic office-based tests are the ice-pack and Tensilon tests. Both need a measurable outcome, such as millimeters of ptosis. Because decreased temperature improves NMJ transmission, ice can be placed over a ptotic eye for 30–60 seconds and the ptosis can be reassessed for improvement. Some believe, however, that the ptosis improves with rest alone. Edrophonium chloride (Tensilon), an acetylcholinesterase inhibitor, can also be given intravenously as the patient is reassessed for improvement of ptosis. Both tests are relatively sensitive (80–95%), but their specificity and positive predictive value are poor. Nerve conduction studies with repetitive nerve stimulation can be performed and may show a decrement of motor amplitude with slow, repetitive stimulation. The sensitivity of NCS is 60–90% in generalized MG but only 10–45% in isolated ocular MG. Although not universally available, the most sensitive test

for MG is single-fiber EMG of weak muscles. A routine EMG scan of patients with MG should be normal. Finally, all patients diagnosed with MG should have a CT scan of the chest to exclude a coexisting thymoma.

Tx—Treatment of MG depends on the acuity and severity of symptoms. All patients are offered symptomatic therapy with acetylcholinesterase inhibitors, such as pyridostigmine. Cholinergic side effects, which include abdominal cramps, diarrhea, nausea, and increased secretions, may be limiting. Oral steroids in low doses are used in isolated ocular MG. Titration up to higher doses of oral steroids can be done for more severe or generalized symptoms. Starting at high doses initially can sometimes precipitate a myasthenic crisis; hence, low-dose initiation is the usual rule. Plasmapheresis or IVIG is used in moderate to severe disease prior to use of oral steroids and to treat myasthenic crisis. Alternative immunosuppressants, such as azathioprine, cyclosporine, or mycophenolate mofetil, are also used as steroid-sparing agents. Certain medications (specifically aminoglycosides, fluoroquinolones, phenytoin, and β blockers) can exacerbate symptoms and should be avoided. Finally, any patient with a thymoma should undergo thymectomy. Treatment of patients with thymic hyperplasia alone is controversial.

Lambert-Eaton Myasthenic Syndrome (LEMS)

D—An antibody-mediated disorder of the NMJ with markedly decreased release of ACh from the presynaptic nerve terminal, resulting in weakness.

Epi—The prevalence is unknown. There is a male predominance. It is estimated that 3% of patients with small cell lung cancer (SCLC) have LEMS, making it the most common paraneoplastic manifestation of SCLC. Half of the patients with LEMS are diagnosed with a malignancy within 2 years of presentation. These patients are typically over the age of 40. Thirty-three percent of cases are not associated with malignancy.

These patients tend to be younger. There is an association with HLA haplotype and auto-immune LEMS.

P—Antibodies are directed against the voltage-gated calcium channel (VGCC) in the presynaptic nerve terminals, resulting in decreased calcium influx. Calcium is necessary for the release of ACh into the NMJ. Approximately half of all cases are associated with malignancy, most commonly SCLC. Rarely, LEMS is associated with a lymphoproliferative disorder, such as Hodgkin's lymphoma. In these paraneoplastic disorders, antibodies directed against the tumor cross-react with the VGCCs. In addition, LEMS may be associated with autoimmune disease, including pernicious anemia.

RF—Known malignancy, especially SCLC, is the most significant risk factor for paraneoplastic LEMS. Risk factors for SCLC (age, smoking) are, by extension, risk factors for paraneoplastic LEMS. Patients with autoimmune LEMS often have other autoimmune diseases or family members with autoimmune disease.

SiSx—Patients invariably complain of fluctuating, symmetric proximal limb weakness, which is worse in the legs. Weakness is present at rest; it may but does not always improve during brief exercise, and fatigue occurs with sustained exercise. Muscles are described as stiff or achy. On confrontational testing, muscle strength appears greater than the patient's description. Mild autonomic symptoms, such as dry mouth and erectile dysfunction, are more common than in MG. The sensory exam is normal. Reflexes are depressed or absent. Ocular and bulbar muscles are typically spared or minimally involved, differentiating LEMS from MG. Although rare, respiratory failure can occur late in the disease course.

Dx—The diagnosis of LEMS can be confirmed by electrophysiologic studies and/or serum antibody tests. Repetitive nerve stimulation must be performed to make the diagnosis. In both postsynaptic (MG) and presynaptic (LEMS) NMJ disorders, there is a decrease in motor amplitude with *slow*, repetitive stimulation. In presynaptic LEMS only, there is a characteristic increase in motor amplitude with either *fast*, repetitive nerve stimulation or after brief exercise. The presence of antibodies to VGCCs is both highly sensitive and specific for LEMS but does not differentiate paraneoplastic from autoimmune LEMS. If a patient with LEMS has other known paraneoplastic antibodies (e.g., anti-HU), then the risk of associated malignancy is markedly increased. Most patients with LEMS should be screened with a CT scan of the chest, abdomen, and pelvis followed by a PET scan if the CT findings are negative.

Tx—For paraneoplastic LEMS, treat the underlying malignancy. Weakness often resolves after successful treatment of the underlying malignancy. Symptomatic improvement can be obtained from 3, 4-diaminopyridine, which increases ACh release from the presynaptic nerve terminal. Low-dose pyridostigmine, an acetylcholinesterase inhibitor, may augment the effects of 3, 4-diaminopyridine when given concurrently. Plasmapheresis and IVIG are reserved for severe weakness. For patients who do not respond to conventional therapies, oral immunosuppressive agents, such as prednisone and azathioprine, can be used.

Myopathies

Myopathies comprise a heterogeneous group of diseases that may be either inherited or acquired. Inherited myopathies can be further divided into muscular dystrophies (most common), congenital myopathies, channelopathies, metabolic myopathies, and mitochondrial myopathies. Acquired myopathies can be further divided into inflammatory myopathies (such as inclusion body myositis, discussed in Chapter 6), endocrine myopathies, drug- or toxin-induced myopathies (such as statin myopathy), and myopathies associated with systemic diseases such as critical illness myopathy. The more common inherited myopathies are shown in Table 11-28.

Inherited Myopathies	P/Epi	SiSx and Dx	Tx
Duchenne Muscular Dystrophy (DMD)/ Becker's Muscular Dystrophy (BMD)	These are conditions caused by mutations in the dystrophin gene on the X chromosome. DMD occurs when the mutation disrupts the amino acid reading frame, resulting in absent or greatly reduced dystrophin. Mutations causing BMD are in-frame mutations resulting in moderately reduced functional dystrophin. DMD is the most common form of muscular dystrophy, with an incidence of 1 in 3500 live male births. The incidence of BMD is 1 in 30,000 live male births.	Patients with DMD present with waddling gait, toe walking, difficulty running, jumping, and climbing stairs, and pseudohypertrophy of the calves (secondary to fatty replacement) by the age of 5 (usually by the age of 3). Patients with classic BMD present with similar symptoms by the age of 15. However, mild BMD may present in 30- to 40-year-old patients. On exam, patients have proximal limb weakness, especially in their lower extremities. A Gower's sign, which is a nonspecific sign of proximal weakness in which patients use their hands to push themselves upright from the floor, is usually present. • After the age of 6, patients with DMD develop progressive weakness and become wheelchair-bound by age 13. In contrast, patients with BMD may become wheelchair-bound by age 16, with some remaining ambulatory into their fifth decade of life. • Both DMD and BMD have significant cardiac involvement (dilated cardiomyopathy and conduction abnormalities). In DMD, these cardiac abnormalities develop after the age of 10. • Patients with DMD develop scoliosis and respiratory failure during their teenage years. • Serum CK is usually elevated >10 times the normal limit, especially early in the disease. Serum CK levels decrease with age. • The diagnosis can be confirmed by genetic testing.	In DMD, steroids (prednisone or deflazacort) transiently improve muscle strength for 3 months and slow disease progression, as manifested by prolonged ambulation. The efficacy of steroids in BMD is unknown. The average life span of DMD patients is 20 years. The average life span of BMD patients is 45 years.
Myotonic Dystrophy Type 1 (DM1)	DM1 is an autosomal dominant disorder caused by a CTG trinucleotide repeat in the 3' untranslated region of the DMPK gene on chromosome 19. The severity of DM1 generally correlates with the length of the CTG repeat. If there are more than 1000 CTG repeats, DM1 presents in neonates. DM1 is the most common adult muscular dystrophy, affecting 1 in 7400 people.	DM1 is a progressive multisystem disease with cataracts, frontal baldness, insulin resistance, cardiac conduction abnormalities, GI symptoms, and myopathy. • The myopathy of DM1 can be recognized from its atypical distribution of weakness and the presence of clinical myotonia (failure of muscle relaxation). • In DM1, there is prominent weakness of the face (ptosis, jaw closure, facial expression) and the distal limb muscles. Patients typically describe myotonia as muscle stiffness. • On examination, myotonia can be demonstrated by asking the patient to squeeze the eyes shut or make a fist for 15 seconds and then rapidly stop. • Clinical myotonia may be seen in other rare muscle diseases, but the combination of facial and distal limb weakness and myotonia is highly suggestive of DM1. • On EMG, patients have both myopathic motor units in affected muscles and myotonia (abnormal high-frequency, spontaneous discharges that vary in amplitude and frequency). • The diagnosis can be confirmed by genetic testing.	No treatment is currently available for the myopathy. Myotonia may be treated with mexiletine or imipramine, but patients with DM1 are not typically bothered by their myotonia. A cardiac evaluation should be performed in all patients, given the risk of cardiac conduction abnormalities, and this should be done prior to starting mexiletine. *continued*

Table 11-28. *(Continued)*

Inherited Myopathies	P/Epi	SiSx and Dx	Tx
Mitochondrial Disease Myopathies	A heterogeneous group of inherited disorders that affect the electron transport chain. They may be caused by mutations of either mitochondrial or nuclear DNA. Mutations of mitochondrial DNA are maternally inherited, while mutations of nuclear DNA follow Mendelian genetics.	• Mitochondrial diseases preferentially affect tissues with high metabolic demand, such as brain, muscle (skeletal and cardiac), retina, nerves, and, less commonly, the GI system. • Symptoms are commonly exacerbated after periods of increased metabolic demands such as infection. The myopathy may present with weakness, exercise intolerance (fatigue the day after exercise), or myoglobinuria. • Based on which tissues are affected and how the disease manifests, most patients may be diagnosed with a specific mitochondrial syndrome, such as chronic progressive external ophthalmoplegia (CPEO), Kearns-Sayre syndrome, myoclonic epilepsy and ragged red fibers (MERRF), mitochondrial encephalomyopathy lactic acidosis and stroke-like episodes (MELAS), and Leigh syndrome. A full discussion of each of these syndromes is beyond the scope of this book. • If a mitochondrial disease is suspected, the evaluation usually includes the serum or CSF lactate/pyruvate ratio, muscle biopsy, and genetic testing. An elevated serum or CSF lactate level and an elevated serum or CSF lactate/pyruvate ratio is often seen in mitochondrial disease. However, a normal serum or CSF lactate level does not exclude mitochondrial disease. • If muscle is involved clinically or electrophysiologically, there is often an abnormal accumulation of mitochondria around the peripheral muscle cell (ragged-red fibers). The muscle biopsy specimen may also be stained for cytochrome oxidase (a protein subunit of the electron transport chain), which is absent in most mitochondrial diseases. • An abnormal muscle biopsy confirms the presence of a mitochondrial disease but does not identify the syndrome or the genetic defect. • Genetic testing based on clinical characteristics will confirm the diagnosis of a specific syndrome.	No treatment is currently available for mitochondrial diseases. A cardiac evaluation should be performed in most patients, especially those with MERRF and Kearns-Sayre syndromes, who have a high frequency of cardiac conduction abnormalities.

The Dementias

Alzheimer's Disease (AD)

D—A progressive neurodegenerative disorder that affects cognition, especially memory and visuospatial perception, causing functional impairment. With disease progression, patients develop behavioral problems and global cognitive dysfunction.

Epi—Alzheimer's disease is the most common dementia syndrome, with an estimated prevalence of 4.5 million cases in the United States. The prevalence of AD markedly increases with age; 10–15% of people over the age of 65 and 35–50% of people over the age of 85 are affected. It is slightly more common in women.

P—The exact pathogenesis of AD is unknown. Accumulation of two different proteins, β-amyloid (1-42) in extracellular amyloid plaques and tau in intraneuronal neurofibrillary tangles, may be causative. Of the two protein aggregates, the density of neurofibrillary tangles correlates with disease severity. These protein aggregates develop first in the hippocampus. The basal forebrain, which contains cholinergic neurons, is usually involved when patients become symptomatic.

RF—Age is the strongest risk factor for AD. A family history is also a risk factor; 20% of patients with AD have a first-degree relative with AD. The most common genetic risk factor identified thus far is a polymorphism in the ApoE gene. The epsilon 4 allele, which is found in 15–20% of the general population, dramatically increases the risk of AD. People who are homozygous for the epsilon 4 allele have a 50% chance of developing AD by the age of 70, while those who are heterozygous have a 50% chance of developing AD by the age of 80. Rare autosomal dominant forms of inherited AD have been linked to genes on chromosomes 21, 14, and 1. As a result, patients with trisomy 21 often develop AD by the age of 40. People with an increased level of education may have a reduced risk of AD.

SiSx—Patients with AD typically have limited insight into their cognitive deficits and may not seek medical attention or accurately describe their difficulties. Information from a family member or close friend is essential for a true assessment of cognitive function. Symptoms of cognitive dysfunction develop gradually. The most prominent symptom in AD is an impairment of recent memory. Patients often forget appointments, conversations, and material they have recently read or watched. Their memory does not improve with prompting. On exam, this is assessed by asking the patient to remember a list of words after a 5-minute delay with distraction. In addition to memory loss, there is often prominent visual-spatial dysfunction. Patients may become lost when driving on familiar roads. They may also have difficulty with calculations or organization. It is particularly important to test calculations and executive function directly because these cognitive domains are not assessed by the mini-mental status exam. Cognitive symptoms may interfere with the patients' ability to care for themselves. With disease progression, patients develop memory impairment for remote events, aggressive behavior, disinhibition, and psychosis (paranoid delusions or hallucinations). Thirty percent of patients have coexistent depression.

Dx—The diagnosis of AD is made from the history and the neurologic exam. The diagnosis is based on the gradual onset of memory impairment and one other area of cognitive dysfunction (language, visuospatial perception, apraxia, or executive function) that interfere with social or occupational function. If there is cognitive dysfunction without functional impairment, the diagnosis is mild cognitive impairment. Mild cognitive impairment typically progresses to AD at a rate of 10–12% of patients per year. All patients should be screened for the rare reversible causes of dementia, such as hypothyroidism, vitamin B_{12} deficiency, depression, normal pressure hydrocephalus, chronic subdural hematomas, and medication toxicity. Neuroimaging in AD is nonspecific, with findings of cortical atrophy and appropriately enlarged ventricles (ex-vacuo dilatation). If patients have parkinsonism on exam, an atypical parkinsonian syndrome should be considered. If patients present with rapid progression of cognitive dysfunction or early myoclonus, Creutzfeld-Jakob disease (CJD) should be considered. The presence of prominent early behavioral symptoms, abrupt onset, abrupt changes, and gait dysfunction suggest an alternative dementia syndrome.

Tx—Currently, there are no disease-modifying therapies. Instead, therapy is aimed at symptomatic improvement of cognition or behavior. Symptomatic therapies for cognition include acetylcholinesterase inhibitors (e.g., donepezil, rivastigmine, galantamine) and memantine, an N-methyl-d-aspartate (NMDA) receptor antagonist. Both donepezil and memantine have been shown to mildly improve cognition, activities of daily living, and behavior in patients with moderate-severe AD. Only acetylcholinesterase inhibitors have shown similar benefits in patients with mild AD. Atypical antipsychotics, antidepressants, and other medications may be helpful in treating the psychiatric manifestations of AD. However, these medications may worsen cognition and thus should be used cautiously.

Vascular Dementia

D—Cognitive dysfunction resulting directly from vascular disease of the brain.

Epi—The exact frequency is unclear. Vascular dementia is considered the second most common dementia by pathologic criteria.

P—There are numerous types that differ in the mechanism of vascular injury, including mild vascular cognitive impairment, multi-infarct dementia, dementia from a hemorrhagic lesion, lacunar lesions, or single large strokes in specific locations, among others.

RF—Vascular disease, a history of stroke, and risk factors for stroke are predisposing conditions.

SiSx—Vascular dementia may present with various manifestations of cognitive dysfunction, depending on the location of the vascular disease/infarct. Cognitive dysfunction may occur after a clinical stroke or develop

insidiously from subclinical ischemic disease. Features suggesting vascular dementia include onset of cognitive deficits with a stroke, abrupt onset, stepwise deterioration, focal neurologic symptoms or signs, and an infarct or severe white matter disease seen on neuroimaging.

Dx—Since AD and vascular disease are relatively common diseases of the elderly, they may coexist, making differentiation impossible.

Tx—Treat the underlying condition and modifiable vascular risk factors (especially hypertension) to prevent new strokes. Acetylcholinesterase inhibitors and NMDA-receptor antagonists likely provide mild symptomatic benefit.

Frontotemporal Lobar Dementia (FTLD)

D—A clinical syndrome caused by degeneration of the frontal and sometimes temporal lobes characterize by progressive change in behavior or loss of language function.

Epi—It is the most common dementia in people <60 years of age.

P—Pathologically, FTLD is divided into two subtypes based on whether the intraneuronal protein aggregates are composed of tau protein (Pick's disease) or TAR DNA-binding protein (TDP-43). These pathologic subtypes cannot be distinguished clinically. Tau and progranulin gene mutations are associated with FTLD.

RF—From 20% to 40% of patients have a family history of FTD (see below).

SiSx—In contrast to AD, memory is relatively spared. Frontotemporal lobar dementia is divided into three clinical subtypes:

1. *Frontotemporal dementia* (FTD): This is the most common subtype, accounting for more than half of FTLD patients, with a male:female ratio of 2:1. Patients present with inappropriate social behavior (disinhibition, lack of empathy), apathy, overeating (especially sweets), repetitive/ritualistic behaviors, and poor judgment. Patients completely lack insight; thus, comorbid depression does not occur. Commonly, these patients present after severe

social dysfunction (e.g., loss of job, divorce). Fifteen percent of these patients develop ALS.

2. *Nonfluent aphasia*: This is marked by focal involvement of the left frontal lobe. Patients present with decreased speech output, difficulty with grammar, and dysarthria. In contrast to FTD, patients are often aware of their language difficulties before others. They may develop atypical parkinsonian syndromes, either progressive supranuclear palsy or corticobasal degeneration

3. *Semantic dementia*: Classically, this is described as focal involvement of the left temporal lobe. Patients present with difficulty finding words and difficulty understanding words. They may also develop compulsions/ritualistic behaviors. As the disease progresses, patients develop deficits in nonlanguage comprehension, such as the recognition of faces or objects.

Dx—Frontotemporal lobar dementia is a clinical diagnosis. Brain imaging may show focal cerebral atrophy of the frontal and/or anterior temporal lobes. Functional brain imaging studies such as a PET scan may demonstrate decreased frontal and/or anterior temporal lobe metabolism.

Tx—No disease-modifying therapy exists. Symptomatic treatment includes antidepressants for compulsive behaviors and atypical antipsychotics for aggressive behavior. Mean survival is 3.4–5.2 years after diagnosis, depending on the presenting syndrome.

Normal Pressure Hydrocephalus (NPH)

D—A reversible cause of dementia due to increased CSF volume (hydrocephalus) with compensatory loss of brain parenchyma resulting in normal intracranial pressure.

Epi—The exact frequency of NPH is unknown. It may be idiopathic or secondary to disorders of the subarachnoid space (e.g., subarachnoid hemorrhage or meningitis).

P—The exact mechanism is unclear. It may be due to impaired CSF reabsorption at the level of the arachnoid villi.

RF—Risk factors include increased age and a history of meningitis or subarachnoid hemorrhage.

SiSx—The classic triad of symptoms is (1) gait dysfunction, (2) cognitive dysfunction, and (3) urinary incontinence. All of these symptoms are common in the elderly, making diagnosis difficult. The classic gait dysfunction is described as difficulty lifting the legs off the ground (magnetic). The cognitive dysfunction is nonspecific, with psychomotor slowing, decreased attention, and poor executive function.

Dx—Diagnosis is based on clinical criteria, neuroimaging findings, and the response to CSF drainage. Neuroimaging shows enlarged ventricles (hydrocephalus) without increased prominence of the cortical sulci. The opening CSF pressure, measured by lumbar puncture, is normal to slightly elevated. A large volume (30–50 mL) of CSF is removed, and the gait is reassessed immediately after lumbar puncture. Improvement of gait has a high positive predictive value for the diagnosis of NPH. However, large-volume lumbar puncture has a poor negative predictive value, which may necessitate further evaluation with repeat large-volume lumbar puncture or continuous CSF drainage.

Tx—Normal pressure hydrocephalus is treated with the placement of a ventriculoperitoneal shunt. Patients with secondary NPH are more likely to respond than those with idiopathic NPH. Patients are more likely to respond if dementia has been present for less than 2 years and if gait dysfunction preceded cognitive dysfunction.

Pseudodementia

D—Depression with a clinical presentation that mimics dementia.

Epi—Estimates range from 10% to 25% of causes of reversible dementia.

RF—Preexisting psychiatric illness or a predisposition to psychiatric illness are risk factors.

SiSx—Depression is a frequent cause of cognitive dysfunction and, when severe, can mimic dementia (pseudodementia). In contrast to most patients with dementia, patients with depression are very concerned about their cognitive difficulties and frequently seek medical attention. Although patients typically report poor memory, on exam the most prominent findings are psychomotor retardation and poor attention. In addition to cognitive dysfunction, patients often have vegetative symptoms and other somatic complaints.

Dx—This is a clinical diagnosis, which sometimes can be difficult to make. Hence, it is important to rule out other causes of dementia.

Tx—Treatment of underlying depression involves antidepressants and psychotherapy. Severe depression may require electroconvulsive therapy.

Creutzfeld-Jakob Disease (CJD) (see Chapter 8)

Demyelinating Diseases

Multiple Sclerosis (MS)

D—A progressive, inflammatory, predominantly demyelinating disease that primarily affects different parts of the CNS (optic nerves, subcortical white matter, brainstem, and spinal cord) at different points in time. It may progress in four different ways:

1. Relapsing-remitting (85% of cases of MS)—recurrent acute exacerbations that completely resolve.
2. Progressive-relapsing—recurrent acute exacerbations without complete resolution of neurologic disease.
3. Secondary progressive (80% of cases of relapsing-remitting MS after 25 years)—progressive neurologic disease without acute exacerbations after a period of relapsing-remitting MS.
4. Primary progressive (10–15% of cases of MS)—progressive neurologic disease without acute exacerbations.

Epi—Multiple sclerosis affects roughly 300,000 people in the United States, with prevalence rising with increasing distance from the equator. The peak onset of symptoms is between the second and fourth decades; symptoms generally present before 55 years of age. The disease is more common in women.

P—The cause of MS is unknown. Both genetic factors (e.g., HLA-DR2) and environmental factors (e.g., Epstein-Barr virus, human herpes virus-6, and distance from the equator) have been associated with MS. In an active MS lesion, there is an autoimmune response against antigens on myelin resulting in inflammation, demyelination, and partial axonal loss.

RF—Twenty percent of patients with MS have a family member with MS. The family members at highest risk are siblings, with a 20–30% risk in an identical twin and a 3–5% risk in nonidentical siblings. Geography is a risk factor, with high prevalence rates (>60/100,000) in Europe, southern Canada, the northern United States, New Zealand, and southeastern Australia. Patients with preexisting autoimmune diseases are more likely to develop MS.

SiSx—The initial presentation of relapsing-remitting MS is highly variable. Most patients present with one of the following syndromes: optic neuritis, myelopathy, or brainstem dysfunction, as described in Table 11-29. Although these syndromes must persist for at least 24 hours to be consistent with an MS exacerbation, most usually last for 1–3 weeks. In addition to the evaluation of the presenting syndrome, the history and exam should focus on the presence of episodes of previous mild neurologic dysfunction, which may not have prompted medical attention. In patients with relapsing-remitting MS, the frequency of exacerbations is highly variable. Some patients experience multiple exacerbations per year, while others remain symptom-free for years. Recrudescence of previous symptoms may occur in the setting of infection or increased body temperature and should be distinguished from new exacerbations. With disease progression, many patients develop progressive neurologic deficits.

Dx—The diagnosis of relapsing-remitting MS is clinical and requires multiple (at least two) distinct episodes of CNS dysfunction that are more than 3 months apart and exam findings consistent with multiple (at least two) distinct locations of CNS dysfunction.

Table 11-29. Clinical Syndromes Seen in Multiple Sclerosis

Condition	SiSx/Dx	Tx
Optic Neuritis	• The presenting symptom in 15–20% of MS patients; 50% of patients with MS develop optic neuritis during their disease course, which presents with painful eye movements followed by subacute (hours to days) central monocular vision loss. • Simultaneous bilateral optic neuritis is atypical in adults with MS and suggests an alternative diagnosis such as neuromyelitis optica (NMO) (see Table 11-30). • Patients may complain of blurry vision or decreased color vision. On exam, patients have decreased visual acuity and an APD. Severe vision loss (no light perception) is not typical of optic neuritis. Only one-third of patients have an abnormal fundus exam with mild disc swelling. A previous episode of optic neuritis may have persistent exam findings such as an APD and optic pallor on fundus exam. • An MRI scan of the brain may show enhancement and swelling of the optic nerve in 95% of patients. • This can be confirmed with visual evoked potentials demonstrating demyelination of the optic nerve.	• Vision loss peaks at 1–2 weeks and begins to recover within 4 weeks of symptom onset. Patient many have complete or nearly complete visual recovery, especially after the first episode of optic neuritis. • IV methylprednisolone increases the rate of visual recovery but does not affect the amount of visual improvement. • For unclear reasons, oral prednisone was shown to increase the risk of recurrent optic neuritis and therefore is avoided in optic neuritis.
Myelopathy	• The classic myelopathy of MS presents subacutely (hours to days) with asymmetric weakness and/or numbness at and below the lesion in the spinal cord. • The weakness and/or loss of vibration/proprioception sensation are ipsilateral to the lesion, while the loss of pain/temperature sensation is contralateral to the lesion. Bowel or bladder dysfunction may accompany these symptoms or, less commonly, is the sole manifestation of myelopathy. • Symmetric weakness or numbness or involvement of the entire cord is not typical of the myelopathy of MS and suggests idiopathic transverse myelitis or NMO (see Table 11-30). • On exam, patients have ipsilateral spasticity, hyperreflexia, and abnormal primitive reflexes (positive Babinski or Hoffman sign). • An MRI scan of the spine shows gadolinium-enhanced signal abnormality. • A previous episode of myelopathy can be confirmed by demonstrating demyelination on somatosensory evoked potentials.	• As in optic neuritis, patients are often treated with IV methylprednisolone to increase the rate of neurologic recovery.
Brainstem Syndromes	• There are two common brainstem manifestations of MS: horizontal diplopia and ataxia. • Develop subacutely (hours to days). Horizontal diplopia is usually caused by demyelination of the medial longitudinal fasciculus producing an internuclear ophthalmoplegia (INO). • On exam, there is outward deviation of the eyes when the patient looks straight ahead (exotropia) and decreased adduction of the eye ipsilateral to the lesion. • An INO is not specific for MS; it also occurs with brainstem infarctions, which present acutely in patients with vascular risk factors. • Ataxia is usually caused by demyelination of the cerebellar peduncles. On exam, patients have dysmetria ipsilateral to the lesion and gait instability.	• As in optic neuritis, patients are often treated with IV methylprednisolone to increase the rate of neurologic recovery.

Table 11-30. Demyelinating Disorders in the Differential with Multiple Sclerosis

Condition	D/Epi	SiSx/Dx	Tx
Transverse Myelitis (TM)	An idiopathic inflammatory process affecting one to two segments of the spinal cord. Some patients have a history of an infection or vaccination within 3 weeks of symptom onset.	• Classically presents subacutely with symmetric weakness and numbness at and below the lesion. An MRI scan of the spinal cord shows a gadolinium-enhanced signal abnormality. • Half of patients with TM have elevated protein and moderate lymphocytosis on CSF evaluation. • Oligoclonal bands are typically absent.	Patients are often treated with corticosteroids without demonstrated efficacy in RCTs. Most patients experience partial recovery within 1–3 months of symptom onset. Forty percent of patients have persistent disability.
Acute Disseminated Encephalomyelitis (ADEM)	A monophasic, multifocal inflammatory disease that may involve the brain (white and gray matter), brainstem, and spinal cord. Fifty percent have a history of an infection or vaccination within 3 weeks of symptom onset.	• Patients present with acute/subacute onset of fever, encephalopathy (ranging from lethargy to coma), seizures, meningeal irritation, weakness, and numbness. • An MRI scan of the brain and spinal cord shows multifocal symmetric lesions, most of which enhance. On CSF examination, there is a marked pleocytosis (>50 WBCs). Oligoclonal bands are usually absent.	ADEM is treated with intravenous steroids. Patients who do not respond to steroids may be treated with plasmapheresis. There is a 10–30% mortality rate in ADEM, and only 50% of patients completely recover.
Neuromyelitis Optica (NMO)	A severe progressive inflammatory disease of the optic nerves and spinal cord. NMO has a strong female predominance. More common in nonwhites.	• Patients may present with routine optic neuritis, bilateral optic neuritis, or severe symmetric myelopathy. • An MRI scan of the brain is classically normal, although a few nonspecific T2 hyperintensities may be present. An MRI scan of the spine demonstrates central T2 hyperintensities that cross more than three spinal levels. • On CSF examination, there may be marked pleocytosis (>50 WBCs). Oligoclonal bands are present in 20–30% of patients. • A serum antibody to aquaporin-4 (NMO antibody) is present in 75% of patients with NMO with a specificity of 90%.	NMO does not respond to MS disease-modifying therapies. Instead, NMO is treated with chronic immunosuppressive therapy such as rituximab.

Ancillary testing, such as MRI, evoked potentials, and lumbar puncture can help fulfill the criteria and find evidence of prior episodes. Classic MRI findings in relapsing-remitting MS include ovoid T2 hyperintensities in the periventricular white matter and corpus callosum. T2 hyperintensities can also be seen in the brainstem and the spinal cord. The CSF exam in relapsing-remitting MS shows slightly increased protein and mild lymphocytosis (<50 WBCs) and can help rule out other conditions. Cerebrospinal fluid electrophoresis shows oligoclonal bands (typically IgG) in 85–95% of patients, but these are not specific for MS. The different forms of MS are diagnosed by their clinical course. Other demyelinating conditions considered in the differential diagnosis are described in Table 11-30.

Tx—Intravenous corticosteroids increase the rate of recovery from an acute demyelinating episode but do not alter the disease course. Several disease-modifying therapies exist. The standard therapy for relapsing-remitting MS is one of three formulations of interferon-β (1a or 1b) or glatiramer acetate (a mixture of polymers simulating the amino acid composition of myelin basic protein). All of them moderately reduce the frequency of exacerbations, the number of new T2 hyperintensities on MRI, and disease progression. The major side effect of interferon-β is flu-like symptoms. Natalizumab, a monoclonal antibody directed against α-4 integrin proteins on leukocytes that mediate margination, also can reduce the frequency of exacerbations and the number of new T2 hyperintensities. However, there is an estimated 0.1% risk of progressive multifocal leukoencephalopathy (PML). Mitoxantrone, a chemotherapeutic agent, can be used in patients with frequent exacerbations despite the use of standard disease-modifying therapy and is the only medication shown to slow disease progression in secondary progressive MS. There is no currently available treatment for primary progressive MS.

Progressive Multifocal Leukoencephalopathy (PML)

D—A progressive demyelinating disease of the brain caused by reactivation of the JC polyomavirus in severely immunocompromised patients.

Epi—It occurs almost exclusively in severely immunocompromised patients. The prevalence of PML in patients with HIV/AIDS is 1–2%.

P—Infection with JC virus occurs during childhood in most people (>80% of adults have antibodies to the virus). The virus remains latent in the kidneys and lymphoid organs, with no clinical significance in immunocompetent patients. In severely immunosuppressed patients, the virus may become reactivated and infect oligodendrocytes (CNS myelin-producing cells), causing demyelination.

RF—Immunosuppression is a risk factor, especially in patients with AIDS and solid organ transplant recipients.

SiSx—Typically, PML presents subacutely (over weeks) with progressive neurologic deficits, depending on the location of the lesion or lesions. Common presenting symptoms include visual field loss, weakness, limb ataxia, or gait dysfunction. Patients may have altered mental status in addition to these symptoms, but isolated altered mental status is unusual in PML. Unlike MS, PML typically does not affect the optic nerves or spinal cord.

Dx—An MRI scan shows classic findings in PML such as multifocal large T2 hyperintensities in the subcortical white matter without mass effect that are not contrast enhancing. Cerebrospinal fluid analysis may be unremarkable. However, polymerase chain reaction (PCR) detection of JC virus in the CSF is highly specific, although it has a sensitivity of only 70%. Brain biopsy in select hard-to-diagnose cases can be done. Pathognomonic features include infected oligodendrocytes with ground glass intranuclear inclusions of JC virus and bizarre reactive astrocytes.

Tx—No specific treatment exists for PML. Improvement of the patient's immune system is the mainstay of therapy. Immunosuppressive therapy should be decreased if possible. Antiretroviral therapy should be considered in HIV patients. Survival is otherwise quite poor overall (months).

Spinal Cord Disorders

- Spinal cord disease (myelopathy) should be suspected when a patient presents with motor or sensory signs or symptoms that do not involve the head or face, paraplegia, quadriplegia, trauma, or hemisensory loss of vibration and proprioception on one side of the body and loss of temperature or pinprick sensation on the other side.
- Focal spinal cord injuries may be localized by sensory loss below the lesion (sensory level), lower motor neuron signs (atrophy, flaccid weakness, hyporeflexia) at the level of injury if the anterior horn cells are involved, or radicular pain at the level of the injury if the nerve roots are involved.
- Spinal cord disease can be caused by numerous different pathologies. Some of the more common etiologies are described below. Transverse myelitis, neuromyelitis optica, and MS affecting the spinal cord are described in the Multiple Sclerosis section.

Traumatic Myelopathy

D—Spinal cord dysfunction following trauma.

Epi—It affects 10,000 patients per year. It is the most common cause of severe disability after traumatic injury.

P—There is mechanical disruption of axons and arterial injury with resultant ischemia.

RF—Trauma is the risk factor.

SiSx—Traumatic spinal cord compression presents acutely. The clinical presentation depends on the location and severity of the spinal cord injury. Injury below T1 causes leg weakness (paraparesis) and numbness, while injury above C5 causes arm and leg weakness (quadriparesis). In the acute setting, patients are flaccid, with absent reflexes (spinal shock). Typical upper motor signs (spasticity,

hyperreflexia) develop over days to weeks. Patients may develop symptomatic hypotension and bradycardia (neurogenic shock) secondary to the loss of sympathetic tone to the blood vessels and heart.

Dx—The evaluation of traumatic spinal cord injury begins with an emergent CT scan of the cervical, thoracic, and lumbar spine for dislocated fractures. An MRI scan of the spine is necessary to exclude spinal cord injury in patients who have sustained trauma and have altered mental status.

Tx—Treatment includes supportive treatment of hypotension with normal saline and pressors as needed. High-dose IV methylprednisolone has been shown to improve recovery but also causes poor wound healing. Traction is indicated for most dislocated cervical fractures, whereas dislocated thoracic and lumbar fractures may require surgical reduction.

Nontraumatic Compressive Myelopathy

D—Cord dysfunction caused by extrinsic compression such as from herniated discs, osteophyte formation, or vertebral metastases. Rarely, an epidural mass (abscess or hematoma) or a meningioma can cause this condition.

Epi—Spinal cord compression due to chronic degenerative changes is the most common cause of myelopathy. The most common metastatic tumors to the spine are breast, lung, prostate, and kidney cancers, lymphoma, and myeloma.

P—Neurologic dysfunction is primarily caused by direct mechanical compression, but secondary ischemia may develop from arterial or venous compression.

RF—Risk factors for chronic degenerative changes include increased age, a history of trauma, coexistent degenerative changes in other spinal segments, and congenital stenosis. The major risk factor for an epidural abscess or hematoma is a recent procedure.

SiSx—An epidural hematoma or abscess presents subacutely (hours to days), whereas degenerative or neoplastic compression occurs gradually. Patients often present with difficulty walking due to leg weakness or stiffness. Since the corticospinal fibers innervating the leg are the most lateral, these fibers are affected first. Hand clumsiness may also be present with cervical compression. Neck or back pain is common and frequently radiates in a dermatomal distribution secondary to nerve root irritation. On exam, patients with metastases often have spinal tenderness. Patients have unilateral or bilateral lower motor neuron signs (hyporeflexia, atrophy, and decreased tone) at the level of compression and upper motor neuron signs (hyperreflexia, spasticity, and the Babinski sign) below the level of compression. Patients have ipsilateral loss of vibration and proprioception sensation and contralateral loss of temperature and pinprick sensation.

Dx—The diagnosis is made by an urgent MRI scan of the spine. A CT myelogram may be performed if MRI is contraindicated.

Tx—The treatment of metastatic spinal cord compression or acutely worsening degenerative changes is dexamethasone 10 mg followed by 6 mg every 6 hours until emergent surgical decompression can be performed. Chronic spinal cord compression is treated with urgent surgical decompression. Radiation therapy is used in conjunction with surgery for metastatic disease. Antibiotics are used in conjunction with surgery for an epidural abscess.

Syringomyelia (Syrinx)

D—A fluid-filled central cavity, usually in the cervical spinal cord. It invariably affects the anterolateral system as it crosses in the anterior commissure.

Epi—There is an estimated prevalence of 8/100,000 patients.

P—The pathogenesis is unclear. Syrinx may be caused by increased CSF pressure in the central canal resulting in compensatory loss of surrounding tissue.

RF—Most commonly, syrinx is associated with congenital malformations, such as an Arnold-Chiari malformation. It may also occur after spinal cord injury from trauma, infection, or neoplasm.

SiSx—A syrinx may be asymptomatic and discovered on neuroimaging. When it is symptomatic, patients develop pain or numbness over the shoulders insidiously between the ages of 25 and 40. On exam, patients have decreased pain and temperature sensation, usually over their shoulders (shawl distribution). If the syrinx enlarges, it may do so in any direction. Lateral enlargement will affect the lateral corticospinal tract, causing weakness and upper motor neuron signs in the legs. Posterior enlargement will affect the posterior columns, causing loss of vibration or proprioception sensation in the legs. Anterior enlargement will affect the anterior horn cells, causing weakness and lower motor neuron signs in the arms. The syrinx may also enlarge rostrally, affecting the brainstem (syringobulbia).

Dx—An MRI scan of the cervical spine will demonstrate a central T2 hyperintensity with the same signal characteristics as CSF. The administration of gadolinium increases the sensitivity of the scan.

Tx—Patients with neurologic deterioration or intractable pain are treated with surgical decompression (fenestration and/or shunt placement). Neurologic deficits usually stabilize and may improve after surgery.

Anterior Spinal Artery Infarction

D—Sudden onset of spinal cord injury caused by decreased spinal perfusion.

Epi—The exact prevalence is unknown. It accounts for 1% of all strokes.

P—The anterior spinal artery supplies the anterolateral system, lateral spinal cord, and anterior horn cells. The anterior spinal artery in the cervical region receives its blood supply from the vertebral arteries. The anterior spinal artery in the thoracic and lumbar regions receives its blood supply from aortic branches. The thoracic spinal cord has the poorest collateral blood supply, making it particularly susceptible to ischemia.

RF—Patients with aortic disease (aneurysm or dissection) and those undergoing aortic surgery are at risk.

SiSx—Symptoms develop acutely. Patients usually present with back pain followed by severe weakness, numbness, and incontinence. In the acute setting, patients are flaccid, with absent reflexes (spinal shock). There is loss of bilateral pain and temperature sensation below the infarction. Proprioception and vibration sensation are spared. Typical upper motor signs (spasticity, hyperreflexia) develop over days to weeks.

Dx—This is a clinical diagnosis. An MRI scan of the spine will demonstrate T2 hyperintensities in two-thirds of patients. A normal MRI scan does not exclude the diagnosis of an anterior spinal artery infarction.

Tx—The goal of treatment is to improve spinal cord perfusion. Blood pressure is allowed to autoregulate. The insertion of a lumbar drain allows for continuous CSF drainage, which decreases the pressure in the spinal canal, optimizing spinal cord perfusion.

Subacute Combined Degeneration

D –Degeneration of the posterior columns and lateral corticospinal tracts due to vitamin B_{12} deficiency.

Epi—The prevalence of vitamin B_{12} deficiency is unknown.

P—Vitamin B_{12} is a cofactor in the formation of myelin. The posterior columns and lateral corticospinal tracts are preferentially affected because these tracts have larger axons with more myelin than the anterolateral system.

RF—Elderly people, vegans, and obese patients treated with gastric bypass are at risk. Nitrous oxide inactivates vitamin B_{12}. A single exposure to nitrous oxide in patients with vitamin B_{12} deficiency can cause an acute myelopathy. Chronic nitrous oxide use also causes myelopathy.

SiSx—Patients present with gradual onset of tingling and sensory ataxia. On exam, patients have loss of vibration and proprioception. If untreated, patients slowly develop progressive weakness. On exam, there are symmetric upper motor neuron signs (hyperreflexia, spasticity, Babinski sign). Cobalamin deficiency also causes peripheral neuropathy, cognitive impairment, optic neuropathy, or anemia. These disease manifestations do not have to be present

for patients to develop subacute combined degeneration syndrome.

Dx—An MRI scan of the spine may demonstrate T2 hyperintensities in the posterior and lateral white matter. The serum cobalamin level is either decreased or in the low normal range, making this test insensitive. Elevated methylmalonic acid and homocysteine levels are more sensitive tests for cobalamin deficiency. Homocysteine levels are also elevated in folic acid deficiency. Once the diagnosis is confirmed, patients are evaluated for abnormal absorption of vitamin B_{12} (pernicious anemia) by testing for antibodies to intrinsic factor, which are present in only 50–70% of patients with pernicious anemia.

Tx—If cobalamin absorption is impaired, patients are treated with IM cobalamin injections. If cobalamin absorption is normal, patients are treated with high-dose oral cobalamin. After supplementation begins, the methylmalonic acid and homocysteine levels should be followed. Neurologic recovery is variable, depending on the duration of disease. Most patients recover within 6 months of the initiation of treatment.

Headache and Facial Pain

Migraine Headache

D—A clinical syndrome characterized by episodic head pain with hypersensitivity to normal sensory stimuli. It is divided into migraine with aura (brief, focal neurologic symptoms that immediately precede the headache) and migraine without aura. Migraine headaches with a motor aura are called *hemiplegic migraines*. Many patients have both types of migraines.

Epi—The prevalence in the United States is 18% of women, 6% of men, and 4% of children. Prior to adolescence, there is a slight male predominance. The disorder typically begins by the third decade of life and is most prevalent between the ages of 25 and 55. Only 30% of patients have an aura.

P—The pathogenesis is unknown but is believed to be both environmental and genetic. The aura of migraine is caused by cortical spreading depression, a propagating self-depolarization of neurons and glial cells. The headache likely has multiple underlying pathologies that involve both the trigeminal nerve and the CNS, especially the thalamus, hypothalamus, and brainstem.

RF—A family history of migraine is a risk factor. Migraine has also been associated with right-to-left cardiac shunts, such as patent foramen ovale (more commonly) or an atrial septal defect.

SiSx—Sixty percent of patients report prodromal symptoms that precede the headache by up to 2 days. Prodromal symptoms occur in patients with and without an aura and include depressed mood, irritability, difficultly concentrating, fatigue, sensitivity to light/sound, yawning, neck stiffness, anorexia, increased thirst, and food cravings. Auras typically last for 4–60 minutes and occur within 60 minutes of headache onset. An aura can present like any focal neurologic deficit. Visual auras are the most common type of aura and patients may describe flashing lights, loss of vision, or zigzagging or colorful lights that migrate across their vision. Paresthesias of the arms and face are the next most common aura. Rare auras include slurred speech, aphasia, or unilateral weakness. Twenty percent of auras actually have no accompanying headache. Migraine headaches themselves are gradual in onset and can last for 4–72 hours. Typically, they are throbbing, moderately severe in intensity, worse with activity, and associated with nausea, light sensitivity (photophobia), and sound sensitivity (phonophobia). Vomiting is frequent. The headache is unilateral in 60% of patients, and 20% have headaches that recurs consistently in the same location. Precipitating factors may include caffeine, chocolate, and onset of menses, among others. On exam, patients may have tenderness to palpation of the scalp, but the neurologic exam is normal.

Dx—The diagnosis of migraine is based entirely on the history, which differentiates migraine headaches from other primary headache syndromes such as tension-type and cluster headaches (described below). Routine neuroimaging should be performed if the headaches are new (especially in patients >50 years of age), if there is a change in headache quality, or if the neurologic exam is abnormal. A patient with a migraine headache that lasts for >72 hours is diagnosed with status migrainosus. With persistent or daily headaches, a detailed history of prescription and over-the-counter medication use should be obtained because headache is a common symptom of withdrawal from analgesic medications (analgesic rebound).

Tx—Patients should avoid triggers if they are identified (alcohol and caffeine use, sleep deprivation, and so forth). The treatment of migraine can be divided into prophylaxis, acute (abortive) therapies, and rescue therapies. These therapies are shown in Table 11-31.

Cluster Headache

D—An extremely painful headache syndrome that occurs periodically or in clusters with spontaneous remissions.

Epi—The prevalence is <1%. There is a male predominance. The mean age of onset is 25.

P—The exact etiology is unclear. Hypotheses include intense pain from dilation of blood vessels or an abnormality in the hypothalamus. Common triggers include chocolate, nicotine, and alcohol, among others.

RF—Patients frequently have a history of alcohol and tobacco abuse. The headache may be precipitated by head trauma.

SiSx—Patients with cluster headaches have brief (15 minutes to 3 hours), very severe unilateral periorbital/retro-orbital stabbing headaches, usually accompanied by autonomic symptoms (lacrimation, conjunctival injection, nasal congestion, rhinorrhea, ptosis, or anisocoria). Photophobia and phonophobia are quite common. Patients have one to three headaches per day that frequently occur in the early hours of the morning (1–2 a.m.). Patients may be headache-free for months or years and then develop a period of daily headaches (clusters). Pain is usually more intense than other headache conditions.

Dx—This is a clinical diagnosis based on the symptoms noted above.

Table 11-31.   Treatment Options for Migraines

Treatment Type	Agents	Comments
Prophylactic Treatment	β-Receptor antagonists (propranolol) Tricyclic antidepressants Anticonvulsants (topirimate, gabapentin, valproic acid)	Offer these agents to patients who have migraine headaches more than 6 days per month or patients with prolonged, severe headaches. Otherwise, therapy depends on patient preference. These agents reduce the frequency of migraine headaches by 30–50%. Agent choice is based on coexisting medical conditions, such as hypertension, depression, and epilepsy, side-effect profiles, and patient preference. Patients who do not respond to one prophylactic medication titrated to a therapeutic dose may respond to a different medication.
Acute (abortive)	5-HT agonist (triptans) Oral, intramuscular, intranasal, and suppository ergot-containing agents (ergotamine, dihydroergotamine) Analgesics (aspirin, acetominophen, NSAIDs, butalbital)	Triptans are the optimal treatment; they should be taken as early as possible and always within 2 hours of headache onset. Response rates for the different triptans vary from 25% to 50%, and individual patients may respond to one triptan after failing to respond to another. Sublingual, nasal, and subcutaneous preparations of triptans are available. Analgesics are also frequently used and are effective in a percentage of patients. Frequent use causes daily headaches (analgesic rebound). Neither ergot-containing agents nor triptans should be used in patients with vascular disease or migraines with motor auras.
Rescue Therapies	Glucocorticoids	Used mainly for status migrainosus after other therapies have failed.

Tx—Headaches respond acutely to subcutaneous or nasal sumatriptan or inhalation of 100% oxygen at a rate of 7–10 L/min via a nonrebreather mask. Headaches may be acutely prevented for 7–10 days with daily triptan use or high-dose glucocorticoids. Verapamil is the primary choice for chronic headache prophylaxis during a cluster. No medications have been shown to prevent recurrent cluster headaches.

Tension-Type Headache

D—Mild to moderate squeezing headache.

Epi—This is the most common type of primary headache, accounting for 90% of all headaches. It may be episodic or chronic. Most people have infrequent episodes. There is a female predominance.

P—The exact etiology is not known but may be due to abnormal interpretation of pain signals by temporal muscles.

RF—Precipitants vary among individuals and include, stress, lack of sleep, hunger, and withdrawal from caffeine use, among others.

SiSx—Patients with tension-type headache have mild to moderate bilateral, constant squeezing ("vice-like") headaches without nausea or vomiting. Photophobia or phonophobia may occur. These headaches may last for 30 minutes to 7 days. Stress is frequently reported as a precipitating factor.

Dx—The diagnosis is made by clinical exam and history when there are no features of other headache syndromes. It is always important to assess for red flag symptoms that suggest another cause of headache, such as meningitis (fever, neck stiffness, focal neurologic deficits), elevated intracranial pressure (that worsens when lying down, awakening with headache or vomiting, focal neurologic deficits), or posttraumatic headaches, among others.

Tx—Tension-type headaches typically respond acutely to over-the-counter analgesics, such as aspirin, NSAIDs, or acetaminophen. Tricyclic antidepressants may be used for prophylaxis if tension-type headaches occur frequently.

Trigeminal Neuralgia (TN)

D—Also called *tic douloureux,* a syndrome of facial pain in the distribution of one or more branches of the trigeminal nerve.

Epi—This is the most common neuralgia syndrome. Annual incidence is 4–13/100,000 and increases with age. It is more common in women.

P—From 80% to 90% of cases are caused by compression of the trigeminal nerve root by an aberrant vascular loop, producing focal demyelination (primary TN). Other cases are caused by various etiologies, such as a mass lesion (vestibular schwannoma, meningioma, epidermoid cyst, aneurysm, dental malignancies) or demyelination from MS (secondary TN).

RF—Age is the main risk factor, with a peak incidence in the sixth and seventh decades of life.

SiSx—Trigeminal neuralgia presents with recurrent episodes of sudden, severe, brief (seconds), stabbing facial pain that is maximal at onset and is often described as electric or lightning-like. It is unilateral in 95% of patients and is usually located in the cheek/upper jaw (second branch of the trigeminal nerve), lower jaw (third branch), or both. Fewer than 5% of cases affect only the forehead or eyebrow (first branch of the trigeminal nerve). Pain can be triggered by talking, chewing, smiling, cold air, or brushing the teeth. In primary TN, the neurologic exam, including facial sensation, is normal. Decreased facial sensation suggests secondary TN.

Dx—The diagnosis of TN is made clinically. An MRI scan of the brain is usually performed to exclude secondary TN, especially in young patients. Magnetic resonance angiography (MRA) may demonstrate vascular compression of the trigeminal nerve, but this finding does not alter the management of primary TN.

Tx—First-line therapy is carbamazepine for primary TN and is effective in 70–80% of patients. Alternative medications include baclofen, oxcarbamazepine, gabapentin, and phenytoin, among others. For nonresponders to medications, ablative procedures, such as alcohol or glycerol rhizotomy or gamma knife radiosurgery, may offer pain relief, but symptoms may recur.

Giant Cell Arteritis (see Chapter 6)

Primary CNS Tumors (see Chapter 10)

Central Nervous System Related Infections (see Chapter 8)

CHAPTER 12

Dermatology

BASIC ANATOMY

The skin is divided into three sections, as shown in Figure 12-1.

Epidermis: The outermost layer of the skin, composed of keratinocytes, melanocytes, and Langerhans cells.

Dermis: Directly beneath the epidermis, the dermis is largely composed of extracellular matrix proteins. Fibroblasts in dermis make collagen, elastic fibers, and ground substance. The dermis also contains vessels, nerves, hair follicles, sweat glands, and mast cells.

Subcutaneous fat: This anchors the dermis to the underlying fascia, lobules of lipocytes separated by fibrous septae.

APPROACH TO COMMON PROBLEMS

Approach to Describing Skin Lesions and Eruptions

First, one must recognize the primary and associated second lesions that are seen. Primary lesions are those directly associated with the disease process. Secondary lesions are those that represent a change in the primary lesion, usually as a result of external factors, injury, or natural evolution of the primary process. These are shown in Table 12-1 and Color Figure 12-2 through 12-10.

Along with a description of primary or secondary lesions, it is helpful to include **color** (pink, red, purple, and so forth), **margination**

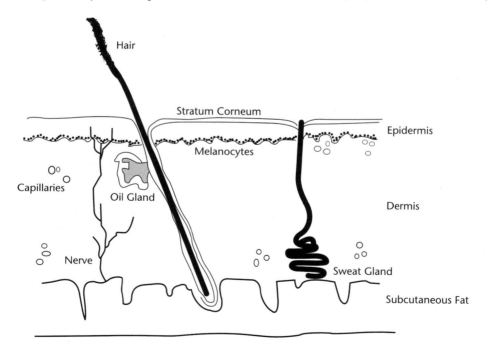

Figure 12-1. Anatomy of the Skin.

Table 12-1. Description of Dermatologic Lesions

(A) Primary Lesions

	Description	Picture
Macule	A circumscribed area of change in skin color <1.0 cm, without elevation or depression	See Color Figure 12-2
Patch	A circumscribed area of change in skin color >1.0 cm, without elevation or depression	See Color Figure 12-3
Papule	A solid, elevated area, usually described as a dome-shaped or flat-topped lesion <0.1 cm	See Color Figure 12-4
Plaque	An elevated, plateau-like lesion >1.0 cm, often formed by confluent papules	See Color Figure 12-5
Nodule	A dome-shaped lesion >1.0 cm	See Color Figure 12-6
Urticaria (hives)	A plateau-like, edematous, red to pink, oval or arcuate lesion; individual lesions lasts <24 hours	See Color Figure 12-7
Vesicle	A circumscribed <1.0 cm lesion filled with clear or red (blood-tinged) fluid	See Color Figure 12-8
Bulla	A vesicle that is >1.0 cm; may be uni- or multiloculated	See Color Figure 12-9
Pustule	A circumscribed, elevated cavity containing pus; various sizes and shapes	See Color Figure 12-10

(B) Secondary Lesions

	Description
Scale	Dry masses of keratin loosely attached to the skin surface
Crust	Dried serum, pus, or blood mixed with epithelial debris on the skin surface
Excoriation	A linear abrasion produced by scratching, usually involving only the epidermis
Fissure	A linear cleft through the epidermis into the dermis; usually occurs in dry, inelastic skin
Erosion	A loss of epidermis only; it heals without scarring
Ulceration	A loss of epidermis and some or all of the dermis; it heals with scarring
Scar	A fibrous tissue that replaces normal skin following an ulceration; it may be depressed, elevated, or flush with the skin surface

(is it well circumscribed?), **shape** (oval, annular, linear, geometric, and so forth), **number** (single or multiple), **arrangement** (grouped, scattered, annular, confluent), **distribution** (localized, regional, generalized), and **pattern** (sun-exposed, sites of pressure, dermatomal, intertriginous).

Approach to Skin Signs in Systemic Disease

A list and discussion of dermatologic conditions associated with common systemic medical conditions is presented below.

Diabetes

- **Diabetic dermopathy:** reddish-brown papules and hyperpigmented brown macules on the lower legs. They are present in more than half of patients with diabetes and are more common in patients with other signs of microvascular disease.
- **Necrobiosis lipoidica diabeticorum:** waxy, orange, atrophic lesions on the lower legs. They are present in many patients who do not have diabetes but only in a small percentage of diabetic patients.
- **Diabetic bullae:** spontaneous, noninflammatory bullae on the lower legs. They are seen in patients with long-standing diabetes and microvascular disease.

Sarcoidosis

This is a chronic systemic granulomatous disease involving skin and internal organs with a wide spectrum of clinical manifestations and prognosis.

Skin involvement can consist of papules, annular lesions, macules of hypopigmentation in dark-pigmented patients, plaques, erythema nodosum, and ichthyosis.

The combination of erythema nodosum, systemic symptoms, and hilar lymphadenopathy as a presentation of sarcoidosis is known as *Löfgren's syndrome* and is associated with a good prognosis.

Amyloidosis

This is a primary systemic amyloidosis characterized by deposition of amyloid material around blood vessels, causing fragility, and in a variety of other organs, including the skin.

Macroglossia can occur due to deposition in the tongue, and the skin can have shiny, firm, skin-colored papules and plaques, often around mucocutaneous junctions.

The blood vessel fragility causes easy bruising in the form of "pinch purpura" and periorbital ecchymoses.

Hyperthyroidism

This condition is characterized by warm skin with increased sweating, pruritus, hypertrichosis, and vitiligo. Patients with Graves' disease can have specific skin changes of pretibial myxedema, exophthalmos, and thyroid acropachy (thickening of the terminal phalanges).

Hypothyroidism

This condition is characterized by cool, pale skin, decreased sweating, poor wound healing, dry, brittle hair, diffuse hair loss, and yellowish skin (carotenemia).

Nutritional Deficiencies

In general, nutritional deficiencies share the following characteristic skin changes: scaling and erythema of the perioral, acral, genital, and perineal areas, with atrophic changes to the tongue, and erosions at the corners of the mouth (angular chelitis) (see Chapter 5 Appendix).

Lupus

- **Chronic Cutaneous Lupus:** discoid lupus—circular, hyper- and hypopigmented macules

with central erythema, most commonly on the head, neck, and ears, exacerbated by ultraviolet light (UV) exposure. If they are located in hair-bearing areas, they lead to scarring alopecia. Lesions are typically limited to just the skin; only 5% of these patients go on to develop systemic lupus erythematosus (SLE).

- **Subacute Cutaneous Lupus:** scaly, annular red lesions or lesions resembling psoriasis, also exacerbated by UV exposure. About 30% of patients meet the criteria for SLE, and many have a positive antinuclear antibody (ANA), as well as anti-Ro and anti-La antibodies. This condition can also be medication-induced.

- **Systemic Lupus Erythematosus:** commonly has cutaneous signs; 4 of the 11 American College of Rheumatology (ACR) criteria for diagnosing SLE are skin-related: **malar rash, discoid rash, photosensitivity, and oral ulcers**. The malar or butterfly rash is erythema in a photo distributed area across the cheeks, classically sparing the nasolabial folds, and at the V of the neck and chest. Other common skin signs of lupus include bullous lesions (bullous lupus), periungal telangiectasias, and scarring or nonscarring hair loss. In patients with antiphospholipid antibody syndrome, livedo reticularis and ulcers can be seen.

Dermatomyositis

This is a syndrome of characteristic skin changes and inflammatory myopathy, often associated with an underlying malignancy. Skin changes include photosensitivity and erythema over the face, chest, and V of the back (called the *shawl sign*). Violaceous papules over the knuckles are called *Gottron's papules*, an area sometimes considered pathognomonic for dermatomyositis. Erythema can develop around the eyes and is called a *heliotrope rash*, and the hands can become scaled and fissured (mechanic's hands) with ragged cuticles (Samitz sign). These skin changes can occur in the absence of myopathy and are then called *amyopathic dermatomyositis*.

Scleroderma

- **Morphea:** sclerosis of the skin and subcutaneous fat resulting in smooth, light-colored, immobile skin. It can be localized to one or two patches, occur in generalized small macules, or have widespread involvement that can cause joint contractures. Internal organs are not affected.

- **CREST Syndrome:** *Calcinosis, Raynaud's phenomenon, Esophageal dysmotility, Sclerodactyly,* and *Telangectasias.* These patients can go on to develop a more progressive scleroderma, but usually this happens very slowly (see Chapter 6).
- **Progressive Systemic Sclerosis:** connective tissue disease involving thickening of the dermal collagen and abnormalities of the vasculature in internal organs. All organs can be affected, but basilar pulmonary fibrosis and esophageal disease are most common. Skin changes are widespread and characteristic, including **sclerodactyly and inability** to open the mouth widely. Patients look younger than their stated age due to smoothing of facial wrinkles.

Graft-versus-Host Disease (GVHD)

- **Acute GVHD:** defined as occurring within the first 100 days after stem cell transplant or donor lymphocyte infusion. It usually begins as a morbilliform rash that can progress to erythroderma and full-thickness skin necrosis. The clinical appearance can be identical to that of a severe drug reaction. Acute skin GVHD is often seen at the same time as gut or hepatic GVHD. This can be a life-threatening condition, and systemic immunosuppression and systemic steroids are the treatment.
- **Chronic GVHD:** skin lesions that can take many different forms, including lichen planus–like lesions, sclerosis resembling scleroderma, and eczematous lesions. Chronic skin GVHD can be disabling but is rarely life-threatening.

Sweet's Syndrome

Also known as *acute febrile neutrophilic dermatosis,* this condition is characterized by acute, tender, red to purple plaques that may develop small pustules or vesicles on the surface, involving the face, upper trunk, and arms. Most patients will also have systemic symptoms of fever, malaise, arthritis, arthralgias, and leukocytosis with a left shift and elevated ESR. The syndrome can be idiopathic, appear after viral infection in women, occur in association with malignancy (most commonly AML), or appear with the use of certain medications, most commonly granulocyte-macrophage colony-stimulating factor (GM-CSF) or granulocyte colony-stimulating factor (G-CSF).

Human Immunodeficiency Virus (HIV)

Skin manifestations depend on the patient's viral load and CD4 count, as well as on the types and duration of antiretroviral medications taken.

- Eosinophilic folliculitis: itchy, red, follicular based papules and pustules on the head, neck and trunk.
- Prurigo nodularis: hyperpigmented papules on the extremities resulting from long-standing scratching and picking.
- Photosensitivity/hyperpigmentation: can be due to HIV itself or to medication.
- Infectious disease: increases in all types of warts, HSV and zoster reactivation, and molluscum contagiosum.
- Oral hairy leukoplakia: white, adherent membrane on the tongue that cannot be scraped off, related to EBV reactivation.
- Angular chelitis: inflammatory lesion at the corner of the mouth that can be superinfected with candida and is associated with thrush.

Disseminated Intravascular Coagulation (DIC)

Abnormalities of the clotting cascade in critically ill patients result in necrotic erosions and ulcerations on a background of purpura called *purpura fulminans.* Lesions occur on acral areas and can lead to loss of digits if the patient recovers from the underlying disease.

Approach to Skins Signs and Infectious Diseases

A list and discussion of dermatologic conditions associated with common infectious conditions is presented below.

Viruses

- **Herpes Simplex Virus (HSV):** causes grouped vesicles on an erythematous base or grouped erosions. The primary infection usually occurs at a young age and is asymptomatic; reactivation can occur at any time in the future and often develops in response to stress or sun exposure. Type 1 HSV reactivates at the mucocutaneous junction of the lips. Type 2 HSV more commonly affects the genital mucosa. Either type can become disseminated in immunosuppressed patients and cause mortality.
- **Varicella-Zoster Virus (VZV):** the initial infection causes chicken pox, with widespread pruritic vesicles on an erythematous base in a systemically ill patient. The virus is then latent in the dorsal root ganglia and can reactivate as zoster (shingles). Vesicles occur on erythematous skin in mainly one dermatome. If lesions appear on more than three dermatomes, the disease is likely to be disseminated VZV, which occurs in immunosuppressed patients. Common, serious morbidity of zoster virus is **postherpetic neuralgia**, which is more likely to occur in older patients. Zoster virus should be treated with acyclovir or valacyclovir in order to prevent this condition.
- **Human Papillomavirus:** infects only skin and mucous membranes, and leads to verruca (warts) including common, flat, plantar, periungal, and genital warts. Long-term infection, infection with certain types, and immunosuppression increase the risk for progression of warts to squamous cell cancer and anal/cervical cancer. Treatment involves destructive methods, including cryotherapy, salicylic acid, and imiquimod.

Bacteria

Localized Bacterial Skin Infections

- Staphylococcal and streptococcal bacteria commonly cause primary skin disease in the following forms:
  - Furunculosis—infection of the hair follicle, commonly presenting as a skin abscess (the most common presentation of community-acquired methicillin-resistant *Staphylococcus aureus*). It is treated with incision and drainage (I&D)and possibly with antibiotics.
  - Cellulitis—infection of the subcutaneous tissue, presenting as an ill-defined area of warmth, erythema, edema, and tenderness in a febrile patient. It is treated with antibiotics.

Systemic Bacterial Infections Causing Skin Lesions

Neisseria meningitis: stellate, gunmetal gray macular lesions and ulcerations over the distal extremities.

Ecthyma gangrenosum: necrotic, punched-out eschars on a background of intense erythema and induration in critically ill patients with *Pseudomonas* septicemia, often seen on extremities, buttocks, and genitals.

Staphylococcus scalded skin syndrome: diffuse erythema with superficial desquamation due to a *Staphylococcus* toxin that causes fever and cleaves the attachment of the upper layer of the skin. It is more common in children but is also seen in adults with renal failure.

Staphylococcus and streptococcus toxic shock syndromes: both syndromes can present with diffuse erythema and desquamation, usually beginning at the flexor areas, due to supertoxins elaborated by the bacteria. Patients are also hypotensive and febrile.

Rocky Mountain spotted fever: due to a rickettsial disease, this condition is typically marked by petechiae or red macules at the wrists and ankles that can spread proximally.

Mycobacteria

- **Tuberculosis (TB):** can disseminate to the skin from underlying disease or spread hematogenously; it can also be inoculated into skin primarily. *Lupus vulgaris* is the name for a single reddish-brown TB plaque in a patient with moderate immunity to TB.
- **Atypical Mycobacteria:** these bacteria, particularly *Mycobacterium marinum, M. ulcerans,* and *M. abscessus,* can cause ulcerated nodules in a sporotrichoid distribution (ascending

along lymphatic vessels) after primary inoculation. *Mycobacterium marinum* typically causes disease after exposure to swimming pools, fish tanks, or other water sources.

Fungi

- **Dermatophytes:** various species of fungi that infect the hair, skin, and nails, causing tinea corporis, tinea cruris, tinea pedis, tinea capitis, and onychomycosis. They are often a significant problem in immunosuppressed hospitalized patients.
- **Candida:** a type of yeast that most commonly causes red, macerated confluent macules and papules, sometimes with pustules and typical "satellite lesions" in the intertriginous areas in hospitalized patients on antibiotics. It can also cause fungemia in immunocompromised patients, especially those having central lines and receiving TPN. In these fungemic patients, one may see widespread red papules and hemorrhagic pustules.
- **Invasive Fungal Infections:** in immunosuppressed patients, certain types of fungi can either enter the bloodstream from a pulmonary or GI source and become disseminated to the skin, or become inoculated into the skin primarily with secondary fungemia. Skin signs and biopsy can provide a rapid diagnosis and a guide to treatment.
  - *Aspergillus, Fusarium, Mucor:* angioinvasive fungi that can cause necrotic eschars, especially if they occur under tape, arm boards, or monitor leads in a neutropenic patient. The eschars require emergent treatment.
  - *Cryptococcus:* fungus that causes various presentations of skin disease in HIV patients with disseminated disease, often umbilicated papules on the head and neck that resemble molluscum contagiosum.
  - **Coccidioidomycosis, Histoplasmosis, Blastomycosis:** diseases that can occur in immunocompetent or suppressed hosts. Disseminated disease can occur with papules, nodules, erythema nodosum, or other skin manifestations. *Candida tropicalis* infection can develop in an immunocompromised host.

Primary Dermatologic Diseases

Commonly Encountered Dermatoses

Irritant Dermatitis

D—A nonspecific inflammation of skin causing redness, scaling, cracking, and erosions.

P—This can occur in anyone if exposure to the irritant is prolonged or at high enough concentrations. Prior sensitization is not required. The condition is not immune-mediated. Common irritants in hospitalized patients include water, feces, or urine in incontinent patients, adhesive tape, povidone iodine, monitoring leads, and alcohol-based or other types of hand sanitizer.

SiSx—Typically, patients report pain, stinging, or burning more often than itching.

Dx—This is a clinical diagnosis based on the typical appearance, symptoms, and response to removal of the irritant.

Tx—Treatment consists of avoidance of irritants, barrier creams (zinc oxide, white petrolatum), and topical steroids.

Pruritus Without Primary Lesions

D—A condition that often presents with acute or chronic itching without a rash.

P—Pruritus is commonly caused by xerosis, or dry skin, especially in elderly patients who have an abnormal skin barrier and do not moisturize, take frequent or hot showers, and live in cold climates. Medications can also cause pruritus; narcotics are a common cause in hospitalized patients.

SiSx—Sometimes patients have excoriations or prurigo nodules (hyperpigmented nodules or papules appearing at sites of chronic picking or scratching) on exam, but there are no primary lesions.

Dx—Internal causes of itching include uremia or chronic kidney disease; liver disease with obstructive jaundice, in particular primary biliary cirrhosis; blood disorders such as polycythemia vera and iron-deficiency anemia; lymphoma, especially Hodgkin's disease; solid malignancies; HIV; intestinal parasites; hepatitis C virus even in the absence of cirrhosis; and hypo- or hyperthyroidism. Initial work-up for a patient with new-onset pruritus without primary skin lesions or dry skin includes a CBC with differential to look for eosinophilia or abnormal cells and evaluation of liver, kidney, and thyroid functions. Depending on the patient, other investigations can include hepatitis C and HIV tests, stool ova and parasite exams, and chest X-ray.

Tx—Treatment is directed at the underlying disease. Phototherapy can be helpful for renal or hepatic pruritus along with aggressive use of moisturizers, decreased bathing, and short courses of topical steroids.

Allergic Contact Dermatitis

D—An immunologically mediated inflammation of the skin that causes redness, vesicles, bullae, crusts, and erosions.

P—This condition occurs only in susceptible patients who have been previously sensitized to the antigen. Common allergens in hospitalized patients include topical antibiotics (polysporin, neomycin), topical anesthetics, tincture of benzoin, rubber or rubber accelerators in respirator masks, and prosthetics or other medical appliances.

SiSx—Typically, patients complain of itching more often than burning or pain.

Dx—Clinical suspicion is based on the appearance of the skin and the presence of itching, the condition can be confirmed with patch testing. It is differentiated from cellulitis by its lack of systemic symptoms, presence of itching, and a history of something being applied to skin.

T—Avoidance of the allergen is key, as is the use of topical steroids to treat the current inflammation.

Atopic Dermatitis/Eczema

D—Dry skin, itching, erythema and lichenification (thickening of the skin in response to chronic rubbing or scratching). It usually begins in childhood and improves with age. Often it is part of the atopic triad with allergic rhinitis and asthma.

P—Defects in profilaggrin, the major epidermal calcium-binding protein, have been shown to lead to abnormal skin barrier function and increased transepidermal water loss.

Epi—The condition is common, with an equal incidence in men and women.

SiSx—Pruritus is a hallmark of atopic dermatitis. Flexural areas frequently are involved in adults, and the face and extensor surfaces are affected in children.

Dx—The diagnosis is clinical, based on a typical personal or family history of atopy, chronicity, itching, and exam.

Tx—Aggressive use of moisturizers and avoidance of irritants to prevent flares is recommended. Topical anti-inflammatories such as topical steroids or topical immunomodulators, oral antihistamines, and phototherapy to control the itch are also used.

Seborrheic Dermatitis

D—A chronic greasy scaling and erythema of the scalp, ears, nasolabial folds, eyebrows, beard, or chest.

Epi—It is very common in older men and is seen in patients with neurologic disease.

P—It may be a reaction to or overgrowth of normal yeast on the skin.

SiSx—Occasionally, patients have itching; otherwise, they are asymptomatic.

Dx—The diagnosis is clinical, based on the typical appearance (see Color Figure 12-11).

Tx—Treatment includes short courses of low-potency topical steroids followed by maintenance therapy with topical antifungals and antidandruff shampoo.

Psoriasis

D—A chronic inflammatory disease causing well-circumscribed red plaques or papules with characteristic silvery scales and nail changes, sometimes accompanied by psoriatic arthritis. It commonly affects extensor surfaces, the scalp, and the buttocks. Other forms include inverse psoriasis and pustular psoriasis; the latter is an acute systemic illness accompanied by fever, leukocytosis, and potential for CHF. A variant form, guttate psoriasis, can be seen after viral infections.

Epi—It affects 1–2% of the North American population, with an equal incidence in men and women.

P—There is evidence for genetic and environmental factors leading to abnormal trafficking, functioning, and interactions of lymphocytes and keratinocytes.

RF—A family history is a risk factor. Disease may also be precipitated or exacerbated by streptococcal infections, β blockers, lithium, or other medications.

SiSx—Pruritus occurs in chronic plaque psoriasis; arthritis develops in psoriatic arthritis; fever, malaise, and even high-output heart failure may be seen in erythrodermic or pustular psoriasis.

Dx—The diagnosis is based on the typical clinical appearance, as shown in Color Figure 12-12 and sometimes in skin biopsy.

Tx—Treatment depends on the type and extent of psoriasis and can include many different topical therapies: UV light therapy; systemic drugs such as methotrexate, acitretin, or cyclosporine; or biologic agents such as etanercept or infliximab.

Pityriasis Rosea

D—An inflammatory, pruritic dermatosis characterized by red to hyperpigmented oval patches that follow the skin lines of cleavage to form a "fir tree" configuration on the back.

Epi—It is seen most commonly in young healthy people, with an equal incidence in men and women.

P—Sometimes it follows a URI; it is often idiopathic.

SiSx—Occasional pruritus is reported.

Dx—The diagnosis is clinical, based on the appearance and history. A lesion called a *herald patch* appears first and is larger than the others. Secondary syphilis can present identically and must be ruled out.

Tx—Topical steroids are given if there is significant itching, but the condition will resolve by itself in weeks to months.

Hidradenitis Suppuritiva

D—A chronic inflammatory disease with comedones and recurrent, usually sterile, abscesses in areas of skin folds, particularly the groin, axillae, and inframammary and perianal areas. Draining sinus tracts and scarring are common.

Epi—It occurs after puberty and affects more women than men.

P—Idiopathic inflammation of the hair follicle and apocrine units is seen, possibly related to hyperandrogenism, friction, or heat.

SiSx—Patients may complain of annoying and/or painful lumps in the associated areas.

Dx—The diagnosis is clinical, based on recurrent abscess and ruling out a primary infection.

Tx—Reduction of friction and moisture is important, along with intralesional steroid injections, topical and oral antibiotics, other medical therapies, and surgical resection of involved areas.

Lichen Planus

D—A chronic idiopathic inflammatory disease that can affect the skin, mucous membranes, hair, and nails.

Epi—It affects men and women equally.

P—It is idiopathic or due to medications: NSAIDS, proton pump inhibitors, antimalarials, gold, and d-penicillamine.

RF—Hepatitis C virus (HCV) infection has been associated with the development of lichen planus; patients with a new diagnosis of lichen planus should be screened for HCV.

SiSx—Skin lesions are classically described as "purple, polygonal, planar (meaning flat-topped), pruritic papules." These lesions commonly occur on the wrists, ankles, thighs, and trunk. They have characteristic gray or white streaks named **Wickham's striae,** and pruritus is usually significant. Fingernails and toenails may be dystrophic and show a variety of abnormalities, and the oral and genital mucosa may exhibit erythema, erosions, or Wickham's striae.

Dx—The diagnosis is based on the clinical appearance and skin biopsy results.

Tx—Treatment consists of topical or intralesional steroids for localized disease, systemic steroids or phototherapy for extensive disease, and removal of offending medications.

If a patient has underlying HCV infection, the lichen planus may or may not be affected by treatment directed at the HCV.

Bullous Skin Disorders

Pemphigus Vulgaris

D—A chronic autoimmune blistering disease affecting the oropharynx and skin.

Epi—Men and women are equally affected, usually in their 50s or 60s. They tend to be slightly younger than patients affected by bullous pemphigoid.

P—Patients have circulating antibodies to components of the desmosome, the structure that attaches adjacent cells in the epidermis. Disruption of the desmosome leads to skin fragility, flaccid blistering, and erosions.

RF—Some medications have been reported to cause or exacerbate pemphigus vulgaris, including ACE inhibitors, nifedipine, penicillin, and rifampin.

SiSx—Patients may note blisters that can be superinfected, causing fluid loss. Eating may become difficult if the oropharynx is heavily involved.

Dx—The diagnosis is based on clinical findings of flaccid blisters and erosions involving the mouth and skin. It is also based on typical findings of "tombstoning" of the epidermal basal layer keratinocytes on histopathologic tests and IgG deposition in an intracellular pattern on direct immunofluorescence, sometimes aided by ELISA for the IgG antibodies.

Tx—The disease was always fatal before oral corticosteroids became available. Now it can be treated with prednisone 1–2 mg/kg/day followed by steroid-sparing agents such as azathioprine, mycophenolate mofetil, cyclophosphamide, and possibly IVIG.

Bullous Pemphigoid

D—A chronic autoimmune blistering disorder affecting the skin.

Epi—It is found in elderly people; men and women are equally affected.

P—Patients have circulating autoantibodies to components of the hemidesmosome, the structural component that anchors the epidermis to the dermis. Disruption of the hemidesmosome leads to separation of the epidermis from the dermis, a deeper split than that seen in pemphigus vulgaris, with resultant tense bullae that can rupture and lead to erosions.

RF—Some medications have been reported to exacerbate or cause bullous pemphigoid, including furosemide, captopril, enalapril, penicillin, and penicillamine.

SiSx—Skin eruptions are often preceded or accompanied by intense pruritus.

Dx—The diagnosis is based on clinical findings of tense blisters and erosions on the skin and supportive findings on skin biopsy of a subepidermal blister, as well as deposition of IgC and C3 seen on direct immunofluorescence.

Tx—As in pemphigus vulgaris, the initial disease is controlled with corticosteroids, followed by long-term steroid-sparing agents such as azathioprine or mycophenolate.

Drug Reactions

Urticaria (Hives)

D—Very pruritic annular or circular pink plaques; individual lesions last <24 hours.

P—Urticaria is seen as part of a type I IgE-mediated allergic reaction that can progress to anaphylaxis, most commonly associated with penicillin and other β-lactam antibiotics. It can also be caused by nonimmunologic means, most commonly NSAIDS or aspirin due to their direct effects on prostaglandins. Angioedema can be seen alone or with urticaria as part of anaphylaxis; it consists of edema of the deeper subcutaneous tissues. Angioedema can be life-threatening if it affects the airway. Hereditary angioedema is a rare but important cause of angioedema seen in young, healthy individuals with a family history of angioedema. An important diagnostic distinction is that these patients do not have urticaria, only angioedema.

SiSx—Individual lesions are very pruritic and come and go.

Dx—The diagnosis is based on the typical appearance and on a history of individual lesions disappearing in 24 hours.

Tx—Treatment involves oral antihistamines, topical steroids, and avoiding or withdrawing the underlying cause.

Morbilliform Eruptions

D—A drug reaction characterized by pruritic red macules and papules that coalesce, usually beginning in the axillae, groin, and trunk and spreading peripherally. Patients lack systemic symptoms or findings such as edema, fever, malaise, arthralgias, leukocytosis, or transaminitis.

Epi—It is the most common drug reaction.

P—Antibiotics are the most common cause of this reaction, although many types of medication have been reported to cause morbilliform rashes. Rash usually develops in the first 2 weeks of treatment. Almost all patients who have EBV or CMV infection and receive amoxicillin develop a morbilliform rash; it is not a true allergy, as it does not appear on rechallenge with the medication.

SiSx—It may be asymptomatic or pruritic.

Dx—The diagnosis is based on the typical clinical appearance and lack of systemic symptoms or mucous membrane involvement

Tx—Treatment involves monitoring patients closely to make sure that they do not develop a more severe drug reaction, as well as giving topical steroids and oral antihistamines for pruritus; often, the medication must be stopped. However, if the medication is necessary and the patient has no systemic symptoms, careful continuation of the medication may be considered.

Systemic Hypersensitivity Reactions

D—An inflammatory reaction, sometimes referred to as DRESS syndrome (drug reaction with eosinophilia and systemic symptoms), that presents with a morbilliform eruption identical to that seen in simple morbilliform exanthems. These patients can also have edema of the hands and face, lymphadenopathy, fever, malaise, pharyngitis, an atypical lymphocytosis, eosinophilia, transaminitis, sterile pyuria, and penumonitis.

P—Common causes include anticonvulsants, sulfonamides such as trimethoprim-sulfamethoxazole, allopurinol, NSAIDS, and semisynthetic penicillins. Systemic hypersensitivity reactions usually occur 2–6 weeks after starting the medication.

SiSx—Symptoms include skin discomfort, pruritus, and the systemic symptoms described above.

Dx—The diagnosis is based on the clinical appearance and a typical history. It can be supported by skin biopsy in unclear situations.

Tx—It is absolutely necessary to stop any possibly offending medications, and patients often require treatment with systemic steroids.

Stevens-Johnson Syndrome (SJS)

D—An acute drug reaction characterized by erosions and edema of the ocular, oral, urogenital, and rectal mucosa, as well as bullous skin lesions ranging from very few lesions to widespread involvement. Skin lesions may have macules of erythema with bullae or necrosis in the center. Most patients also have fever and flu-like symptoms.

P—Common causes of SJS include anticonvulsants, trimethoprim-sulfamethoxazole, NSAIDs, and aminopenicillins. Infection with *Mycoplasma pneumoniae* can also cause SJS.

SiSx—Symptoms include skin pain and tenderness, oral and esophageal pain limiting swallowing, and eye pain, as well as systemic symptoms of fever and malaise.

Dx—The diagnosis is based on the clinical appearance and typical history and is supported by typical skin biopsy findings of necrotic keratinocytes (see Color Figure 12-13).

Tx—Treatment includes stopping the offending agent, aggressive supportive care, wound care and ophthalmologic evaluation, urogenital evaluation to prevent stricture formation, and nutritional supplementation if patients cannot swallow. Corticosteroid and IVIG treatment remain somewhat controversial but are usually employed.

Toxic Epidermal Necrolysis

D—Stevens-Johnson syndrome with skin lesions that cover more than 30% of the patient's body surface area.

P—The causative medications are the same as those seen in SJS.

SiSx—Early on, skin pain and tenderness appear, progressing to large areas of skin necrosis and sloughing. There is a high risk of mortality and long-term disability.

Dx—The diagnosis is based on the clinical appearance and supported by a skin biopsy demonstrating full-thickness necrosis of the epidermis. Early intervention with IVIG is often indicated, and skin biopsy sent for a frozen specimen in order to hasten diagnosis is common (see Color Figure 12-14).

Tx—Treatment requires care in the ICU with fluid resuscitation, electrolyte monitoring, meticulous skin care, and infection prevention. Patients are sometimes cared for in burn units, and the use of IVIG for treatment is common. Epidermal regrowth is seen in 3 weeks, but long-term complications related to ocular scarring are common.

Primary Skin Cancers

Melanoma

D—A malignancy of melanocytes. There are different types, including the following:

Superficial spreading—common, seen in patients of all ages, as well as on the upper back of both men and women and on the legs of women.

Lentigo maligna—common, seen in elderly patients in areas of significant sun exposure, affecting the head, neck, and hands.

Acral lentiginous—uncommon, seen on the hands and feet; the most common type is seen in darkly pigmented patients.

Nodular—arises with no radial growth phase, forming a dome-shaped, sometimes friable, nodule, or papule.

Epi—Melanoma is the most common cause of skin cancer–related death. Twenty-five

percent of patients are <40 years old. There are 55,000 cases per year.

P—The disease is due to a malignant transformation of melanocytes; metastases occur via lymph nodes and blood.

RF—Risk factors include a personal history of frequent sun burning and/or clinically or pathologically atypical nevi. There is also a family history, specifically familial atypical mole and melanoma syndrome.

SiSx—Pain, itching, and bleeding are possible but not necessary. Many patients are asymptomatic in early-stage disease.

Dx—Any suspicious lesions require a biopsy. The clinical appearance of suspicious lesion is a dark papule or macule that is new, changing, has bled, or has the ABCDE characteristics (see Table 12-2): **A**symmetry, **B**orders are irregular, **C**olor is not uniform, **D**iameter is larger than 5 mm, and the lesion is **E**volving. The diagnosis is based on biopsy results. Depending on the depth of invasion of the primary lesion, regional lymph nodes may be evaluated using a sentinel lymph node biopsy. If this biopsy is positive, completion lymphadenectomy is performed to evaluate the entire nodal basin. Imaging of the chest, abdomen, and pelvis to look for distant metastatic disease is indicated in the case of a deep primary lesion or nodal metastases.

The primary lesion is staged based on its:

Breslow depth: the depth (measure in millimeters) from the top of the granular layer to the bottom of the tumor. Breslow depth determines the surgical margins for excision of the primary tumor.

Table 12-2. Assessment of Melanoma

Asymmetry
Borders—irregular?
Color—nonuniform?
Diameter >5 mm?
Elevation/evolving
Family history
Growth
History of previous cancer or moles

Table 12-3. Clark's Levels for Assessment of Melanoma

Clark's Level	Location of Tumor
I	Fills epidermis
II	Involves upper dermis
III	Involves lower dermis
IV	Fills entire dermis
V	Involves subcutaneous fat

Clark's level: location of the tumor in relation to the normal structures of the skin (see Table 12-3).

Ulceration: the presence of microscopic ulceration increases the stage of the primary tumor.

Tx—Treatment is based on the stage. A primary lesion is excised based on Breslow's depth. Adjuvant therapy such as interferon-α is offered based on the presence of metastases or the high likelihood of metastases based on the primary lesion.

Basal Cell Carcinoma

D—A tumor of basal layer keratinocytes.

Epi—It is the most common form of skin cancer as well as the most common cancer in general. There are 900,000 cases per year. The estimated lifetime risk is about 33%.

P—Malignant transformation of basal layer keratinocytes occurs, probably in response to UV exposure. Basal cell carcinoma can be locally invasive and destructive, but it rarely metastasizes.

RF—Risk factors include sun exposure, skin that sunburns easily, and a family history.

SiSx—Pain, itching, and bleeding are possible but not necessary.

Dx—The diagnosis is based on biopsy of a suspicious lesion. Clinical, a suspicious lesion appears as a pearly papule or nodule. It is translucent and may have a red, smooth surface, classically with telangiectasias, as shown in Color Figure 12-15. It can also be ulcerated or pigmented or look like a superficial scar, and can be confused clinically with a melanoma.

Tx—Surgical excision, radiation therapy, electrodesiccation and curettage, and immunomodulating topical therapies are all options based on the size and location of the tumor. Mohs micrographic surgery is removal of the tumor followed by immediate frozen section histopathologic examination of 100% of the margins with subsequent reexcision of tumor-positive areas and final closure of the defect; it results in the highest cure rates. There is a high rate of development of future skin cancers, so continued skin exams are needed regularly.

Squamous Cell Carcinoma

D—A tumor of keratinocytes.

P—Malignant transformation of keratinocytes occurs, probably in response to UV or other radiation, viral infection, or immunosuppression. It has the capacity to be locally destructive and to metastasize.

RF—Risk factors include sun exposure, skin that sunburns easily, immunosuppression, human papillomavirus (HPV) infection, and chronic inflammation from a chronic ulcer or burn scar (known as Marjolin's ulcer).

SiSx—Pain, itching, and bleeding are possible but not necessary.

Dx—Diagnosis is based on a biopsy of a suspicious lesion. The clinical appearance of a suspicious lesion varies. Commonly, it is an indurated red papule or nodule with an overlying crust or scale; sometimes it is ulcerated. There can be a precursor lesion: an actinic keratosis, which is a red macule with adherent scale that may infrequently progress to become a squamous cell cancer.

Tx—Surgical excision, radiation therapy, electrodesiccation and curettage, and immunomodulating topical therapies are all options based on the size and location of the tumor. Mohs micrographic surgery is removal of the tumor followed by immediate frozen section histopathologic examination of 100% of the margins with subsequent reexcision of tumor-positive areas and final closure of the defect; it results in the highest cure rates. There is a high rate of development of future skin cancers, so continued skin exams are needed regularly.

APPENDIX A

Quick Guide to ECG Usage

ECG LEADS

- Leads measure electric activity from depolarization of cells in the heart.
- There are 12 leads.
  - ◘ Three are limb leads labeled I, II, and III. These are bipolar leads. They are made up of the right and left arm leads and the foot leads alone.
  - ◘ Three are augmented limb leads labeled AVR, AVL and AVF (made from combinations of leads I, II, and III). These are also bipolar leads.
  - ◘ Six are precordial leads labeled V1 through V6. These are unipolar leads.
- All of the limb leads measure activity in the coronal plane. The precordial leads measure activity in the sagittal plane.

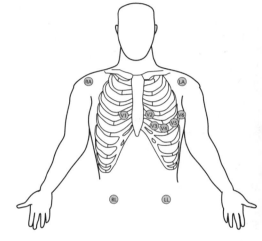

Figure A-1. Twelve-Lead ECG Lead Placement.

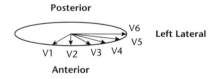

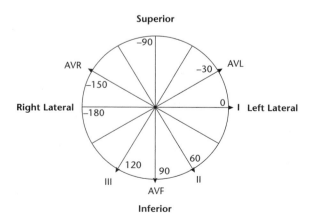

Figure A-2. Relationship of Lead Position and Coronary Anatomy. II, III, and AVF relate to the inferior heart border. V1 through V4 deal with the anterior myocardium. V6, I, and AVL concern the lateral heart border since they are the lateral leads. Numbers represent degrees.

- V1 and V2 are placed in the fourth intercostal space. V4 is placed in the midclavicular line. V6 is placed in the midaxillary line. V3 and V5 fall in between. Limb leads can be placed on the arms and legs or as shown in Figure A-1.
- The leads are arranged in a standard way on tracing paper that approximates the representation of the heart, with groups of leads providing specific types of information based on the direction of their vectors, as shown in Figure A-2.

LEAD DEFLECTION TRACING NOMENCLATURE

- Waves of depolarization coming toward the lead give a positive (upward) deflection on the ECG tracing, and those going away from the lead give a negative (downward) deflection.
- Standard electrical waves on the ECG are labeled P, Q, R, S, and T.
- The P wave represents atrial depolarization. Atrial systole occurs immediately afterward.
- The QRS wave represents ventricular depolarization, and ventricular systole occurs directly afterward.
- The T wave represents ventricular repolarization. Atrial repolarization waves are not seen, as atrial repolarization occurs at the same time as the QRS.
- For definitional purposes, a Q wave is the first negative downward deflection. An R wave is the first upward deflection and an S wave is the first downward deflection following an upward deflection if there is one (see Figure A-3).

A systematic approach to ECG interpretation is useful to prevent missing important findings. The following approach is fairly common, as shown in Table A-1.

SCALE

- A small box is 1 mm square. A large box is 5 mm square. The ticker speed is 25 mm/sec. Therefore, five large boxes make 1 second, each large box is 200 ms, and each small box is 40 ms.

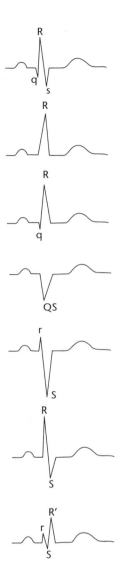

Figure A-3. Nomenclature of ECG Lead Deflection An uppercase letter means that the wave is the dominant deflection in the QRS complex; a lowercase letter means that the wave is not the dominant deflection.

- The standardization preceding the ECG shows the scale. It is 10 mV high and one box wide. This changes based on the computer's attempt to fit the patient's voltage on the page. Variations in the vertical scale are shown in Figure A-4.

Table A-1. Algorithm for ECG Interpretation

Identification and Scale	Is this the correct patient? Are the leads at full or half standard?
Rate	Normal, >100 (tachycardic), or <60 (bradycardic)?
Rhythm	Regular? Dropped beats? Sometimes this may be deferred until the waveform and intervals are assessed.
Axis	Normal, left or right axis deviation? Or rarely, extreme axis deviation?
Intervals	PR (>200 ms?), QRS (>440 corrected in men, >460 in women?), QT (>120 ms?)
Waveform	Hypertrophy (atrial and ventricular) or low voltage ST segments (elevated, depressed, down- or upsloping) T waves (inverted, biphasic, peaked) Q waves (present?) R wave progression? P waves (present everywhere?) Paced beats?

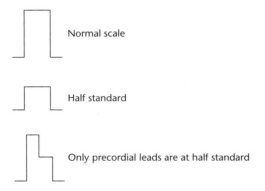

Figure A-4. Differences in the ECG Vertical Scale.

RATE

- To get the rate in a regular rhythm, divide 300 by the number of boxes between QRS complexes. Thus, a separation of one box between QRS waves gives a rate of 300 bpm; two boxes, 150 bpm; three boxes, 100 bpm; four boxes, 75 bpm; and so forth.
- This works because in 1 minute the machine traces out 300 large boxes (25 mm/sec or 5 large boxes per second)
- If the rate is irregular or very bradycardic, then count the number of beats over 6 seconds (30 large boxes) and multiply by 10.
- Tachycardia is defined as a rate >100 bpm. Bradycardia is defined as a rate <60 bpm. Any rate in between is normal.

- Dropped beats are indicative of possible heart block (see Chapter 2) or blocked conduction.

RHYTHM

- If the rhythm is regular, a P wave precedes every QRS. If the P waves are upright in I and II and biphasic in V₁, then this is likely sinus rhythm.
- If either rate is irregular, if the QRS intervals and P intervals are irregular, or if there are dropped beats, then it is likely not sinus rhythm and you need more information to determine the rhythm. Continue with the algorithm and come back to this.
- If P waves seem absent, consider atrial fibrillation, junctional rhythm, or buried Ps within the QRS (as with atrioventricular nodal reentrant tachycardia).
- If you see dropped beats (which come after normally timed P waves), consider second-degree heart block (early P waves or PACs may block if they occur too early because the ventricle is refractory).
    - Mobitz I—also called *Wenckebach block*. Here the PR interval is gradually prolonged until finally there is a dropped beat. They key is that PR intervals are not uniform. Their cycle is described by the number of P waves that accompany a number of QRS waves where the latter are always one less than the former: 2:1, 3:2, 4:3, and so on. This is generally a benign rhythm.

◌ Mobitz II—there are dropped beats, but the PR intervals are constant. These are named by the ratio of the number of P waves to the number of QRS waves. Sometimes multiple QRS waves will be dropped in a row. Mobitz II is usually an indication for a pacemaker.

◌ Note that a 2:1 block cannot be easily distinguished as a type I or II since each second beat is dropped.

◌ Third degree—there is no correlation of the P and QRS waves, but each marches out at regular intervals. In addition, there should be more P waves than QRS complexes. The ventricles have their own intrinsically slower pacer that fires at its own rate independent of what the atria are doing. The defect may not be in the AV node but rather anywhere distal up to the point of ventricular activation before the bifurcation into right and left bundles.

AXIS

- Usually the QRS wave axis is determined, but the T wave and P wave axes are sometimes important.
- The normal QRS axis ranges from –30° to +90°.
- As a quick assessment, if the QRS waves in leads I and II are both positive, then the axis is within normal limits. However, this should be compared to a previous tracing to assess for change.
- Use leads I and II (some people use AVF; however, lead II is better) first to determine the quadrant in which the axis lies (see Table A-2).

Table A-2. Determination of the ECG Axis

Lead I	Lead II	Quadrant
Positive	Positive	Normal quadrant
Positive	Negative	Left axis deviation
Negative	Positive	Right axis deviation
Negative	Negative	Extreme axis quadrant

- Once the quadrant is found, find what is called an *isoelectric lead* (a lead in which the positive area equals the negative area under the waveform), if one exists. If an isoelectric lead is found, the true axis lies perpendicular to it. Exact axis determination can be made by vector analysis based on how many millivolts positive the R wave is in particular leads. The computer generally does a good job of determining the axis, however, as it does with the P and T waves. The P wave axis should be between 0° and 90°. The T wave axis should be within 60° of the QRS.
- Common reasons for left axis deviation include the presence of an inferior infarct or a left anterior fascicular block (LAFB). Left bundle branch block (LBBB) should not give a left axis deviation, nor should left ventricular hypertrophy (LVH) in most people.
  ◌ Left anterior fascicular block is defined as (1) left axis deviation and (2) small q's in lead I and a small R in lead III.
- Common reasons for a right axis deviation include left posterior fascicular block (LPFB), right ventricular hypertrophy, or dextrocardia. Note that a right bundle branch block (RBBB) does not cause axis deviation, so if you see this, consider a concomitant fascicular block (called bifascicular block).
  ◌ Left posterior fascicular block is defined as (1) right axis deviation and 2) small q's in lead III and a small R in lead I.

INTERVALS

- **PR**
  ◌ If PR is >200 ms, then this is first-degree atrioventricular block (AVB).
  ◌ If PR is 80–200 ms, then it is normal.
  ◌ If PR is <80 ms, then consider either preexcitation (i.e., the ventricle is activated faster than the AV node) or that the P wave is not related to the QRS.
- **QRS:** If this is >120 ms, it is prolonged. Think of RBBB, LBBB, an accessory pathway, or a ventricular focus. An RBBB is upright in lead V_1 with an rSR′ morphology (see Figure A-3) with

a deep S wave in lead I. An LBBB is negative in lead V_1 and upright in lead V_6.

- **QT:** This interval changes with the rate; therefore, the corrected QT interval is used (it is called QTc and defined as QT interval/[Square Root of RR interval]), which corrects to a rate of 60. As a rule of thumb, in a patient who is not tachycardic, if the QT is less than half of the QRS—QRS distance, then it is normal.

WAVEFORM

Hypertrophy

Left ventricular hypertrophy (LVH)—There are multiple criteria and scoring systems, but in general, this is either obvious or it is not. If the scale is normal and the QRS complexes in the precordial leads are touching each other, there is LVH. Other simple rules of thumb are:

- R or S in any lead of 20 mm or more.
- R of V_5 plus S of V_1 >35 mm.
- AVL has R >11 mm (tends to be more specific).

Right ventricular hypertrophy (RVH)—There are large R waves in the early precordial leads where normally S >> R. Then, in the later precordial leads, the S wave persists where it normally should be absent, mostly by V_6. Right axis deviation may also be present.

Left atrial enlargement/abnormality (LAE)—The ECG findings are hard to correlate with the actual left atrium (LA) size. However, there are two ECG-defined patterns that may imply pathology:

- *P mitrale* with notched P waves in leads II and III AVF and a P wave in lead I that is greater than that in lead III.
- A predominantly negative second portion of the biphasic P wave in V_1 or V_2. The width of the P wave in leads I and II is more than two boxes.

Right atrial enlargement/abnormality—There are tall-peaked P waves in the inferior leads, and a large initial positive P wave component is seen in V_1.

ST Segment Deviation

Acute Myocardial Injury Patterns

ST elevation: This is pathologic if it is flat or has a "tombstone shape." Sharp ST elevation in multiple leads implies infarction. There may be associated reciprocal changes in other leads (the ST changes seen from the opposite side of the heart).

J point elevation: This is seen mainly in V_1 through V_3. It occurs as a smooth, upsloping curve takeoff of 2 to 3 mm elevation at inflection point transition from the S wave to the T wave. *Benign early repolarization* is another name for this condition.

ST depression: A flat or downsloping curve that implies ischemia and is more specific for this condition than ST elevation. Upsloping ST depression is usually seen with tachycardia and in most cases is benign.

T Waves Changes

Inversions usually are nonspecific; however, deep, symmetric T wave inversions in V_1 and V_2 suggest a proximal LAD lesion. The asymmetric "hockeystick"-type pattern (where the initial downward segment is long, and the rise back to the baseline is short) is common and signifies a repolarization abnormality, as seen with LVH. Peaked T waves may be hyperacute, implying early ischemia, or may signify hyperkalemia.

Q Waves

A *diaphragmatic Q wave* in lead III is allowed without anything in the other leads.

Significant pathologic Q waves are those that are more than *one small box wide* (most important criterion) and more than one-third of the total QRS length. They must also be present in more than one lead. Otherwise, non pathologic Q waves seen on the ECG may represent normal depolarization of the septum.

R Wave Progression

An R wave may or may not be present in V_1 and may then be maximal in V_3 or V_4, where the transition point occurs. Thereafter, the R:S ratio should continue becoming larger. An R wave greater than S wave in V_1 is always abnormal and may indicate RVH, RBBB, posterior infarction, or an accessory pathway. Early R wave progression is considered a transition point between V_2 and V_3, meaning that leads are placed too far left or that the left ventricle is farther to the right in the chest than normal. With a late R wave progression, the R wave is less than the S wave in V_4 and beyond. This can be because the leads are placed too far to the right, or because there is less LV muscle mass, as occurs after an infarction.

U Waves

These are extra humps after the T waves, seen in delayed repolarization in hypokalemia and ischemia.

Figure A-5 shows several examples of the above findings.

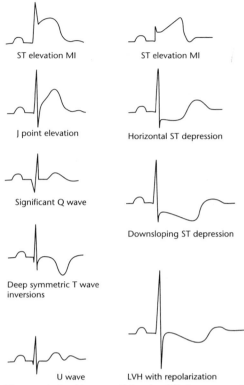

Figure A-5. Abnormalities in ST Segments, T Waves, Q Waves, and U Waves.

APPENDIX B

Reading Chest X-rays

BASICS OF READING CHEST FILMS ON ROUNDS

As with ECGs, have an algorithm so that you are systematic and do not miss anything. A sample algorithm is shown here.

1. **Orientation and Location**

   - Are the name and date correct for the study?
   - Is the right or left side labeled, and is the film oriented this way?
   - Is the film anterior–posterior (AP), usually taken with the patient in bed, or posterior–anterior (PA), usually taken with a lateral film with the patient standing?

2. **Rotation:** Is the patient straight or rotated, either forward, backward, or sideways?

   - Lateral rotation is seen by looking at the clavicular ends in the front to see if the thoracic spine lines up in the middle of them. If it does not, then the patient is rotated with either the right or left shoulder forward.
   - For AP rotation (i.e., if the patient is tilting forward or backward during the film), look at the amount of lung above the clavicle. It should be about two intercostal spaces. If it is more than this, then the patient is leaning forward. If it is less, then the patient is leaning backward.

3. **Penetration:** Are the X-rays adequate to give you the needed information?

   - The vertebral bodies should be barely visible at the heart shadow.
   - If they are not visible, the film is underpenetrated.

   - If they are completely visible and most of the structures look dark on the film, it is overpenetrated.

4. **Structures:** Go through the ABCs

   Airway
   - If the film is taken at full inspiration, one should usually be able to count 10 ribs posteriorly or 6 anteriorly.
   - If the film is not taken at full inspiration, fewer ribs will be seen.
   - Assess the trachea to see if it is in the midline and not shifted.

   Bones
   - Look for fractures, evidence of osteoporosis, cervical ribs, metastases, and so forth.

   Circulation/Heart
   - Is the heart size normal? Is there chamber enlargement or pericardial effusion or calcification?
   - The size of the heart on a PA film should be less than half the width of the mediastinum.
   - An enlarged cardiac silhouette from cardiomegaly or pericardial effusion is less reliably demonstrated on an AP film.

   Diaphragm and Below
   - Is there tenting or flattening, as seen in COPD or are the diaphragms normally curved? Are the hemidiaphragms symmetric?
   - The right hemidiaphragm is usually a little higher than the left as it sits under or over the liver.
   - Look carefully for free air under the diaphragm in an upright film.

Equipment

- Any there any lines or tubes?
- Central lines should not be farther in than the right atrium. The exact position of a Swan-Ganz catheter is sometimes hard to judge on a film.
- A right internal jugular line or subclavian line should not cross the midline.
- Nasogastric or orogastric tubes may go off the screen into the stomach but are radiopaque.
- Chest tubes usually have a marker with lines and an interruption where a main side hole occurs.
- Endotracheal tubes should be a few centimeters just above the carina.
- Implantable cardiac defibrillators (ICDs) are differentiated from pacemakers by their thick shocking coil and large "can," which holds the generator. Be sure to count the number of leads of any ICD or pacemaker device.

Fields of Lung

- Go lobe by lobe and always compare both sides, looking for asymmetry.
- If the right heart border is obscured, then something is wrong with the right middle lobe (i.e., an infiltrate).
- If the left heart border is obscured, there is an infiltrate in the lingula.
- Use the lateral film, if available, to confirm findings suspected in the lower lobes. Infiltrates will usually have a positive *spine sign*—normally, the spine is darker on the way down on a lateral film. If the spine gets brighter as one looks downward, then this suggests pathology.

APPENDIX C

Antibiotics Guide

Class	Mechanism	Sensitive Organisms	Clinical Uses	Toxicities/Comments
Penicillins (PCNs)	Cell wall synthesis inhibitors; stop peptido-glycan cross-linking. Bactericidal because they initiate autolytic systems that initiate programmed cell death.	Mostly strep infections, with later generations having better gram-negative coverage and better staphylococcus coverage.	Many. See below, as it depends on the specific class.	1. Hypersensitivity drug reaction (common, ranging from rash to anaphylaxis). 2. Renal toxicity. 3. Serum sickness. 4. Neurotoxicity in certain cases.
Natural PCNs PCN G (IV) PCN V (oral) Procaine PCN (IM) Benzathine PCN (IM and repository)	Cell wall synthesis inhibitors.	1. β-hemolytic streptococci (groups A, B, C, D) 2. *Treponema pallidum* 3. *Neisseria* 4. *Streptococcus pneumoniae* and *Strep. viridans* 5. *Bacteriodes/Fusobacterium, Pasteurella* 6. *Borrelia burgdorferi* 7. *Erysipelothrix* 8. *Actinomyces*	1. *Streptococcus pyogenes* pharyngitis 2. Skin and soft tissue infections 3. Drug of choice for syphilis 4. *Strep. pneumoniae* respiratory infections if sensitive. Not good for *Staphylococcus* because it makes β-lactamase.	Eliminated by kidney, so redosing needed in renal insufficiency.
Amino PCNs (second-generation PCNs) Amoxicillin Ampicillin	Cell wall synthesis inhibitors.	The above plus *Listeria, Haemophilus influenzae, Escherichia coli, Proteus, Salmonella, Shigella,* and *Enterococcus*	1. Otitis media caused by *Strep. pneumoniae* or *H. influenzae.* 2. Endocarditis prophylaxis. 3. *Listeria* meningitis. 4. Susceptible *E. coli* infections.	Amoxicillin is better absorbed if given orally.

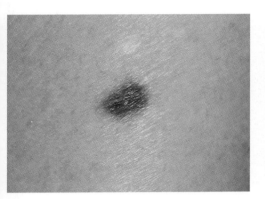

Color Figure 12-2. Macule.
Courtesy of the Dermatology Department,
Hospital of the University of Pennsylvania.

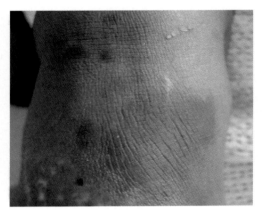

Color Figure 12-3. Patch.
Courtesy of the Dermatology Department,
Hospital of the University of Pennsylvania.

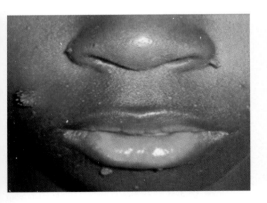

Color Figure 12-4. Papule.
Courtesy of the Dermatology Department,
Hospital of the University of Pennsylvania.

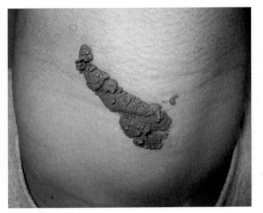

Color Figure 12-5. Plaque.
Courtesy of the Dermatology Department,
Hospital of the University of Pennsylvania.

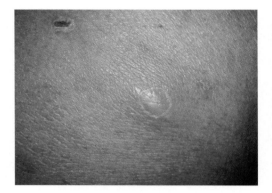

Color Figure 12-6. Nodule.
Courtesy of the Dermatology Department,
Hospital of the University of Pennsylvania.

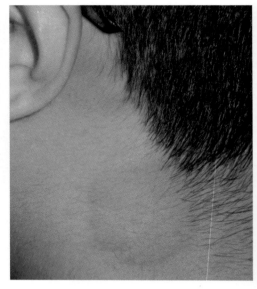

Color Figure 12-7. Urticaria.
Courtesy of the Dermatology Department,
Hospital of the University of Pennsylvania.

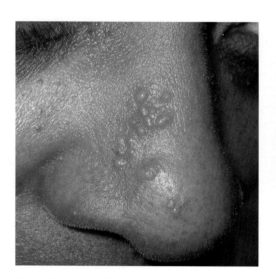

Color Figure 12-8. Vesicle.
Courtesy of the Dermatology Department,
Hospital of the University of Pennsylvania.

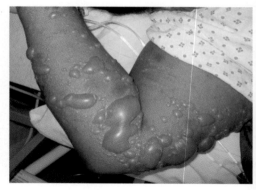

Color Figure 12-9. Bulla.
Courtesy of the Dermatology Department,
Hospital of the University of Pennsylvania.

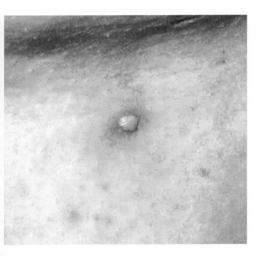

Color Figure 12-10. Pustule.
Courtesy of the Dermatology Department,
Hospital of the University of Pennsylvania.

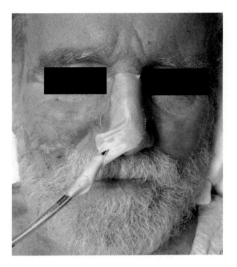

Color Figure 12-11. Seborrheic Dermatitis.
Courtesy of the Dermatology Department,
Hospital of the University of Pennsylvania.

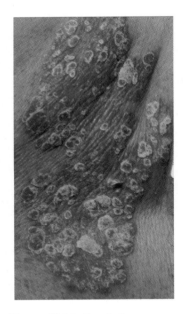

Color Figure 12-12. Psoriasis.
Courtesy of the Dermatology Department,
Hospital of the University of Pennsylvania.

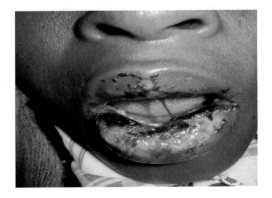

Color Figure 12-13. Stevens-Johnson
Syndrome.
Courtesy of the Dermatology Department,
Hospital of the University of Pennsylvania.

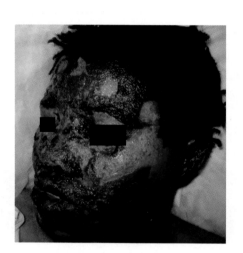

Color Figure 12-14. Toxic Epidermal
Necrolysis.
Courtesy of the Dermatology Department,
Hospital of the University of Pennsylvania.

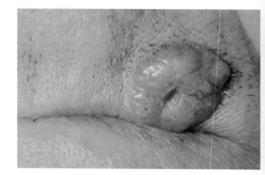

Color Figure 12-15. Basal Cell Carcinoma.
Courtesy of the Dermatology Department,
Hospital of the University of Pennsylvania.

Drug Class	Mechanism	Coverage	Clinical Uses	Side Effects
Carboxy PCNs (third-generation PCNs) Carbenicillin Ticarcillin	Cell wall synthesis inhibitors.	1. *Pseudomonas* 2. Other gram-negative rods (have broader gram-negative coverage than amino PCNs). Overall poor activity against *Streptococcus* and *Staphylococcus*, however.	Used with an aminoglycoside or quinolone for double coverage of *Pseudomonas*.	Sodium overload, hypokalemia, platelet dysfunction (novel to this class).
Ureido PCNs (fourth-generation PCNs) Piperacillin Azlocillin	Cell wall synthesis inhibitors.	1. Great gram-negative coverage. 2. Good pseudomonal coverage (especially Piperacillin). 3. Some anaerobic activity, such as against *Bacteroides fragilis*. Less *Streptococcus* and *Enterococcus* coverage.	Hepatobiliary infections, nosocomial gram-negative infections/sepsis.	Hypernatremia, hypokalemia, bleeding (novel to this class).
Penicillinase-Resistance PCNs Cloxacillin (PO) Dicloxacillin (PO) Methacillin (IV) Nafcillin (IV) Oxacillin (IV)	Cell wall synthesis inhibitors.	1. Methicillin-sensitive *Staph. aureus* (MSSA). 2. Group A streptococcus. No gram-negative coverage. No enterococcal coverage.	1. Skin and soft tissue infections. 2. MSSA infections such as endocarditis.	These are not cleared by the kidney, but rather by hepatobiliary elimination. Therefore, take care in patients with liver disease.
β-Lactam with β-Lactamase Inhibitors Amoxicillin-clavulanate (Augmentin) Ampicillin-sulbactam (Unasyn) Piperacillin-tazobactam (Zosyn) Ticarcillin-clavulanate (Timentin)	Cell wall synthesis inhibitors.	1. MSSA 2. *Bacteriodes fragilis* 3. *Klebsiella* 4. *Haemophilus influenzae* 5. *Moraxella catarrhalis* 6. Good for *Pseudomonas* if parent compound covered this before. Not for methicillin-resistant *Staphylococcus aureus* (MRSA).	1. Community-acquired pneumonia 2. Aspiration PNA. 3. UTI. 4. Skin and soft tissue infections. 5. Community-acquired abdominal infections. 6. Broad polymicrobial coverage.	Mostly GI side effects.

(continued)

Class	Mechanism	Sensitive Organisms	Clinical Uses	Toxicities/Comments
Cephalosporins	Similar mechanism to PCN with β-lactam ring and cell wall inhibition.	Early generations are more gram-positive and later generations are more gram-negative.	Varies significantly by class.	Ten percent cross-reactivity with PCN reactions; therefore, do not give if PCN reaction was severe (e.g., anaphylaxis).
First Generation (cefazolin, cephapirin, cephalexin, cefadroxil)	Cell wall synthesis inhibitors.	1 Gram-positive cocci, MSSA. 2. A few gram-negatives such as *Proteus, E. coli, Klebsiella*. No other gram-negative coverage.	1. Cellulitis or superficial skin infections. 2. Surgical prophylaxis.	Does not cross blood-brain barrier
Second Generation (cefamandole, cefuroxime and cefoxitin, cefotetan)	Cell wall synthesis inhibitors.	1. Gram-positive cocci. 2. Gram-negatives such as *H. influenzae* (especially cefuroxime), *Bacteroides* (especially cefoxitin), *Enterobacter, Neisseria, Proteus, E. coli, Klebsiella, Serratia*.	1. Community-acquired PNA. 2. UTIs. 3. Some intra-abdominal infections. 4. Surgical prophylaxis for obstetric-gynecologic procedures.	All but cefuroxime have a side chain that can inhibit vitamin K action in increased PT and that is also associated with a disulfuram-like reaction.
Third Generation (cefotaxime, ceftriaxone, ceftizoxime, (ceftazidime)	Cell wall synthesis inhibitors.	1. *Proteus, Serratia, Citrobacter*. 2. *Pseudomonas* (ceftazidime only). IV formulations have the best pneumococcal activity. Not for *Enterobacter* or *Enterococcus*.	1. Ceftriaxone: meningitis, Lyme disease of the CNS. 2. Gonorrhea. 3. Community-acquired PNA. 4. UTIs. 5. Used in combination with metronidazole for intra-abdominal infections.	Ceftriaxone—biliary tract sludging. More stable against β-lactamases of GNRs. Ceftriaxone has the longest half life.

Drug	Mechanism	Coverage	Clinical Use	Adverse Effects
Fourth Generation (cefepime)	Cell wall synthesis inhibitor.	1. *Pseudomonas* 2. Enterobacteriaceae 3. *Neisseria* 4. *H. influenzae, Proteus, Citrobacter, Serratia* (enteric gram-negatives).	1. Nosocomial infections of almost any sort. 2. Febrile neutropenia.	GI intolerance. Penetrates into the CSF. Has positively charged NH_4^+ on its ring that allows better penetration through a gram-negative rod's outer membrane.
Carbapenems Imipenem-cilastatin Meropenem Ertapenem	Given with cilastatin to decrease activation in renal tubules.	1. Gram-positive cocci, gram-negative rods, anaerobes 2. MSSA, *Enterococcus*. 3. *H. influenzae, Nocardia, Pseudomonas, Acinetobacter.* 4. Good anaerobic coverage (e.g., *Bacteriodes, Clostridium, Peptostreptococcus*). Slight better gram-negative coverage with meropenem.	1. Broad coverage for polymicrobial infections (intra-abdominal, pelvic, pulmonary, soft tissue). 2. Febrile neutropenia	Rash, seizures at high levels. GI distress.
Aztreonam	Similar to penicillin; inhibits mucopeptide synthesis in the bacterial cell wall. Bactericidal.	Most aerobic gram-negatives, including *Pseudomonas*. No gram-positive aerobic or anaerobic coverage.	Alternative to aminoglycosides, usually in PCN-allergic patients.	Rash. GI side effects (diarrhea, nausea, vomiting). Rarely, toxic epidermal necrolysis.
Aminoglycosides Amikacin Gentamicin Kanamycin Neomycin Streptomycin Netilmicin Tobramycin	Binds 30S ribosomal subunit and inhibits translocation. Synergistic effect with β-lactam agents. Decreased effect at low pH. Bactericidal	Aerobic gram-negative bacilli, including Enterobacteriaceae, *Pseudomonas* (tobramycin is most potent against this), *H. influenzae*.	Empiric therapy in presumed gram negative rod septicemia, complicated UTI, gram-negative osteomyelitis, endocarditis. In cases where synergy with β lactams is useful. Synergistic with certain β lactams and vancomycin (for endocarditis).	Nephrotoxicity. Ototoxicity. Neuromuscular toxicity (diagnosis of myasthenia gravis is an absolute contraindication).

(continued)

Class	Mechanism	Sensitive Organisms	Clinical Uses	Toxicities/Comments
Tetracyclines Demeclocycline Tetracycline Doxycycline Minocycline Oxytetracycline Tigecycline	Reversibly binds the 30S transport system and block the tRNA acceptor site. Bacteriostatic. Tigecycline is a newer 30S inhibitor tetracycline analogue called a *glycylcycline* that has broader-spectrum activity.	1. *Rickettsia* 2. *Chlamydia* 3. *Mycoplasma pneumoniae* 4. *Vibrio cholerae/vulnificus* 5. *Brucella* 6. *Borrelia* 7. *Actinomyces* 8. *Campylobacter* 9. Syphilis 10. *Nocardia* 11. *Helicobacter pylori* (in combination therapy)	1. Rickettsial infections (Rocky Mountain spotted fever, scrub and endemic typhus, Q fever). 2. STDs (chlamydia, lymphogranuloma venereum, syphilis, nongonococcal urethritis, pelvic inflammatory disease). 3. Spirochetes (Lyme disease). 4. Acne 5. MRSA and *Acinetobacter* (Tigecycline).	Avoid combination with PCNs, as the combination has a decreased effect. GI-related conditions are most common (nausea, vomiting, pain). Photosensitivity. Discoloration of teeth in children. Rash.
Clindamycin	Blocks peptide bond formation at the 50S ribosomal subunit. Bacteriostatic.	Good anaerobic activity (*B. fragilis, Clostridium perfringens*), though some are resistant. Some gram positives.	1. Intra-abdominal infections: appendicitis, diverticulitis, perforated ulcer, abscesses, anaerobes in fecal matter (but usually with an aminoglycoside). 2. Skin/soft tissue infections: cellulitis, folliculitis, impetigo, carbuncles, hidradenitis suppurativa, necrotizing fasciitis, diabetic foot ulcers, osteomyelitis. 3. GU: pelvic inflammatory disease, bacterial vaginosis. 4. Pulmonary: aspiration, lung abscesses.	Pseudomembranous colitis. Fever, diarrhea.

Drug	Mechanism	Spectrum	Uses	Adverse Effects
Linezolid	Binds 23S RNA and prevents formation of the 70S complex, stopping bacterial translation. Bacteriostatic for *Staphylococcus* and *Enterococcus* and bactericidal for *Streptococcus*.	1. Many gram-positive, including MRSA and Vancomycin-resistant enterococci (VRE). 2. Useful against some mycobacteria. No gram-negative activity.	Soft tissue, bloodstream with resistant gram-positive organisms.	Oral or IV. Myelosuppression. A weak monoamine oxidase inhibitor as well.
Vancomycin	Bactericidal. Inhibits cell wall mucopeptide formation. Resistance when change of D-ala D-ala to D-ala D-lac.	Gram-positive drug-resistant organisms like MRSA (IV) and *Costridium difficile* (given orally).	IV for most gram-positive infections, endocarditis, line infections. Oral for *C. difficile*.	Few. Red man syndrome prevented by slow infusion and pretreatment with antihistamines.
Macrolides Erythromycin Azithromycin Clarithromyin	Blocks the 23S rRNA of the 50S subunit. Bacteriostatic.	Most beta β-hemolytic streptococci. There is widespread macrolide resistance in *Staph. aureus*.	1. URIs: especially for atypical diseases like *Mycoplasma*, *Legionella*, *C. pneumonae* 2. STDs (*Neisseria*, *Chlamydia*). 3. Streptococcal infections (in PCN-allergic patients).	GI discomfort, cholestatic hepatitis, eosinophilia, skin rashes.
Trimethoprim-Sulfamethoxazole (Bactrim)	Two compounds that inhibit bacterial synthesis of tetrahydrofolic acid sequentially. Bactericidal.	1. UTI organisms: *E. coli*, *Klebsiella*, *Proteus*, *Enterobacter*. 2. *Pneumocystis* infections. 3. GI organisms: *Shigella*, *Salmonella*, *Vibrio*, *Yersinia*. 4. *Nocardia*, *Listeria*, *Mycobacterium marinum*, some protozoa. Clarithromycin is superior for *Strep. pneumoniae* and beta β-hemolytic streptococci.	1. UTIs—acute symptomatic. 2. Chronic bacterial prostatitis. Strong resistance to *Pneumococcus*, so not good for URIs. 3. *Pneumocystis*—first drug of choice. 4. GI—infectious diarrhea 5. *Listeria* meningitis in PCN-allergic patients. 6. Second-line drug for osteomyelitis. 7. Spontaneous bacterial peritonitis prophylaxis. 8. Toxoplasmosis prophylaxis.	GI intolerance. Severe rashes. Do not give to patients with G6PD deficiency, can cause hemolytic episode, folate deficiency Pancytopenia. Hyperkalemia. Hypoglycemia. Affects other medications, including warfarin, sulfonylureas, phenytoin. Hypersensitivity.

(continued)

Class	Mechanism	Sensitive Organisms	Clinical Uses	Toxicities/Comments
Chloramphenicol	Binds the 50S subunit and prevents amino acid addition to growing peptide chains, inhibiting protein synthesis. Bacteriostatic.	1. Most important aerobic and anaerobic bacteria. 2. *H. influenzae* 3. *Neisseria* 4. *Salmonella* 5. *Rickettsia* 6. *Chlamydia* Not MSSA. Not *Klebsiella, Pseudomonas*.	In the United States, rarely used except in circumstance where there are highly resistant organisms (such as for *Neisseria meningitides* in a PCN-allergic patient or for VRE when other options are limited).	Aplastic anemia and reversible bone marrow suppression. Rare backup drug.
Metronidazole (Flagyl)	Interacts with DNA to cause strand breakage and loss of structure resulting in cell death. Bactericidal.	1. Most facultative anaerobic bacteria, including *H. pylori, Gardnerella vaginalis, Bacteroides, C. perfingens, Prevotella,* and protozoa. 2. *Trichomonas vaginalis*. Resistance to metronidazole is rare but has been reported with *Actinomyces*.	1. *C. difficile* infection. 2. Aspiration PNA. 3. Intra-abdominal infections in combination with quinolones. 4. *H. pylori* (as part of triple therapy). 5. Some GU conditions, like bacterial vaginosis and trichomoniasis. 6. Sepsis coverage of anaerobes.	GI intolerance. Metallic taste. Rash. Darkening of the urine. Reaction with disulfiram, causing psychosis. Cleared hepatically. Excellent penetration, including into CSF.

Drug	Mechanism	Spectrum	Clinical Uses	Adverse Effects
Quinolones Ciprofloxacin Levofloxacin Moxifloxacin Gemifloxacin	DNA gyrase and topoisomerase IV inhibitors that inhibit bacterial DNA synthesis. Bactericidal.	1. Gram-negative bacilli (*Enterobacter, H. influenzae*). 2. Gram-negative cocci (*Neisseria, M. catarrhalis*) 3. Atypicals 4. *Strep. pneumoniae* (Ciprofloxacin is not appropriate for Pneumococcus; others are active against it in an appropriate dose.)	1. Community-acquired PNA. 2. UTI. 3. Sinusitis. 4. COPD exacerbation.	GI intolerance, rash. Arthropathy QT prolongation.
Daptomycin (Cubicin)	Disrupts bacterial cell membrane function, causing rapid cell depolarization and halting protein, DNA, and RNA synthesis, causing cell death.	Gram-positive organisms only, including *Staphylococcus* (MRSA), *Streptococcus*, and *Enterococcus* (including VRE).	Skin infections caused by MRSA and right-sided endocarditis.	GI (diarrhea, vomiting, or constipation). Anemia. Myopathy.

APPENDIX D

Medical Abbreviations

AAA	abdominal aortic aneurysm
ABG	arterial blood gas
ABI	ankle-brachial index
ABPA	allergic bronchopulmonary aspergillosis
ACE	angiotensin converting enzyme
ACL	anterior cruciate ligament
ACLS	Advanced Cardiac Life Support
ACS	acute coronary syndrome
ACTH	adrenocorticotropic hormone
ADEM	acute disseminated encephalomyelitis
ADH	antidiuretic hormone
ADL	activities of daily living
AED	antiepileptic drug
AF	atrial fibrillation
AFP	α-fetoprotein
AI	adrenal insufficiency
AIDP	acute inflammatory demyelinating polyneuropathy
AIDS	acquired immunodeficiency syndrome
AIN	acute interstitial nephritis
AIP	acute interstitial pneumonia
AIVR	accelerated idioventricular rhythm
ALL	acute lymphoblastic leukemia
ALS	amyotrophic lateral sclerosis
ALT	alanine aminotransferase
AMA	antimitochondrial antibody
AML	acute myelogenous leukemia
ANA	antinuclear antibody
ANC	absolute neutrophil count
ANCA	antineutrophil cytoplasmic antibody
APC	activated protein C
APD	afferent papillary defect
APML	acute promyelocytic leukemia
APS	antiphospholipid antibody syndrome
AR	aortic regurgitation
ARB	angiotensine receptor blocker
ARDS	acute respiratory distress syndrome
AS	aortic stenosis

ASD	atrial septal defect
AST	aspartate aminotransferase
ATIII	antithrombin III
ATN	acute tubular necrosis
ATRA	all-trans-retinoic acid
AV	atrioventricular
AVB	atrioventricular block
AVNRT	atrioventricular nodal reentrant tachycardia
AVRT	atrioventricular reciprocating tachycardia
AZT	Zidovudine
BiPAP	bi-level positive airway pressure
BMD	bone mineral density
BMI	body mass index
BMP	basic metabolic panel
BMT	bone marrow transplant
BNP	brain natriuretic peptide
BO	bronchiolitis obliterans
BOOP	bronchiolitis obliterans organizing pneumonia
BP	blood pressure
BPH	benign prostatic hyperplasia
BUN	blood urea nitrogen
CABG	coronary artery bypass grafting
CAD	coronary artery disease
CAP	community-acquired pneumonia
CBC	complete blood count
CCK	cholecystokinin
CCP	cyclic citrullinated peptide
CDI	central diabetes insipidus
CEA	carcinoembryonic antigen
CHF	congestive heart failure
CIDP	chronic inflammatory demyelinating polyneuropathy
CIN	contrast-induced nepropathy
CJD	Creutzfeldt-Jakob disease
CK	creatine kinase
CKD	chronic kidney disease
CK-MB	creatine kinase with muscle and brain subunits
CLL	chronic lymphocytic leukemia
CML	chronic myelogenous leukemia
CMV	cytomegalovirus
CNS	central nervous system
COPD	chronic obstructive pulmonary disease
CPAP	continuous positive airway pressure
CPPD	calcium pyrophosphate deposition disease
CPR	cardiopulmonary resuscitation
CRP	C-reactive protein
CRT	chronic resynchronization therapy
CSF	cerebrospinal fluid

CT	computed tomography
CTCL	cutaneous T-cell lymphoma
CTS	carpal tunnel syndrome
CVA	cerebrovascular accident
CVID	common variable immunodeficiency
CVVHD	continuous venovenous hemodialysis
DCIS	ductal carcinoma in situ
DCT	distal collecting tubule
DDAVP	1-deamino(8-D-arginine) vasopressin
DEXA	dual-energy x-ray absorptiometry
DFT	defibrillator function threshold
DGI	disseminated gonococcal infection
DHEA	dehydroepiandrosterone
DHEAS	dehydroepiandrosterone sulfate
DIC	disseminated intravascular coagulation
DIP	desquamative interstitial pneumonia
DKA	diabetic ketoacidosis
DOE	dyspnea on exertion
DRE	digital rectal examination
DTR	deep tendon reflex
DVT	deep vein thrombosis
EBUS	endobronchial ultrasound
EBV	Epstein-Barr virus
ECF	extracellular fluid
ECG	electrocardiogram
ECHO	echocardiogram
EEG	electroencephalogram
EF	ejection fraction
EGD	esophagogastroduodenoscopy
ELISA	enzyme-linked immunosorbent assay
EM	electron microscopy
EMG	electromyography
EP	electrophysiology
ER	emergency room
ERCP	endoscopic retrograde cholangiopancreatography
ESLD	end-stage liver disease
ESR	erythrocyte sedimentation rate
ESRD	end-stage renal disease
ESWL	extracorporeal shock wave lithotripsy
ETEC	enterotoxigenic Escherichia coli
ETOH	ethyl alcohol
FDPs	fibrinogen degradation products
FEV_1	forced expiratory volume at 1 second
FFP	fresh frozen plasma
FISH	fluorescent in situ hybridization
FOBT	fecal occult blood testing
FRC	functional residual capacity

FSGS	focal segmental glomerulosclerosis
FSH	follicle stimulating hormone
FTLD	frontotemporal lobar dementia
FUO	fever of unknown origin
FVC	forced vital capacity
G6PD	glucose-6-phosphate dehydrogenase
GABA	gamma-aminobutyric acid
GBM	glomerular basement membrane
GBS	Guillain-Barré syndrome
GCA	giant cell arteritis
GCT	germ cell tumor
GE	gastroesophageal
GERD	gastroesophageal reflux disease
GFR	glomerular filtration rate
GGT	gamma-glutamyl transpeptidase
GH	growth hormone
GHRH	growth hormone releasing hormone
GI	gastrointestinal
GIB	gastrointestinal bleed
GIST	gastrointestinal stromal tumor
GN	glomerulonephritis
GNB	Gram-negative bacilli
GPC	Gram-positive cocci
GU	genitourinary
GVHD	graft-versus-host disease
HAART	highly active antiretroviral therapy
HAV	hepatitis A virus
HBV	hepatitis B virus
HCC	hepatocellular carcinoma
hCG	human chorionic gonadotropin
HCTZ	hydrochlorothiazide
HCV	hepatitis C virus
HD	hemodialysis
HDL	high-density lipoprotein
HDV	hepatitis D virus
HEV	hepatitis E virus
HHS	hyperosmolar hyperglycemic state
HIT	heparin-induced thrombocytopenia
HIV	human immunodeficiency virus
HNPCC	hereditary nonpolyposis colorectal cancer
HOA	hypertrophic osteoarthropathy
HOCM	hypertrophic obstructive cardiomyopathy
HPLC	high-performance liquid chromatography
HPV	human papillomavirus
HRCT	high-resolution CT
HRT	hormone replacement therapy
HSP	Henoch-Schonlein purpura

HSV	herpes simplex virus
HTLV	human T-cell lymphoma/leukemia virus
HUS	hemolytic-uremic syndrome
I&D	incision and drainage
IBD	inflammatory bowel disease
ICD	implantable cardiac defibrillator
ICF	intracellular fluid
ICH	intracerebral hemorrhage
ICP	intracranial pressure
ICS	intercostal space
IFA	immunofluorescence assay
IGF	insulin-like growth factor
IL	Interleukin
ILD	interstitial lung disease
IM	intramuscular
IMA	inferior mesenteric artery
INO	internuclear ophthalmoplegia
INR	international normalized ratio
IPAH	idiopathic pulmonary arterial hypertension
IPF	idiopathic pulmonary fibrosis
ITP	idiopathic thrombocytopenic purpura
IUD	intrauterine device
IV	intravenous
IVC	inferior vena cava
IVDU	intravenous drug use
IVIG	intravenous immune globulin G
IVP	intravenous pyelogram
JIA/JRA	juvenile idiopathic arthritis/juvenile rheumatoid arthritis
JNC-7	Joint National Committee
JVP	jugular venous pressure
KUB	Kidney's ureter bladder X ray
LA	left atrium
LAD	left anterior descending artery
LAE	left atrial enlargement
LAFB	left anterior fascicular block
LAM	lymphangioleiomyomatosis
LBBB	left bundle branch block
LCA	left coronary artery
LCIS	lobular carcinoma in situ
LCL	lateral collateral ligament
LCX	left circumflex artery
LDH	lactic dehydrogenase
LDL	low-density lipoprotein
LEMS	Lambert-Eaton myasthenic syndrome
LFT	liver function test
LGIB	lower GI bleed
LGV	lymphogranuloma venereum

LIMA	left internal mammary artery
LLQ	left lower quadrant
LMWH	low molecular weight heparin
LOC	loss of consciousness
LP	lumbar pucture
LPFB	left posterior fascicular block
LPS	lipopolysaccharide
LR	lactated Ringer's
LUL	left upper lobe
LUQ	left upper quadrant
LV	left ventricle
LVEDP	left ventricular end-diastolic pressure
LVH	left ventricular hypertrophy
LVOT	left ventricular outflow tract
MAC	mycobacterium avium complex
MAHA	microangiopathic hemolytic anemia
MAI	Mycobacterium avium-intracellulare
MALT	mucosa-associated lymphoid tissue
MAP	mean arterial pressure
MAT	multifocal atrial tachycardia
MCA	middle cerebral artery
MCL	midclavicular line
MCP	metacarpophalangeal
MCTD	mixed connective tissue disease
MCV	mean corpuscular volume
MDS	myelodysplastic syndrome
MELAS	mitochondrial encephalomyopathy lactic acidosis and stroke-like episodes
MEN	multiple endocrine neoplasia
MERRF	myoclonic epilepsy and ragged red fibers
METS	metabolic equivalents
MG	myasthenia gravis
MGN	membranous glomerulonephritis
MGUS	monoclonal gammopathy of uncertain significance
MI	myocardial infarction
MODY	maturity-onset diabetes of youth
MPGN	membranoproliferative glomerulonephritis
MPO	myeloperoxidase
MR	mitral regurgitation
MRA	magnetic resonance angiography
MRCP	magnetic resonance cholangiopancreatography
MRI	magnetic resonance imaging
MRSA	methicillin-resistant *Staph. aureus*
MRV	magnetic resonance venography
MS	mitral stenosis
MSSA	methicillin-sensitive *Staph. aureus*
MTC	medullary thyroid carcinoma
MTP	metatarsophalangeal

MVP	mitral valve prolapse
MVR	mitral valve replacement
NASH	nonalcoholic steatohepatitis
NCS	nerve conduction studies
NDI	nephrogenic diabetes insipidus
NG	nasogastric
NGU	nongonococcal urethritis
NHL	non-Hodgkin's lymphoma
NMJ	neuromuscular junction
NNRTI	nonnucleoside reverse transcriptase inhibitors
NPH	neutral-protamine-Hagedorn
NRTI	nucleoside reverse transcriptase inhibitor
NSAIDs	nonsteroidal anti-inflammatory drugs
NSCLC	non–small cell lung cancer
NSIP	nonspecific interstitial pneumonia
NSTEMI	non–ST elevation MI
NSVT	nonsustained ventricular tachycardia
NTP	neutropenic
NYHA	New York Heart Association
OA	osteoarthritis
OCP	oral contraceptive pill
OGTT	oral glucose tolerance test
OM	obtuse marginal
ORT	orthodromic reciprocating tachycardia
OSA	obstructive sleep apnea
PAC	premature atrial contraction
PAF	paroxysmal atrial fibrillation
PAH	pulmonary arterial hypertension
PAN	polyarteritis nodosa
PAS	periodic acid–Schiff
PASP	pulmonary artery systolic pressure
PBC	primary biliary cirrhosis
PCA	posterior cerebral artery
PCI	percutaneous coronary intervention
PCL	posterior cruciate ligament
PCN	penicillin
PCOS	polycystic ovary syndrome
PCP	*Pneumocystis carinii* pneumonia
PCR	polymerase chain reaction
PCT	proximal convoluted tubule
PCV	pressure-controlled ventilation
PCWP	pulmonary capillary wedge pressure
PD	peritoneal dialysis
PDA	posterior descending artery
PE	pulmonary embolus
PEEP	positive end expiratory pressure
PEG	percutaneous endoscopic gastrojejunostomy

PERC	percutaneous stone extraction
PET	positron emission tomography
PFO	patent foramen ovale
PFT	pulmonary function test
PICA	posterior inferior cerebellar arteries
PID	pelvic inflammatory disease
PIGN	acute postinfectious GN
PIP	proximal interphalangeal
PKD	polycystic kidney disease
PMI	point of maximal impulse
PML	progressive multifocal leukoencephalopathy
PMN	polymorphonuclear leukocyte
PMR	polymyalgia rheumatica
PND	paroxysmal nocturnal dyspnea
PNH	paroxysmal nocturnal hemoglobinuria
PPD	purified protein derivative
PPI	protein punp inhibitor
PR	progesterone receptor
PSA	prostate-specific antigen
PSC	primary sclerosing cholangitis
PTCA	percutaneous transluminal coronary angioplasty
PTH	parathyroid hormone
PTU	propylthiouracil
PVC	premature ventricular contraction
PVD	peripheral vascular disease
PVR	pulmonary vascular resistance
RA	rheumatoid arthritis
RAI	radioactive iodine
RAP	right atrial pressure
RAS	renal artery stenosis
RBBB	right bundle branch block
RBC	red blood cell
RBILD	respiratory bronchiolitis-associated interstitial lung disease
RCA	right coronary artery
RCT	random controlled trial
RDW	RBC distribution width
RFA	radiofrequency ablation
RLQ	right lower quadrant
RLS	restless legs syndrome
RLSB	right lower sternal border
RMSF	rocky mountain spotted fever
RPGN	rapidly progressive (crescentic) GN
RPR	rapid plasma reagin
RSV	respiratory syncytial virus
RTA	renal tubular acidosis
RUL	right upper lobe
RUQ	right upper quadrant

RVH	right ventricular hypertrophy
RVVT	Russell viper venom time
SA	Sinoatrial
SAAG	serum-ascites albumin gradient
SAH	subarachnoid hemorrhage
SARS	severe acute respiratory syndrome
SBE	subacute bacterial endocarditis
SBP	systolic blood pressure
SCC	squamous cell cancer
SCLC	small cell lung cancer
SCM	sternocleidomastoid
SIADH	system of inappropriate antidiuretic hormone
SIRS	systemic inflammatory response syndrome
SJS	Stevens-Johnson syndrome
SLE	systemic lupus erythematosus
SLL	small lymphocytic lymphoma
SLNTG	sublingual nitroglycerin
SMA	superior mesenteric artery
SOB	shortness of breath
SPEP	serum protein electrophoresis
SSA	sulfosalicylic acid
SSRI	selective serotonin reuptake inhibitor
STD	sexually transmitted disease
STEMI	ST elevation MI
SVC	superior vena cava
SVG	saphenous vein graft
SVR	systemic vascular resistance
TALH	thick ascending loop of Henle
TBW	total body water
TCA	tricyclic antidepressants
TCD	transcranial doppler
TEE	transesophageal echocardiography
TFT	thyroid function test
TGF	transforming growth factor
TIA	transient ischemic attack
TIBC	total iron binding capacity
TLC	total lung capacity
TMG	toxic multinodular goiter
TMP-SMX	trimethoprim-sulfamethoxazole
TNF	tumor necrosis factor
TPA	tissue plasminogen activator
TR	tricuspid regurgitation
TRALI	transfusion-related acute lung injury
TRH	thyroid releasing hormone
TSH	thyroid stimulating hormone
TTE	transthoracic ECHO
TTP	thrombotic thrombocytopenic purpura

TWI	T wave inversion
UC	ulcerative colitis
UES	upper esophageal sphincter
UGIB	upper GI bleed
UIP	usual interstitial pneumonia
UPEP	urinary protein electrophoresis
URI	upper respiratory infection
UTI	urinary tract infection
UV	ultraviolet light
V/Q	ventilation-perfusion
VAD	ventricular assist device
VATS	video-assisted thorascopic surgery
VC	vital capacity
VDRL	Venereal Disease Research Laboratory
VEGF	vascular endothelial growth factor
VF	ventricular fibrillation
VLDL	very low density lipoprotein
VMA	vanillylmandelic acid
VSD	ventricular septal defect
VST	venous sinus thrombosis
VT	ventricular tachycardia
VZV	varicella-zoster virus
WBC	white blood cell
WHO	World Health Organization
WPW	Wolfe-Parkinson-White
ΔMS	change in mental status

INDEX

Note: Page numbers followed by "*f*" and "*t*" denote figures and tables, respectively.